RADIOGRAPHY ESSENTIALS
FOR LIMITED PRACTICE

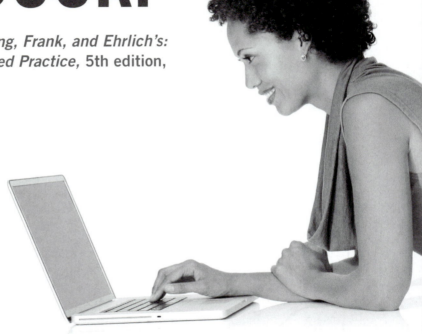

RADIOGRAPHY ESSENTIALS
FOR LIMITED PRACTICE

Fifth Edition

BRUCE W. LONG
MS, RT(R)(CV), FASRT, FAEIRS
Director and Associate Professor
Radiologic and Imaging Sciences Programs
Indiana University School of Medicine
Indianapolis, Indiana

EUGENE D. FRANK
MA, RT(R), FASRT, FAEIRS
Associate Professor Emeritus
Mayo Clinic College of Medicine
Rochester, Minnesota

RUTH ANN EHRLICH
RT(R)
Retired, Radiology Faculty
University of Western States
Portland, Oregon;
Adjunct Faculty
Portland Community College
Portland, Oregon

ELSEVIER

ELSEVIER

3251 Riverport Lane
St. Louis, Missouri 63043

RADIOGRAPHY ESSENTIALS FOR LIMITED PRACTICE,
FIFTH EDITION

ISBN: 978-0-323-35623-7

Notices

Knowledge and best practice in this field are constantly changing. As new research and experience broaden our understanding, changes in research methods, professional practices, or medical treatment may become necessary.

Practitioners and researchers must always rely on their own experience and knowledge in evaluating and using any information, methods, compounds, or experiments described herein. In using such information or methods they should be mindful of their own safety and the safety of others, including parties for whom they have a professional responsibility.

With respect to any drug or pharmaceutical products identified, readers are advised to check the most current information provided (i) on procedures featured or (ii) by the manufacturer of each product to be administered, to verify the recommended dose or formula, the method and duration of administration, and contraindications. It is the responsibility of practitioners, relying on their own experience and knowledge of their patients, to make diagnoses, to determine dosages and the best treatment for each individual patient, and to take all appropriate safety precautions.

To the fullest extent of the law, neither the Publisher nor the authors, contributors, or editors, assume any liability for any injury and/or damage to persons or property as a matter of products liability, negligence or otherwise, or from any use or operation of any methods, products, instructions, or ideas contained in the material herein.

Previous editions copyrighted 2013, 2010, 2006, and 2002.

Library of Congress Cataloging-in-Publication Data
Names: Long, Bruce W., author. | Frank, Eugene D., author. | Ehrlich, Ruth
  Ann, 1938- author.
Title: Radiography essentials for limited practice / Bruce W. Long, Eugene D.
  Frank, Ruth Ann Ehrlich.
Description: Fifth edition. | St. Louis, Missouri : Elsevier, [2017] |
  Includes bibliographical references and index.
Identifiers: LCCN 2016015047 | ISBN 9780323356237 (pbk. : alk. paper)
Subjects: | MESH: Radiography—methods | Technology, Radiologic | Allied
  Health Personnel
Classification: LCC RC78 | NLM WN 200 | DDC 616.07/572—dc23 LC record available at
  https://lccn.loc.gov/2016015047

Executive Content Strategist: Sonya Seigafuse
Content Development Manager: Billie Sharp
Associate Content Development Specialist: Laurel Shea
Publishing Services Manager: Jeff Patterson
Book Production Specialist: Carol O'Connell
Design Direction: Ashley Miner

Printed in the United States of America

Last digit is the print number: 10 9 8 7 6 5 4 3 2 1

Review Board

Since the publication of the first edition of *Radiography Essentials for Limited Practice*, information has been continually gathered about the education and work of the limited x-ray machine operator (LXMO). The term "limited operator" and the acronym "LXMO" will be used throughout this book, since these have become the generally accepted terms. However, each state with a licensure law may use different terms. We have included a list of these most current terms, by state, in Appendix A near the end of this book.

Several significant events have impacted the limited operator's status in the diagnostic imaging profession. The 2004 publication by the American Society of Radiologic Technologists (ASRT) of the Limited X-ray Machine Operator Curriculum was intended to establish national standardized educational guidelines for LXMOs, including clinical and didactic components. An updated ASRT Limited X-ray Machine Operator Curriculum was adopted in 2009. In 2013, the American Registry of Radiologic Technologists (ARRT) adopted a new set of Content Specifications for the Limited Scope of Practice in Radiography examination. A new version is scheduled for adoption in 2018. This examination is used by nearly all states with LXMO licensure laws as their validation of a LXMO's competency to hold that license. The material in this fifth edition of *Radiography Essentials for Limited Practice* has been updated to encompass all the concepts included in the current ARRT Content Specifications, providing the most up-to-date learning source for LXMO examination candidates.

National accreditation of LXMO educational programs is now a reality. In January 2012, the Joint Review Committee on Education in Radiologic Technology (JRCERT) began to accredit these programs. This national organization, itself accredited by the U.S. Department of Education, serves as the programmatic accreditation agency for radiography education programs. It now offers accreditation services to LXMO education programs to promote academic excellence, patient safety, and quality health care delivery. Since the JRCERT will require accredited LXMO programs to adhere to the ASRT LXMO Curriculum, *Radiography Essentials for Limited Practice* will meet the educational content needs of these programs.

The radiography profession is accepting the limited operators as an integral part of the radiology department by hiring them and allowing them to perform a limited range of radiography examinations. Although many LXMOs work alone or with other LXMOs in small clinics and hospitals, chiropractic clinics, and so forth, an increasing number of them are working alongside radiologic technologists in large clinics, imaging centers, and hospitals throughout the United States. As this new health care worker emerges, strong emphasis is being placed on the education and certification of these individuals. The need for a comprehensive textbook written specifically for limited practice has never been greater.

For this fifth edition we worked with an advisory board and instructors in limited operator schools throughout the United States to determine the content needed to educate limited operators and were challenged by our discovery of the extremely wide range of curriculums. We found schools whose didactic curriculum presentation ranged from as few as 3 days to as many as 9 months. Many had clinical components, and many had none. Obviously, the lack of a national standardized curriculum made our revision work all the more difficult. As we revised the text, we determined that it was best to produce a comprehensive text that would serve the schools that had the most comprehensive curriculums. We used the latest ASRT Limited X-ray Machine Operator Curriculum as a guide. Schools with abbreviated curriculums can use this textbook by selecting those chapters or sections of chapters that apply to their programs.

Our foremost goal for this edition was to ensure that the content of this book matches that of the textbooks used in the JRCERT-accredited radiography or radiologic technology programs. Information taught to LXMOs should not differ from that taught to radiographers. The same technical exposure factors, radiation protection, and positioning of body parts should be used by both LXMOs and radiographers when performing radiographic procedures. Therefore we strove to make sure that the content of this text paralleled the mainstream radiography textbooks. This also ensures that those graduates of limited schools who must take a limited scope state licensure examination will be prepared to pass the Limited Scope of Practice in Radiography examination administered by the ARRT.

For instructors who teach limited operators, the comprehensive coverage of radiographic topics in this book should facilitate the teaching of any aspect of limited practice. However, because of the wide range of limited operator curriculums, it is up to the instructor, or more specifically the school or its curriculum committee, to determine the scope of what is taught. Some will present all the chapters in this book, whereas others will have time to cover only selected chapters or portions of chapters. To assist instructors, we have developed a comprehensive workbook and licensure exam prep that will help students learn radiologic concepts and prepare for a limited scope state licensure examination. A comprehensive test bank is also available for instructors to use in evaluating student outcomes.

CONTENT AND ORGANIZATION

Radiography Essentials for Limited Practice is organized in five parts, each with a different focus.

- Part I, *Introduction to Limited Radiography*, covers the role of the LXMO as a health care worker, introduces radiographic equipment, and includes material to refresh or improve math skills needed later in the book.
- Part II, *X-ray Science*, contains clear and concise discussion of all physical principles related to the production or control of the x-ray exposure needed to create medical radiographs. The expanding world of digital radiography has prompted many updates to chapters in this section.
- Part III, *Radiographic Anatomy, Positioning, and Pathology*, presents the essential procedural steps required to produce quality radiographs of all body structures.
- Part IV, *Professionalism and Patient Care*, covers the attitudes, behaviors, knowledge, and skills required to deliver safe and effective patient care.
- Part V, *Ancillary Clinical Skills*, includes chapters presenting other diagnostic and patient care skills that may be needed in the practice environment where the limited operator frequently works.

In addition, a collection of appendices has been included to provide information that an instructor or limited operator may find useful during the educational program or during performance of job duties.

FEATURES

Simplified Concepts

Simplified math and physics concepts are presented throughout the text. Many chapters were written to ensure that students focus on the most relevant information. Added art and radiographs augment the text for ease of learning. Over 900 illustrations are provided for reference purposes.

Special Boxes

Throughout the text, special boxes are inserted that contain information to reinforce important points in the text. The addition of many new boxes ensures that important concepts are identified.

Step-by-Step Procedures

The position and procedures chapters contain step-by-step instructions on how to perform each projection. The projections have been completely revised in this edition to provide quick, easy-to-understand reference. All the projections were revised to ensure consistency with radiologic technologist textbooks and to ensure that LXMOs perform x-ray procedures exactly the same way.

Learning Objectives, Key Terms, Glossary

Learning objectives and key terms highlight important information in each chapter and can be used as review tools. The key terms are bolded throughout the text. Definitions for these terms can be found in the glossary at the end of the book.

NEW TO THIS EDITION

The fifth edition incorporates many outstanding features. Up-to-date information from the new ASRT Limited X-ray Machine Operator Curriculum covers limited practice radiography and state-by-state guidelines for licensure and testing.

ARRT Limited Scope of Practice in Radiography Examination

The text was revised so that complete coverage of all the subjects students need to know to pass the ARRT Limited Scope of Practice in Radiography examination is included. Although the text covers the Content Specifications of the Limited Scope of Practice in Radiography examination, most chapters contain additional relevant information for limited practice.

New Content

The introductory and x-ray science sections of the book have been extensively updated to reflect the current practice environment of the Limited Operator, the latest ASRT Limited X-ray Machine Operators Curriculum, and the latest ARRT Content Specifications for the Limited Scope of Practice in Radiography examination. Photos of modern digital radiography equipment have been added to augment the more extensive coverage of digital imaging principles. All chapters have been updated with the international system of units (SI), which is broadly used. All screen-film imaging and film processing material has been moved to an appendix, if needed. It should be noted that screen-film imaging and film processing will be removed from the ARRT Contents in 2018.

The radiographic positioning material has been updated to include the latest recommendations of image receptor and radiation field sizes. All positioning instructions reflect the latest material contained in the mainstream positioning and procedures textbooks used in accredited radiography programs. Recommendations have been added for modifications to procedures needed to properly image the obese patient. Positioning photographs in Chapters 13, 14, and 15 have been updated to reflect use of digital image receptors.

The patient care and ancillary skills sections have been entirely updated to reflect current national standards and recognized best practices.

A final note on the use of this text: The ARRT does not review, evaluate, or endorse publications. Permission to reproduce ARRT copyrighted material should not be construed as an endorsement of the publication by the ARRT.

LEARNING AIDS FOR THE STUDENT

Workbook and Licensure Examination Prep for *Radiography Essentials for Limited Practice*

This workbook matches the textbook chapter for chapter, challenging students with a variety of exercises. Included are multiple-choice and fill-in-the-blank questions, matching exercises, and numerous labeling exercises of illustrations and radiographic images. The workbook is designed specifically to focus on the most important concepts contained in each chapter of the textbook. A Challenge Exercise is featured at the end of most chapters to assist the student in reviewing the key concepts presented in the workbook chapter. In addition, a Study Plan has been added to help students stay organized and on track as they prepare for their state licensure examination. The workbook also contains full-length, simulated limited licensure examinations to provide practice and identify deficiencies in knowledge for students preparing to take a state licensure examination. The answers for the workbook questions can be found on the free Evolve site.

TEACHING AIDS FOR THE INSTRUCTOR

Evolve

Evolve is an interactive learning environment designed to work in coordination with *Radiography Essentials for Limited Practice*. This website contains the Image Collection (all images in book), Microsoft PowerPoint slide presentations (for each book chapter), Test Bank, and the answers for the workbook questions. In addition, instructors may use Evolve to provide an Internet-based course component that reinforces and expands on the concepts delivered in class. Evolve may be used to publish the class syllabus, outlines, and lecture notes; set up "virtual office hours" and email communication; share important dates and information through the online class calendar; and encourage student participation through chat rooms and discussion boards. Evolve allows instructors to post examinations and manage their grade books online. For more information about how to register for access to these free Evolve resources, visit http://evolve.elsevier.com/Long/radiographylimited or contact an Elsevier sales representative.

Contents

PART I

Introduction to Limited Radiography

Chapter 1

Role of the Limited X-ray Machine Operator

At the conclusion of this chapter, you will be able to:

- Compare the role of the limited x-ray machine operator with that of the registered radiologic technologist
- Identify the discoverer of x-rays and the date of the discovery
- Explain the primary purposes of the American Registry of Radiologic Technologists, American Society of Radiologic Technologists, and Joint Review Committee on Education in Radiologic Technology
- Determine the legal requirements for the practice of radiography in your state
- Describe the typical work environment of the limited x-ray machine operator
- Describe in a general way the duties of a limited x-ray machine operator

Key Terms

American Registry of Radiologic
  Technologists (ARRT)
American Society of Radiologic
  Technologists (ASRT)
back office
front office
Joint Review Committee on Education
  in Radiologic Technology (JRCERT)

limited operator
limited x-ray
limited x-ray machine operator (LXMO)
medical assistant (MA)
radiograph
radiographer
radiologist
reciprocity

Welcome to the fascinating field of radiography! You are beginning a study of the art and science needed to create images of the internal structures of the human body. The images you create will aid physicians in diagnosis and will help patients receive treatment needed to promote or regain health. This is a vital role in the health care delivery system, one that requires knowledge, skill, judgment, integrity, and dedication.

RADIOGRAPHY

X-rays were discovered on November 8, 1895, by Wilhelm Conrad Roentgen (Fig. 1-1) at the University of Würzburg in Germany. Roentgen was a teacher and researcher with a special interest in the conduction of high-voltage electricity through low-vacuum tubes. His discovery of the x-ray during his regularly planned experiments was accidental. The first x-ray image by Roentgen was of his wife Bertha's hand using a 15-minute exposure (Fig. 1-2). The first radiographers were scientists and physicians who experimented with primitive x-ray apparatus to make x-ray images of the human body (Fig. 1-3). Soon these pioneers trained their assistants to make these "x-ray pictures," now

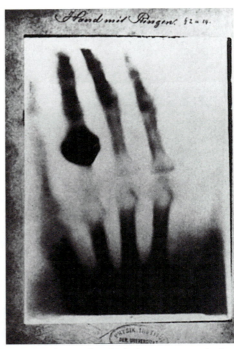

Fig. 1-2 The first radiograph, which demonstrates the bones of the hand of Roentgen's wife Bertha with a ring on one finger.

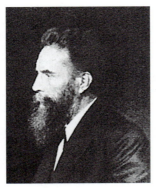

Fig. 1-1 Wilhelm Conrad Roentgen (1845-1923). He discovered x-rays on November 8, 1895.

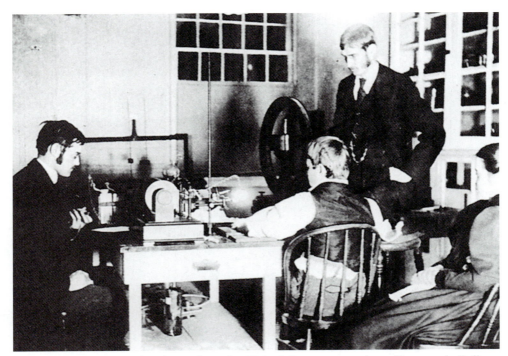

Fig. 1-3 The first clinical radiograph in the United States was made at Dartmouth College in 1896.

called **radiographs,** and the profession of radiography was born.

American Society of Radiologic Technologists

Early radiographers soon began meeting to share their knowledge. The organization, now called the **American Society of Radiologic Technologists (ASRT),** was founded in Chicago in 1920. It is the world's oldest and largest professional radiologic science organization. The ASRT provides many services to its members, including continuing education, a professional journal, a newsletter, guidelines and assistance for radiography educators, and an annual national meeting. The ASRT publishes a *Code of Ethics* that can be found at *www.asrt.org.*

American Registry of Radiologic Technologists

Through the efforts of this organization, the **American Registry of Radiologic Technologists (ARRT)** was formed in 1922 to establish standards and examinations necessary to certify radiologic technologists. Radiologic technologists certified by ARRT use the initials RT(R) after their names. This abbreviation means *registered technologist (radiography).* Registered technologists who have passed the ARRT examination in radiography are referred to as **radiographers.** Do not get radiographer mixed up with radiologist. A **radiologist** is a physician who specializes in radiography. Radiographers and radiologists work together in radiology departments. The ARRT publishes a *Code of Ethics,* which are aspirational statements. This can be found in Chapter 20 or at *www.arrt.org.* It also publishes an important document called the *Rules of Ethics,* which are mandatory and enforceable statements. This document, found in Appendix B, discusses the minimally acceptable professional conduct that those in radiology should adhere to. An important document, the *Task Inventory for Limited Scope of Practice*

in Radiography, is also published by the ARRT. This document, which identifies for the limited operator all the tasks that are tested on the certification examination, can be found in Appendix M.

The profession of radiography has expanded to include a variety of imaging and treatment modalities, including those listed in Box 1-1. Many of these modalities require specialized training beyond that needed for certification by the ARRT in radiography. The newest role for the radiographer is that of radiologist assistant (RA). These radiographers obtain additional schooling, usually at the graduate level, and perform limited duties that a radiologist typically carries out, such as fluoroscopy and initial readings of radiographs.

Joint Review Committee on Education in Radiologic Technology

The **Joint Review Committee on Education in Radiologic Technology (JRCERT)** is the national organization that formally conducts the accreditation of schools of radiologic technology. The JRCERT was formed in 1969 and accredits, as of this printing, 637 radiography programs in the United States. The JRCERT publishes the *Standards for an Accreditation Program in Radiography* document, which tells colleges what standards are required to be accredited. Certification in radiography requires at least 2 years of education (six college semesters) in an accredited program that includes comprehensive academic coursework in the sciences. These programs are affiliated with acute care general hospitals to provide extensive clinical experience in the care of patients who are severely ill or injured. A growing number of programs are changing to a 4-year bachelor's degree curriculum.

Effective January 1, 2012, the JRCERT began to accredit limited scope x-ray machine operator educational programs. This accreditation is designed to promote academic excellence, patient safety, and quality health care.

 **Box 1-1**

Imaging and Treatment Modalities in Radiology

Angiography: imaging of blood vessels with the injection of special compounds called *contrast media*

Bone densitometry (BD): art and science of measuring the bone mineral content and density of specific skeletal sites or the whole body

Computed tomography (CT): computerized x-ray system that provides axial images (transverse "slices") of all parts of the body

Fluoroscopy: real-time viewing of x-ray images in motion

Magnetic resonance imaging (MRI): computerized imaging system that uses a powerful magnetic field and radiofrequency pulses to produce images of all parts of the body

Mammography: x-ray imaging of the breast using a special x-ray machine

Nuclear medicine (NM): injection or ingestion of radioactive materials and recording of their uptake in the body using a gamma camera

Positron emission tomography (PET): highly sophisticated computerized form of nuclear medicine imaging

Radiation therapy: treatment of malignant diseases using radiation

Sonography: imaging of soft tissue structures using sound echoes. This modality is also referred to as "ultrasound"

Many states currently have limited x-ray machine operator programs of anywhere from 10 weeks to 9 months. Many of these programs are expected to apply for this national accreditation and recognition. Documents from the JRCERT can be obtained at *www.jrcert.org*.

To understand how these three organizations work together to develop a professional radiographer, the following scenario is provided. Individuals interested in becoming a radiographer must qualify and enter a JRCERT-accredited radiography program. While in the program they complete a comprehensive curriculum developed by the ASRT. On graduation, these students take the certification examination in radiography given by the ARRT. ARRT-registered technologists can perform all diagnostic x-ray examinations and operate complex radiography equipment in all 50 states. The titles *registered technologist* and *radiographer* are used throughout this text to denote these professionals.

LIMITED X-RAY MACHINE OPERATOR

The ASRT recently published the *Limited X-ray Machine Operator Curriculum* to support the education of limited operators of x-ray equipment. The curriculum allows states and faculty flexibility in the development of limited curricula to meet the needs of individuals performing diagnostic x-ray procedures within a limited scope. The ASRT officially terms the limited operator, a **limited x-ray machine operator (LXMO).** The titles **limited operator** and LXMO are used throughout this text to denote limited operators of x-ray equipment. The ARRT and JRCERT also use these titles in their publications. LXMOs are encouraged to join the ASRT to support the profession and to obtain continuing education.

Limited x-ray work is regulated within the offices of each state's Department of Health. The majority of states that have regulations for those who operate x-ray equipment use the above titles for individuals who perform limited x-rays. However, a few states use other terms such as *basic x-ray machine operator*, *practical x-ray machine operator*, *limited radiologic technologist*, or *limited radiographer*.

Limited x-ray is practiced primarily in clinics and physicians' offices (Fig. 1-4). In some areas, however, limited operators are employed in hospitals, a practice that is expanding.

Limited x-ray developed as nurses, medical assistants, chiropractic assistants, laboratory technologists, and health care office personnel were trained to perform limited aspects of radiography in addition to their primary duties. It is called *limited* because the scope of practice is restricted compared with that of registered technologists. Limited x-ray practice does not involve the use of contrast media for the imaging of blood vessels and abdominal organs or the operation of complex radiographic equipment such as computed tomography (CT) and

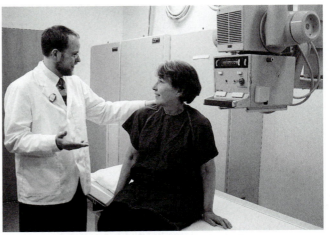

Fig. 1-4 Limited operator at work.

magnetic resonance imaging (MRI) scanners and angiography equipment.[a]

Additional restrictions may be applied because the scope of practice varies among the states. In contrast to registered technologists, limited operators are often educated as certified **medical assistants (MA)** and perform a variety of office procedures that do not involve imaging, such as drawing blood samples, performing diagnostic tests, and assisting the physician with treatments and patient care procedures. Information about some of these duties is included in the final chapters.

CERTIFICATION

Certification in radiography by the ARRT has been accepted as the minimum credential for radiographers for many years. No legal requirements were applied to the practice of radiography until the early 1970s, when licensure laws for radiologic technologists were passed in New York and New Jersey. California passed licensing legislation shortly thereafter. Today, most states have laws requiring some type of licensure to practice radiography, and at least half of these include provision for limited x-ray practice. State licensure is not ARRT credentialing. Currently, depending on the state, limited x-ray may be prohibited, permitted without restriction, or regulated quite specifically. For example, New York prohibits limited x-ray, whereas Missouri has no requirements for certification and Wisconsin restricts limited x-ray to only the limbs, chest, and spine. Oregon issues eight different categories of limited permits based on the specific procedures for which the radiographer is qualified.

Legal requirements are subject to change, so it will be necessary for you to inquire directly of the appropriate

---

[a]One exception to this statement is the granting of limited permits in California that allow qualified limited operators to use contrast media for examinations of the gastrointestinal tract and the urinary system.

agency in your state to determine whether limited x-ray is permitted, whether its practice is regulated, and how to obtain the necessary certification. Appendix A provides additional information on where to obtain information.

Most states that regulate limited x-ray also regulate the education necessary to qualify. The student who plans to obtain a limited license or permit must be certain that the planned education meets state requirements. These requirements may include the need for clinical experience and clinical supervision. Some states also have continuing education requirements for renewal of licenses or permits. **Reciprocity** is common in many states. This means that the education and credential issued in one state is approved in another state.

Each state that regulates limited x-ray has established standards for the scope of practice allowed. There are serious sanctions for practicing radiography outside the boundaries defined by state laws and regulations. Practicing without a valid license or permit or practicing outside the scope of one's credentials may result in fines, imprisonment, or both. In addition, a license or permit may be suspended or permanently revoked. Employers may also be penalized if their employees practice radiography in violation of regulations. *All radiographers and limited operators must be aware of the legal standards that apply to them and take care that their practice conforms to these standards.* This information also is available from the agencies listed in Appendix A.

The practice of radiography involves a variety of knowledge and skills. Although the *scope of practice* may be limited, there is no restriction on the knowledge and skill necessary for the practice. In other words, the limited operator is held to the same high standards as a registered radiologic technologist in performing procedures within the permitted scope of practice.

American Registry of Radiologic Technologists Limited Scope Examination

The ARRT provides the examination for all the states that require limited x-ray operators to be certified. Thirty-five states utilize the ARRT limited scope examination for state licensing purposes. The examination, entitled "Limited Scope of Practice in Radiography," is completed on a computer at an ARRT-approved testing site. The ARRT's detailed *Content Specifications* document for this examination can be found in the *Workbook and Licensure Prep* for this text. The document identifies the various areas of limited practice that are tested, along with an outline of what is contained in each area. The limited scope examination contains a core module of 100 questions. The questions for this section come from Chapters 1 through 11. The limited scope examination also contains the following procedure modules: chest, skull/sinus, spine, and extremities, which contain 90 questions total. The questions for these sections come from Chapters 12 through 22. Individuals do not have to

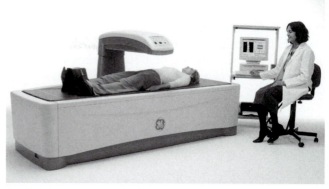

Fig. 1-5 Patient on a GE Lunar bone densitometry machine. Limited operator is controlling the scan using a computer.

write each procedure module, only those that contain the x-ray procedures they perform. There is also a specialty podiatry module specifically for those who work in that area. The podiatry module contains 20 questions. The ARRT also provides a *Limited Scope Exam Handbook* that explains the process and contains the application. The Handbook can be found at www.arrt.org.

The ARRT's limited scope examination is the same for all states that require licensure for limited operators. An important aspect of this examination is that all x-ray projections of the abdomen, pelvis, hips, ribs, and sternum are not tested. X-ray projections using contrast media, such as the stomach, colon, and kidneys, are also not tested.

Bone Densitometry

Bone densitometry (BD) is a specialized area of radiography. A separate x-ray machine is used to measure the bone mineral content and density of various bones in the body. Many diseases affecting the bones, especially osteoporosis, are diagnosed using this machine (Fig. 1-5). Each state will have its own regulations regarding the operation of BD x-ray machines. Many states allow limited x-ray operators to perform BD examinations. However, separate ARRT certification may be required. The ARRT provides states with the "Bone Densitometry Equipment Operators Examination." This examination contains 60 questions covering the equipment and procedures performed. The ARRT's *Content Specifications* document for this examination is also found in the *Workbook and Licensure Prep* for this text. Chapter 26 provides the introductory information needed to understand BD and prepare for the examination.

WORK ENVIRONMENT

As a limited operator, your direct supervisor may be a physician, a nurse, a registered technologist, an office manager, or a radiology administrator. In most instances your supervisor will be a radiologic technologist. Work environments vary greatly, depending on the type of organization, its size, and its organizational structure. You will often work directly with one or more physicians (Fig. 1-6). These physicians may be primary-care physicians whose

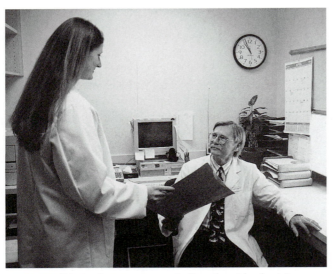

Fig. 1-6 Limited operators work directly with physicians.

specialty is general practice and who see both adults and children for a wide variety of complaints. On the other hand, you may work for a specialist, a physician who has completed extensive additional training to qualify as an expert in a particular aspect of medical or chiropractic care. Box 1-2 lists health care specialists and describes their areas of clinical interest. It will be helpful to understand these terms because you will encounter them frequently in various aspects of your work.

The work of outpatient clinic facilities is divided into two general areas, often referred to as the **front office** and the **back office.** The front office (Fig. 1-7) is a public area and includes the reception desk, the patient waiting area, and the desks or offices of those who deal with medical records, billing, and insurance claims. The back office (Fig. 1-8), the area where patients are examined and treated, includes consulting rooms, examination rooms, treatment rooms, laboratory facilities, and the x-ray department. Utility and storage areas are also found there.

The radiography suite will include one or more x-ray rooms, a computer room or station to view and process digital images and access electronic records, a desk or countertop with various computers, a film viewing area for looking at older film x-rays, and a film storage area. Dressing rooms and restrooms are usually convenient to x-ray rooms. The limited operator is a *back office employee*

Box 1-2

Abbreviated Listing of Health Care Specialists

Anesthesiologist: administers anesthetics and monitors patient during surgery

Dermatologist: diagnoses and treats conditions and diseases of the skin

Emergency department physician: specializes in treating trauma and emergency situations; a triage expert in disaster situations

Family practice physician: treats individuals and families in the context of daily life

Gastroenterologist: diagnoses and treats diseases of the gastrointestinal tract

Geriatrician: specializes in problems and diseases of elderly persons

Gynecologist: treats problems and diseases of the female reproductive system

Internist: specializes in diseases of the internal organs

Neurologist: specializes in functions and disorders of the nervous system

Obstetrician: specializes in pregnancy, labor, delivery, and immediate postpartum care

Oncologist: specializes in tumor identification and treatment

Ophthalmologist: diagnoses and treats problems and diseases of the eye

Pathologist: specializes in the scientific study of body alterations caused by disease and death

Pediatrician: treats and diagnoses disorders and diseases in children

Podiatrist: diagnoses and treats disorders and diseases of the feet

Psychiatrist: specializes in diagnosis, treatment, and prevention of mental illness

Radiologist: specializes in diagnosis by means of medical imaging

Surgeons:

Abdominal: specializes in surgery of the abdominal cavity

Neurologic: specializes in surgery of the brain, spinal cord, and peripheral nervous system

Orthopedic: diagnoses and treats problems of the musculoskeletal system

Plastic: restores or improves the appearance and function of body parts

Thoracic: specializes in problems of the chest

Urologic: diagnoses and treats problems of the urinary tract and the male reproductive system

Chiropractic specialties: specialty certification is available to chiropractic physicians in the fields of radiology, orthopedics (nonsurgical), neurology, nutrition, sports medicine, and other fields

Both medical and chiropractic physicians may limit their practices to specific areas of interest with or without certification. Those with certification may have a general practice outside the scope of their specialty.

Modified from Ehrlich RA, Coakes D: *Patient care in radiography,* ed 9, St Louis, 2016, Mosby.

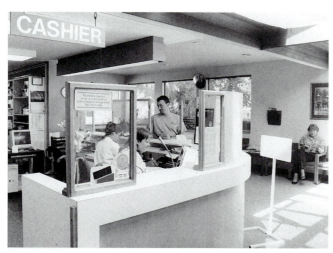

Fig. 1-7 The front office includes the waiting room and reception area.

and may be assigned other back office duties in addition to radiography.

Limited operators employed by hospitals will work in a much different environment. The radiology department is supervised by a director, usually a registered radiologic technologist. Limited operators, like radiographers, work directly with radiologists, the physician specialists who interpret the radiographs and perform special imaging procedures. There will be less contact with the patients' primary care physicians, although some will visit the radiology department. The duties are likely to be limited to radiographic procedures, with other personnel handling paperwork, patient transportation, and much of the communication with physicians' offices and other hospital departments. On the other hand, limited radiographers who also have medical assisting skills may also be employed in ways that use these skills.

The hospital radiology staff may also include a number of limited operators with assignments involving specific procedures or work areas and some with responsibility for supervision or quality control. The staff may be scheduled in three shifts around the clock. In small institutions, the department may be closed during late night hours and on Sundays and holidays. When the department is closed, limited operators may take turns being "on call," that is, available by telephone or pager to come to the hospital when necessary.

Hospitals are complex, highly structured institutions. Each has many rules and procedures that must be mastered for the safety of patients and the efficient performance of the health care team. It is beyond the scope of this text to prepare limited operators to cope with all the situations and judgments they might face in an acute care hospital setting. A thorough orientation to the institution is necessary, and the use of additional texts and references is highly recommended.

TYPICAL DUTIES OF A LIMITED X-RAY MACHINE OPERATOR

The limited operator encounters the patient after he or she has been admitted to the clinic or radiology department. A physician will have examined the patient, and one or more specific x-ray procedures will have been ordered. The physician may give the order directly to the limited operator or may instruct a nurse or medical assistant to communicate the order. The order may be verbal or in the form of a written requisition. The necessary x-ray paperwork may be completed by a clerical employee but is often the radiographer's responsibility.

Once the paperwork is completed, the limited operator greets the patient and determines whether the patient

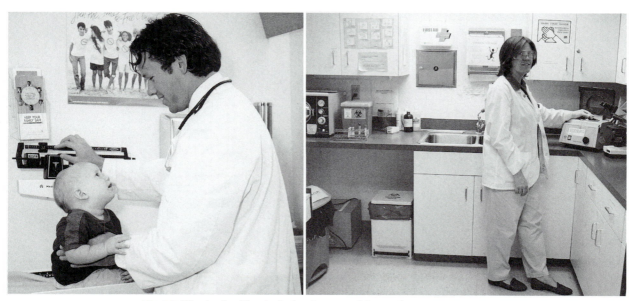

Fig. 1-8 The back office includes the consulting and treatment areas.

will need to undress and don a gown before radiography. A dressing room or examining room is usually used for this purpose. The exact clothing to be removed is determined according to the examination. Generally, patients must remove outer clothing from the body area to be examined. Specific instructions for patient preparation are included in the appropriate sections of the text.

The patient is then taken into the x-ray room. At this point, the limited operator provides a brief explanation and answers any questions about the procedure. When you have completed this text, you should be prepared to respond appropriately to most patient questions and concerns. Very often the limited operator will have to discuss the examination with a radiographer or work directly with the radiographer to ensure that the appropriate x-ray projections are done and the correct exposure techniques used (Fig. 1-9).

The next step is to assist the patient into the general position required for the x-ray examination (Fig. 1-10).

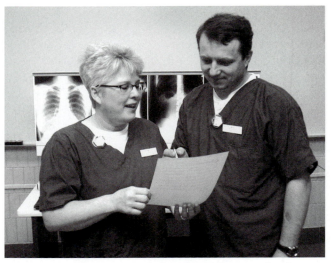

Fig. 1-9 Limited operator *(right)* discussing a patient's x-ray projections with a registered technologist *(left)*.

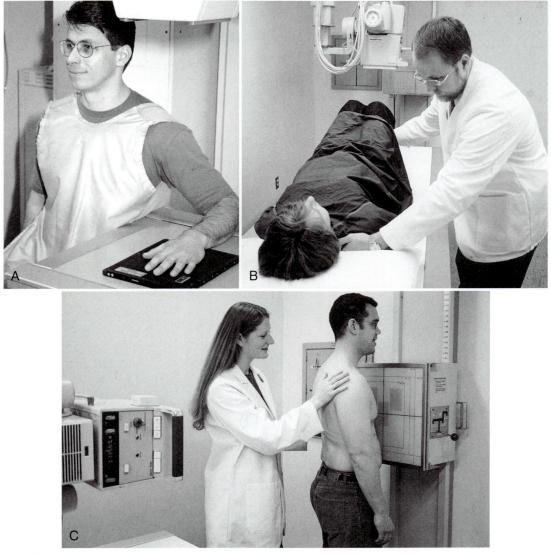

Fig. 1-10 A, Patient seated at table for hand radiograph. **B,** Limited operator assisting patient to lie on radiographic table. **C,** Limited operator assisting patient into position at upright cassette holder.

For example, if a hand is to be x-rayed, the patient can be seated at the end of the x-ray table. For a spine examination, the patient may need to lie on the table. If a chest examination is ordered, the patient will stand at an upright cassette holder. The limited operator then selects the correct cassette and places it in position. Next, the patient is positioned precisely, and the x-ray tube is aligned with the body part and the film at a specific distance. The body part must be measured to determine the proper exposure factors from a technique chart. At this point, lead shields are positioned for radiation protection. The limited operator then goes to the control booth, consults the technique chart, and sets the x-ray control panel to the desired exposure. Final instructions are given to the patient, and the exposure is made. If more than one exposure is needed, the cassette is changed, the patient repositioned, and the steps repeated until the examination is complete.

After ensuring that the patient is safe and comfortable, the limited operator takes the cassette to the processing and reader device. Once the image is viewed on the computer monitor and approved, it can be sent for reading by the radiologist or stored. The processing and management of digital images are detailed in Chapter 8. If the image is satisfactory and no further exposures are needed, the patient is returned to an examining room or dressing room. The limited operator then readies the x-ray room for the next examination and prepares the films for reading.

The exact nature of a limited operator's duties will vary with the place of employment, the size of the staff, and the equipment available.

SUMMARY

Limited x-ray is a relatively new professional role in the field of health care. Similar to radiographers, limited x-ray operators work closely with general physicians and work directly with radiologists, and their duties involve direct patient contact. Most limited operators are employed in outpatient facilities such as clinics, but some are employed by hospitals, and their work may vary considerably, depending on their place of employment. Many limited operators enjoy their work and later enter JRCERT programs to become radiologic technologists.

Requirements and credentials for limited operators differ greatly from state to state, and limited operators are responsible for knowing and following the regulations that apply to them.

Chapter 2

Introduction to Radiographic Equipment

Learning Objectives

At the conclusion of this chapter, you will be able to:

- Use correct terminology when discussing x-ray equipment and its parts
- Demonstrate the radiation field and define the central ray
- Explain the differences between primary radiation, scatter radiation, and remnant radiation
- List two effects of scatter radiation
- List the components of the image receptor system
- List the essential features of a typical x-ray room
- Explain the purposes of the control booth and the transformer cabinet
- Safely change the positions of the radiographic table and the x-ray tube
- Demonstrate a detent and explain its function
- Explain the purpose of a collimator
- Describe precautions to be taken to ensure personnel safety from radiation exposure

Key Terms

adverse incident
attenuation
Bucky
cassette
central ray
collimator
computed radiography (CR)
control booth
control console
CR reader
detent
grid
image receptor (IR)
latent image
phosphor imaging plate

plate
primary radiation
radiation field
remnant radiation
scatter radiation
scatter radiation fog
tissue density
Trendelenburg position
tube housing
tube port
upright cassette holder
visible image
x-ray beam
x-ray tube

This chapter introduces the useful x-ray beam, discusses the equipment found in a typical x-ray room, and provides some fundamentals of radiation safety. Many of these topics are covered in greater detail later in the text, but it will be helpful for you at this point to have an orientation to the equipment and safety considerations that are central to your work as a limited x-ray operator.

PRIMARY X-RAY BEAM

The source of x-rays is the **x-ray tube.** The internal structure and function of the tube are discussed in Chapter 5. X-rays are formed within a very small area inside the tube. From this point, the x-rays diverge into space. The x-ray tube is surrounded by a lead-lined **tube housing.** Some of the scattered x-rays are absorbed by the tube housing. X-rays that are created, exit the housing through an opening called the **tube port.** These x-rays form the triangular-shaped **x-ray beam** (Fig. 2-1). The radiation that leaves the tube is called **primary radiation.** The squared area of the x-ray beam that strikes the patient and x-ray table is called the **radiation field.** An imaginary line in the center of the x-ray beam and perpendicular to the long axis of the x-ray tube is called the **central ray.** The central ray is important in positioning the patient because this point is used to align the x-ray tube to the body part to be imaged.

During a radiographic exposure, x-rays from the tube are directed through the patient to the **image receptor (IR)** (Fig. 2-2). As the x-rays pass through the patient, some of them are absorbed by the patient and others are not. Anatomic structures that have greater **tissue density** (mass), such as bone, will absorb more radiation than less dense tissue, such as muscle. This results in a pattern of varying intensity in the x-ray beam that exits on the opposite side of the patient. This radiation, called **remnant radiation** or exit radiation, then passes through to the IR. The IR now contains an "unseen" image called a **latent image.** This image remains stored in the IR phosphors until it is processed. Processing will convert the latent image into a **visible image.**

SCATTER RADIATION

When the primary x-ray beam strikes matter, such as the patient or the IR, a portion of its energy is absorbed within the matter. Absorption of the x-ray beam is called **attenuation.** Attenuated x-rays can be totally absorbed within the body, reduced in energy, or scattered outside of the body. *The patient is the primary source of scatter.* This **scatter radiation** generally has less energy than the primary x-ray beam, but it is not as easily controlled. It travels out from the absorbing matter in all directions, causing unwanted exposure to the IR and to anyone who is in the room. This is an important reason why the study of radiation safety is so essential to the limited operator. Radiation safety is discussed briefly at the end of this chapter and more extensively in Chapter 11. The unwanted image exposure caused by scatter radiation is called **scatter radiation fog.** The production of scatter radiation and the control of the fog it produces are addressed in Chapter 9.

See Box 2-1 for a summary of primary, remnant, and scatter radiation.

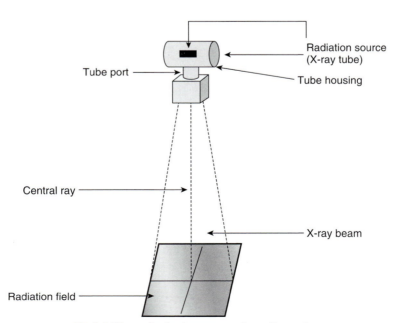

Fig. 2-1 Terms for basic concepts in radiography.

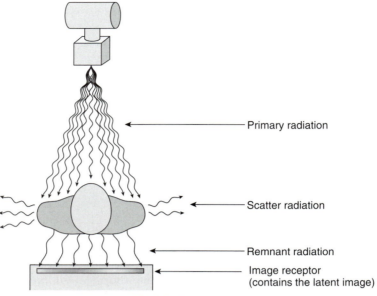

Primary radiation

Scatter radiation

Remnant radiation

Image receptor
(contains the latent image)

Fig. 2-2 X-ray beam.

Box 2-1

Synopsis of Primary, Remnant, and Scatter Radiation

Primary Radiation
- Definition: the x-ray beam that leaves the tube and is unattenuated, except by air.
- Its direction and location are predictable and controllable.

Remnant (Exit) Radiation
- Definition: what remains of the primary beam after it has been attenuated by matter (the patient).
- Tissues of different density, or atomic number, in the body absorb x-rays differently and therefore emit x-rays differently. The remnant beam contains a varied pattern of x-ray energies that reflects the different absorption rates.
- The pattern of the remnant radiation creates the x-ray image.

Scatter Radiation
- Definition: radiation from the primary beam that is randomly scattered within or outside of the body.
- Scatter radiation travels in all directions from the patient and is very difficult to control.
- Generally, it has less energy than the primary beam.

IMAGE RECEPTOR SYSTEM

The IR system consists of a **cassette** that contains a **phosphor imaging plate.** In the radiology department today, the IR is part of the digital imaging system. One component is a cassette (Fig. 2-3, *A*). The cassette contains a **plate** with special phosphors that store the x-ray image until it is processed. The cassette protects the plate's phosphors from damage and dirt. IR plates come

Table 2-1

Most Common Computed Radiography Cassette Sizes

Inches	Centimeters
8 × 10	18 × 24
10 × 12	24 × 30
14 × 14	35 × 35
14 × 17	35 × 43
14 × 36	35 × 91

in standard sizes. The most common sizes are listed in Table 2-1. They are manufactured in both English and metric sizes, with most sizes stated in English. In the radiology department, the terms *cassette* and *plate* are often used to mean IR.

Most departments in which limited operators work use the **computed radiography (CR),** a digital imaging system. The x-ray image is produced in digital format using computer technology (see Chapter 8). When CR systems are used, the conventional radiography machine, positioning of the patient, and setting of technical parameters remain the same. However, the image is obtained from a phosphor material inside the CR plate. After the exposure is made, the CR cassette is inserted into a **CR reader** (Fig. 2-3, *B*) where the phosphor on the plate is scanned by a laser beam and the final image appears on a computer monitor. The image can then be adjusted for final density and contrast and stored in an electronic file or printed out on laser film (Fig. 2-3, *C*). The image is read directly from the monitor by the radiologist.

Throughout this text, *IR* is used to refer to the device that receives the remnant x-ray beam and stores the image of the body part until it is processed.

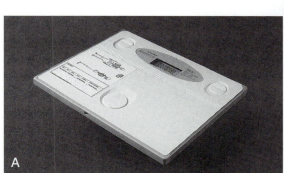
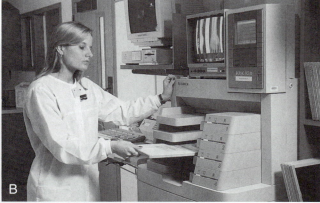
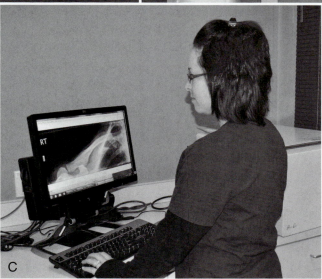

Fig. 2-3 A, Computed radiography cassette containing a phosphor imaging plate. **B,** Limited operator inserting a computed radiographic plate into an image reader device. The unit scans the plate with a laser beam and places the digitized image in a computer for reading. **C,** A computer and monitor are used to view the image and make final adjustments.

X-RAY ROOM

The x-ray room (Fig. 2-4) includes the x-ray equipment itself, a counter area, and a protective **control booth.** The x-ray machine consists of the x-ray tube, the tube support, the **control console** (located in the control booth), and the transformer cabinet. There is usually also a radiographic table and a wall-mounted cassette holder for upright studies. In chiropractic offices, there may not be an x-ray table because chiropractic radiography is often done with the patient upright to provide weight-bearing information (Fig. 2-5).

Radiography involves positioning the patient, the IR, and the x-ray tube, and setting the control panel and making the exposure. Before you learn the specifics of radiographic positioning, it is important to understand how the equipment works so that you can position it safely and efficiently.

X-ray equipment may vary considerably, depending on age, manufacturer, and the complexity of procedures for which it was designed. The equipment descriptions provided here highlight the important features of most general-purpose x-ray machines and some of the common variations. If you are currently associated with a clinical facility that has x-ray equipment, it will be helpful to consider the information that follows in relation to the equipment you will be using. When you have learned to use several different x-ray machines, it will be relatively easy to orient yourself to new equipment.

POSITIONING OF THE X-RAY TUBE

As stated earlier, the x-ray tube is encased in a barrel-shaped tube housing (Fig. 2-6). This housing is lead-lined for radiation control. The housing protects and insulates the tube and provides a mounting for attachments, which the limited operator uses to position the x-ray tube and to control the size of the radiation field.

The tube housing may be attached to a ceiling mount or to a tube stand. Both types of mountings provide

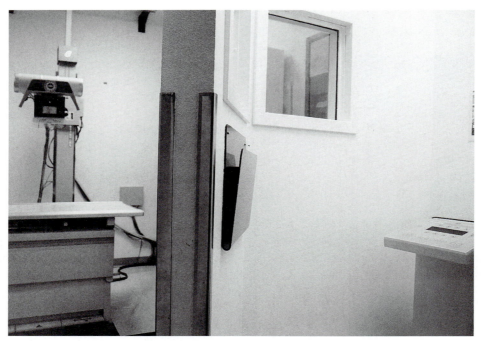

Fig. 2-4 X-ray room and control booth.

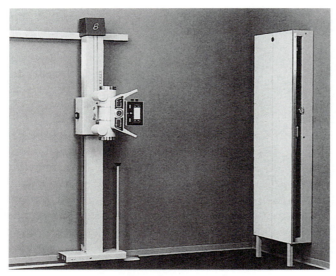

Fig. 2-5 Upright x-ray machine.

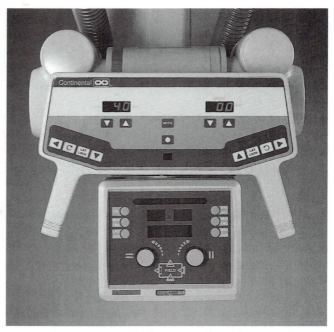

Fig. 2-6 X-ray tube housing and attachments.

support and mobility for the tube. These tube supports allow the operator to move the tube, to align it to the patient and the IR, and to adjust its height. A ceiling-mounted tube support (Fig. 2-7), sometimes called a *ceiling crane* or *tube hanger*, suspends the x-ray tube from a system of tracks, allowing it to be moved to locations throughout the room. A tube stand (Fig. 2-8) is a vertical support with a horizontal arm that suspends the tube over the radiographic table. The tube stand rolls along a track that is secured to the floor (and sometimes also to the ceiling or wall), parallel to the x-ray table. This enables the tube to move longitudinally along the length of the table.

Typical tube motions (Fig. 2-9) include the following:
- *Longitudinal*—along the long axis of the table
- *Transverse*—across the table, at right angles to longitudinal
- *Vertical*—up and down, increasing or decreasing the distance between the tube and the table
- *Rotational*—allows the entire tube stand to turn on its axis, changing the angle at which the tube arm is extended
- *Angular* (tilt, roll)—permits angulation of the tube along the longitudinal axis of the table and allows the tube to be aimed at the wall, rather than at the table

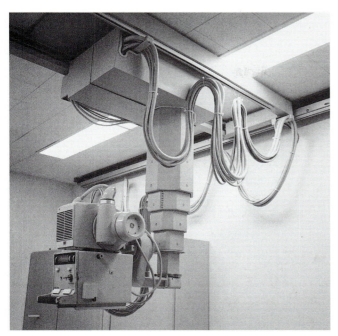

Fig. 2-7 Ceiling-mounted tube support.

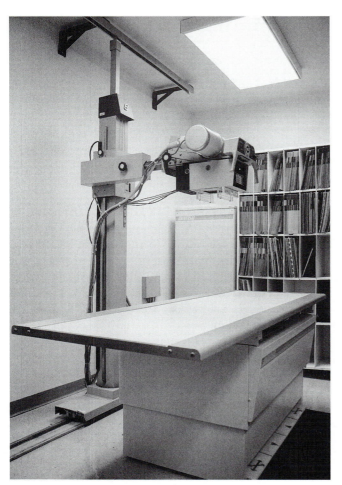

Fig. 2-8 Tube stand.

A system of electric and/or mechanical locks holds the tube in position. The control system for all, or most, of these locks is usually an attachment on the front of the tube housing (see Fig. 2-6). To move the tube in any direction, a locking device must be released. It is sometimes possible to force tube movement without first releasing the lock, but this practice will damage the lock, making it impossible to secure the tube in position. *Do not attempt to move the tube without first releasing the appropriate lock.*

The tube stand and/or the movable portion of the **upright cassette holder** may move unexpectedly when the electric supply to electric locks is turned off. To avoid damaging the equipment, you must be certain that these units are safely positioned before turning off the power to the locks. One way to accomplish this is to position the x-ray tube immediately above a pillow on the tabletop before shutting down the power supply to the tube support locks.

A **detent** is a special mechanism that tends to stop a moving part in a specific location. Detents are built into tube supports to provide ease in attaining placement at standard locations. For example, a vertical detent may indicate when the distance from tube to film is 40 inches, a common standard distance. Other detents provide "stops" when the transverse tube position is centered in relation to the table and when the tube tilt position is such that the central ray is perpendicular to the table or to the wall.

COLLIMATOR

The **collimator** is a boxlike device attached under the tube housing (see Fig. 2-6). It allows the limited operator to vary the size of the radiation field. The collimator includes a light that indicates the beam size and location and the center of the field. There is usually a centering light that aids in aligning the central ray to the **Bucky** tray (Fig. 2-10). Controls on the front of the collimator allow adjustment of the size of each dimension of the radiation field. These dimensions are indicated on a scale on the front of the collimator. A timer controls the collimator light, turning it off after a certain length of time, usually 30 seconds. This helps to avoid accidental overheating of the unit by prolonged use of its high-intensity light.

RADIOGRAPHIC TABLE

The radiographic table is a special unit that is more than just a support for the patient. Although the table is usually secured to the floor, it may be capable of three types of motion: vertical, tilt, and "floating tabletop."

For vertical table motion, a hydraulic motor, activated by a hand, foot, or knee switch, raises or lowers the height of the table. The table may be lowered so that the patient can sit on it easily and then elevated to a comfortable working height for the limited operator. There will

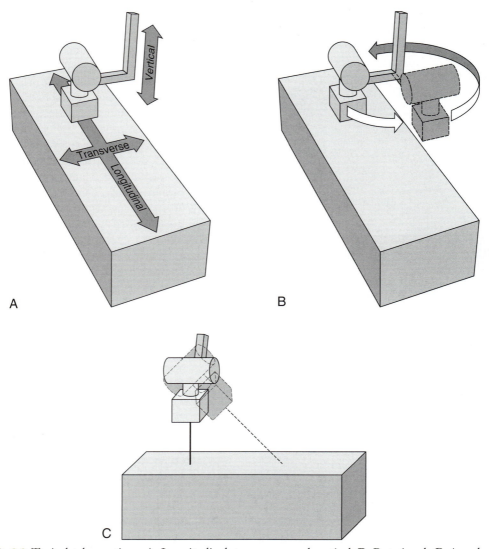

Fig. 2-9 Typical tube motions. **A,** Longitudinal, transverse, and vertical. **B,** Rotational. **C,** Angular.

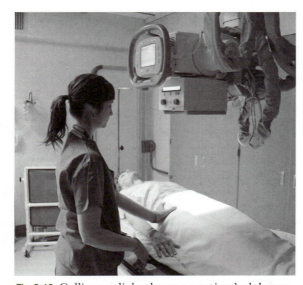

Fig. 2-10 Collimator light shown on patient's abdomen.

be a detent that stops the table in the standard position for routine radiography. This standard table height corresponds to indicated distances from the x-ray tube. It is important that standard tube-to-film distances be used, so it is necessary to return the table to the detent position after lowering it for patient access. Not all tables are capable of vertical motion.

A tilting table (Fig. 2-11) also uses a hydraulic motor to change position. In this case, the table turns on a central axis to attain a vertical position. This allows the patient to be placed in a horizontal position, in a vertical position, or at any angle in between. The table may also tilt in the opposite direction, allowing the head end to be lowered at least 15 degrees into the **Trendelenburg position** (Fig. 2-12). A detent stops the table in the horizontal (level) position.

Special attachments for the tilting table include footboards and shoulder guards for patient safety when the table is tilted (Fig. 2-13). You should pay particular

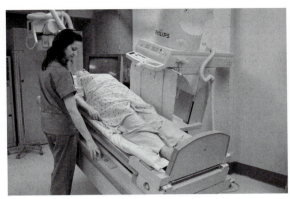

Fig. 2-11 Tilting table.

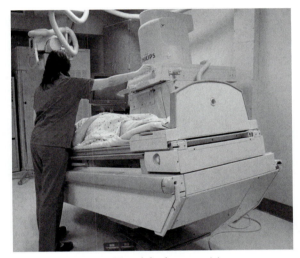

Fig. 2-12 Trendelenburg position.

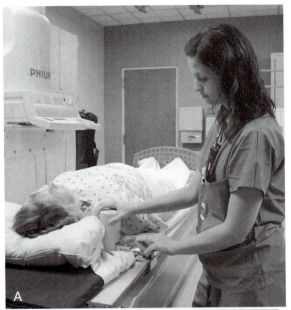

A

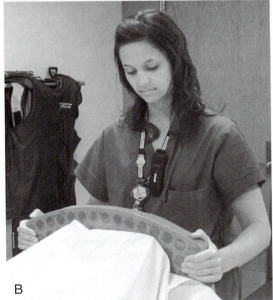

B

Fig. 2-13 Shoulder guards and footboards should be attached securely for patient safety.

attention to the locking mechanisms on these attachments so that you will be able to apply them correctly when needed. *Always test the footboard and shoulder guards to be certain that they are securely attached before tilting the table with a patient on it.*

The motor that tilts the table is quite powerful and can overcome the resistance of obstacles placed in the way. Step stools and other movable equipment have been crushed because they were under the end of the table and out of view when the table motor was activated. Such a collision can also damage the table. *Be certain that the spaces under the table are clear before tilting the table.*

The majority of **adverse incidents** that occur in the radiology department will happen at the x-ray table and upright Bucky (described next). *The most frequent adverse incident is a patient falling.* Never leave a patient alone on the x-ray table. When making the exposure from behind the control console, always have the patient in eyesight. Box 2-2 lists important safety precautions when moving x-ray equipment.

A floating tabletop allows the top of the table to move independently of the remainder of the table, which makes it easy to align the patient to the x-ray beam. This is a common feature of modern tables. This motion may involve a mechanical release that allows the tabletop to be

Box 2-2

Safety Precautions When Moving X-ray Equipment

- Be sure that footboard and shoulder guard are secure before tilting a table with a patient on it.
- Check that no equipment is under the table before tilting it.
- Release locks before attempting to move the x-ray tube.
- Move the x-ray tube out of the way before assisting a patient to or from the table to avoid injuring the patient.
- Be sure that equipment is in a safe position before shutting off power to the locks.
- Ensure that the patient cannot or will not fall off the table.

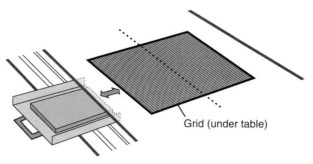

Fig. 2-14 The Bucky, with its cassette tray, is mounted under the tabletop for scatter radiation control.

shifted manually, or the movement may be power-driven, activated by a small control pad with directional switches.

Mounted under the tabletop surface is a **grid** device that absorbs most of the scatter radiation coming off the patient and tabletop and prevents it from reaching the IR. Most of these devices include a small motor that moves the grid during the exposure. The device also includes a pull-out tray to hold the IR plate and center it to the central ray. The grid and tray device is called a Bucky (Fig. 2-14), named after its inventor, American radiologist Gustav Bucky. Some tables may have a stationary grid that does not move during the exposure. The entire Bucky unit can be moved along the length of the table and locked into position where desired. The Bucky and grid are generally used only for radiography of body parts that measure 10 to 12 cm or more in thickness (about the size of the average adult neck or knee) or when the kilovoltage (kVp) is greater than 60. When the grid is not needed, the IR is placed on the tabletop or in an upright cassette holder that does not incorporate a grid. Fig. 2-15 shows a patient having an x-ray taken on the tabletop without the Bucky and a patient having an x-ray that utilizes the Bucky. Grids are discussed in Chapter 9.

UPRIGHT CASSETTE HOLDER

The upright cassette holder, as its name implies, is a device that holds the IR in the upright position for radiography (Fig. 2-16). All x-ray rooms contain an upright holder because many x-rays are done with the patient standing or sitting upright. The holder is usually mounted on a wall and is adjustable in height. It will usually incorporate a Bucky. This unit is typically referred to as the *upright Bucky*. When the patient is to be sitting or standing at the upright cassette holder for radiography, the tube is angled to face the wall and cassette holder. The distance may be adjusted to 40 inches or to 72 inches, depending on the requirements of the procedure (Fig. 2-17). Similarly to the x-ray table, patient falls can occur at the upright Bucky. Ensure that the patient is able to stand and remain standing for the x-ray exposure, or seat the patient. Often someone may have to hold the patient.

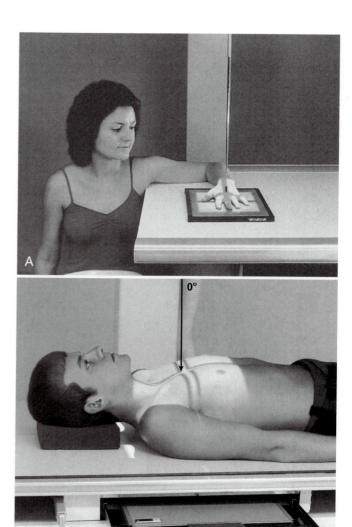

Fig. 2-15 A, Patient having a hand x-ray with cassette placed on the tabletop. **B,** Patient having an x-ray of the chest. Note cassette is placed in the Bucky tray to utilize the grid.

CONTROL CONSOLE

The control console is located in the control booth. This area is separated from the x-ray room by a lead barrier to protect the limited operator from scatter radiation during exposures. There is usually a lead glass window so that the limited operator can observe the patient from the control booth. The control console, or "control panel," is the access point at which the limited operator sets the exposure factors and initiates the exposure (Fig. 2-18). A typical radiographic control console has buttons or switches for controlling the exposure and dials or digital readouts that indicate the settings. Details of the control panel are discussed in Chapter 6.

TRANSFORMER CABINET

The transformer is an essential part of the x-ray machine. Its function is to produce the high voltage

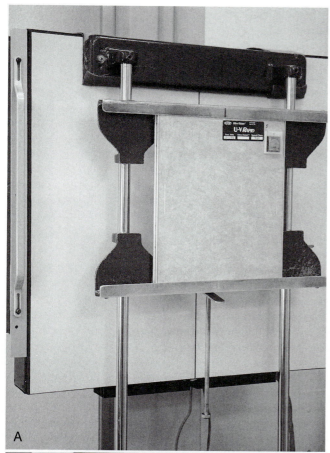

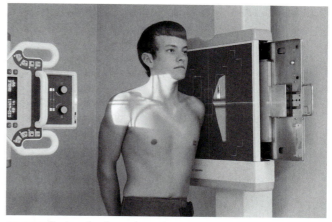

Fig. 2-17 Patient having a lateral trachea x-ray using the upright Bucky. Note cassette in the tray and x-ray tube angled 90 degrees to the unit.

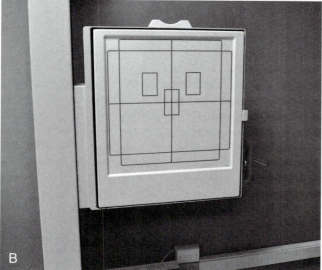

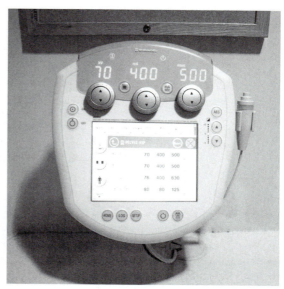

Fig. 2-18 Control console.

Fig. 2-16 Upright cassette holders. **A,** Nongrid cassette holder with cassette in place. **B,** Upright Bucky unit.

PODIATRIC RADIOLOGY

Podiatric radiology is defined as radiography of the ankle and foot. Podiatrists typically have their own private offices and need to have x-ray equipment available to image the foot and ankle. Podiatric x-ray machines have all the components of conventional x-ray machines but are specially designed for imaging these parts of the body (Fig. 2-20). The kVp on a podiatric machine is typically the same as on a conventional machine; however, the mA is considerably lower.

FUNDAMENTAL RADIATION SAFETY

Radiation exposure may pose a health hazard to radiographers if proper safety precautions are not observed. This subject is treated in greater depth in Chapter 11.

required for x-ray production as well as the low milliamperage (mA) needed in the x-ray tube. These are discussed in Chapter 5. The limited operator's work does not involve contact with the transformer. It is a large square unit standing in a corner of the x-ray room, connected by cables to both the control console and the x-ray tube (Fig. 2-19).

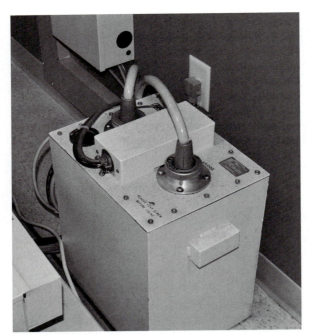

Fig. 2-19 X-ray transformer unit. From this unit, the kVp and mA are sent to the x-ray tube.

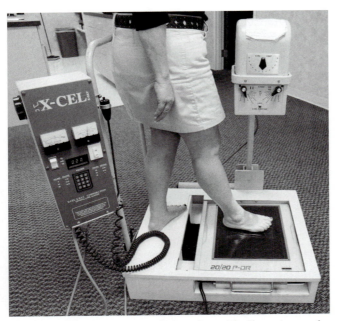

Fig. 2-20 Podiatric x-ray unit designed specifically to image the foot and ankle. This is a self-contained x-ray machine. Note the control console behind the patient and the x-ray tube and collimator above the foot.

The potential hazard is greater for the limited operator than for the patient because the limited operator is in frequent daily contact with the possibility of exposure. At this point, you need to feel confident that you are not endangering yourself or others as you become acquainted with the radiography department.

As stated earlier in this chapter, scatter radiation is present throughout the x-ray room during an exposure. Be aware that x-rays travel at the speed of light, do not

Box 2-3

Preexposure Safety Check

Before making an exposure, be *certain* that:
- The x-ray room door is closed.
- No nonessential persons are in the x-ray room.
- All persons in the control booth are completely behind the lead barrier.
- No image receptors are in the room except the one in use.

linger in the room after the exposure, and are not capable of making the objects in the room radioactive. The only time that a radiation hazard exists is during the x-ray exposure itself.

The sources of radiation are the x-ray tube and any matter that is in the path of the primary x-ray beam. The principal source of scatter radiation is the patient. When a safety barrier such as a lead wall is placed between the sources of radiation and the limited operator, the limited operator is safe from exposure. X-rays travel in straight lines and do not turn corners. Scatter radiation is not powerful enough to generate additional radiation of concern when it interacts with matter, so it is not necessary for the control booth to be sealed.

Limited operators should always be completely behind the lead barrier of the control booth during exposures. They should not be involved in holding patients who are unable to cooperate during the exposure. Immobilization devices should be used or, if necessary, assistance should be obtained from the patient's family. Before making an exposure, the limited operator should perform a safety check (Box 2-3) to ensure that only the required persons are in the x-ray room (usually this means only the patient), that everyone in the control booth is safely behind the lead barrier, and that the x-ray room door is closed. It is also wise to make sure that no IRs have been left lying about. Only the IR that is in immediate use should be in the x-ray room because scatter radiation fog will negatively affect the image.

SUMMARY

The primary x-ray beam originates at a tiny point within the x-ray tube. It exits in one general direction through the tube port and diverges into space. Objects in its path attenuate the beam, forming scatter radiation. This scatter radiation is present throughout the x-ray room during the exposure, creating a potential radiation hazard that requires proper precautions for safety.

The x-ray table, tube support, and cassette holder are capable of many possible motions, allowing alignment of the tube and IR for radiography of all body parts in many positions. Special care is needed to move equipment correctly so that patients will not be injured and the equipment will not be damaged.

Chapter 3

Basic Mathematics for Limited Operators

Learning Objectives

At the conclusion of this chapter, you will be able to:

- Demonstrate calculations involving the use of fractions, decimals, percentages, exponents, ratios and proportions, and simple algebraic equations
- Identify and use standard measurement units, state equivalent values for measurements in both the English and metric systems, and convert measurements from one unit to another
- When given two of the milliampere-second (mAs) values (milliampere [mA], time, mAs), calculate the third
- Calculate changes in radiation intensity and required mAs for changes in source–image receptor distance (SID)
- Given a set of exposure factors, calculate the changes needed to change contrast levels using the 15% rule
- Given a set of exposure factors, make appropriate adjustments for differences in patient part thickness using both kilovolt peak (kVp) and mAs
- Perform routine medication dose calculations accurately

Key Terms

algebra
base number
cubed
decimal
decimal point
denominator
difference
dividend
divisor
equation
exponent
lowest terms
mixed number
numerator
percentage
power
product
proportion
quotient
ratio
remainder
squared
square root
sum

With the rapidly advancing use of digital radiographic systems in limited practice, limited operators are required to perform fewer mathematical calculations than they were in the past. Still, determining measurements, exposure factors, radiation doses, and medication doses requires skill in using units of measurement and the ability to manipulate these numbers accurately (Fig. 3-1). Although the increasing use of computers and computerized equipment has reduced the amount of routine calculation required in radiography, an understanding of these functions helps you recognize errors when they occur and make mathematical adjustments when necessary. Certification examinations frequently test these skills by including problems that must be solved without the aid of a computer or calculator.

This chapter consists of two distinct sections: the first section addresses basic mathematical principles; the second section applies these principles to a variety of practical problems that may be encountered in radiography. How you use the first portion of this chapter will depend on your current skill level. For example, some students may be able to solve some or all of the basic math problems immediately with little or no practice, whereas others may need more intensive study to achieve the same level of competence. It is assumed that the reader can perform basic arithmetic functions: adding, subtracting, multiplying, and dividing whole numbers. At this point in the course, your instructor may want you to demonstrate a mastery of the basic mathematics used in radiography. Alternatively, you may turn to this chapter when you are presented with mathematical concepts later in the text.

In the second section of this chapter, in which mathematical skills are applied to practical problems, you will find that the content is easier to understand when you are familiar with the circumstances in which these calculations are needed. Although brief explanations are provided in this chapter, the references to later chapters will be very important if you are not already familiar

with these situations. For example, formulas for calculating x-ray exposure factors and for preparing medications will be easier to grasp if you are familiar with these activities or have studied the relevant chapters. How you use this portion of the chapter will also depend on your instructor's course design. It may be especially helpful to refer to this chapter in conjunction with your study of Chapter 10.

There are many approaches to solving mathematical problems, and this chapter shows only one approach in most cases. If you are more familiar with another method, there is no reason why you should not continue to use it. The methods given can be used to perform common radiographic calculations, with or without using a calculator. Solutions to the practice problems are in Appendix C.

FUNDAMENTAL MATHEMATICAL PRINCIPLES

Terminology

Discussion of calculations is facilitated by naming the various parts of the problems. New terms are introduced throughout this chapter, but defining a few basic terms at the beginning will assist in your understanding of the sections that follow:

- **Sum:** total, the answer to an addition problem
- **Difference:** the answer to a subtraction problem
- **Product:** the answer to a multiplication problem
- **Dividend:** the number divided into in a division problem
- **Divisor:** the number that is divided into the dividend
- **Quotient:** the answer to a division problem
- **Remainder:** the number that is "left over" when the dividend cannot be evenly divided by the divisor

Fractions and Decimals

Fractions

Fractions are parts of whole numbers. They are commonly used in our everyday lives. For example, you can easily relate to the concept of one half (½) of an orange or one quarter (¼) of a dollar. Older x-ray control panels with synchronous timers have exposure times that are expressed in fractions of seconds.

The lower number of a fraction is called the **denominator.** The denominator indicates the number of equal parts into which the whole has been divided. The upper number is called the **numerator.** The numerator indicates the number of parts or "pieces" of the divided whole. For example, if you cut a sheet of paper into eight equal parts, one of the parts would be ⅛ of the page. Three parts would be ⅜ of the page.

When both the numerator and the denominator of a fraction can be divided evenly by the same number, the resulting fraction is equal to the original fraction. This is

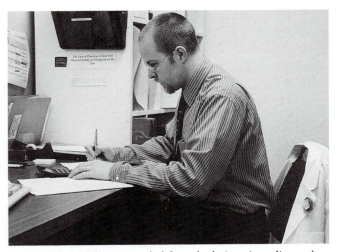

Fig. 3-1 Math skills are needed for calculations in radiography.

called "reducing the fraction to lower terms." For example, if you divide both the numerator and denominator of $\frac{10}{20}$ by 5, the result is $\frac{2}{4}$, lower terms of the fraction $\frac{10}{20}$ and equal to it. The most usual or common form of a fraction is one in which there is no number except one that can be divided evenly into both the numerator and the denominator. Such a fraction is said to be in its **lowest terms.** For example, the numerator and denominator of the fraction $\frac{2}{4}$ can be further divided by 2, resulting in $\frac{1}{2}$, the lowest terms of both $\frac{10}{20}$ and $\frac{2}{4}$.

To reduce a fraction to its lowest terms, divide both the numerator and the denominator by the largest number that will divide evenly into both of them.

Example: Reduce $\frac{9}{12}$ to its lowest terms.

The largest number that can be divided evenly into both the numerator and the denominator is 3.

Divide the numerator by 3: $9 \div 3 = 3$, the numerator of the new fraction.

Divide the denominator by 3: $12 \div 3 = 4$, the denominator of the new fraction.

Therefore $\frac{9}{12} = \frac{3}{4}$.

Because there is no number except 1 that can be divided evenly into both 3 and 4, $\frac{3}{4}$ is the lowest term of $\frac{9}{12}$.

The process of determining the value of a fractional portion of a whole number is calculated by multiplying the fraction times the whole number. The most common calculation of this type in radiography involves the determination of milliampere-seconds when the exposure time is expressed as a fraction of a second.

To multiply a whole number by a fraction, multiply the whole number by the numerator of the fraction and then divide the product by the denominator of the fraction.

Example: How much is $\frac{3}{5}$ of 200? This question can also be expressed as:

$$\frac{3}{5} \times 200 = ?$$

First, multiply the whole number (200) times the numerator of the fraction (3).

$$200 \times 3 = 600$$

Then, divide the product (600) by the denominator of the fraction (5).

$$600 \div 5 = 120$$

Therefore $\frac{3}{5}$ of 200 equals 120.

Decimals

A **decimal** is actually a fraction with a denominator of 10, 100, 1000, or any number that consists of a 1 followed by one or more zeros. With these specialized fractions, the denominator is not written. Its value is indicated by the position of the numerator in reference to a dot or period called the **decimal point.** Figures to the left of the decimal point are whole numbers. Figures to the right of the decimal point represent the numerator of the fraction. The unseen denominator of

the decimal fraction is determined by the number of figures to the right of the decimal point. The first place to the right of the decimal point is 10ths, the second place 100ths, the third place 1000ths, and so on. For example, 0.1 indicates one tenth ($\frac{1}{10}$) and 2.05 indicates two and five hundredths ($2\frac{5}{100}$). You are familiar with the use of decimals to indicate and calculate dollars and cents. In this case, the two figures to the right of the decimal point indicate cents, or hundredths of a dollar.

Zeros between the decimal point and the figures change the places of the figures and change the value of the decimal. For example, 0.3 equals three tenths ($\frac{3}{10}$), whereas 0.003 equals three thousandths ($\frac{3}{1000}$). Zeros added to the right of all other figures in a decimal do not change the value of the decimal. For example, 0.08 is equal to 0.0800. The first is read as eight hundredths ($\frac{8}{100}$) and the second as eight hundred ten thousandths ($\frac{800}{10,000}$). It is customary to drop (eliminate) zeros that are to the right of all other figures in a decimal.

To add or subtract decimals, the numbers must be placed so that the decimal points form a vertical line, both in the problem and in the answer.

Example:

1. $3.4 + 3.04 + 3.004 = ?$

$$\begin{array}{r} 3.4 \\ 3.04 \\ + \ 3.004 \\ \hline 9.444 \end{array}$$

2. $7.3 - 4.7 = ?$

$$\begin{array}{r} 7.3 \\ - \ 4.7 \\ \hline 2.6 \end{array}$$

For easier subtraction, add zeros as needed, so that both numbers have the same number of decimal places.

Example: $6.85 - 2.4315 = ?$

$$\begin{array}{r} 6.8500 \\ - \ 2.4315 \\ \hline 4.4185 \end{array}$$

When multiplying decimals, place the decimal point in the product so that the number of decimal places is equal to the total number of decimal places in the numbers being multiplied. If the product ends in one or more zeros, place the decimal point correctly before dropping the zeros.

Example: $3.271 \times 2.16 = ?$

$$\begin{array}{r} 3.271 \\ \times \ 2.16 \\ \hline 19626 \\ 3271 \\ 6542 \\ \hline 7.06536 \end{array}$$

To divide *into* a decimal, place the decimal point of the quotient in direct alignment with the decimal point of the dividend.

Example: 15.15 ÷ 3 = ?

$$\begin{array}{r} 5.05 \\ 3\overline{)15.15} \end{array}$$

To divide *by* a decimal, move the decimal point to the right of the divisor and move the decimal point of the dividend the same number of places to the right. Align the decimal point in the quotient with the new position of the decimal point in the dividend.

Example: 37.3 ÷ 0.25 = ?

$$\begin{array}{r} 149.2 \\ 0.25.\overline{)37.30.0} \\ 25 \\ \hline 123 \\ 100 \\ \hline 230 \\ 225 \\ \hline 50 \\ 50 \\ \hline 0 \end{array}$$

Although there are methods for performing all calculations using fractions, most people find it simpler to work with decimals. This is especially true when using a calculator, because calculators are designed to use decimals for the expression of all values that are less than 1. For these reasons, this text deals with fractions principally by converting them into decimals and performing any needed calculations using the methods just described for decimals. When a calculation involves fractions, or both decimals and fractions, convert the fractions to decimals and then perform the calculation.

To convert a fraction to a decimal, divide the numerator by the denominator.

Example: Convert ¾ into a decimal.

$$\begin{array}{r} 0.75 \\ 4\overline{)3.00} \\ 28 \\ \hline 20 \\ 20 \\ \hline 0 \end{array}$$

Therefore, the fraction ¾ is equal to the decimal 0.75.

A **mixed number** consists of a whole number and a fraction. For example, 1½ and 8¾ are mixed numbers.

To convert a mixed number to a decimal, calculate the decimal value of the fraction and add it to the whole number. If the fraction is a proper fraction (meaning that the denominator is greater than the numerator and therefore its value is less than 1), the decimal value of the fraction will be to the right of the decimal point and the whole number will be to the left of it.

Example: Convert 5³⁄₁₀ to a decimal.

First, convert ³⁄₁₀ to a decimal. Divide the numerator (3) by the denominator (10).

$$\begin{array}{r} 0.3 \\ 10\overline{)3.0} \end{array}$$

Then, add the whole number (5) to the decimal fraction (0.3). 5 + 0.3 = 5.3

Therefore 5³⁄₁₀ equals 5.3.

Some calculations involving decimals will result in numbers with many decimal places. For example, when the fraction ⅓ is converted into a decimal, a "repeating decimal" is created, in this case an infinite series of threes: 1 ÷ 3 = 0.33333. . . . If two numbers, each having three decimal places, are multiplied together, the product will have six decimal places. Most decimals used in radiography are sufficiently accurate when limited to two, three, or at the most four decimal places. When a decimal has too many places for convenience, it can be shortened by the process of "rounding off."

To round off a decimal, simply drop the excess figures from right to left. If the last figure dropped is 5 or greater, increase the final remaining figure by 1; if the last figure dropped is 4 or less, no change is necessary.

Examples:
1. Round off 3.1416 to three decimal places.
   Drop the excess figure. 3.141~~6~~
   Increase the final figure (1) by 1 because the dropped figure (6) is greater than 5: 3.142
2. Round off 3.1416 to one decimal place.
   Drop the excess figures. 3.1~~416~~
   There is no need to increase the final figure (1), because the last figure dropped (4) is not 5 or greater. The result is 3.1.

Practice Problems Using Fractions and Decimals

1. **Reducing to lowest terms.** Reduce the following fractions to their lowest terms:
   a. ⁵⁄₁₅
   b. ³⁄₉
   c. ¹²⁄₁₈
   d. ¹⁸⁄₂₀
   e. ¹⁶⁄₂₄
   f. ²⁰⁄₂₅
   g. ⁸⁄₁₀
2. **Multiplying whole numbers by fractions.** Multiply the following whole numbers by the indicated fractions:
   a. ¹⁄₁₀ × 300 = ?
   b. ⅕ × 200 = ?
   c. ³⁄₂₀ × 100 = ?
   d. ⅔ × 300 = ?
   e. ¹⁄₃₀ × 100 = ?

3. **Rounding off decimals.** Round off each of the following decimals to the number of decimal places indicated in parentheses:
   a. 0.66666 . . . (2)
   b. 7.711 (2)
   c. 5.55 (1)
   d. 0.0101 (2)
   e. 10.2498 (3)

4. **Converting fractions and mixed numbers to decimals.** Express the following fractions and mixed numbers as decimals with up to three decimal places:
   a. $\frac{1}{20}$
   b. $\frac{2}{5}$
   c. $\frac{1}{4}$
   d. $\frac{3}{8}$
   e. $\frac{7}{15}$
   f. $2\frac{3}{4}$
   g. $10\frac{2}{3}$
   h. $1\frac{1}{8}$

5. **Addition.** To add the fractions, first convert them to decimals with two decimal places.
   a. $0.78 + 0.01 = ?$
   b. $0.24 + 0.17 + 0.06 = ?$
   c. $3.2 + 1.04 + 0.722 = ?$
   d. $31.3 + 5.007 + 0.516 = ?$
   e. $20 + 1.9 + 0.838 = ?$
   f. $\frac{1}{2} + \frac{1}{4} = ?$
   g. $\frac{2}{5} + \frac{3}{10} + \frac{3}{20} = ?$

6. **Subtraction.** To subtract the fractions, first convert them to decimals with two decimal places.
   a. $1.42 - 0.23 = ?$
   b. $2.008 - 0.71 = ?$
   c. $4.7 - 0.528 = ?$
   d. $3 - 0.54 = ?$
   e. $6.911 - 1.0007 = ?$
   f. $\frac{7}{8} - \frac{1}{4} = ?$
   g. $\frac{2}{5} - \frac{1}{20} = ?$

7. **Multiplication.** To multiply the fractions, first convert them to decimals with two decimal places.
   a. $0.33 \times 0.75 = ?$
   b. $0.2 \times 0.934 = ?$
   c. $0.03 \times 82 = ?$
   d. $0.17 \times 8524 = ?$
   e. $50 \times 0.7872 = ?$
   f. $\frac{1}{5} \times 25 = ?$
   g. $\frac{2}{3} \times 18 = ?$
   h. $\frac{4}{5} \times 0.16 = ?$

8. **Division.** To divide the fractions, first convert them to decimals with two decimal places.
   a. $0.216 \div 3 = ?$
   b. $0.12 \div 5 = ?$
   c. $36 \div 0.09 = ?$
   d. $0.49 \div 0.007 = ?$
   e. $3.44 \div 1.6 = ?$
   f. $47 \div \frac{1}{4} = ?$
   g. $\frac{1}{2} \div \frac{2}{5} = ?$

Percentages

A **percentage** is a form of fraction with a denominator of 100. The term *percent* means "per hundred" and is indicated by the % sign. For example, the statement that "52% of the population is female" means that out of every 100 people in the population, 52 of them are females. One hundred percent indicates the whole and is equal to the number 1 in fractional terms.

Addition or subtraction involving only percentages may be performed as with whole numbers or decimals. A percent sign (%) is added to the answer.
   Examples:
1. $4\% + 8\% = 12\%$
2. $35\% - 15\% = 20\%$

When multiplying or dividing percentages or performing calculations that involve a percentage and a whole number or decimal, the percentage must first be converted to a decimal. To convert a percentage to a decimal, move the decimal point two places to the left and drop the percent sign.
   Examples:
1. $76\% = 0.76$
2. $4\% = 0.04$
3. $150\% = 1.50 = 1.5$

To convert a decimal to a percentage, move the decimal point two places to the right and add a percent sign.
   Examples:
1. $0.23 = 23\%$
2. $0.08 = 8\%$
3. $1.7 = 170\%$
4. $0.177 = 17.7\%$

To determine a percentage *of* a number means to multiply the number times the percentage. The percentage is first converted to a decimal.
   Example: How much is 25% of 300?
   Convert the percentage to a decimal: $25\% = 0.25$
   Multiply the number by the decimal: $300 \times 0.25 = 75$
   Therefore 75 equals 25% of 300.

To determine what percentage one number is in relation to another, divide one number by the other. The dividend is the number whose percentage you are determining, the portion. The divisor is the whole. (Note that the portion may be greater than the whole, resulting in a percentage that is greater than 100%.)
   Examples:
1. 15 is what percentage of 75?
   Divide the portion (15) by the whole (75): $15 \div 75 = 0.2$
   Convert the decimal into a percentage: $0.2 = 20\%$
   Therefore 15 equals 20% of 75.
2. 75 is what percentage of 15?
   Divide the portion (75) by the whole (15): $75 \div 15 = 5$
   Convert the answer to a percentage: $5 = 500\%$
   Therefore 75 equals 500% of 15.

To increase a number by a certain percentage, add the percentage to 100% and multiply the sum times the number to be increased.

Example: Increase 60 by 30%.

Add the percentage increase (30%) to 100%: 30% + 100% = 130%

Convert the sum of the percentages to a decimal: 130% = 1.3

Multiply the number to be increased (60) by the converted sum of the percentages (1.3): 60 × 1.3 = 78

Therefore 60 plus 30% of 60 equals 78.

To decrease a number by a certain percentage, subtract the percentage from 100% and multiply the difference times the number to be decreased.

Example: Decrease 60 by 20%.

Subtract the percentage decrease (20%) from 100%: 100% − 20% = 80%

Convert the difference between the percentages to a decimal: 80% = 0.8

Multiply the number to be decreased (60) by the converted difference between the percentages (0.8): 60 × 0.8 = 48

Therefore 60 minus 20% of 60 equals 48.

Practice Problems Using Percentages

1. Convert the following percentages to decimals:
   a. 7%
   b. 8.5%
   c. 59%
   d. 99.44%
   e. 140%
   f. 300%
   g. 21%
   h. 2.3%
   i. 100%
2. Convert the following decimals to percentages:
   a. 0.2
   b. 0.19
   c. 0.91
   d. 1.65
   e. 1.2
   f. 6.0
   g. 20.5
   h. 0.03
   i. 0.008
3. Perform the following calculations involving percentages:
   a. 37% + 33% = ?
   b. 100% + 65% = ?
   c. 25% − 13% = ?
   d. 20% × 80% = ?
   e. 150% ÷ 30% = ?
   f. ½ of 40% = ?
   g. 1.10 of 80% = ?
   h. 80% − 10% = ?

4. Calculate the value of the following percentages:
   a. 20% of 88
   b. 90% of 200
   c. 50% of 61
   d. 130% of 40
   e. 300% of 12
   f. 3% of 50
   g. 29% of 1000
   h. 15% of 90
5. Determine the following percentages. Express your answers to the nearest tenth of a percent.
   a. 13 = ? % of 63
   b. 29 = ? % of 80
   c. 43 = ? % of 200
   d. 40 = ? % of 160
   e. 50 = ? % of 35
   f. 20 = ? % of 2
   g. 100 = ? % of 25
   h. 25 = ? % of 1000
6. Calculate the solutions to the following problems that involve increasing and decreasing numbers by a percentage:
   a. Increase 100 by 15%
   b. Increase 30 by 250%
   c. Increase 150 by 25%
   d. Decrease 85 by 10%
   e. Decrease 20 by 12%
   f. Increase 15 by 40%
   g. Increase 46 by 100%
   h. Decrease 200 by 50%

Equations

Algebra is a branch of mathematics that provides a useful method of solving certain kinds of problems. Algebra problems are stated in the form of equations. An **equation** is a mathematical declaration that two mathematical statements (groups of numbers, together with their signs or mathematical functions) are equal to each other. Equations can be very complex, and it is this complexity that causes many students to feel intimidated by the thought of equations. Equations can also be quite simple. For example, 3 + 1 = 4 is an equation. The equations used in radiography are relatively simple ones.

The equations used in arithmetic are always stated so that the unknown quantity is to the right of the equal sign, for example, 3 + 1 = ? In algebra, the unknown quantity is usually indicated by a letter, often x, and may be at any position in the equation. The same symbols for mathematical operations used in arithmetic are also used in algebra: plus (+), minus (−), times (×), divided by (÷ or /), and equal (=). For example, 3 + x = 4 is an algebraic equation. When a number and a letter are adjacent to each other, this indicates multiplication. For example, $5x$ means 5 times the value of x (x × 5). A horizontal line in an equation means "divided by." For example, $\frac{2x}{3} = 6$ means 2 times x divided by 3 equals 6.

When solving algebraic problems, the equation must be kept in balance. That is, the mathematical statements on both sides of the equal sign must always be equal to each other. Operations are performed on both sides of the equation to "isolate" the unknown and determine its value. When the unknown is isolated, it is alone on one side of the equal sign and its value is on the other side.

Balance is maintained in an equation by performing the same operation on both sides of the equation.

Example: $3 + x = 4$

To isolate x on one side of the equation, subtract 3 from both sides of the equation:

$$3 - 3 + x = 4 - 3$$

To determine the value of x, perform the mathematical operations: $3 - 3 = 0$; $4 - 3 = 1$;

$$0 + x = 1$$

Therefore $x = 1$.

Other mathematical operations may be performed on both sides of an equation, depending on what is needed to isolate the unknown.

Examples:
1. $3x = 27$

To isolate x, divide both sides of the equation by 3:
$3x \div 3 = 27 \div 3$
Therefore $x = 9$.

2. $\frac{x}{12} = 3$

To isolate x, multiply both sides of the equation by 12:

$$\frac{x}{12} \times 12 = 3 \times 12$$

Perform the calculations: $12 \div 12 = 1$;
$3 \times 12 = 36$
Therefore $1x = 36$ or $x = 36$.

3. $x - 10 = 17$

To isolate x, add 10 to both sides of the equation:

$$x - 10 + 10 = 17 + 10$$

Perform the calculations:

$$-10 + 10 = 0$$
$$17 + 10 = 27$$

Therefore $x = 27$.

To save steps when an equation consists of two fractions, you can eliminate the denominators from consideration by using the method of cross multiplication.

In cross multiplication, each numerator is multiplied by the denominator on the opposite side of the equation.

Example: $\frac{16}{4} \bowtie \frac{8}{x}$

Cross multiply: $16x = 4 \times 8$
Perform calculation: $16x = 32$
To isolate x, divide both sides of the equation by 16:
$16x \div 16 = 32 \div 16$

Perform the mathematical operations: $16x \div 16 = x$;
$32 \div 16 = 2$
Therefore $x = 2$.

Ratios and Proportions

A **ratio** expresses the operation in which one number is divided by another. A ratio may be written using a colon (3:4), a division symbol (3 ÷ 4), or a slanted line (3/4), or by placing the dividend over the divisor with a line between them: $\frac{3}{4}$.

A **proportion** is a statement that two ratios are equal to each other. An example of a proportion is 3:4 :: 9:12. This is read, "3 is to 4 as 9 is to 12." It could also be written 3/4 = 9/12.

Many mathematical relationships in radiography are proportional to each other, so you may need to solve ratio and proportion problems in which one quantity of the proportion is unknown. These problems are set up in the format $a/b = c/d$. Numerical values that are known are substituted in the formula and the rules of algebra explained in the previous section are used to solve the problem.

Example: If you walk at the rate of 3 miles/hr, how far can you go in an hour and a half?

The known ratio is 3 miles/1 hr. In the second ratio, the time is known and the distance is not.

Therefore, the problem looks like this:

$$\frac{3 \text{ miles}}{1 \text{ hr}} \times \frac{x \text{ miles}}{1.5 \text{ hr}}$$

Cross multiply: $1x = 3 \times 1.5$
Perform calculation: $x = 4.5$ miles

Proportions are often designated as either *direct* or *inverse*. In a direct proportion, when one of the values increases, the other also increases. For instance, when food intake increases, body weight increases. This statement indicates that the relationship between food intake and weight gain is a direct proportion. On the other hand, if one value increases when the other decreases, this is termed an *inverse proportion*. For example, as exercise decreases, body weight increases, so this would indicate an inverse proportion between exercise and weight gain. Later in this chapter you will note both kinds of proportions in the formulas used to solve technical problems.

Practice Problems Involving Equations

Determine the value of x in each of the following equations:
1. $3x + 6 = 10 + 2$
2. $21/x = 8 - 1$
3. $x - 17 = 13$
4. $20 = 3x - 4$
5. $2x = 18/2$
6. $45 = 9x$
7. $30/x = 6/2$

8. $x/7 = 36/6$
9. $56/8 = 49/x$
10. $12/4 = x/15$

Exponents and Square Roots

Exponents

When a number is multiplied by itself, this operation may be expressed as an **exponent.** An exponent is a small superscript number (in elevated type position) that indicates how many times the number is multiplied by itself. For example, the number 64 equals $2 \times 2 \times 2 \times 2 \times 2 \times 2$. The number 2 is multiplied by itself 5 times and the number 2 is used as a multiplication factor 6 times. Using an exponent, 64 can be expressed as 2^6. In this case the repeated number, or **base number,** is 2, and the exponent or **power** of the base number is 6. This is read as "2 to the sixth power," or simply as "2 to the sixth." When the exponent is 2 or 3, special terms are commonly used. The number is said to be **squared** when it is multiplied by itself once and the exponent is 2. When the exponent is 3, the number is multiplied by itself twice and is said to be **cubed.**

Examples:

1. What is the value of 12 squared?

$$12^2 = 12 \times 12 = 144$$

2. What is the value of 2 cubed? $2^3 = 2 \times 2 \times 2 = 8$

Square Roots

The **square root** of a number is the value that, when multiplied by itself, equals the original number. The square root is represented by the radical sign, $\sqrt{\ }$.

Examples:

1. $\sqrt{4} = 2$
2. $\sqrt{100} = 10$

Square roots that are small, whole numbers, such as those in the examples given, can be easily perceived. It is a complex mathematical operation to extract square roots that are not whole numbers. Fortunately, today simple math calculators provide this function.

Practice Problems Involving Exponents and Square Roots

1. Calculate the value of the following exponential terms:
   a. 5^3
   b. 2^4
   c. 9^2
   d. 10^4
   e. 4^3
2. Determine the square roots of the following numbers:
   a. $\sqrt{49} = ?$
   b. $\sqrt{36} = ?$
   c. $\sqrt{64} = ?$
   d. $\sqrt{400} = ?$

Measurement Units and Their Conversion

In the United States many measurements are made using the English system that involves such units as pounds, feet, and gallons. Scientists worldwide prefer measurements made in the metric system, mainly because it is based on the number 10, which simplifies many calculations. You will encounter measurements in both systems and must be able to convert measurements readily from one system to the other. If you need to understand or convert measurements not found in this chapter, you can find information on measurement units used in health care in almost any medical dictionary. The Internet also provides this information; for example, *www.allmath.com* provides comprehensive English-to-metric conversion tables, or if you wish, you can enter your own measurements and have them converted for you at *www.sciencemadesimple.com/conversions.html*.

Metric System

The basic units of the metric system are the gram for measuring weight, the liter for measuring liquid volume, and the meter for measuring length. Various prefixes are used with these units to specify measurements that are larger or smaller than the basic units by factors that are multiples of 10. For example, *kilo* is a prefix meaning 1000. You may already be familiar with the fact that 1 kilovolt equals 1000 volts. A kilometer is equal to 1000 meters. The prefix *milli* indicates $\frac{1}{1000}$ or 0.001 times the basic unit. For example, 1 milliliter equals 0.001 liter. The basic units of the metric system are summarized in Table 3-1. Metric prefixes are summarized in Table 3-2.

English System

The relationships between measurements in the English system are far less orderly than those in the metric system. As stated before, the basic units are the pound (weight), the foot (length), and the gallon (liquid volume), but a number of other units are also used to measure these same parameters in the English system. For example, the ounce and the ton are also common weight measurements, the inch and the mile are also used to measure length, and liquids may be measured in ounces, pints, quarts, or gallons. Table 3-3 lists common measurement units of the English system and their relationships to one another. Table 3-4 compares the

Table 3-1

Base Units in the Metric System

Unit	Used to Measure	Abbreviation
Meter	Length	M or m
Liter	Liquid	L or l
Gram	Weight	g or gm

Table 3-2
Metric Prefixes

Prefix	Meaning	Abbreviation
Kilo-	1000	K
Hecto-	100	H
Deka-	10	da
Deci-	$\frac{1}{10}$ (0.1)	d
Centi-	$\frac{1}{100}$ (0.01)	c
Milli-	$\frac{1}{1000}$ (0.001)	m
Micro-	$\frac{1}{1,000,000}$ (0.000001)	μ or mc
Nano-	$\frac{1}{1,000,000,000}$ (0.0000000001)	n

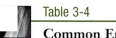

Table 3-3
English Units

Type of Unit	Unit	Abbreviation	Equivalents
Length	inch	in	0.0833 ft
	foot	ft	12 in
	yard	yd	3 ft
	mile	mi	5280 ft
Liquid	ounce	oz	0.0625 pt
	pint	pt	16 oz
	quart	qt	2 pt
	gallon	gal	4 qt
Weight	ounce	oz	0.0625 lb
	pound	lb	16 oz
	ton	T	2000 lb

Table 3-4
Common English/Metric Equivalents

Type of Unit	English Units	Metric-Equivalents
Length	inch	2.54 cm
	yard	1.0926 m
Liquid	ounce	30 ml
	quart	0.946 L
Weight	pound	2.2 kg

most common English measurements with their counterparts in the metric system.

Conversions Between Measurement Units

Table 3-5 provides shortcuts for conversions between units that are commonly used. For example, to change from inches to centimeters, simply multiply the number of inches by 2.54, the number of centimeters in an inch.

Table 3-5
Common Unit Conversion Guide

Length	millimeters × 0.04 = inches
	inches × 2.54 = centimeters
	centimeters × 0.39 = inches
	inches ÷ 12 = feet
	feet × 12 = inches
	feet ÷ 3 = yards
	feet × 0.305 = meters
	meters × 3.28 = feet
	yards × 0.91 = meters
Weight	pounds × 0.45 = kilograms
	kilograms × 2.2 = pounds
	grams × 0.0022 = pounds
	kilograms × 35.27 = ounces
Volume	cm³ = milliliters
	ounces × 30 = milliliters
	ounces ÷ 16 = pints
	pints × 16 = ounces
	quarts × 2 = pints
	ounces × 0.0624 = pints
	gallons × 4 = quarts
	liters × 0.26 = gallons
	liters × 2.11 = pint
Time	seconds ÷ 60 = minutes
	minutes × 60 = seconds
	minutes ÷ 60 = hours
	hours × 60 = minutes
	hours ÷ 24 = days
	days × 24 = hours

You can also use the proportion formula that follows. The method for solving proportion problems is explained earlier in this chapter.

Proportion problems for converting measurements from one unit to another are set up in this format:

$$\frac{A\ units}{B\ units} = \frac{1\ A\ unit}{B\ units\ per\ unit\ A}$$

Examples:
1. Convert 10 kilometers into meters.
   In this problem we designate kilometers as the A unit and meters as the B unit.
   Substitute values in the proportion formula above:

$$\frac{10\ Km}{x\ M} = \frac{1\ Km}{1000\ m\ per\ Km}$$

Cross multiply: $1 \times x = 10 \times 1000 = 10{,}000$ m
2. Convert 300 milliamperes (mA) into amperes (A).
   In this problem we designate milliamperes as the A unit and amperes as the B unit.
   Substitute values in the proportion formula:

$$\frac{300\ mA}{x\ A} = \frac{1\ mA}{0.001\ A\ per\ mA}$$

Cross multiply: $x = 300 \times 0.001 = 0.3$ A

3. Convert 1 foot into centimeters.

In this problem we designate inches as the A unit and centimeters as the B unit. Because we do not have a factor for converting feet directly into centimeters, we must first convert feet into inches. This is easily accomplished using Table 3-3, where we see that 1 foot = 12 inches.

Substitute values in the proportion formula:

$$\frac{12 \text{ in}}{x \text{ cm}} = \frac{1 \text{ in}}{2.54 \text{ cm/in}}$$

Cross multiply: $x = 12 \times 2.54$
Calculate: $x = 30.48$ cm

Units of Time

Units that measure time are universal, and there is only one system, which is a mixture of the English and metric systems. The base unit for measuring time is the second. Milliseconds and nanoseconds are short time periods using metric prefixes to indicate thousandths and billionths of a second, respectively.

The time units greater than a second are probably quite familiar to you. Sixty seconds equal 1 minute, there are 60 minutes in an hour, and 24 hours constitute 1 day.

You can use the proportion formula from the previous section to convert from one time unit to another. Table 3-5 contains some shortcuts for converting between common units of time.

Units of Temperature

There are two common scales for measuring temperature. The English system uses the Fahrenheit scale (F). Using this scale, water freezes at 32° F and boils at 212° F.

The Celsius (C) temperature scale is used in the metric system. At one time this scale was called *centigrade*, and you may still encounter this term. Each degree on the Celsius scale represents a greater quantity of temperature change than a degree on the Fahrenheit scale. Water freezes at 0° C and boils at 100° C.

The following formulas are used to convert between the Fahrenheit and Celsius temperature scales:

$$F = (C \times 1.8) + 32°$$
$$C = F - 32° \div 1.8$$

Examples:

1. Convert normal body temperature (98.6° F) to the Celsius scale.

Substitute the known Fahrenheit value in the formula for obtaining Celsius units:

$$C = (98.6°F - 32°) \div 1.8$$

Perform calculations: $C = 66.6° \div 1.8 = 37°$ C

2. Convert 25° C to the Fahrenheit scale.

Substitute the known Celsius value in the formula for obtaining Fahrenheit units:

$$F = (25°C \times 1.8) + 32°$$

Perform calculations: $F = 45° + 32° = 77°$ F

Practice Problems Using Measurement Units

1. Conversions from one metric unit to another
   a. Convert 75 kilovolts to volts.
   b. Convert 3 meters to centimeters.
   c. Convert 10 milliliters to liters.
   d. Convert 20 grams to kilograms.
   e. Convert 15 centigrams to grams.
2. Conversions from one English unit to another
   a. Convert 16 inches to yards.
   b. Convert ½ pint to fluid ounces.
   c. Convert 84 inches to feet.
   d. Convert 18 quarts to gallons.
   e. Convert 4.8 pounds to ounces.
3. Conversions between English and metric units
   a. Convert 3 fluid ounces to milliliters.
   b. Convert 0.25 pound to grams.
   c. Convert 5 inches to meters.
   d. Convert 30 millimeters to inches.
   e. Convert 40 grams to ounces.
4. Time and temperature conversions.
   a. Convert ½₀ second to milliseconds.
   b. Convert 330 seconds to hours.
   c. Convert 3.4 days to hours.
   d. Convert 19° C to the Fahrenheit scale.
   e. Convert 50° F to the Celsius scale.

MATHEMATICS APPLIED TO RADIOGRAPHY

Milliampere-seconds

The concept of milliampere-seconds as an exposure factor in radiography is introduced in Chapter 5 and further expanded in Chapters 7 and 10. The unit called *milliampere-seconds*, abbreviated *mAs*, is the product of milliamperage and exposure time (seconds). Milliamperage (mA) is a unit that represents the rate at which x-rays are produced. When this number is multiplied by the exposure time in seconds, the resulting quantity is expressed in units of mAs and indicates the total quantity of radiation involved in an exposure. Several possible combinations of mA and time may be used to obtain a given mAs quantity. The manipulation of these three quantities is part of the everyday work in radiography.

The formula for determining mAs is:

$$mA \times seconds = mAs$$

Example: Determine the mAs of an exposure made using 300 mA and 0.4 sec

$$300 \text{ mA} \times 0.4 \text{ sec} = 120 \text{ mAs}$$

According to the principles of algebra explained earlier in this chapter, this formula can be rearranged to isolate any of its three parts.

Examples:

1. Using the mAs formula, derive a formula for determining the exposure time when the values of mA and mAs are known.

$$\frac{\cancel{mA} \times sec}{\cancel{mA}} = \frac{mAs}{mA}$$

Divide the first fraction by mA, thus reducing it to isolate seconds.

Therefore the exposure time in seconds equals the mAs divided by the mA. The formula can be stated:

$$mAs/mA = T \text{ (sec)}$$

2. If the desired mAs is 20 and you wish to use 200 mA, what should be the exposure time?

$$20 \text{ mAs} \div 200 \text{ mA} = 0.1 \text{ sec or } \frac{1}{10} \text{ sec}$$

NOTE: When calculating exposure time for controls that have exposure times in decimals, it is best to divide so as to obtain a decimal. For controls that have exposure times in fractions, formulate the problem as a fraction and reduce the fraction, if needed, to obtain a fractional exposure time. See the instructions earlier in this chapter for reducing fractions to their lowest terms.

The diagram in Fig. 3-2 is a handy reminder of the relationships among mA, exposure time, and mAs. When you cover the factor you wish to obtain, the calculation needed is apparent. For example, when mAs is covered, mA and time are separated by a vertical line indicating that these factors should be multiplied to obtain mAs. When mA is covered, time is beneath the horizontal line and mAs is over it, indicating that mAs is divided by time in seconds to calculate mA.

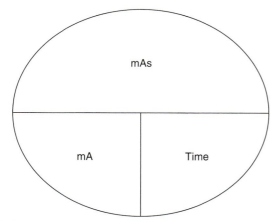

Fig. 3-2 The relationships among milliamperes (mA), time, and milliampere-seconds (mAs).

It will often be the case that you will calculate values for mA, time, or mAs that are not available on your control console. It is helpful to remember that variations in exposure of less than 20% are scarcely noticeable on the image. When the ideal exposure factor is not available, simply select the factor that is closest to the value you want. Most control consoles are designed to provide settings within a 20% range of any specific goal you may calculate.

Practice Problems Involving Milliampere-Seconds

1. Calculate the mAs for the following exposures. Round any extended decimals to two decimal places.
   a. 200 mA, $\frac{1}{40}$ sec
   b. 300 mA, $\frac{1}{20}$ sec
   c. 100 mA, $\frac{2}{15}$ sec
   d. 500 mA, 0.02 sec
   e. 50 mA, 0.3 sec
   f. 150 mA, $1\frac{1}{4}$ sec
   g. 400 mA, 2 msec
   h. 300 mA, $\frac{1}{120}$ sec
   i. 1200 mA, 0.005 sec
   j. 600 mA, 0.04 sec
   k. 750 mA, 0.1 sec
   l. 300 mA, 0.3 sec
   m. 13200 mA, 0.4 sec

2. Calculate the exposure time for the following exposures. Round any extended decimals to three decimal places.
   a. 50 mA, 40 mAs
   b. 200 mA, 25 mAs
   c. 300 mA, 10 mAs
   d. 100 mA, 1 mAs
   e. 400 mA, 8 mAs
   f. 500 mA, 50 mAs
   g. 800 mA, 20 mAs
   h. 150 mA, 300 mAs
   i. 25 mA, 150 mAs
   j. 1000 mA, 5 mAs

3. Calculate the mA for the following exposures:
   a. 10 mAs, $\frac{1}{30}$ sec
   b. 25 mAs, $\frac{1}{2}$ sec
   c. 40 mAs, $\frac{2}{15}$ sec
   d. 5 mAs, 0.01 sec
   e. 8 mAs, 0.02 sec
   f. 100 mAs, 0.5 sec
   g. 20 mAs, 0.2 sec
   h. 3 mAs, 0.01 sec
   i. 60 mAs, 0.3 sec

Source–Image Receptor Distance and Radiation Intensity

Source–image receptor distance (SID) is the distance in inches between the radiation source in the x-ray tube and the imaging plane. Chapter 7 explains and illustrates the relationship between radiation intensity and SID according to the inverse square law:

Radiation intensity is inversely proportional to the square of the distance.

$$\frac{I_1 \,(\text{Original intensity})}{I_2 \,(\text{New intensity})} = \frac{SID_2^2 \,(\text{New distance, squared})}{SID_1^2 \,(\text{Original distance, squared})}$$

Example: When the SID is changed from 30 inches to 90 inches, what is the relationship between the original radiation intensity and the intensity at the new distance?

Substitute the distances in the formula. The original intensity is assigned a relative value of 1. The new intensity is unknown:

$$\frac{I_1}{I_2} = \frac{90^2}{30^2}$$

The calculation is greatly simplified if you first reduce the fraction. $90^2/30^2$ can be reduced by dividing both the numerator and the denominator by 30:

$$\frac{I_1}{I_2} = \frac{3^2}{1^2}$$

Calculate the squares: $3^2 = 3 \times 3 = 9$; $1^2 = 1 \times 1 = 1$
Substitute these values in the formula:

$$\frac{I_1}{I_2} = \frac{9}{1}$$

Cross multiply: $9 \times I_2 = 1$
To isolate I_2, divide both sides by 9:

$$\frac{9 \times I_2}{9} = \frac{1}{9}$$

Therefore $I_2 = \frac{1}{9}$. That is, the new intensity is one ninth of the original intensity.

Although knowing this relationship enhances understanding, it is not of great practical value. Assuming that the original radiation intensity was satisfactory, the more important question is how to maintain a constant radiation intensity when the distance changes. The mAs is used to compensate for changes in distance. The correct change in mAs enables you to maintain the same radiation intensity when the distance is changed. Because the intensity decreases when the distance increases (an inverse proportion), the mAs must be *increased* when the distance increases (a direct proportion).

To maintain a constant radiographic intensity, the mAs must be directly proportional to the square of the distance. The formula for changing mAs to maintain a constant radiation intensity when the distance changes is as follows:

$$\frac{mAs_1 \,(\text{Original})}{mAs_2 \,(\text{New})} = \frac{SID_1^2 \,(\text{Original distance, squared})}{SID_2^2 \,(\text{New distance, squared})}$$

Example: A satisfactory radiograph is made using 20 mAs at 40 inches SID. How much mAs is required to produce a similar radiograph at 60 inches SID?

Substitute in the formula:

$$\frac{20 \text{ mAs}}{mAs_2} = \frac{40^2}{60^2}$$

To simplify the calculation, reduce the fraction (divide both numerator and denominator on the right side of the equation by 20):

$$\frac{20 \text{ mAs}}{mAs_2} = \frac{2^2}{3^2}$$

Calculate the squares: $2^2 = 2 \times 2 = 4$; $3^2 = 3 \times 3 = 9$
Substitute these values in the formula:

$$\frac{20 \text{ mAs}}{mAs_2} = \frac{4}{9}$$

Cross multiply: $4 \times mAs_2 = 20 \text{ mAs} \times 9$
Perform the calculation: $4 \times mAs_2 = 180 \text{ mAs}$
To isolate mAs_2, divide both sides by 4:

$$\frac{4 \times mAs_2}{4} = \frac{180}{4} \quad 45 \text{ mAs}$$

Therefore the new mAs required at 60 inches SID is 45 mAs.

Practice Problems Involving Distance Changes

1. What is the relative change in radiation intensity when the distance changes from 40 inches SID to 30 inches SID?
2. What is the relative change in radiation intensity when the distance is changed from 72 inches SID to 40 inches SID?
3. A satisfactory radiograph is made using 15 mAs at 40 inches SID. How much mAs is needed to produce a similar radiograph at 48 inches SID?
4. A satisfactory radiograph is made using 40 mAs at 72 inches SID. How much mAs is needed to produce a similar radiograph at 84 inches SID?
5. A satisfactory radiograph is made using 10 mAs at 40 inches SID. How much mAs is needed to produce a similar radiograph at 72 inches SID?
6. What is the relative change in radiation intensity when the distance is changed from 72 inches SID to 40 inches SID?
7. A satisfactory radiograph is made using 25 mAs at 40 inches SID. How much mAs is needed to produce a similar radiograph at 60 inches SID?
8. A satisfactory radiograph is made using 100 mAs at 72 inches SID. How much mAs is needed to produce a similar radiograph at 60 inches SID?
9. A satisfactory radiograph is made using 20 mAs at 60 inches SID. How much mAs is needed to produce a similar radiograph at 48 inches SID?
10. A satisfactory radiograph is made using 8 mAs at 72 inches SID. How much mAs is needed to produce a similar radiograph at 40 inches SID?

Exposure Adjustments for Patient Size

Alteration of Kilovoltage for Patient Part Size Changes

A single set of exposure factors is not adequate for all sizes of patients. For the purpose of determining correct exposure factors, body parts are measured with calipers in centimeters. Adjustments in kilovoltage for variations in part size are discussed in Chapter 10. As stated there, kilovolts peak (kVp) is a useful adjustment only for relatively small variations from normal because large changes in kVp cause significant alteration in the appearance of the image.

Below 85 kVp, an adjustment of 2 kVp/cm will compensate for small changes in part size. Above 85 kVp, a change of 3 kVp/cm is necessary.

> **Example:** A wrist measures 4 cm in posteroanterior diameter, and an exposure of 5 mAs at 56 kVp produces a satisfactory radiograph. How much kVp adjustment is needed for the lateral projection, which measures 6 cm?
>
> The kVp range is below 85, so the adjustment is 2 kVp/cm.
>
> The size difference is 2 cm (6 cm − 4 cm = 2 cm).
>
> 2 cm × 2 kVp/cm = 4 kVp increase.
>
> The original kVp (56) plus the increase (4) equals the new kVp (60).
>
> Therefore the exposure for the lateral wrist projection is 5 mAs at 60 kVp.

Alteration of Milliampere-Seconds for Patient Part Size Changes

As explained in Chapter 10, mAs is the usual and best choice of factors to adjust when compensating for differences in patient part size. The mAs is increased by 30% for a 2-cm increase in part size and decreased by 20% for a 2-cm decrease in part size. These percentages may be added or subtracted, respectively, from 100% and the result multiplied by the original mAs. *These changes compound, much like compound interest, and must be applied 2 cm at a time.*

For a 2-cm increase in patient part size, increase the mAs by 30% (multiply the mAs by 1.3). For a 2-cm decrease in patient part size, decrease the mAs by 20% (multiply the mAs by 0.8).

> **Examples:**
> 1. If 20 mAs is a satisfactory exposure for a patient part measuring 20 cm, how much mAs is needed to produce a similar image of a patient part measuring 24 cm?
>
> Multiply the mAs by 1.3 for the first 2-cm increase:

$$20 \text{ mAs} \times 1.3 = 26 \text{ mAs for a } 22\text{-cm patient part}$$

> Multiply the mAs for 22 cm (26) by 1.3 to obtain the mAs for 24 cm:

$$26 \text{ mAs} \times 1.3 = 33.8 \text{ mAs for a } 24\text{-cm patient part}$$

> 2. If 60 mAs is a satisfactory exposure for a patient part measuring 28 cm, how much mAs is needed for a patient part measuring 26 cm?
>
> Multiply the mAs by 0.8 for a 2-cm decrease:

$$60 \text{ mAs} \times 0.8 = 48 \text{ mAs for the } 26\text{-cm patient part}$$

Practice Problems Involving Patient Part Size Changes

1. A satisfactory radiograph is made using 96 kVp on a body part measuring 30 cm. Adjust the kVp to compensate for a body part size decrease to 27 cm.
2. A satisfactory radiograph is made using 74 kVp on a body part measuring 16 cm. Adjust the kVp to compensate for a body part size increase to 18 cm.
3. A satisfactory radiograph is made using 50 mAs on a body part measuring 24 cm. Adjust the mAs to compensate for a body part size decrease to 18 cm.
4. A satisfactory radiograph is made using 30 mAs on a body part measuring 19 cm. Adjust the mAs to compensate for a body part size increase to 25 cm.
5. A satisfactory radiograph is made using 10 mAs on a body part measuring 12 cm. Adjust the mAs to compensate for a body part size increase to 16 cm.
6. A satisfactory radiograph is made using 55 kVp on a body part measuring 4 cm. Adjust the kVp to compensate for a body part size increase to 7 cm.
7. A satisfactory radiograph is made using 100 mAs on a body part measuring 36 cm. Adjust the mAs to compensate for a body part size decrease to 30 cm.
8. A satisfactory radiograph is made using 4 mAs on a body part measuring 19 cm. Adjust the mAs to compensate for a body part size increase to 21 cm.
9. A satisfactory radiograph is made using 40 mAs on a body part measuring 20 cm. Adjust the mAs to compensate for a body part size increase to 24 cm.

Alteration of Contrast With Kilovoltage: The 15% Rule

Kilovoltage may be altered to modify the appearance of the radiographic image by changing the scale of contrast. Radiographic contrast is discussed in Chapter 7 and its relationship to kilovoltage is explained in Chapter 10. The kVp is *increased* to lengthen the scale of contrast; this change decreases contrast, increases latitude, and creates a grayer image. The kVp is *decreased* to shorten the scale of contrast; this change increases contrast, producing a more black-and-white appearance. When kVp is changed, however, the radiographic density, or darkness of the image, is also affected. If the original radiographic density was satisfactory and you wish only to change the level of contrast, mAs must be used to compensate for the density change that occurs when kVp is altered. An increase in kVp with a corresponding decrease in mAs results in a lower patient dose. As explained in Chapter 10, the 15% rule provides guidelines for altering the kVp while maintaining a constant radiographic density.

To use the 15% rule to increase contrast, decrease the kVp by 15% and multiply the mAs by 2.

> **Example:** A radiograph made using 40 mAs and 90 kVp has satisfactory radiographic density but is lacking in contrast. Suggest a new technique that will provide more contrast with similar radiographic density.
>
> To decrease kVp by 15%, multiply by 0.85 (100% − 15% = 85% or 0.85):
>
> 90 kVp × 0.85 = 77 kVp
>
> *NOTE: When calculating kVp changes, round off to the nearest whole kilovolt.*
>
> Multiply the mAs by 2: 40 mAs × 2 = 80 mAs
>
> Therefore the new technique is 80 mAs at 77 kVp.

To use the 15% rule to decrease contrast, increase latitude, lower patient dose, increase the kVp by 15%, and divide the mAs by 2.

> **Example:** A satisfactory radiograph is made using 60 mAs and 76 kVp. Suggest a new technique that will provide more latitude and lower the patient dose.
>
> To increase kVp by 15%, multiply by 1.15 (100% + 15%): 76 kVp × 1.15 = 87 kVp
>
> Divide the mAs by 2: 60 mAs ÷ 2 = 30 mAs
>
> Therefore the new technique is 30 mAs at 87 kVp.
>
> *NOTE: The 15% rule may be reapplied to the new technique if the first calculation does not produce sufficient change.*

Practice Problems Using the 15% Rule

(When changing kVp, round off your answers to the nearest whole number.)

1. An exposure made using 25 mAs and 86 kVp has satisfactory radiographic density. Suggest a new technique that will provide more contrast.
2. An exposure made using 100 mAs and 80 kVp has satisfactory radiographic density. Suggest a new technique that will decrease the patient dose.
3. An exposure made using 10 mAs and 66 kVp has satisfactory radiographic density. Suggest a new technique that will provide more latitude.
4. An exposure made using 40 mAs and 94 kVp has satisfactory radiographic density. Suggest a new technique that will provide more contrast.
5. An exposure made using 60 mAs and 72 kVp has satisfactory radiographic density. Suggest a new technique that will provide less contrast.
6. An exposure made using 80 mAs and 96 kVp has satisfactory radiographic density. Suggest a new technique that will provide more contrast.
7. An exposure made using 20 mAs and 70 kVp has satisfactory radiographic density. Suggest a new technique that will decrease the patient dose.
8. An exposure made using 5 mAs and 54 kVp has satisfactory radiographic density. Suggest a new technique that will provide more latitude.
9. An exposure made using 30 mAs and 120 kVp has satisfactory radiographic density. Suggest a new technique that will provide more contrast.
10. An exposure made using 50 mAs and 68 kVp has satisfactory radiographic density. Suggest a new technique that will provide less contrast.

Medication Dosage Calculations

Calculation of medication dosage is discussed in Chapter 23. This section highlights that information and provides practice problems.

Medications are provided in many forms, but the most common forms are tablets and liquids. Regardless of form, each medication is provided in specific strengths. The strength of the medication indicates the amount of active drug contained in a certain volume of the medication. For example, a liquid medication may have 5 mcg of solid dissolved in each milliliter of liquid and the strength would be stated as 5 mcg/mL. A tablet may contain 2 mg of the active drug and would be labeled simply as 2 mg/tablet.

The basic formula for determining the correct quantity of any drug is as follows:

$$\frac{\text{Dose}}{\text{Strength}} = \text{Volume}$$

In this formula, *dose* refers to the prescribed amount of the active ingredient in the medication. *Strength* refers to the amount of active ingredient per unit of volume as described in the preceding paragraph. *Volume* refers to the total quantity of medication that is administered.

Examples:

1. The physician has prescribed a dose of 50 mg of meperidine (Demerol) intramuscularly. The available stock has a strength of 20 mg/mL. How much of this solution should you draw up into the syringe?

   Substitute the known quantities in the formula and perform a calculation to determine the volume.

   $$\frac{50 \text{ mg}}{20 \text{ mg/mL}} = 2.5 \text{ mL} \left(\text{Volume to be injected} \right)$$

2. A toddler got into the medicine cabinet and ate 4 acetaminophen tablets. The strength of the tablets is 500 mg. What dose did the toddler receive?

   Substitute the known quantities in the formula:

   $$\frac{x \text{ mg}}{500 \text{ mg/tablet}} = 4 \text{ tablets} \left(\text{Volume taken} \right)$$

   To isolate the dose, multiply both sides of the equation by 500:

   $$\frac{x \text{ mg} \times \cancel{500 \text{ mg/tablet}}}{\cancel{500 \text{ mg/tablet}}} = 500 \text{ mg} \times 4 \text{ tablets}$$

   Dose = 500 mg × 4 = 2000 mg (2 g)

Practice Problems Calculating Medication Dosage

1. The prescribed dose is 100 mg. The available stock is in the form of 25-mg tablets. How many should be given?
2. The prescribed dose is 250 mg. The available stock has a strength of 50 mg/mL. How much should be given?
3. The prescribed dose is 40 mcg. The available stock has a strength of 80 mcg/tablet. How much should be given?
4. The prescribed dose is 5 mg. The available stock has a strength of 1 mg/mL. How much should be given?
5. A patient reports taking 8 tablets of ibuprofen (Advil) a day. The tablets have a strength of 200 mg. What is the patient's daily dose?

SUMMARY

The information in this chapter supplements that in later chapters regarding mathematical relationships and technique formulation.

Fractions are portions of whole numbers and are sometimes used to measure exposure times. They are most commonly reduced to lowest terms and can easily be calculated when converted to decimals. Decimals are fractions with denominators of 10, 100, 1000, and so on, and are written differently from other fractions. The most familiar decimals are those used to indicate dollars and cents. Percentages are specific decimals with denominators of 100.

Exponents are used to shorten the notation of very large and very small numbers. A positive exponent indicates the number of times the base number is multiplied by itself. Negative exponents designate quantities smaller than 1.

Equations are numerical expressions of two quantities that are equal to each other. They can be manipulated to determine the value of an unknown quantity, but the balance of the equation must be maintained. Special equations of the type $a/b = c/d$ are called *proportions*. They represent relationships between quantities that may be either direct or inverse and are a common way of expressing relationships between technical factors in radiography.

These problem-solving skills are important, whether or not you need to use them every day. They are used to calculate mAs values and to adjust exposure factors for changes in patient size, source–image receptor distance, and kVp, as well as to accurately determine dose for medication administration.

PART II
X-ray Science

Chapter 4

Basic Physics for Radiography

Learning Objectives

At the conclusion of this chapter, you will be able to:

- Define matter and list its three forms
- Name the fundamental particles of the atom and list characteristics of each
- Draw or describe a conceptual model of atomic structure
- List and describe five forms of energy
- Draw a sine wave and measure its amplitude and its wavelength
- Relate the wavelength of a sine wave to its velocity and frequency
- Compare and contrast the characteristics of x-rays with the characteristics of visible light
- Explain the relationships between potential difference, current, and resistance in an electric circuit and state the units used to measure each
- State the frequency of alternating current in the United States and Canada using the correct units
- Describe the process of electromagnetic induction
- Draw simple diagrams of a step-up transformer and a step-down transformer

Key Terms

ampere (A)	kilovolt peak (kVp)
atom	mass
atomic number	matter
binding energy	milliampere (mA)
chemical compound	molecules
circuit	neutron
conductor	nucleus
current	photon
electromagnetic energy	potential difference
electromagnetic induction	proton
electron	rectification
element	resistance (R)
frequency	sine wave
ion	transformer
ionization	volt (V)
K-shell	wavelength

Limited operators do not require an extensive background in physics, but some basic principles of physical science are essential to an understanding of x-rays and their use. This chapter covers the basic concepts of matter, energy, and electricity and relates these principles to radiography. It also discusses the nature of radiation.

If your educational background includes coursework in physics or chemistry, this chapter will provide a comprehensive review of the pertinent material. If you are unfamiliar with these subjects, it will be important for you to master them so that you can relate well to the material that follows.

Everything of a physical nature in the universe can be classified as either **matter** or energy. Both matter and energy can exist in several forms.

MATTER

Matter is defined as anything that occupies space and has shape or form. The three basic forms of matter are solids, liquids, and gases. The quantity of matter that makes up any physical object is called its **mass.** Although the scientific definitions differ somewhat, mass is essentially the same thing we think of as "weight." An object may change in form, but its mass is unchangeable. For example, a 20-lb bucket of water may freeze into a 20-lb bucket of ice or it may evaporate, resulting in 20 lb of water vapor. The form changes, but the mass remains the same.

Laws of Conservation

Matter can be neither created nor destroyed, but it can change form.
Energy can be neither created nor destroyed, but it can change form.

Atoms

All matter is composed of "building blocks" called **atoms.** Scientists have determined that atoms may be made up of nearly 100 different subatomic particles, but only three basic particles concern us here. The fundamental particles that compose atoms are **neutrons, protons,** and **electrons.** All neutrons are identical, as are all protons and all electrons. It is the number and arrangement of these particles in the atom that account for the differences in matter.

The neutrons and protons together form the **nucleus** of the atom, its center. The electrons circle the nucleus in orbits called *shells.* A useful model for visualizing atomic structure is that of the solar system, with the nucleus as the sun and the electrons as planets in orbit around the sun (Fig. 4-1). This model was first described by Niels Bohr in 1913 and is referred to as *Bohr's atom.*

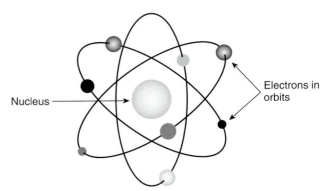

Fig. 4-1 Bohr's concept of the atom.

Atomic particles differ from one another with respect to electric charge. Neutrons are electrically neutral (0); that is, they have no electric charge. Protons have a positive charge (+). Electrons have a negative charge (−); that is, their charge is equal to, but opposite, the charge of a proton. A particle's charge is important because it results in a magnetic effect. Opposite charges attract one another, seeking a neutral state. Like charges repel one another. Neutral particles neither attract nor repel and are not attracted or repelled by charged particles. Table 4-1 contains a summary of the characteristics of the fundamental atomic particles.

In its "normal" or neutral state, an atom has an equal number of protons and electrons, so the electric charges are balanced and the atom as a whole has no charge. The electrons are arranged in their orbits, with a specific number of electrons allotted to each shell. The shells are lettered alphabetically, beginning with the letter K nearest the nucleus (Fig. 4-2). From the nucleus outward, each additional shell is greater in size and can accommodate a larger number of electrons than the previous shell. Table 4-2 lists atomic shells with their letter symbols and the maximum number of electrons in each. Different types of atoms will have different numbers of electrons in their shells up to the maximum shown. From a radiography standpoint, the most important shell is the **K-shell.** The removal of electrons in this shell is one way in which x-rays are created.

Each of the electrons around the nucleus is in continuous motion. The distance that the shell is from the nucleus determines the energy level of the electron. The electrons are held in place by a **binding energy.** Electrons near the nucleus are attached with greater binding energy than those in outer shells. The binding energy of

  Table 4-1

Fundamental Atomic Particles

Particle	Location	Mass Number	Charge
Proton	Nucleus	1	+1
Neutron	Nucleus	1	0
Electron	Orbital shells		−1

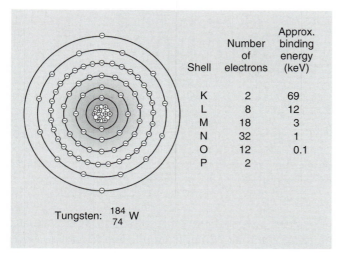

Tungsten: $^{184}_{74}$W

Shell	Number of electrons	Approx. binding energy (keV)
K	2	69
L	8	12
M	18	3
N	32	1
O	12	0.1
P	2	

Fig. 4-2 Atomic configuration for tungsten. Note shell number and number of electrons in each shell. Binding energy is higher for shells closer to the nucleus.

Table 4-2

Electron Shells

Shell Number	Shell Symbol	Maximum Number of Electrons
1	K	2
2	L	8
3	M	18
4	N	32
5	O	50
6	P	72
7	Q	98

each shell varies for different atoms; larger atoms have greater binding energy than smaller ones.

Elements

The essential characteristic of an atom that determines its type is the number of protons in the nucleus. An **element** is a substance made up of only one type of atom; that is, all atoms of an element have the same **atomic number.** Scientists have identified 118 different elements. Many of these are rare, and some of them are human made. Each element has a name and a chemical symbol consisting of one or two letters. Three common elements we may be familiar with are calcium (Ca), iodine (I), and lead (Pb). Each element also has an atomic number that represents the number of protons in the nucleus. The atomic numbers for the three elements described are 20, 53, and 82. The greater the atomic number, the greater is the element's mass and density. In radiology, a lead bullet inside a body would be easier to see on an x-ray than a calcium stone because of lead's greater atomic number and density. The mass number of the element is the combined total of the protons and

neutrons in the nucleus. One of the most important elements used in the production of x-rays is tungsten. Tungsten is the element inside the x-ray tube where the x-rays are created (discussed in Chapter 5). Tungsten (see Fig. 4-2) is represented by the symbol W and its atomic number is 74. Its mass number is 184, indicating that the nucleus contains 74 protons and 110 neutrons. The number of neutrons is determined by subtracting the atomic number from the mass number.

Two or more atoms may combine chemically to form **molecules.** This combination occurs with the sharing of one or more outer shell electrons between atoms. A substance that consists of only one type of molecule is called a **chemical compound.** Water is an example of a chemical compound. Its chemical symbol is H_2O, indicating that it is made up of two atoms of hydrogen and one atom of oxygen. Substances that contain more than one type of molecule are called *mixtures.*

Ionization

When a neutral atom gains or loses an electron, it is called an **ion** and the atom is said to be ionized. This process, which is called **ionization,** produces an atom with an electric charge. If an electron is added to a neutral atom, electrons will outnumber the protons and the atom will have a negative charge. If an electron is removed, there will be more protons than electrons, so the atom will have a positive charge. Because the outer orbital electrons are not tightly bound to the nucleus, the application of a small amount of energy can remove an outer orbital electron from the atom (Fig. 4-3).

A familiar example of ionization is the "bad hair day" that occurs when the weather is cold and dry. The friction of a hairbrush removes electrons from atoms in the hair. In very dry air, the electrons cannot readily return to their orbits, and each hair is left with a positive charge. Because like charges repel each other, the hairs are repelled from one another and will not lie smoothly together.

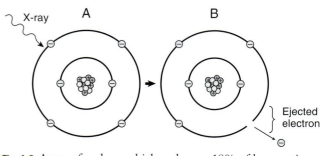

Fig. 4-3 Atom of carbon, which makes up 18% of human tissue. During an x-ray many carbon atoms will be ionized. **A,** X-ray entering the neutral atom. **B,** An outer shell electron is ejected, leaving more protons than electrons. This atom is positively charged and ionized. The x-ray is scattered to another atom or outside the body.

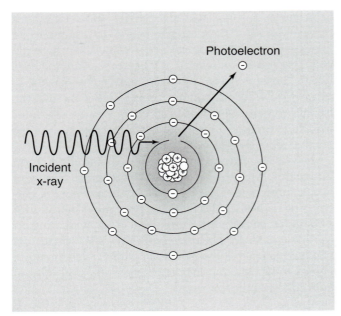

Fig. 4-4 X-ray entering an atom in the human body and interacting with an inner shell electron (K-shell) and causing ionization. The x-ray becomes totally absorbed. The K-shell electron is ejected from the atom.

The term ionization is very important in the field of radiology. X-rays cause ionization in the atoms of the human body (Fig. 4-4), a fact that explains many of the negative effects of radiation discussed later in the text.

ENERGY

Energy is defined as the ability to do work. It occurs in several forms and can be changed from one form to another. Some familiar forms of energy include heat, light, and electricity. Scientists have categorized energy in various ways. One method classifies energy into the following types: mechanical, chemical, thermal, nuclear, electric, and electromagnetic.

Mechanical energy can be further classified as either kinetic energy or potential energy. Kinetic energy is energy of motion, the ability of a moving object to do work. For example, a bowling ball in motion has energy to knock down the pins. Potential energy can be thought of as "stored" energy. When a bowling ball has been lifted, the work required to raise it is "stored" in the ball because of its position. When the ball is released, its potential energy is also released and is converted into kinetic energy. In a later chapter you will learn that the x-ray tube has a very high potential energy before the exposure is made.

Chemical energy is released through chemical changes in atoms or molecules. An example of chemical energy is fire. A gasoline engine converts the chemical energy of gasoline into mechanical energy. Chemical energy from the food we eat produces the energy needed for muscle movement and many other vital processes.

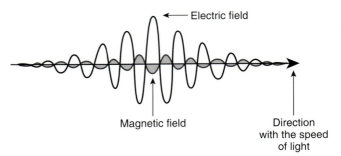

Fig. 4-5 An x-ray photon can be visualized as two sine waves travelling in a straight line at the speed of light.

Thermal energy is commonly called *heat*. It is the result of atomic motion. As temperature rises, electrons move faster in their orbits and the orbits expand, which causes the electrons to move farther from the nucleus. This phenomenon explains why matter expands in size when heated and contracts when cooled. In a later chapter you will learn that the majority of energy created in the x-ray tube is converted to heat.

Nuclear energy is the energy released by radionuclides. This is the energy used to produce electricity in a nuclear power plant or the explosion of a nuclear bomb.

Electric energy, or electricity, is the ability of electric charges to do work. Although this process may seem mysterious, it is familiar to all of us. We use it to light our homes, run our computers, and make toast. Electric energy also may exist in the form of potential energy. Potential electric energy exists in a battery or at an unused wall socket. When we turn on a flashlight or plug in an appliance, this potential energy is converted into electricity. Electric energy is important in producing x-rays because the standard low electric voltage is raised to very high levels in the x-ray machine.

Electromagnetic energy is the important energy we deal with every day in radiology. This energy consists of light, x-rays, radio waves, microwaves, and other forms of energy. These energies have both electric and magnetic properties, changing the field through which they pass both electrically and magnetically (Fig. 4-5). These changes in the field occur in the form of a repeating wave, a pattern that scientists call a *sinusoidal form* or **sine wave** (Fig. 4-6).

A more comprehensive understanding of electric energy and electromagnetic energy is essential to the limited operator. These energy forms are discussed in greater detail in the sections that follow.

ELECTROMAGNETIC ENERGY

As stated earlier, electromagnetic energy occurs in the form of a sine wave. Several characteristics of this waveform are significant. The distance between the crest and the trough of the wave (its height) is called the amplitude (Fig. 4-7). More important in radiology is the distance

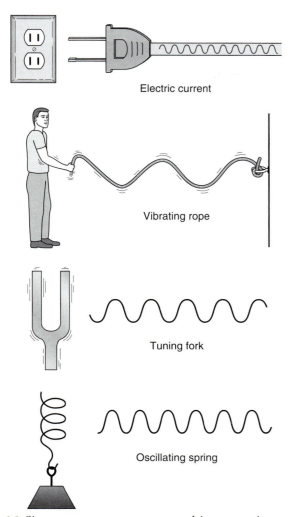

Fig. 4-6 Sine waves are energy expressed in a recurring waveform. Sine waves are associated with many naturally occurring phenomena, including electromagnetic radiation.

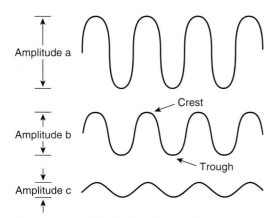

Fig. 4-7 Sine wave amplitude, the distance from crest to trough. These three sine waves are identical except for their amplitude.

from one crest to the next, or **wavelength** (Fig. 4-8). The **frequency** of the wave is the number of times per second that a crest passes a given point (Fig. 4-9).

Electromagnetic energy moves through space at the velocity (speed) of approximately 186,000 miles/second.

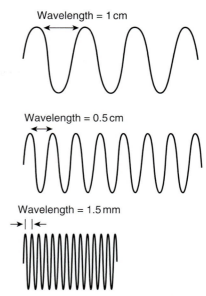

Fig. 4-8 Sine wave wavelength, the distance from crest to crest. These three sine waves have different wavelengths. The shorter the wavelength, the higher the frequency. An x-ray would appear like the bottom wavelength.

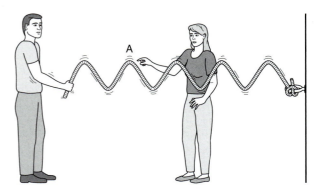

Fig. 4-9 Sine wave frequency, the number of crests or troughs that pass a fixed point per unit of time. The unit of time is typically 1 second.

All electromagnetic energy moves at the same velocity. When the wavelength is short, the crests are closer together, so more of them will pass a given point in a second, resulting in a higher frequency. Longer wavelengths will have a lower frequency. This may be expressed mathematically as follows:

$$\text{Velocity} = \text{Wavelength} \times \text{Frequency}$$

The more energy the wave has, the greater its frequency and the shorter its wavelength. We can therefore use either wavelength or frequency to describe the energy of the wave. In radiology, wavelength is more often used to describe the energy of the x-ray beam. The average wavelength of a diagnostic x-ray beam is about a billionth of an inch. *X-rays with greater energy have shorter wavelengths, have higher frequencies, and are more penetrating.*

Applications:	Wavelength:	
Therapeutic x-ray	1/100,000 nm	
	1/10,000 nm	
Gamma rays	1/1000 nm	Ionizing
	1/100 nm	
Diagnostic x-ray	1/10 nm	
	1 nm	
Ultraviolet rays	10 nm	
	100 nm	
Visible light	1000 nm	
Infrared rays	10,000 nm	
	100,000 nm	
	1/1000 m	
Radar	1/100 m	Nonionizing
	1/10 m	
	1 m	
Television	10 m	
Radio	100 m	
	1 nanometer = 0.000000001 meter	

Fig. 4-10 Electromagnetic spectrum. The applications below the bold line are nonionizing because they have longer wavelengths. Note x-rays appear above the bold line. X-rays' very short wavelength enables them to ionize tissues.

The wavelength of electromagnetic radiation varies from exceedingly short (even shorter than that of diagnostic x-rays) to very long (more than 5 miles). This range of energies is known as the *electromagnetic spectrum*. It includes x-rays, gamma rays, visible light, microwaves, and radio waves (Fig. 4-10). Radiation with a wavelength shorter than 1 nm (0.000000001 m) is often called *ionizing radiation* because it has sufficient energy to remove an electron from its atomic orbit. X-rays are one type of ionizing radiation.

The smallest possible unit of electromagnetic energy is the **photon,** which may be thought of as a tiny "bundle" of energy. Photons come out of the x-ray tube as discrete bundles of energy.

Sine Wave Velocity

Wavelength × Frequency = Velocity

The velocity of electromagnetic radiation is 186,000 miles/sec. Note that *all* electromagnetic radiation has the same velocity.

Sine Wave Energy

- Sine waves with shorter wavelengths (higher frequency) have more energy.
- X-rays with shorter wavelengths are more penetrating.

Ionizing Radiation

- Sufficient energy to remove an electron from its orbit
- Wavelength of 1 nm or less
- X-rays are one form of ionizing radiation

Box 4-1
Characteristics of X-rays

- Have no mass
- Are highly penetrating and invisible
- Are electrically neutral
- Are polyenergetic and heterogeneous
- Travel in straight lines at the speed of light
- Can ionize matter
- Produce biologic changes in tissues
- Produce secondary and scatter radiation

CHARACTERISTICS OF X-RAYS

X-rays have very unique characteristics, which are summarized in Box 4-1. Because x-rays and visible light are both forms of electromagnetic energy, they have some similar characteristics. Both travel in straight lines at the same velocity and both have an effect on photographic film.

Both x-rays and light have a biologic effect; that is, they can cause changes in living organisms. For example, excessive exposure to either sunlight or x-rays may cause burns to the skin. X-rays are capable of producing more harmful effects than light because of their greater energy.

Unlike light, x-rays cannot be detected by the human senses. This fact may seem obvious, but it is important to consider. If x-rays could be seen, felt, or heard, we would have an increased awareness of their presence, and radiation safety might be much simpler. Because x-rays are undetectable, safety requires that you learn to know when and where x-rays are present despite being unable to perceive them.

X-rays can penetrate matter. This penetration is differential, depending on the mass, atomic number, and thickness of the matter. For example, x-rays penetrate air in the lungs very readily. There is less penetration of muscle or bone.

Unlike light, x-rays cannot be refracted by a lens. The x-rays come out of the x-ray tube and into space until they are absorbed or go through the human body.

ELECTRICITY

X-ray energy is human made and is produced electrically. To understand this process, it is helpful to know something about electric current. Electric current will flow in a vacuum, in certain liquids (saltwater, for example), and through certain metals called **conductors.** Copper wire is an excellent conductor and is commonly used for electric wiring. It is connected to form a **circuit,** a continuous path. Current will flow in the circuit when there is a difference in electric charge, a potential difference, between two points in the circuit. Current is produced when negatively charged electrons flow toward a positive charge. A positive potential can be maintained at one point in the circuit by means of electric energy from a battery or a public utility.

Electric Units

Three electric factors are part of an electric circuit: resistance, current, and potential difference. Practically, only current and potential difference are important in our understanding of how x-rays are created from an electric circuit.

Resistance is any property of the circuit that opposes or hinders the flow of current. The unit used to measure resistance is the ohm, represented by the Greek letter omega (Ω). Resistance depends on several factors: the material of the conductor, its length, and its diameter. The longer the conductor, the more resistance it will provide. Resistance is decreased when the wire diameter is greater.

Current is the *quantity* of electrons flowing in a circuit. The **ampere,** abbreviated **A,** is the unit used to measure the *rate,* or *volume,* of *current flow* in the circuit. In your home the electric circuit to the toaster may require 8 amps and the circuit to a lamp may require only 1 amp. In radiology, every body part will require a different amperage setting on the generator.

Potential difference is the *force,* or *speed,* of the electron flow in the current. The **volt,** abbreviated **V,** is the unit used to measure potential difference. In your home the electric circuit to the stove or dryer that contains 220 V has twice as much electricity as the 110-V circuit going to your television. In radiology, every body part will require a different voltage setting on the generator.

In our daily work in the radiology department we never use the terms current and potential difference. Instead, the units amp and volt are used in every x-ray we take because these are two of the factors set on the x-ray generator to send electricity to the x-ray tube. Limited operators can separately control the volts and amps.

The electric requirements for x-ray tubes are much different from those for household appliances (Table 4-3). The voltage provided by public utilities for general household use is 120 V, and a common household circuit has a current of 15 to 30 A. X-ray tubes use much greater voltage and less amperage. A typical x-ray tube operates at a range of 40,000 to 125,000 V (very high numbers). The x-ray tube current is less than 1 A at about 0.025 to 0.5 A

Table 4-3		
Electric Supply Requirements: Household vs. X-ray Tube		
	Volts	**Amps**
Household circuit:	120 V	30.0 A
X-ray circuit:	120,000 V	0.3 A

Table 4-4		
Electric Units		
Measurement	**Unit**	**Abbreviation**
Current	Ampere	A
	Milliampere	mA
Kilovoltage	Volt	V
	Kilovolt peak	kVp

(very low numbers). For this reason, it is convenient to use the **kilovolt peak (kVp),** equal to 1000 V to measure the voltage across an x-ray tube, and the **milliampere (mA),** equal to $\frac{1}{1000}$ of an ampere (0.001 A), to measure x-ray tube current. Using kVp and mA enables much easier to relate to values. For example, for the typical x-ray tube voltages described earlier, the range would be described as 40 to 125 kVp. Note the smaller numbers used. For the amperages described above, the range would be 25 to 500 mA. Note the lack of decimal points and zeros. The volt and amp numbers are to relate to when using kilovolts and milliamps. The significance of these units in x-ray production is discussed in Chapter 5.

Table 4-4 lists units of electric measurement that are important for radiographers to remember.

Electric Circuits

An electric circuit is a continuous path for the flow of electric charges from the power source through one or more electric devices and back to the source (Fig. 4-11).

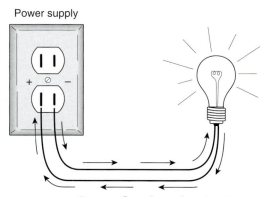

Fig. 4-11 Current flow through a circuit.

Table 4-5

Electric Circuit Elements: Their Symbols and Functions

Circuit Element	Symbol	Function
Ammeter	(A)	Measures electric current
Voltmeter	(V)	Measures electrical potential
Transformer		Increases or decreases voltage by fixed amount (AC only)
Diode		Allows electrons to flow in only one direction

AC, Alternating current.
Modified from Bushong SC: *Radiologic science for technologists,* ed 10, St Louis, 2013, Mosby.

Electric circuit diagrams are "maps" of circuits that show how current flows through the devices connected in the circuit. Table 4-5 contains some common symbols used in these diagrams. Circuit diagrams are used in this text to demonstrate electric principles and to explain the function of the x-ray machine, so it will be helpful for you to become familiar with these symbols.

Direct Current and Alternating Current

The electric service provided by a public utility is in the form of alternating current (AC). The polarity (positive or negative electric potential) of the power source reverses at regular intervals, causing the current to flow first in one direction, then in the opposite direction (Fig. 4-12). The change is not instantaneous. In a household circuit, for example, the electric cycle begins with the voltage at 0, increases to a *positive* 120 V, where it peaks, and then declines to 0 again. At this point the polarity changes and the voltage increases from 0 to a *negative* 120 V, peaks, and again returns to 0 (Fig. 4-13). In the United States and Canada, public utilities deliver

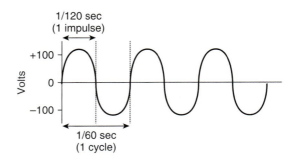

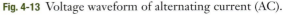

AC in U.S. and Canada: 60 cycles/sec (60 Hz)

Fig. 4-13 Voltage waveform of alternating current (AC).

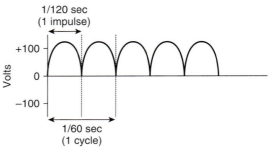

Fig. 4-14 Voltage waveform of rectified alternating current.

alternating current at a frequency of 60 cycles/second. The unit of electromagnetic frequency is the *hertz (Hz)*. Thus the duration of each cycle is $\frac{1}{60}$ second. Half a cycle is called an *impulse*. There are 120 impulses/second with 60 Hz AC, so the duration of one impulse is $\frac{1}{120}$ second. In radiology, high-frequency generators are used and for these the frequency is increased from 60 Hz to as high as 6000 Hz. These are described in Chapter 6.

This alternating polarity produces electric current that is constantly changing. The current flow increases, peaks, and declines as the voltage changes. The current flow changes direction when the polarity changes.

Alternating current can be converted so that it flows in one direction only. This process is called **rectification.** The x-ray tube cannot produce x-rays unless the current is rectified. Rectified alternating current is sometimes also referred to as *direct current*; it differs from DC produced by a battery in that it is pulsating rather than constant (Fig. 4-14). In the x-ray room, electricity comes in as AC, 120 V, 90 As, 60 Hz. The transformer of the x-ray machine will change this to DC, variable 40 to 125 kVp, variable 50 to 500 mA, and up to 6000 Hz. This transformation of electricity is discussed in Chapter 6.

ELECTROMAGNETIC INDUCTION AND TRANSFORMERS

Magnetic fields and electric energy are interrelated. Magnetic fields can be used to produce electricity, and conversely, electric currents create magnetic fields.

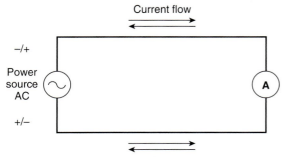

Fig. 4-12 Simple electric circuit, alternating current (AC). The polarity of the power source alternates between positive and negative at regular intervals. *A,* Ammeter.

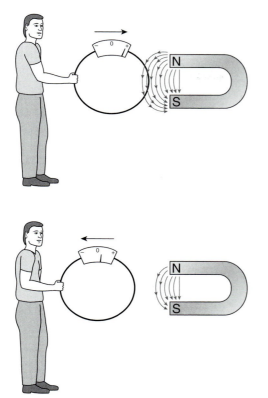

Fig. 4-15 When a conductor moves in and out of a magnetic field, alternating current will flow in the conductor. *N*, North magnetic pole; *S*, south magnetic pole.

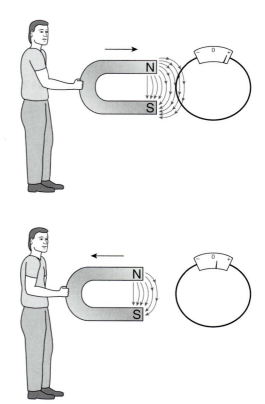

Fig. 4-16 When a magnetic field moves in relation to a conductor, alternating current will flow in the conductor. *N*, North magnetic pole; *S*, south magnetic pole.

When a conductor is placed in a magnetic field and there is movement between the lines of magnetic force and the conductor, current will flow in the conductor. This principle can be demonstrated by moving a circuit in and out of the force field surrounding a magnet (Fig. 4-15). The same result is obtained by moving the magnet in relation to the conductor (Fig. 4-16). This process is called **electromagnetic induction.** When the direction of the movement changes, the direction of the current flow is reversed, creating alternating current. This effect also occurs with a change in the influencing pole of the magnet. For these reasons, *induced current is always alternating current.* This is the principle used to generate electric power. Public utilities use some other form of energy (steam generated by coal, gas, or nuclear energy, or water flowing over a dam) to move either the magnet or the conductor.

When current is flowing through a circuit, it creates a magnetic field surrounding the conductor (Fig. 4-17). If this current is alternating, its magnetic field will be in constant motion. This moving magnetic field can be used to *induce* current to flow in another conductor (Fig. 4-18). The circuit that is connected to the power supply is called the *primary circuit.* The circuit that carries the induced current is called the *secondary circuit.* Note that the two circuits are not connected to each other.

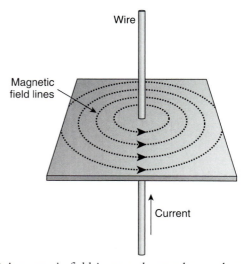

Fig. 4-17 A magnetic field is created around a conductor when current flows through the circuit. When the current is alternating, the magnetic field is in constant motion.

Electromagnetic induction is the basis for the **transformer,** the device used to produce the high voltage needed for x-ray production. A transformer consists of primary and secondary coils, usually surrounding an iron core (Fig. 4-19). The iron core further enhances the magnetic fields of the coils. Electric current always flows from the primary to the secondary coils.

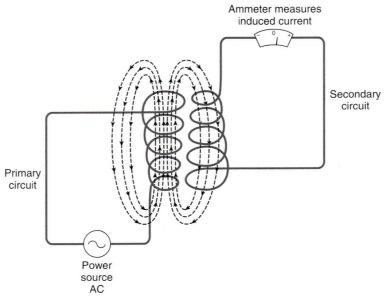

Fig. 4-18 When a conductor is placed in the magnetic field of an alternating current (AC) circuit, induced current will flow through the conductor.

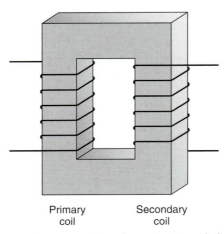

Fig. 4-19 A transformer consists of two circuits coiled around an iron core that enhances the magnetic fields. Because the circuits are insulated from the core, current cannot flow directly between the circuits.

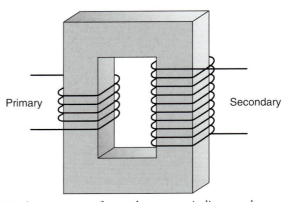

Fig. 4-20 A step-up transformer has more windings on the secondary side. This type of transformer is used in x-rays to increase the volts to kilovolts.

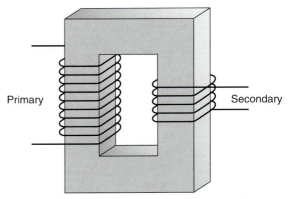

Fig. 4-21 A step-down transformer has fewer windings on the secondary side. This type of transformer is used in x-rays to reduce the amperage down to milliamperage levels.

When different numbers of turns, or "windings," are used in the coils of the primary and secondary circuits, the kilovolt peak across the two coils will also be different. This makes it possible to change voltage by means of electromagnetic induction, which is the primary purpose of a transformer. When there are more windings in the secondary coil than in the primary coil, the voltage on the secondary side is greater, and the transformer is called a *step-up* transformer (Fig. 4-20). On the other hand, if the secondary side has fewer turns, the secondary voltage will be less than the primary voltage and the transformer is called a *step-down* transformer (Fig. 4-21). The voltage increase or decrease produced by a transformer is *directly* proportional to the number of turns in each coil. For example, if the secondary side has twice as many turns as the primary side, the secondary voltage will be twice the primary voltage.

A transformer always increases or decreases the incoming voltage by a set multiple called the *transformer ratio*. The first number in the ratio is always the number of windings on the secondary side. For example, if the voltage across the primary side were 200 V and the transformer had 500 secondary turns for each primary turn, the ratio would be *500:1* and the secondary voltage would be 200 × 500, or stepped up to 100,000 V (100 kVp). On the other hand, a transformer with 90 turns on the primary side and 30 turns on the secondary side would have a *1:3* ratio. If the primary voltage were 150 V, the secondary voltage would be 150 ÷ 3 or stepped down to 50 V. Mathematical calculations involving transformer ratios and voltage are covered in Chapter 3.

It is helpful to remember that both voltage and amperage flow in an electric circuit. Therefore amperage also flows through the transformer. However, kilovoltage and amperage are *inversely* proportional while flowing through the transformer. It is important to remember that as a step-up transformer increases voltage from primary to secondary, amperage is decreased. Conversely, as a step-down transformer decreases voltage from primary to secondary, amperage is increased. An x-ray machine uses both step-up and step-down transformers.

SUMMARY

The atom is the basic building block of all matter, consisting of positively charged protons and uncharged neutrons in its nucleus and negatively charged electrons in orbits around the nucleus. Ionization takes place when a neutral atom or molecule gains or loses an electron, which results in one or two charged particles.

Energy exists in many forms and can be converted from one form to another. X-rays are one form of electromagnetic energy. Electromagnetic energy exists in the form of sine waves, whose energy is a function of their wavelength. X-rays have no mass and are not visible. They travel in straight lines at the speed of light and can penetrate matter. They have a very short wavelength and very high frequency.

Electric current is the flow of electric charges in a circuit. Potential difference (voltage) causes current (amperage) to flow through resistance. A conductor in which alternating current flows is surrounded by a moving magnetic field. This field can induce current to flow in a circuit that is adjacent to it. This electromagnetic induction is the principle of the transformer, a device used to change voltage in the x-ray circuit.

Chapter 5

X-ray Production

Learning Objectives

At the conclusion of this chapter, you will be able to:

- Draw a simple x-ray tube and label its parts
- Describe both the composition and the function of the basic parts of the x-ray tube
- Associate the terms *anode* and *cathode* with the appropriate parts of the x-ray tube
- Describe the production of both bremsstrahlung and characteristic radiation
- Explain what is meant by a dual-focus tube and describe its advantages
- Explain the significance of the target angle with respect to the line focus principle and the maximum field size
- Define "effective focal spot" and state its significance with respect to the radiographic image
- Explain the function of a rotating anode and state its purpose
- State the effect of changes in milliampere (mA) and kilovolt (kVp) levels on the resulting x-ray beam

Key Terms

actual focal spot
anode heel effect
bremsstrahlung radiation
characteristic radiation
dual-focus
effective focal spot
electron stream
exposure time
filament
filtration
focal spot
focal track
focusing cup

heterogeneous
kilovolts peak (kVp)
line focus principle
milliampere-second (mAs)
millisecond (msec)
photon
rotating anode
space charge
spatial resolution
target
target angle
thermionic emission
tungsten

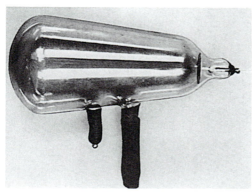

Fig. 5-1 Crookes tube used by Roentgen, 1895.

This chapter is about x-ray tube structure and function and how these factors affect the primary x-ray beam. The electric factors that control x-ray production are introduced in this chapter. Chapters 4 and 5 contain a tremendous amount of detail, and most of it is probably unfamiliar to you. Although it is all interrelated and is presented in a logical order, you may feel a bit overwhelmed if you try to comprehend it too quickly. Do not attempt to assimilate it all at once. When this material is taken in small bites and reviewed as needed, the entire process of creating and controlling x-rays will gradually come into focus.

Roentgen discovered x-rays while working with a Crookes tube (Fig. 5-1), a cathode ray tube that was the forerunner of the fluorescent tube and the neon light. These tubes were used in physics laboratories in the late nineteenth century for the investigation of electricity. In 1913, the General Electric Company introduced the Coolidge tube (Fig. 5-2), a "hot cathode tube" that was the prototype for modern x-ray tubes.

X-RAY TUBE

Fig. 5-3 illustrates a simple x-ray tube with its principal parts labeled. There are four essential requirements for the production of x-rays: (1) a vacuum, (2) a source of electrons, (3) a **target,** and (4) a high potential difference (voltage) between the electron source and the target.

A Pyrex glass envelope forms the basic structure of the x-ray tube. It is made of strong, heat-resistant glass and contains both the source of electrons and the target. The air is removed from the glass envelope to form a near-perfect vacuum so that gas molecules will not interfere with the process of x-ray production. The tube is fitted on both ends with connections for the electric supply.

The source of electrons is a **filament** at one end of the tube. The filament consists of a small coil of **tungsten** wire. Tungsten (chemical symbol W) is a metal element; it is a large atom with 74 electrons in orbit around its nucleus. An electric current flows through the filament to heat it. An advantage of using tungsten is that it has a high melting point, which enables it to last through thousands of exposures. As explained in Chapter 4, heat speeds up the movement of the electrons in their orbits and increases their distance from the nucleus. Electrons in the outermost orbital shells move so far from the nucleus that they are no longer held in orbit but are flung out of the atom, forming an "electron cloud" around the filament (Fig. 5-4). This process is called **thermionic emission.** The electron cloud is called a **space charge** and is the source of free (in air) electrons for x-ray production.

At the opposite end of the tube is the anode (also referred to as the target), a hard, smooth, slanted metal surface that is also made of tungsten. The electrons are directed toward the target, which is the place where x-rays are generated.

A high-voltage electric source provides acceleration of the electrons. A large step-up transformer supplies the voltage (40 to 125 kVp) required for x-ray production. The two ends of the x-ray tube are connected in the transformer circuit so that the filament end is negative and the target end is positive during an exposure. The positive, target end of the tube is called the *anode;* the negative, filament end is called the *cathode.*

The high positive electric potential at the target attracts the negatively charged electrons of the space charge, which move rapidly across the tube, forming an **electron stream.** When these fast-moving electrons collide with the target, the kinetic energy of their motion is

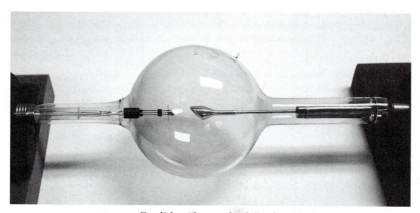

Fig. 5-2 Coolidge "hot cathode" tube, 1913.

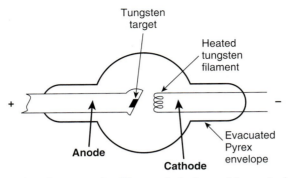

Fig. 5-3 Simple x-ray tube. The anode is the positive end of the tube; the target is part of the anode. The cathode is the negative end of the tube; the filament is part of the cathode.

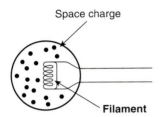

Fig. 5-4 Thermionic emission. As tungsten is heated, electrons in the tungsten atom's orbits spin faster, moving farther from the nucleus. Electrons in outer orbits are flung out of the atom, forming an "electron cloud," or space charge. The space charge provides the electron source for x-ray production.

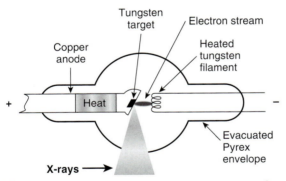

Fig. 5-5 The energy of the electron stream is converted at the anode into heat (>99%) and x-rays (<1%).

converted into a different form of energy. The great majority of this kinetic energy (>99%) is converted into heat, and only a small amount is converted into the energy form that we know as x-rays (Fig. 5-5).

BREMSSTRAHLUNG AND CHARACTERISTIC RADIATION

X-rays are produced at the target as a result of either a sudden deceleration or an absorption of the electron stream. These interactions of electrons with tungsten atoms may occur in one of two ways (Box 5-1).

 **Box 5-1**

Tungsten Target Interactions That Produce X-rays

Bremsstrahlung radiation: created when an incoming electron is suddenly slowed down, changes direction, and leaves the tungsten atom. The kinetic energy of the electron is converted into an x-ray photon.

Characteristic radiation: created when an incoming electron interacts with the K-shell electron and knocks it out of orbit. When the electron void is filled with an outer shell electron, an x-ray photon is created.

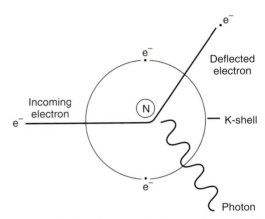

Fig. 5-6 Bremsstrahlung is created when an incoming electron slows suddenly near the nucleus (N) of the tungsten atom and abruptly changes direction, resulting in the creation of an x-ray photon.

Bremsstrahlung Radiation

X-rays are produced when an incoming electron misses all the electrons in the tungsten atom, gets very close to the nucleus, and then suddenly slows down and abruptly changes direction. As a result, the electron loses energy. This sudden energy change is converted into an x-ray **photon** (Fig. 5-6). The photon produced is a small "bundle" of electromagnetic energy. X-rays created by this interaction are called **bremsstrahlung radiation.** Bremsstrahlung is a German word that means braking or slowing. The short term "brems" is often used instead of the long word. Every x-ray exposure will contain photons produced from bremsstrahlung interactions in the anode. Below 70 kVp, 100% of the photons in the x-ray beam are from bremsstrahlung interactions. Above 70 kVp, about 85% of the beam is bremsstrahlung. Therefore it is evident that the majority of all x-ray photons produced are from the bremsstrahlung interactions.

Characteristic Radiation

X-rays are also produced when an incoming electron collides with the K-shell (inner shell) electron of the

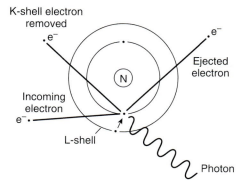

Fig. 5-7 Formation of characteristic radiation. An incoming electron removes an inner orbital electron from the tungsten atom, creating a "hole" in the K-shell. When an outer-shell electron drops to fill the hole, a characteristic photon is emitted. *N*, Nucleus.

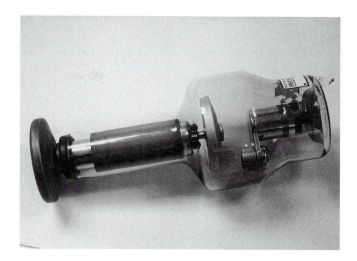

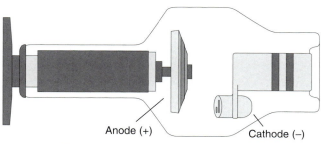

Fig. 5-8 Modern, dual-focus x-ray tube.

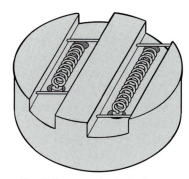

Fig. 5-9 Dual filaments in their focusing cups.

tungsten atom and ejects it out of orbit. Both the incoming electron and the K-shell electron are removed. The void in the K-shell is filled with an electron from any of the other orbits. X-rays created by this interaction are called **characteristic radiation** (Fig. 5-7). Below 70 kVp, there are no characteristic photons produced. Above 70 kVp, about 15% of the beam is characteristic. This is because the binding energy of a K-shell is 69.5 and it takes at least a 70-kVp exposure to eject this electron.

In terms of producing x-ray images, there is no difference between a bremsstrahlung and characteristic photon. They are simply produced by different interactions of the incoming electrons in the anode. Technically, this cannot be controlled. The primary x-ray beam is made up of both bremsstrahlung and characteristic radiation.

The wavelength and energy of the x-ray beam is said to be **heterogeneous.** This means that it is made up of many different wavelengths and energies. X-ray energy is measured in kiloelectron volts (keV).

CHARACTERISTICS OF THE CATHODE AND THE ANODE

Cathode

Although it is essential to have at least one filament for x-ray production, modern multipurpose x-ray tubes are **dual-focus** tubes (Fig. 5-8). They contain two filaments, one large and one small. Only one filament is used at a time.

Each filament is situated in a hollow area in the cathode called a **focusing cup** (Fig. 5-9). The focusing cup has a slight negative charge. The shape of the focusing cup and its negative electric charge cause the electrons to be repelled in the direction of a very precise area on the target called the **focal spot** (Fig. 5-10).

Focal Spot Size

Actual
- Measurement of focal spot on target surface
- Affects tube heat capacity
- *Bigger* is better!

Effective
- Measurement of vertical projection of actual focal spot
- Affects image resolution
- *Smaller* is better!

When the small filament is activated, its electrons are directed to a small focal spot on the target. The small filament and focal spot provide much better **spatial resolution.** Spatial resolution is the new digital term used to

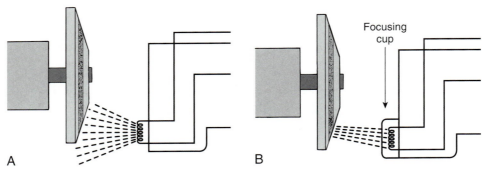

Fig. 5-10 A, Without a focusing cup, the electron stream spreads beyond the target area. **B,** Negatively charged focusing cup repels electrons, focusing them on a small target area, the focal spot.

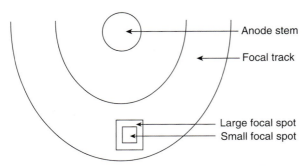

Fig. 5-11 Actual focal spot on lower part of anode. This is the area on the target where the electron stream is focused. Dual-focus tubes have two focal spots: one large and one small.

describe the sharpness of the structures recorded in the image. Generally speaking, it simply refers to the amount of detail seen on the visible x-ray image. The small focal spot should be used for most body parts on small- to average-size patients to obtain the best resolution. The exposure factors (kVp, mA, and exposure time) on these patients will be low to moderate. The large filament provides more electrons and strikes a larger target area. The large focal spot is used on larger patients or thick and dense body parts. The large focal spot can better absorb the heat generated by the increased exposure technique required for these patients. The two focal spots have the same center on the target and strike the same area (Fig. 5-11). If the small focal spot is selected and the exposure technique is too high, most modern x-ray generators will automatically switch to the large focal spot. If the large focal spot is selected and the exposure technique is too high (this would be on very dense body parts or obese patients), the exposure cannot be made and the x-ray not taken. This is occurring more often today because of the growing number of obese and morbidly obese patients.

Anode

As stated earlier in this chapter, the vast majority of the energy of the electron stream is converted into heat. This energy conversion takes place at the target, *so the anode tends to get very hot.* Anodes are therefore constructed to dissipate heat. Tungsten is an excellent material for x-ray tube targets because it has a very high melting point and it is efficient at conducting heat away from the anode.

Early x-ray tubes had, and current dental tubes have, a solid, stationary copper anode with a slanted tungsten face (Fig. 5-12). Modern tubes for general radiography have a **rotating anode** (Fig. 5-13). The rotating anode is in the form of a solid disk, with a beveled-edge target. This disk spins during the exposure, so the heat is distributed all around the circumference of the disk (Fig. 5-14). An electromagnetic *induction motor* is used to rotate the anode. Because this motor is sealed inside the x-ray tube, it works through electromagnetic induction, similar to a transformer.

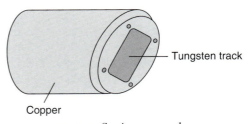

Fig. 5-12 Stationary anode.

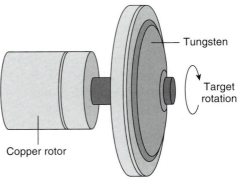

Fig. 5-13 Rotating anode. The copper rotor stem is part of the induction motor used to turn the anode disk.

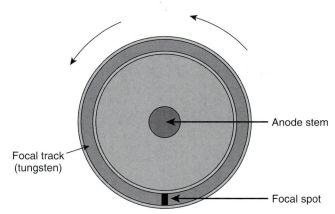

Fig. 5-14 Rotating anode face. The electrons strike the anode in the tiny focal spot area, but the heat is spread around the entire focal track of the spinning anode face.

The tungsten focal area all around the beveled edge of the rotating anode is called a **focal track.** The focal spot remains in the same location in space, but the target metal is spinning. The tungsten struck by the electron stream is constantly rotating during the exposure, distributing the anode heat over a larger area and increasing the heat capacity of the tube. X-ray tubes rotate at a standard speed of about 3600 revolutions per minute (rpm) during the exposure. Most x-ray tubes in use today also have a high-speed rotation at 10,000 rpm. The high-speed rotation automatically engages when high exposure factors (kVp, mA, and exposure time) are reached. The high-speed rotation enables the anode to dissipate the heat generated by the high technical factors more efficiently. When the operator pushes the exposure button on the generator, there is a short delay before the exposure is made. This delay allows the rotor to accelerate to its designated rpm while, at the same time, the filament is heated. Only then is the kVp applied to the x-ray tube. An audible sound is made during the exposure. When the sound ends, the exposure ends and the operator releases the button or switch. When the exposure is completed, the rotor slows down quickly.

Both the slanted face of the stationary anode and the beveled edge of the rotating anode present an angled surface to the oncoming electron stream. The slant of the anode surface is called the **target angle** (Fig. 5-15). X-ray tube target angles are between 7 and 17 degrees,

with 12 degrees being most common. The target angle is built into the x-ray tube and cannot be changed. The target angle affects the tube's heat capacity, the sharpness of the radiographic image, and the maximum size of the x-ray beam. These effects of the target angle are discussed in the following section.

Line Focus Principle

The term **actual focal spot** refers to the area on the target surface that is struck by the electron stream. The **effective focal spot** refers to the *vertical projection* of the actual focal spot onto the patient and image receptor (IR) (Fig. 5-16). The size of the *effective* focal spot influences resolution in the image. This fact is called the **line focus principle.** When vertical lines are drawn from each corner of the slanted actual focal spot, these lines define an "image" of the focal spot as viewed from the IR. The effective focal spot is always smaller than the actual focal spot. If the electron stream is reduced to half its size, the actual focal spot will be half its size and the effective focal spot will also be halved. This smaller focal spot would then produce greater resolution.

Focal spots are rectangular as seen on the face of the target. Most x-ray tubes used today contain a 0.6-mm

Line Focus Principle
• The size of the *effective* focal spot determines image resolution.
• The relative size of the effective focal spot is determined by the target angle.
• The steeper the target angle, the greater the difference between the actual and the effective focal spot sizes.

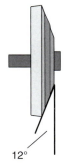

12°

Fig. 5-15 Target angle.

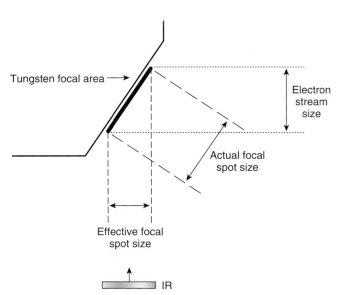

Fig. 5-16 The effective focal spot is the vertical projection of the actual or "true" focal spot.

small focal spot and a 1.2-mm large focal spot. The small focus is half the size of the large but will provide double the resolution (Fig. 5-17). Some x-ray tubes may be purchased with larger focal spots of 1.0 mm for the small and 2.0 mm for the large.

Just how the effective focal spot influences resolution is explained in Chapter 7. At this point, simply note the fact that a smaller effective focal spot size will result in greater resolution in the image and that a larger effective focal spot will have the opposite effect.

The angle of the target face determines the size difference between the actual focal spot and the effective focal spot. Fig. 5-18 shows two targets with the same-size actual focal spot but different target angles. It demonstrates that the "steeper" (more vertical) target has a smaller effective focal spot. *The smaller the target angle, the greater the size difference between the actual and effective focal spots.*

Although a *small effective* focal spot is desirable for greater resolution, a large actual focal spot is desirable to dissipate the heat of large exposures. The best solution would seem to be to use the smallest possible target angle. There is a practical limit, however, on how steep the target angle can be. As you can see in Fig. 5-19, a

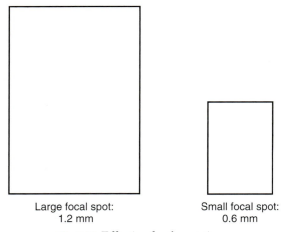
Fig. 5-17 Effective focal spot sizes.

Large focal spot: 1.2 mm

Small focal spot: 0.6 mm

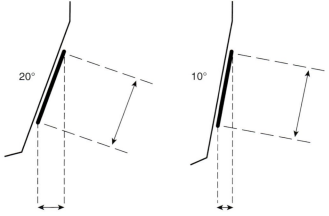
Fig. 5-18 A smaller target angle results in a smaller effective focal spot with a given actual focal spot size.

20°   10°

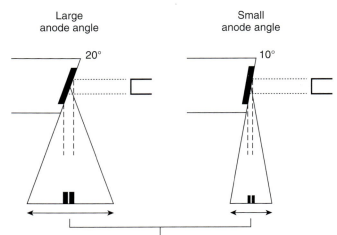

Large anode angle   20°

Small anode angle   10°

Field coverage at same image distance

Fig. 5-19 The anode angle controls the maximum field size. The anode margin of the field extends from the anode face at the same angle. The cathode side is the mirror image of the anode side. A 12-degree target angle is needed to cover a 14- × 17-inch image receptor at a 40-inch distance from the source.

straight line extended from the target face defines the margin of the x-ray beam on the anode side and, by default, the opposite margin of the beam. Thus the target angle determines the maximum possible size of the x-ray beam and the radiation field. A target angle of at least 12 degrees is needed to produce a radiation field that will cover a 14- × 17-inch IR at a distance of 40 inches; the largest IR in general use and a common, convenient working distance. Understand that once a given x-ray tube is purchased, the two focal spot sizes and the angle of the anode cannot be changed. Therefore the amount of resolution needed for the x-ray projections that are done in the room has to be determined in advance.

Anode Heel Effect

Most x-rays are not produced on the absolute surface of the target. Incoming electrons may penetrate the target to a depth of several layers of atoms before interacting with the target material. X-rays produced *within* the target must then pass through a portion of the target to get out (Fig. 5-20). Some of the x-rays will be absorbed by the

Anode Heel Effect

- Variation in radiation intensity across the length of the radiation field
- Greater radiation intensity toward the cathode end of the field
- Only significant when using the whole beam (14- × 17-inch IR at 40 inches or full spine at 72 inches)
- Place thinner portion of body part toward anode end of tube

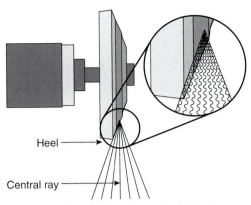

Fig. 5-20 Anode heel. X-rays are formed within the target material and are absorbed by the target as they exit. The sloping target face causes uneven absorption of the primary beam.

target in this process. Because of the slanted face of the target, some x-rays will have to pass through more target material than others, depending on their direction. Those x-rays that are directed away from the cathode are more likely to be absorbed than those that are directed toward it. This results in uneven distribution of radiation intensity in the x-ray beam and is called the **anode heel effect.**

Fig. 5-21 illustrates the relative intensity of the x-ray beam from one end to the other. If the intensity of the beam is measured at the central ray and that intensity is designated as 100%, the intensity at the cathode end can be as high as 120%. At the anode end, it can be as low as 75%—a 45% difference.

The anode heel effect is only significant in radiography when the entire beam is in use. This is the case when a large IR (14 × 17 inches) is used at a distance of 40 inches. Examples include examinations of the femur (thigh bone), the thoracic spine and chest, and the lumbar spine and abdomen. The anode heel effect is also important when an extra-long (14 × 36 inches) IR is used for radiography of the full spine or the entire leg. In these cases, it is advantageous to place the patient so that the

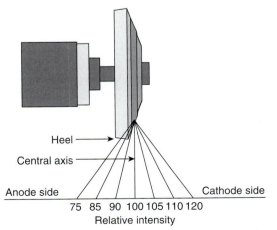

Fig. 5-21 Anode heel effect. The intensity of the x-ray beam is least toward the anode end of the field.

thinnest portion of the anatomy to be radiographed is toward the anode end of the tube. If the anode heel effect is not used correctly, the result will be that the thinner portions of the anatomy appear too dark on the IR and the thicker portions will be too light. It is not always practical to position the x-ray tube so the anode end is at the thinner portion of the anatomy. Compensating wedge filters are often used to prevent thinner areas from being overexposed.

Obviously, to effectively use the anode heel effect, the limited operator must know which end of the tube is which. Sometimes this is easily determined by examining the tube housing. The cable connections to the housing are often labeled. If no labels are apparent on or near the tube housing, try following the cables to their connections at the other end, the transformer cabinet, and check for labels there. A definitive determination can be made by taking a radiograph. Expose a 14- × 17-inch IR at a 40-inch distance using approximately 1 mAs and about 40 to 44 kVp. Open the collimator so that the radiation field covers the IR. Place a lead marker at one end so that you will be able to tell from the finished radiograph how it was placed during the exposure. The radiograph will demonstrate the anode heel effect because one end will be lighter than the other. The light end will signify the anode end of the tube.

ELECTRIC CONTROL OF X-RAY PRODUCTION

Kilovoltage

Voltage is measured at the *peak* of the electric cycle. When the voltage across the x-ray tube is measured, the units are often stated as **kilovolts peak,** abbreviated **kVp**. The terms *kV* and *kVp* are used interchangeably in radiography, with kVp being the preferred term.

The voltage applied to the x-ray tube controls the speed and power of the electrons in the electron stream. As stated earlier, the electrons move faster when the voltage is increased, producing x-rays with shorter wavelengths and greater energy. Therefore kVp controls the energy (wavelength) of the x-ray beam. Because x-rays with shorter wavelengths are more penetrating, *the penetrating power of the x-ray beam is controlled by varying the kVp.* Larger and denser body parts will require higher kVp settings than small or low-density body parts. *The contrast in the radiographic image is also controlled by the kVp.* High kVp creates low contrast, and low kVp creates high contrast.

Milliamperage

Milliamperage (mA) is a measure of the *rate of current flow* across the x-ray tube, that is, the number of electrons flowing from filament to target *each second.* The number of available electrons is determined by the filament heat.

When filament heat is increased, more electrons are available each second to cross the tube. Thus increasing the filament heat increases the mA in the x-ray tube circuit. When more electrons strike the target, more x-rays are produced, so *mA controls the volume, or quantity, of x-ray production* and thus also the *rate of exposure*. High mA settings produce more x-rays, and low mA settings produce fewer x-rays. Stated differently, mA controls the intensity of the x-ray beam, determining the number of photons that will strike the patient and IR. *The density in the radiographic image is controlled by the mA, exposure time, or the mAs.* In radiology the mA is directly proportional. If the mA is doubled, the x-rays are doubled, and if the mA is halved, the x-rays are reduced by 50%. In later chapters you will learn that mA, because it controls the volume of x-rays in the beam, affects the density of the x-ray image.

Exposure Time

Exposure time refers to the length of time that the x-rays are turned on. It is the duration of the x-ray exposure. Exposure time is measured in units of seconds (sec). Most x-ray exposure times are less than 1 second, and therefore **milliseconds (msec)** are used: 1 millisecond equals 0.001 second. A timer in the x-ray circuit terminates the exposure after a preset length of time. Like the mA, the quantity of x-rays produced is directly proportional to the exposure time. If the exposure time is doubled, the x-rays are doubled, and if the time is halved, the x-rays are reduced by 50%. One can see that a change in mA or exposure time will produce the same effect on the image. In later chapters there will be a discussion of when to choose mA and when to choose exposure time to change the quantity of x-rays (or density on the IR).

Milliampere-seconds

In radiography it is often useful to know the *total quantity* of an exposure. The quantity of x-ray photons in an exposure cannot be determined by either the mA or the exposure time alone. Although mA determines the *quantity* of x-ray production, it does not indicate the total quantity because it does not indicate how long the exposure time lasts. Exposure time does not indicate the total quantity either because it does not measure the rate of x-ray production. To determine the total quantity of

radiation involved in an exposure, both mA and time must be considered. The unit used to indicate the quantity of exposure is **milliampere-seconds,** abbreviated **mAs**. This unit is the product of mA and exposure time:

$$mA \times Time\ (seconds) = mAs$$

To better understand the concept of mAs, imagine for a moment that the x-ray beam consists of only a few hundred photons and that each mA of current produces only one x-ray photon per second. If this were true, an exposure rate of 100 mA would produce 100 photons per second. If the exposure time were 2 seconds, the mAs would equal 200 and the total number of photons in the exposure would be 200.

A desired quantity of exposure may be obtained by any combination of mA and time that multiplied together equals the desired mAs. In the previous example, for instance, 200 photons could also be obtained using 200 mA and an exposure time of 1 second.

Each of the following mA and time combinations will produce the same number of x-rays and an identical image density because the mAs is the same:

    100 mA, 0.40 sec = 40 mAs
    200 mA, 0.20 sec = 40 mAs
    400 mA, 0.10 sec = 40 mAs
    800 mA, 0.05 sec = 40 mAs

In the radiology department today, most generators are designed so that the operator sets the kVp and the mAs (Fig. 5-22). The operator always has the advantage of adjusting either the mA or the exposure time separately if needed. For example, if a crying baby's chest x-ray required 40 mAs from the four example techniques above, one would choose the last technique, 800 mA and 0.05 sec, because it has the shortest exposure time. A short exposure time would enable considerably less motion in the x-ray image.

X-RAY BEAM FILTRATION

As explained earlier in this chapter, the x-ray beam is heterogeneous, consisting of photons with many different energy wavelengths. Those photons with long wavelengths are easily absorbed by the body and are unlikely to penetrate the subject and expose the IR. They do not

---

Milliampere-seconds (mAs)

Measure of total quantity of electrons involved in exposure

$$mA \times Time\ (seconds) = mAs$$

Indicative of total quantity of photons produced by an exposure

---

X-ray Beam Filtration

- Filter material placed between the tube housing port and the patient removes the long-wavelength radiation from the primary beam.
- Because this radiation does not have sufficient energy to penetrate the patient, the cassette, and the table, it does not contribute to the image.
- Filtration lowers patient dose significantly.
- Filtration decreases the average wavelength of the x-ray beam.

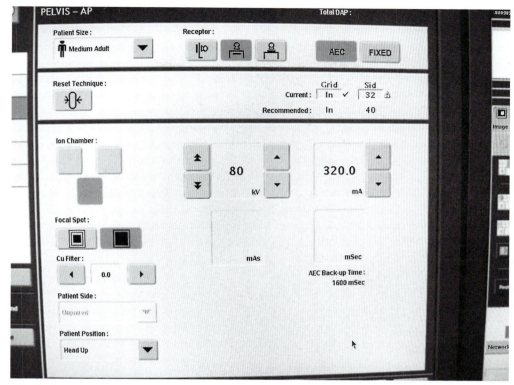

Fig. 5-22 Computer monitor on the x-ray generator. Note near the center of the monitor that the exposure technique is set for 80 kVp and 320 mAs.

contribute to the x-ray image. If these photons are not eliminated from the x-ray beam, they will be absorbed by the patient. To prevent this unnecessary radiation dose to the patient, the primary x-ray beam is filtered. **Filtration** is the process of removing the long-wavelength photons from the x-ray beam. Filtration material placed between the x-ray tube and the patient absorbs these long-wavelength photons (Fig. 5-23). *The primary purpose of filtration is to reduce patient dose.*

The material commonly used to filter the x-ray beam is aluminum. This is considered *added filtration.* One or more aluminum plates installed between the tube port and the collimator serve this purpose (Fig. 5-24). Any other material through which the beam passes also provides filtration. This includes the Pyrex glass of the tube itself, the oil that surrounds the tube, and the mirror that shines the light onto the patient. Because aluminum is the primary filtration material, all filtration is measured in units of millimeters of aluminum equivalents (mm Al equiv), the amount of filtration provided by a millimeter of aluminum.

Low-energy photons   High-energy photons

Aluminum

Fig. 5-23 Filtration absorbs long-wavelength photons and reduces dose to the patient.

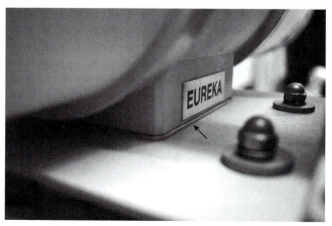

Fig. 5-24 Photograph of the port of the x-ray tube. *Arrow* is pointing to the added aluminum inserted in the port.

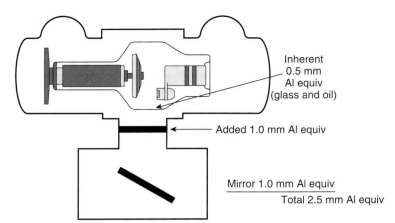

Inherent
0.5 mm
Al equiv
(glass and oil)

Added 1.0 mm Al equiv

Mirror 1.0 mm Al equiv
Total 2.5 mm Al equiv

Fig. 5-25 Total filtration equals inherent filtration plus added filtration. *Al equiv*, Aluminum equivalent.

The filtration provided by the glass of the tube and the surrounding oil is called *inherent (built-in) filtration* and is approximately equal to 0.5 mm Al equiv. Filtration from the mirror is also considered *inherent* and equal to about 1.0 mm Al equiv. All other filtration is referred to as *added filtration*. The total filtration is equal to the inherent filtration plus the added filtration (Fig. 5-25). Radiology departments must follow the federal law with regard to filtration of x-ray machines. *X-ray equipment capable of producing 70 kVp or more* (all general-purpose equipment) is required to have total filtration of at least 2.5 mm Al equiv permanently installed. The required added filtration is an important safety feature in radiography. It significantly reduces the dose to the patient by removing the low-energy (long-wavelength) photons. Because the long wavelengths are removed from the x-ray beam, the filtered beam has a much shorter average wavelength.

SUMMARY

X-rays are produced in a vacuum tube when high-speed electrons suddenly decelerate at the tube target. The electrons are liberated by heating the tungsten filament and are accelerated by high voltage from a step-up transformer.

Modern x-ray tubes for general radiography are dual-focus tubes, with rotating anodes. Focusing cups that are part of the cathode assembly direct the electrons to the focal area on the target. The small filament and focal spot are used to provide better-recorded detail. The large filament and focal spot provide more electrons and greater heat capacity for large exposures. According to the line focus principle, the effective focal spot is always smaller than the actual focal spot, and its size affects the spatial resolution. The rotating anode increases tube heat capacity.

The intensity of the radiation field varies from one end to the other because of the anode heel effect. The radiographer must know which end of the x-ray tube is the anode end and position the patient so that the anode heel effect is applied correctly when using large IRs at a 40-inch distance.

The penetrating power of the x-ray beam is controlled by the kVp. The *quantity* of the exposure is indicated by the mAs, the product of the mA and exposure time.

Filtration of the x-ray beam significantly reduces the patient's dose, decreases the average wavelength, and increases the average energy of the x-ray beam. A total of 2.5 mm Al equiv filtration is required to be permanently installed on all equipment capable of operating above 70 kVp.

X-ray Circuit and Tube Heat Management

At the conclusion of this chapter, you will be able to:

- Explain the x-ray circuit, label the principal parts, and state the function of each
- Explain what is meant by rectification and compare the three basic types
- Draw the voltage waveform for each of the following types: unrectified, half-wave rectified, full-wave rectified, three-phase rectified, and high frequency
- List the primary features of all x-ray control panels and discuss the principal differences between conventional and computerized control consoles
- Describe the components of the automatic exposure control system and anatomically programmed exposure system
- List five possible causes of x-ray tube failure and describe methods to prevent each

Key Terms

anatomically programmed radiography (APR)
automatic exposure control (AEC)
autotransformer
back-up time
control console
density control
diode
electronic timer
exposure switch
exposure timer
full-wave rectification

half-wave rectification
heat unit (HU)
high-frequency (HF)
mA selector
phototimer
rectification
rectifier
rotor switch
single-phase current
synchronous timer
three-phase current
tube rating chart

This chapter centers on a greatly simplified diagram of an x-ray circuit and is intended to aid your understanding of the various components of the circuit and how they work together to produce and control x-rays. The various features of the x-ray circuit and the x-ray control panel are discussed. *It is not necessary to memorize or understand the circuits in detail.* The circuits help you to understand how three relatively complex electric circuits are integrated to produce x-rays. Because x-ray tubes may be damaged by improper use and are expensive to replace, this chapter provides guidelines for the safe operation of tubes and suggestions for prolonging tube life.

X-RAY CIRCUIT

As indicated in Fig. 6-1, the x-ray circuit is divided into three sections or subcircuits: the *low-voltage circuit*, the *filament circuit*, and the *high-voltage circuit*. Each circuit contains a specialty transformer. The various components of each section are numbered so that you can easily refer to them in the discussion that follows.

Low-voltage Circuit

The low-voltage circuit is illustrated in the upper left portion of Fig. 6-1 and is expanded in Fig. 6-2, *A*. It is the subcircuit between the alternating current (AC) power supply (1) and the primary (input) side of the high-voltage (step-up) transformer (7). If you trace this circuit beginning at the AC power supply, you will note that current flows through several devices before reaching the primary

side of the step-up transformer. From the transformer, it returns to the power source, forming an enclosed loop. With the exception of the step-up transformer, all of the devices in this subcircuit are actually located within the **control console.** The control console is the unit where the operator sets all of the exposure techniques, such as kilovolts peak (kVp), milliamperes (mA), and exposure time. They include the main switch (2), autotransformer (3), kVp selectors (4), exposure switch (5), and exposure timer (6).

The AC power supply (1) is wired into the building, providing electric power from the local power company. Most outpatient facilities have a 220-V power supply going into the x-ray room. Hospitals with more powerful equipment may have a larger supply. The main switch (2) controls the power to the control console. Many of the components in this circuit operate at the standard 120 V.

Although the power supply may be rated at 220 V, the actual voltage can vary as much as ±5%, depending on the demand for power in the building or the neighborhood. Small variations in the incoming line voltage may cause large variations in the kVp to the x-ray tube. For this reason, the incoming voltage is monitored and stabilized by a voltage compensator.

The **autotransformer** (3) is a single-coil transformer that serves three functions: it provides the means for kVp selection, it provides compensation for fluctuations in the incoming line voltage, and it supplies power to other parts of the x-ray circuit.

The autotransformer's primary purpose is to vary the voltage to the primary side of the step-up transformer. This is

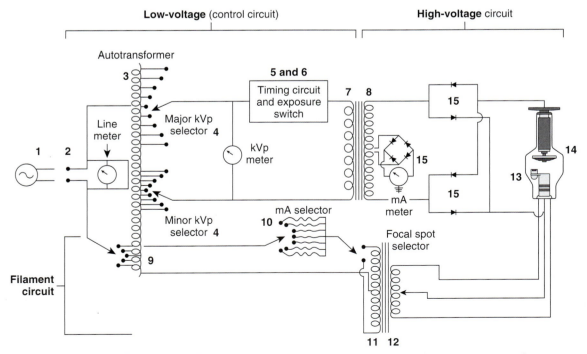

Fig. 6-1 Simplified diagram of an x-ray circuit. Electric circuit going into the x-ray room is at far left (1) and circuit ends at x-ray tube far right (14).

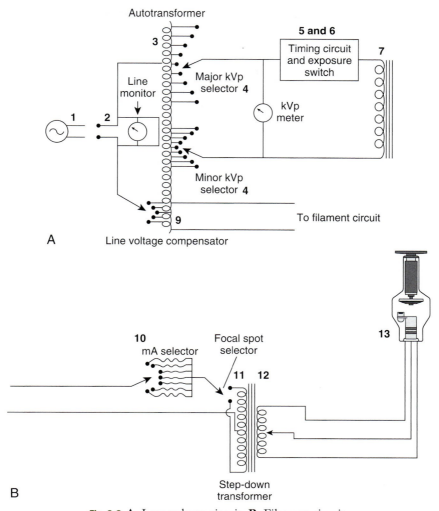

Fig. 6-2 A, Low-voltage circuit. **B,** Filament circuit.

accomplished by the kVp selector (4), which is on the secondary (output) side of the autotransformer. The autotransformer varies the kVp to the tube by controlling the input to the step-up transformer.

The **exposure switch** (5) closes the circuit, allowing electric current to flow through the primary side of the step-up transformer. When this occurs, current is *induced* to flow through the secondary side of the transformer, creating voltage across the x-ray tube. As discussed earlier, this voltage causes the electron stream to flow across the tube, producing x-rays. The **exposure timer** (6) is a device that terminates the exposure and is set by the operator on the control console.

Filament Circuit

The filament circuit is the subcircuit of the main x-ray circuit shown as the lower portion of Fig. 6-1. It is expanded in Fig. 6-2, *B*. This circuit is divided into two parts by the *step-down* transformer (11 and 12). *The primary purpose of the filament circuit is to supply a low current to heat the x-ray tube filament for thermionic emission of*

electrons. The filament circuit is activated any time the operator adjusts the mA on the generator.

The primary side of this circuit begins and ends with the contacts on the autotransformer (9). Current in this circuit flows from the autotransformer, through the mA selector (10) and the primary side of the *step-down* transformer (11), and back to the autotransformer. The secondary side begins and ends with the secondary side of the step-down transformer (12) conducting current through the x-ray tube filament (13). The step-down transformer reduces the voltage on the secondary side, providing an appropriate current to heat the filament.

The **mA selector** (10) controls amperage in the filament circuit. Because the current through this circuit controls filament heat, this setting determines the number of available electrons at the x-ray tube filament and thus determines the mA in the high-voltage circuit that includes the x-ray tube.

High-voltage Circuit

The high-voltage circuit is the subcircuit shown in the upper right portion of Fig. 6-1. It is expanded in Fig. 6-3.

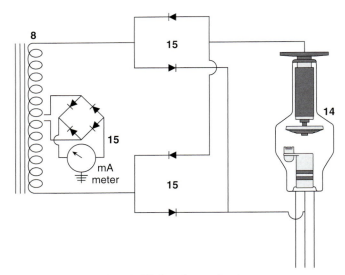

Fig. 6-3 High-voltage circuit.

This circuit begins and ends with the secondary side of the *step-up* transformer (8). It includes the x-ray tube (14) and the rectifier unit (15). *Current flows in this circuit only during an exposure.* This is a dangerous circuit because of the very high voltage. The high-voltage cables going to the x-ray tube are very thick because of their high insulation requirement (Fig. 6-4).

The step-up transformer is also referred to as the *high-voltage* or *high-tension* transformer. As explained in Chapter 4, it increases the incoming voltage by the value of the *transformer ratio*. This transformer has a very high ratio of at least 500:1. For example, if the primary side of the step-up transformer receives 180 V from the auto-transformer, and the ratio is 500:1, the voltage induced on the secondary side will be 90,000 V, or 90 kVp.

The primary purpose of the high-voltage circuit is to supply the x-ray tube with voltage high enough to create x-rays.

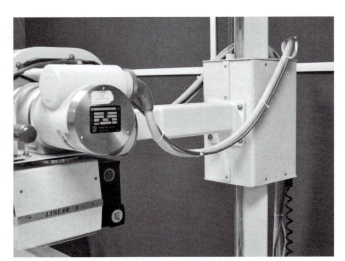

Fig. 6-4 High-voltage cables going into the x-ray tube. Note their large size because of the high-voltage electricity moving in the copper wire.

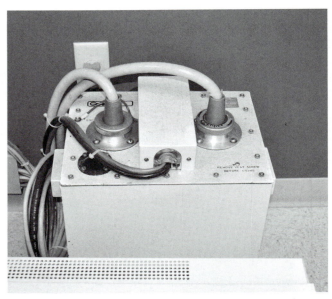

Fig. 6-5 X-ray transformer tank containing the autotransformer, filament transformer, high-voltage transformer, and rectifier. The transformers are immersed in oil.

The autotransformer, step-down transformer, and high-voltage transformer are all located in a tank near the x-ray machine (Fig. 6-5). Oil surrounds the transformers inside the tank for heat dissipation.

Rectification

The process of changing alternating current into direct current so it flows in one direction only.

RECTIFICATION

The primary purpose of the **rectifier** *unit (15) is to change the alternating current (AC) into direct current (DC).* The process of **rectification** prepares the current for x-ray production by ensuring that it flows in the right direction, in this case from the filament to the target. There are three ways in which current is rectified: *self-rectification, half-wave rectification,* and *full-wave rectification.* Self-rectification was an inefficient form of rectification and is no longer used. Half-wave rectification and full-wave rectification are described next.

Half-wave Rectification

AC electrical current travels in the copper wire as a sine wave. It moves in a pulsating manner from positive to negative at a rate of 60 pulses, or waves, per second and is stated as 60 Hz (Fig. 6-6). Rectifiers use diodes to convert the circuit from AC to DC. A **diode** is an electronic device that permits current to flow in one

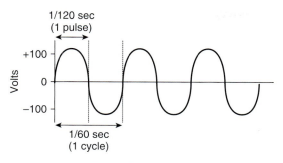

AC in U.S. and Canada: 60 cycles/sec (60 Hz)

Fig. 6-6 Electric current moves in a copper wire as a series of alternating (AC) waves called a sine wave. One positive and negative pulse equals one cycle or 1 Hz. U.S. current contains 60 Hz per second.

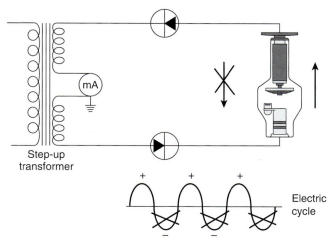

Fig. 6-7 Voltage waveform for half-wave rectification. NOTE: Negative phase (X) is eliminated.

direction only. Two diodes are used in **half-wave rectification** (Fig. 6-7). Diodes prevent "backflow" of current during the negative half of the electric cycle. This causes the negative half of the cycle to be eliminated. Note that the arrow direction of the diode symbol indicates the direction of current flow permitted by the diode.

In half-wave rectification the negative phase of the electric cycle is totally eliminated and a gap remains. The x-rays are turned off during the eliminated (negative) phase. With only the positive phase remaining, the electric current is "direct" only, or DC. The x-rays are pulsating on, off, on, off, and so forth at a rate of 60 pulses per second.

Full-wave Rectification

By employing four diodes in the circuit, the current can be "redirected" during the negative half of the electric cycle so that current will flow in the same direction during both the positive and negative halves of the cycle. This process is called **full-wave rectification**

because it utilizes the entire electric cycle for x-ray production. The negative impulses are made positive during full-wave rectification rather than being eliminated (Fig. 6-8). The pulsed x-ray output of a full-wave rectified machine occurs 120 times each second compared with 60 times a second for half-wave rectification. This results in a doubling of the x-ray output. The waveform of full-wave rectified current is shown in Fig. 6-9. Note there are twice as many impulses in the cycle compared with Fig. 6-7. All modern general-purpose x-ray machines are full-wave rectified. *The main advantage of full-wave rectification is that the exposure time can be cut in half because of the doubling in x-ray output compared with half-wave rectification.*

GENERATORS

Single-phase Generators

Single-phase x-ray generators are powered by a single source of AC current. Single-phase generators produce a pulsating current that alternates from positive to negative during each electric cycle (Fig. 6-6). Therefore **single-phase current** results in a pulsating x-ray beam. The three voltage waveforms and rectifications described earlier were produced by single-phase electric power. In single-phase current with full-wave rectification, there are 120 pulses of electricity per second that create 120 pulses of x-rays per second. Single-phase generators are considered the lowest power and most basic x-ray machines. These are also the least expensive, which makes them a popular choice in small clinics and physician offices.

Three-phase Generators

Three-phase x-ray generators are powered by three separate sources of AC current at the same time. A more constant and efficient voltage source is provided by a three-phase power supply. Alternating current is generated in three overlapping cycles that produce the waveform illustrated in Fig. 6-10. When this current is rectified, its waveform has the appearance of a "ripple" with no real low points. In **three-phase current** with full-wave rectification there are 360 pulses of electricity per second that create 360 pulses of x-rays per second. The resulting waveform is shown in Fig. 6-11. *A major advantage of three-phase current is that it is more efficient and produces approximately 40% more x-rays than single-phase current.* This greater output enables exposure times to be decreased by 40%. The purchase and installation of three-phase x-ray equipment is very expensive compared with that of single-phase equipment. The three-phase generator is the predominant type of x-ray machine in hospitals and large clinics because of its increased power.

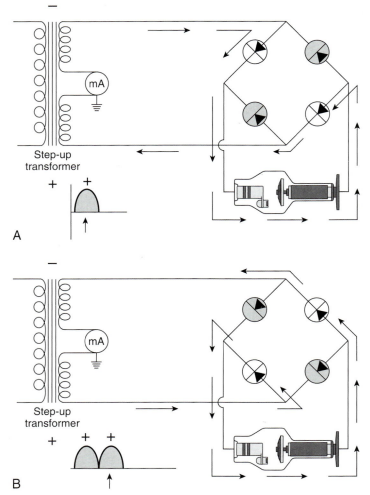

A

B

FIG. 6-8 Full-wave rectification. **A,** First half of cycle *(arrows)*. **B,** Second half of cycle *(arrows)* rectified from negative to positive. This more complex rectification unit electrically moves the negative pulse above the line, changing it to positive in the process.

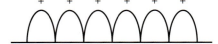

Fig. 6-9 Full-wave rectification voltage waveform produces 120 impulses (x-rays) per second compared with 60 impulses in half-wave rectification.

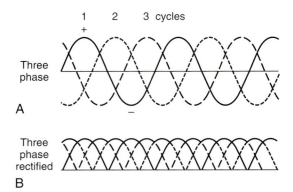

Fig. 6-10 Three-phase current voltage waveform. **A,** Unrectified. **B,** Rectified. Note how the negative pulses are moved above the line to positive.

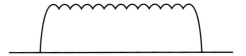

Fig. 6-11 Rectified three-phase voltage waveform.

High-frequency Generators

High-frequency (HF) x-ray generators are the most common generators used today. They produce x-rays much more efficiently than single-phase or three-phase generators. A single source of AC current, similar to single-phase, is used to power the generator. *The primary function that occurs in the complex HF circuitry is that the 60 Hz full-wave rectified circuit is converted to a significantly higher frequency of about 6000 Hz* (Fig. 6-12) for most general use generators. The highest-powered HF units can convert the frequency to as high as 100,000 Hz. Inverter circuits bring the frequency up to the high level, and several layers of smoothing capacitors assist in creating the HF current. The inverter circuit changes the

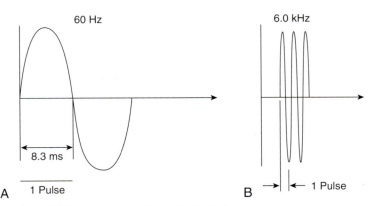

Fig. 6-12 **A,** Standard 60 Hz electric waveform. **B,** High-frequency waveform. An inverter circuit has increased the frequency to 6500 Hz (labeled 6.5 kHz).

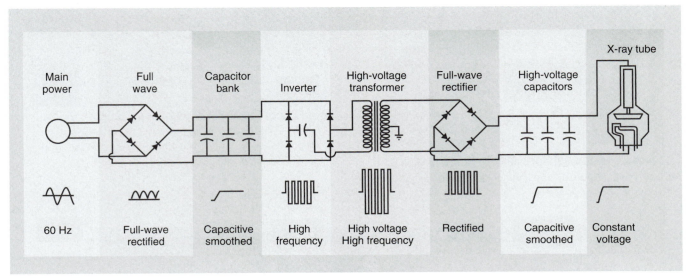

Fig. 6-13 Complex electric circuit for a high-frequency transformer. Note 60 Hz AC power entering the circuit at left, undergoing six conversions, and achieving a constant voltage before entering the x-ray tube.

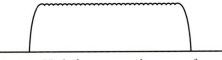

Fig. 6-14 High-frequency voltage waveform.

wave-like current into a square pulse. The steps in the production of HF are shown in Fig. 6-13. High-frequency generators produce a near-constant voltage waveform, which results in even less exposure time compared with three-phase (Fig. 6-14). They produce the greatest amount of x-rays for the same exposure technique. The very high frequency produced in an HF generator can sometimes be heard as a singing sound.

High-frequency generators are not only used because of their efficient x-ray production, but also because their overall size is smaller. The high-voltage step-up transformer tank is about one-tenth the size of that in a three-phase generator because it produces x-rays more efficiently at high frequencies (Fig. 6-15). This reduces the overall cost of the system.

X-RAY CONTROL PANEL

The devices of the x-ray control panel were introduced in the section on the control circuit. At this point, we consider how these devices appear on the control console and how the limited operator uses them.

X-ray control panels and the labels of their components vary depending on age and manufacturer. Newer, computerized models have button-like controls and digital readouts (Fig. 6-16). Some control panels are operated by touch-control on a computer monitor (Fig. 6-17). These computerized consoles automatically perform some functions that were previously done manually.

All control panels provide some means for selecting kVp, mA, exposure time, and focal spot size, and all indicate

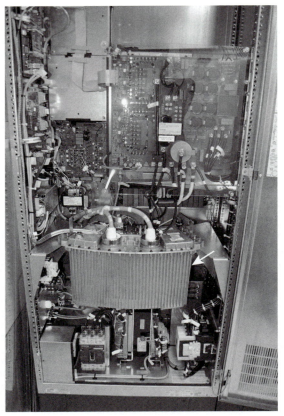

Fig. 6-15 High-frequency circuitry. Note the smaller size high-voltage transformer *(arrow)*.

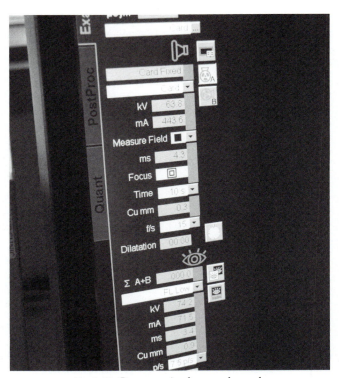

Fig. 6-16 Computerized control panel.

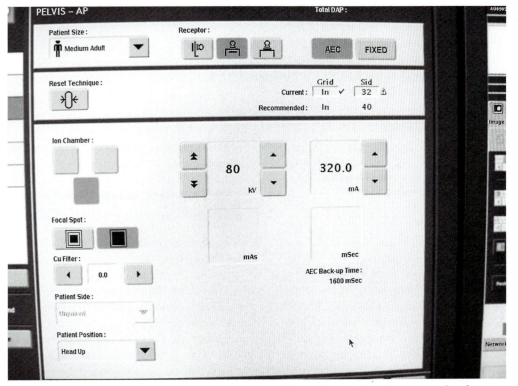

Fig. 6-17 Computer monitor showing x-ray controls. This is from a digital system and is finger-touch controlled. Note kVp major and minor controls, mA control next to it, and Grid In/Out near top right. Large and small focal spot setting is shown at center left. The back-up time of 1600 msec is set near bottom right.

the current settings. There will also be switches to control power to the console and the Bucky, plus rotor and exposure switches.

Power Control

The on/off switch on the console corresponds to the main power switch in the circuit diagram (see Fig. 6-1, *2*). This switch controls the power to the control panel and the entire x-ray generator. There is usually an electric panel in the wall of the control booth that contains one or more circuit breakers. The appropriate circuit breaker must be turned on for the machine to receive power.

Milliamperage Control

Conventional control panels have a mA selector, which provides several choices of mA, often called *mA stations.* The selector may be in the form of a knob or a series of buttons. The number of possible mA settings is limited, and each is usually a whole number. For example, a typical radiographic unit may have the following mA stations: 50, 100, 150, 200, 300, 400, and 500. Three-phase and HF x-ray machines are capable of producing as much as 1500 mA. Single-phase machines are often able to achieve a maximum mA of 500.

Each cathode filament in a dual-focus tube is connected to specific mA stations. The filament and its associated focal spot are chosen automatically when the mA is selected. The control panel will indicate which stations use which filament. For example, a setting marked "200 L" or "200 Large" signifies 200 mA with the large filament and large focal spot. Usually mA settings of 200 to 250 or less employ the small filament; the large filament supplies mA requirements of 250 or more. The rationale for selection of mA stations is discussed in Chapter 12.

Some computerized control consoles do not have mA selectors. These units provide variable mA that is computer controlled according to the selection of the desired milliampere-seconds (mAs) and focal spot size (see Fig. 6-17). Digital readouts on the console will state the mAs setting and the exposure time.

Exposure Time Control

All control consoles contain an exposure timer, whether it is set directly by the limited operator or not. The time set is the length of time the x-rays are turned on. Two types of manually set timers are used for x-ray exposure control: **synchronous timers** and **electronic timers** (Table 6-1).

Computerized controls may select the exposure time on an electronic timer when the mAs is set. In addition, some units have automated exposure controls, which are discussed in the following section.

Table 6-1

Types of Timers

Type	Minimum Exposure Time
Synchronous	17 msec ($\frac{1}{60}$ sec)
Electronic	1 msec (0.001 sec)
Automated	Depends on back-up timer (may be synchronous or electronic)

A synchronous timer is controlled by a small electric motor rotating at 60 revolutions/second. Each of the 60 impulses in the electric cycle can be used as an exposure time. The time settings available will be stated in fractions, and all will be multiples of $\frac{1}{60}$ second, the duration of an electric impulse ($\frac{1}{30}$ second, $\frac{1}{20}$ second, and $\frac{1}{15}$ second). The range of time settings is between $\frac{1}{60}$ second and several seconds.

Electronic timers are more sophisticated devices designed for use with three-phase and high-frequency generators. Electronic timers are more capable of ultrashort exposure times (1 millisecond or less) than are synchronous timers, and exposure times are expressed in decimals (0.03 second, 0.05 second, and 0.07 second). These are the most accurate timers. The range of exposure times on a generator will be from 0.005 milliseconds to as high as 4.0 seconds. The synchronous timer system and exposure times expressed in fractions are found in older x-ray machines that may be in use. Electrical service personnel will regularly perform a quality control (QC) check on the exposure timers to ensure they are accurate.

Kilovoltage Control

Conventional control panels have two kVp selector dials: a major selector that changes kVp by 10 kVp at a time and a minor selector that has increments of 1 or 2 kVp. For example, if the major kVp selector is set at 70 and the minor selector is set at 4, the total kVp will be 74 kVp. This dual-selector system facilitates large changes in kVp. Most general use generators will have kVp settings from about 40 to 125 kVp. The kVp setting on a conventional control panel may be indicated on the selector dials or may be read from a kVp meter.

Computerized controls will have a digital read-out for the current kVp setting and arrow buttons that can be pressed to increase or decrease the kVp (see Fig. 6-17). The rationale for changes in kVp is discussed in Chapter 5. Electric service personnel will regularly perform a QC check on the kVp settings to ensure accuracy.

Bucky Control

As mentioned in Chapter 2, the Bucky is a moving grid that is used for radiography of the larger parts of the body. The Bucky device incorporates a motor to oscillate the grid. A switch on the control panel activates the motor circuit so that the grid will oscillate during the exposure. The control panel may have a three-position switch so that it can control two Buckys, one in the table and one in the upright Bucky. The three positions are usually labeled "Bucky 1," "Bucky 2," and "Off." The grid is sometimes turned off for tabletop exposures of the limbs. On the new digital radiography (DR) x-ray tables, the grid can be physically removed for nongrid exposures. The computerized control panel will indicate if the grid is in place or not (see Fig. 6-17). The limited operator has to know if the grid is being used or not because it affects the exposure technique used.

Manual Exposure Control

Every x-ray exposure that is made will have had three prime factors set on the control panel: *mA, kVp,* and *exposure time*. In many basic x-ray systems, the limited operator "manually" sets these three factors on the control panel. For example, an anteroposterior (AP) knee might require 200 mA, 80 kVp, and 0.20 seconds, and these technical factors will come from the exposure technique chart. The technique is set by simply pushing the three buttons. Two automated exposure systems are described next; however, even with these sophisticated systems, many of the x-ray images will still have to be set with a manual technique.

Automatic Exposure Control

Many x-ray machines provide **automatic exposure control (AEC),** terminating the exposure time when a certain quantity of radiation has been detected at the IR. The AEC system is a complex microprocessor circuit built into the generator and x-ray table and tied directly to the mA, kVp, and exposure time controls. When activating the AEC system on the generator, the mA and kVp values are set as usual; however, *the exposure time is automatically determined.* This eliminates the need to know in advance just how much exposure time a radiograph will require.

A sensing device is located under the x-ray table and detects when a given amount of x-ray photons has been reached. When this happens, the sensor will terminate the exposure time. There are two types of automated exposure control sensors: **phototimers** and *ionization chambers* (Fig. 6-18). It is not important to know details of these two sensing systems. The sensors under the table are referred to by several names: *phototimers, detectors,* and *sensors.* Most of these sensors are located between the grid and the IR. As the Bucky moves along the table, the AEC system moves with it.

The AEC system will usually have three detectors so that limited operators can select the specific location or locations within the radiation field where the radiation quantity will be measured (Fig. 6-19). The selection of

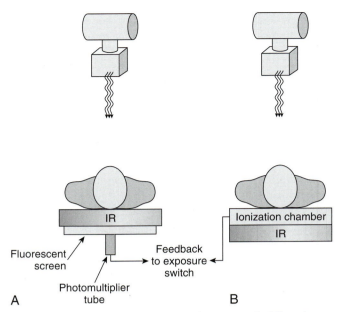

Fig. 6-18 Automatic exposure control systems. **A,** The photomultiplier tube system. **B,** Ionization chamber system. These systems automatically terminate the exposure time. *IR,* Image receptor.

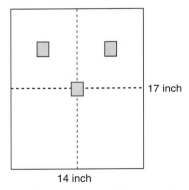

Fig. 6-19 Automated exposure control systems have three detectors below the tabletop. Detectors are positioned as shown relative to a 14- × 17- inch image receptor (IR). NOTE: Center detector is in the center of the image receptor.

active detectors is determined by the image receptor (IR) size and the specific radiographic examination. For example, a knee radiograph will use a central detector, whereas a chest film requires activation of the two upper detectors with positions that correspond to the lungs. The center detector is always in the center of the IR at the central ray. With three detectors, the operator can select from seven different combinations. The kVp and mA are set manually. When using an AEC system, patient positioning *must be absolutely accurate.* Because a sensor under the table will be determining the exposure, positioning to the wrong anatomy or having primary beam reach the detector from overcollimation could cause overexposure or underexposure. The operator must have the ability to override the AEC in the event of an overexposure or underexposure. All AEC systems will have on the control panel a **density control** selection. This enables the density to be increased or decreased by preset amounts. The density control should not be used to compensate for patient part thickness or kVp changes. It is used only after an image is evaluated and a density adjustment needs to be made.

Although the AEC system determines the correct exposure time, a **back-up time** must be set manually. This means that the exposure timer is set to a time that is *greater* than the anticipated exposure time. If the automated system fails for any reason, the back-up timer will terminate the exposure. If the back-up time setting is not long enough, the back-up timer will terminate the exposure prematurely. Setting a back-up time will prevent overexposure to the patient and prevent damage to the x-ray tube in the event that the circuits fail to terminate. Back-up times cannot exceed the tube heat limit (see Fig. 6-17). X-ray operators should voluntarily set the back-up time at 150% more than the anticipated exposure. This means that if an exposure time is typically 0.10 second, the back-up timer should be set at 0.25 second. There is a federal law that applies to maximum exposure times. Public Law 90-602 states that generators must terminate the exposure at *600 mAs* for exposures above 50 kVp.

Anatomically Programmed Radiography Control

One of the most widely used electronic techniques for exposure control is called **anatomically programmed radiography (APR).** With this system, a microprocessor controls the exposure technical factors. These systems are essentially the exposure technique chart stored in the computer memory. By typically selecting only one or two controls, usually the body area and the projection, the kVp, mA, time, AEC detectors, body habitus, Bucky, and source–image receptor distance (SID) will be selected automatically (Fig. 6-20). For example, if the physician

orders an x-ray of the pelvis, the operator selects "Pelvis" and then selects "AP-Projection" and the exposure is ready to be made. The limited operator does have the option to override the automated factor selection for specific patient situations. When an APR system is used, a technique chart may not need to be posted in the room, except for manual exposure techniques. The AEC system described above is utilized within the APR system. With proper and accurate positioning, APR systems can produce excellent radiographs and fewer repeat examinations.

Exposure Controls

Until about 25 years ago, exposure switches were incorporated into a hand switch that was attached to the control panel by a cable. Some of this equipment is still in use, but regulatory agencies now require that it be permanently fastened to the control console so that exposures cannot be made from a position outside the control booth. More modern equipment has exposure switches in the form of buttons or toggle switches, which are mounted on the control panel.

Two separate switches are necessary to make an exposure. The first is the **rotor switch,** which may be labeled "Rotor," "Prep," "Ready," or "Standby." This switch has two functions. When it is activated, the rotating anode begins to spin, and heat is applied to the filament to create electrons via thermionic emission. When this switch has been held in the "on" position for several seconds, a signal will indicate that the tube is ready for an exposure. The signal may be a particular sound or a light on the control panel or both. Making an exposure before the tube is ready may damage the tube. Nearly all x-ray machines in current use have a lockout feature that prevents the initiation of an exposure before the rotor has reached operating speed and the filament has reached operating temperature.

When the tube is ready, *the limited operator initiates the exposure by continuing to hold the rotor switch and also pressing the second switch, the exposure switch* (Fig. 6-21). An exposure indicator on the control panel will indicate when the timer has terminated the exposure. Only then are the two switches released. *Premature release of either the rotor switch or the exposure switch will abort the exposure before it is complete.*

On older equipment, the exposure indicator will be an mA meter on the control panel. It will indicate the mA during the exposure and return to zero as soon as the exposure is complete. Newer models will have an exposure light, usually red, that is on during the exposure. When the light goes off, the exposure is complete and an audible beep will be heard.

The process of setting a *modern* control panel may take place in any order. It is wise to form a habit of setting the controls in the same order each time so that nothing is overlooked. Box 6-1 lists, in order, the steps

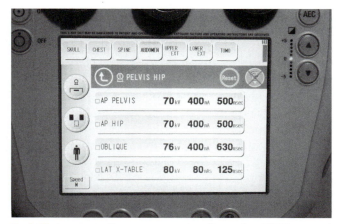

Fig. 6-20 Anatomically programmed radiography (APR) control on the generator. Note body part selection at the top, different projections shown on the screen along with pre-programmed exposure techniques.

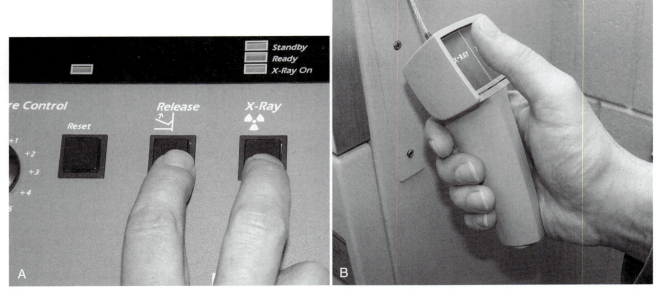

Fig. 6-21 Exposure devices. **A,** Two-button finger exposure device. The left finger activates the rotor and, when ready, the right finger initiates the x-ray exposure. **B,** Handheld device. The four fingers depress the rotor activator and, when ready, the thumb initiates the x-ray exposure.

Box 6-1

Setting Control Panel and Making an Exposure (Traditional X-ray Control)

- Select milliamperes (mA).
- Select exposure time.
- Select kilovolts peak (kVp) major first, then minor.
- Set Bucky switch.
- Activate and hold rotor switch.
- On signal, activate and hold exposure switch.
- Observe exposure indicator to validate exposure and to determine when it is complete.
- Release rotor and exposure switches.

---

for setting the controls and making an exposure with a conventional control console.

PROLONGING X-RAY TUBE LIFE

The anode of the tube accumulates enormous heat during exposures, and this is a primary cause of problems that may shorten tube life. The design of modern tubes incorporates several features for the purpose of rapid heat dissipation. The rotating anode prevents excess heat in any one area of the target, spreading it around the focal track. The anode disk consists of several layers of material (tungsten, molybdenum, and graphite) chosen for their heat-management characteristics. The stem of the anode conducts heat to a copper mass surrounding the rotor mechanism. Also, the space between the tube

and the tube housing is filled with oil. This feature provides electric insulation and also disperses heat from the glass envelope.

X-ray tubes that receive good care provide many years of service. Careless use, however, can significantly shorten the life of a tube and may result in sudden tube failure. Tube replacement is expensive and may cause the x-ray equipment to be out of service for some time. *The factors that affect tube life are controlled by the limited operator.* Responsible operators take care to ensure that x-ray tubes are not abused.

An excessive exposure on a cold tube will cause the anode to expand too rapidly and may cause it to crack and to fail. For this reason, a cool tube should be warmed up before any large exposure. The manufacturer may specify the warm-up procedure. Warm-up settings are preprogrammed into some computerized controls. In the absence of an established warm-up procedure, three exposures—30 seconds apart, at a setting of 200 mA, 0.5 second, and 80 kVp—will safely distribute heat throughout the anode. The warm-up procedure must be repeated if the tube has been idle for more than an hour. Exposures smaller than prescribed warm-up settings may be made without warming the tube. Warm-up exposures must be done before the patient enters the x-ray room. *Do not forget to do a preexposure safety check before doing warm-up exposures.*

A rapid series of large exposures or a single excessive exposure may damage the tube by melting the tungsten surface of the focal track. This melted tungsten boils and then cools to an irregular, pitted surface (Fig. 6-22). A tube that has been damaged in this way provides inconsistent

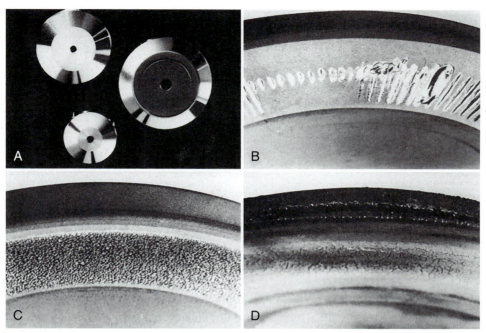

Fig. 6-22 Comparison of smooth, shiny appearance of rotating anodes when new (**A**) and their appearance after failure (**B** through **D**). Examples of anode separation and surface melting shown were caused by slow rotation due to bearing damage (**B**), repeated overload (**C**), and exceeding of maximum heat storage capacity (**D**).

radiation output and does not produce sharp images because of changes in the focal spot.

Nearly all x-ray generators in use today have lockout circuits that prevent single exposures beyond the tube's maximum heat capacity, but this feature should not be relied on as the only measure for tube heat protection. Tubes that are frequently used at or near their capacity will not last as long as tubes that are operated consistently at 80% of capacity or less. Generators today will have a red indicator light that will turn on if the exposure technical factors are too high for the tube rating.

Maximum tube capacity for a single exposure is determined by consulting the **tube rating chart** (Fig. 6-23).

The chart is supplied by the tube manufacturer and is specific for each tube model. Today, rating charts do not have to be reviewed before each exposure because of the automated circuits that do not allow the wrong factors to be set. However, tube rating charts are used when creating exposure technique charts or when programming the APR system. The chart is read by noting the point on the graph at which the horizontal line representing the kVp setting intersects with the vertical line representing the exposure time. If this point is below the curved line that represents the mA setting, the exposure is *safe*. If it is above the mA line, the exposure *exceeds* tube capacity.

The maximum heat capacity of the anode is rated in **heat units (HU).** The heat units produced by an exposure are determined by multiplying the kVp × mA × time. The heat unit formula varies depending on the design of the generator. Note there is an added multiplication factor for the three-phase and the high-frequency generators. The high-frequency generator will produce the most heat for the same technical factors. Specifically, it will produce 40% more heat than a single-phase. The HU factors are:

Single phase:

$$HU = mA \times Time \times kVp$$

Three phase:

$$HU = mA \times Time \times kVp \times 1.35$$

High frequency:

$$HU = mA \times Time \times kVp \times 1.40$$

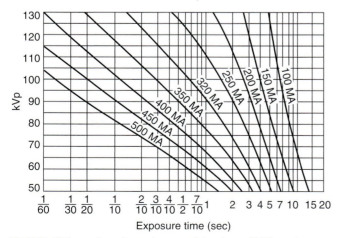

Fig. 6-23 Tube rating chart. Any combination of kVp and exposure time below the curved mA line in the chart will be safe.

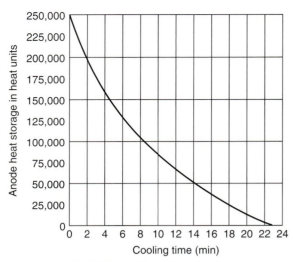

Fig. 6-24 Anode cooling chart.

Box 6-2

Extending X-ray Tube Life

- Warm up the anode according to the manufacturer's instructions.
- Do not hold down the rotor switch for long periods of time.
- Use low mA settings whenever possible.
- Use the low-speed rotor whenever possible.
- Do not make repeated exposures near the tube limits.
- Do not use a tube when you can hear the rotor bearings (call a service engineer).

An exposure of 70 kVp, 0.15 second, 300 mA using a three-phase generator would produce 4253 HU.

Heat units are used to calculate tube cooling time using a cooling chart (Fig. 6-24). Cooling charts also are provided by the tube manufacturer and are specific for each tube model. You will note that the chart in Fig. 6-24 was made for a tube with an anode heat capacity of 250,000 HU. If this tube were heated to its maximum capacity, half of the heat units would be dissipated within a period of 6 minutes. Cooling charts are used by service engineers but they are seldom needed by limited operators.

It is important to note that tubes that are never overheated will eventually fail. With moderate use, an x-ray tube can last up to 8 years. The reason for failure is almost always related to the events that occur when the rotor switch is activated. The anode rotor turns on precision ball bearings that are essential to its operation. These bearings wear out with use, and when this occurs, the tube must be replaced. During rotor activation, the filament is maintained at a high heat, resulting in tiny amounts of vaporization of the filament material. Over time, the diameter of the filament decreases until it is so thin that it breaks, similar to the failure of a light bulb filament that "burns out." The filaments are under greatest stress when used at the highest mA station to which they are connected. Using these settings only when needed will reduce filament wear and prolong tube life.

The life of rotor bearings and filaments can be greatly extended by minimizing the time that the rotor switch is activated. *Do not activate the rotor switch before you are completely ready to make the exposure.* Continuing to hold this switch, rather than proceeding with the exposure as soon as the tube is ready, increases wear on both bearings and

filament, shortening tube life. Many radiographers develop the bad habit of starting the rotor switch before they begin to give breathing instructions to the patient. These instructions and their implementation take more time than is needed by the rotor, so this practice results in unnecessarily prolonged rotor time for every exposure. Most patients can easily hold their breath for the few seconds of preliminary rotor time, so it is best to start the rotor *after* the patient is ready. An exception to this rule is made when the patient is unable to cooperate and the radiographer must have instantaneous control over the timing of the exposure. This is often the case when performing radiography on infants and children. Box 6-2 gives recommendations for prolonging tube life.

SUMMARY

A simplified x-ray circuit diagram provides a means for studying the devices that make up the x-ray generator and the way they work together to meet the requirements of radiography. The limited operator controls the function of these devices by means of a conventional or computerized control console. The control console provides the means for selecting the kVp and mAs and for making the x-ray exposure.

Rectification of alternating current is necessary for x-ray production. Although x-ray tubes tend to be self-rectifying, diodes in the high-voltage circuit provide more reliable rectification, preventing tube damage and increasing the efficiency of x-ray production. X-ray production is most efficient when the voltage waveform is nearly constant, as provided by three-phase and high-frequency generators.

The limited operator is responsible for implementing good practices to prolong x-ray tube life. These practices involve protecting the tube from sudden or excessive heating and minimizing the time that the rotor switch is activated.

Chapter 7

Principles of Exposure and Image Quality

At the conclusion of this chapter, you will be able to:

- List the prime factors of exposure
- State the formula for determining milliampere-seconds (mAs) and explain how this unit is useful to the radiographer
- Explain the radiographic effect caused by changes in each of the four prime factors of exposure
- Recognize changes in radiographic density and state the exposure factors used to control radiographic density
- Identify high, low, and optimum contrast on a radiograph and state the exposure factor that primarily controls radiographic contrast
- Define radiographic distortion and explain the difference between magnification and shape distortion
- Define spatial resolution and list factors that influence it
- List and explain the geometric factors that affect spatial resolution and explain why magnification affects resolution
- List and discuss methods for minimizing motion blur on radiographs

Key Terms

brightness
collimation
contrast
density
distortion
elongation
fog
foreshortening
high-contrast
inverse square law
involuntary motion
long-scale contrast
low-contrast
magnification
object-image receptor distance (OID)
overexposed
penetrometer
penumbra

prime factors
quality
quantity
quantum mottle
radiographic contrast
shape distortion
short-scale contrast
size distortion
source-image receptor distance (SID)
spatial resolution
subject contrast
tissue density
umbra
underexposed
voluntary motion
window level
window width

This chapter explains the prime factors of radiographic exposure and their radiographic effects. You have already been introduced to some of them. In addition, it introduces the four primary factors of radiographic quality and the principal methods for controlling them. You will begin to observe the effects of exposure on radiographs and to understand how the various factors controlled by the limited operator affect the final image.

Prime Factors of Radiographic Exposure

Milliamperes (mA)
- Controls radiographic density
- Controls quantity of x-rays produced
- Controlled by adjusting the mA
- Quantity of exposure is directly proportional to mA

Exposure Time (Seconds)
- Controls radiographic density
- Controls quantity of x-rays produced
- Controlled by adjusting the timer in x-ray circuit
- Controls duration of exposure
- Quantity of exposure is directly proportional to exposure time

Kilovolts (kVp)
- Controls radiographic contrast
- Controls x-ray penetration
- Controls the quantity and quality of the x-ray beam
- Increased kVp results in increased quantity of photons
- Increased kVp results in increased penetration of the body part

Source–Image Receptor Distance (SID)
- Affects the density and intensity of the x-ray beam
- Quantity of exposure is inversely proportional to the square of the distance

Each dimension of the radiation field is proportional to the SID. Therefore the field area is proportional to the square of the SID and the radiation intensity is inversely proportional to the square of the SID.

PRIME FACTORS OF RADIOGRAPHIC EXPOSURE

Exposure is a broad term used to describe the x-rays that the patient is exposed to, the amount of x-rays in the primary beam, and also the amount of x-rays that reach the image receptor (IR). The x-ray beam is often described in terms of its quantity and its quality. The prime factors that affect x-ray **quantity** are *milliamperage-seconds* (mAs), *kilovoltage* (kVp), *source-image receptor distance* (SID), and *filtration*. The factors that affect x-ray **quality** are kilovoltage and filtration. Note that kilovoltage and filtration affect both quantity and quality (Box 7-1). Filtration was discussed in Chapter 5.

Box 7-1

X-ray Beam Quantity and Quality

Quantity Factors	Quality Factors
mA	
Exposure time	
mAs	
kVp	kVp
SID	
Filtration	Filtration

The quantity and quality of the x-ray beam are controlled by four **prime factors.** These factors are under the direct control of the limited operator. The prime factors of exposure are milliamperage (mA), exposure time (S), kVp, and SID.

Milliamperage

As explained in Chapter 5, changes in mA affect the rate of exposure, that is, the number of photons produced per second during an exposure. For this reason, a change in mA will alter the quantity of exposure to the IR. An increase in mA will increase the quantity of exposure; decreased mA will reduce the quantity of exposure. Exposure is *directly proportional* to mA; that is, if the mA doubles, the quantity of exposure also doubles. Technically, when the mA is doubled, the number of electrons at the filament doubles. During the exposure, the number of photons emitted from the tube doubles as well. The opposite is true if the mA decreases by 50%. The electrons at the filament and the photons emitted will be halved. Dose to the patient is also directly proportional. For example, if the mA is doubled, the dose to the patient is doubled.

Exposure Time

Exposure time also controls the exposure to the IR. This factor affects the exposure by determining how long the exposure will last. Obviously a longer exposure time will increase the exposure to the IR, and a decrease in exposure time will reduce the IR exposure. Like the mA described earlier, the quantity of exposure is also *directly proportional* to the exposure time. Dose to the patient is also directly proportional. For example, if the exposure time is doubled, the dose to the patient is doubled.

Milliampere-seconds

As stated in Chapter 5, the unit used to indicate the total quantity of x-rays in an exposure is milliampere-seconds, abbreviated mAs. This unit is the product of mA and exposure time (mA × time = mAs). For example, if the control panel were set at 200 mA and 0.2 second, the mAs would equal 200 × 0.2:

$$200\,mA \times 0.2\,sec\ =\ 40\,mAs$$

A desired quantity of exposure may be obtained by any combination of mA and time that, multiplied together, equals the desired mAs. For example, 40 mAs could be obtained using any of the following combinations:

50 mA, 0.80 sec = 40 mAs
100 mA, 0.40 sec = 40 mAs
200 mA, 0.20 sec = 40 mAs
400 mA, 0.10 sec = 40 mAs

The quantity of exposure and the patient dose are directly proportional to the mAs. For each of the four exposure techniques listed earlier, the volume of photons emitted and the dose to the patient will be equal. The density or blackening effect on the image will also be equal. *The unit mAs is the primary controller of radiographic density.*

Understand that the mA, exposure time, or the equivalent, mAs, all follow the same directly proportional rule in terms of exposure and dose. If any of these three factors are doubled, both the exposure and the dose are doubled. If any of the three are cut in half, the exposure and dose are cut in half.

Kilovoltage

The kVp controls both the quality and the quantity of the x-ray beam. As the kVp is increased, the energy of the photons in the beam is increased, changing its quality. As the photon energy increases, the *penetrating ability* of the photons increases. When larger or denser body parts are x-rayed, the kVp is increased so that the photons can get through the part and reach the IR. If the kVp is set too low, the photons may not all get through the body part to form the image. Setting the correct kVp for each body part is very important so that the correct number of photons reach the IR. *The kVp is the primary controller of the penetration of x-rays.*

The kVp also has an effect on the quantity of exposure to the IR. When the kVp is increased, the electrons from the filament reach the anode with more energy. More interactions then occur in the anode and more x-rays are emitted. When kVp is increased, density is increased; however, mAs is the primary controller of density. Unlike the effects of mA, exposure time, or mAs, changes in exposure are *not* directly proportional to kVp. *The kVp is never doubled.* A doubling of the kVp would result in four times more photons being emitted! Conversely, the kVp would never be halved because four times fewer photons would result. These would be extreme changes in exposure. Although kVp will affect density, kVp should not be used to control radiographic density.

The **contrast** of the image is directly affected by kVp. High kVp produces a **low-contrast** image and low kVp produces a **high-contrast** image. Each body part that is radiographed will have a kVp assigned to it via the exposure technique chart. This kVp is predetermined based on the penetration needed for the part and the contrast required. Often the physician may request that an additional radiograph be taken at a different contrast level in order to see the anatomy differently. *Therefore kVp is the primary controller of radiographic contrast.*

Source–image Receptor Distance

The distance between the tube target and the IR is called the **source–image receptor distance,** abbreviated **SID.** Because the x-ray beam diverges, forming the shape of a cone, the photons get farther apart as they get farther from the target (Fig. 7-1). Thus the SID affects the *intensity* of the x-ray beam and the quantity of x-rays.

The relationship between the SID and the intensity of the beam is expressed by the **inverse square law,** which states that the intensity is *inversely proportional* to the square of the distance. The inverse square law is expressed mathematically as a formula:

$$\frac{I_1}{I_2}\ =\ \frac{D_2^2}{D_1^2}$$

In this formula, *I* represents radiation intensity and *D* represents SID. For all SID calculations, the distance is always squared. As the distance increases, the intensity decreases and vice versa. For example, if the distance were doubled, the intensity would decrease to one fourth of the original intensity. If the distance were reduced 50%, the intensity would increase by four times. In

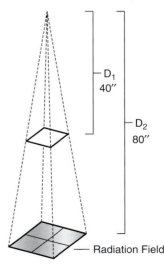

Fig. 7-1 Source–image receptor distance affects both maximum field size and radiation intensity. At 80 inches the field size is four times as large and the x-ray intensity is four times less than at 40 inches.

Fig. 7-1, suppose D_1 is 40 inches and D_2 is 80 inches, or twice as great. If the original intensity at D_1 had a value of 100 mR, the intensity at D_2 would be 25 mR. This value is determined by using the inverse square law formula as follows:

Insert values:

$$\frac{100}{x} = \frac{80^2}{40^2}$$

Square distances:

$$\frac{100}{x} = \frac{6400}{1600}$$

Cross multiply:

$$1600 \times 100 = 160,000$$

Divide by x:

$$160,000 \div 6400 = 25 \text{ mR}$$

In daily x-ray work, the limited operator seldom must make calculations using the inverse square law. As long as it is known that the quantity of x-rays is *reduced 4×* when the SID doubles and that the quantity is *increased 4×* when the SID is halved, it is relatively easy to work with adjustments in the SID. The SID is a prime factor and it must always be set at the correct distance. In practice, the SID is seldom changed and it most often is set at 40 inches. Many departments now use an SID of 48 inches. For chest x-rays done using the upright Bucky, the SID is always set at 72 inches.

It should be evident that the four prime factors are important technical factors in the production of an x-ray image. If the mA, exposure time, mAs, kVp, and SID are not set correctly based on the technique chart, the image of the body part will not have the correct density and contrast.

Chapter 3 contains instructions and practice problems for working with squared numbers and for solving equations of this type.

PHOTOGRAPHIC AND GEOMETRIC FACTORS

There are four primary factors that directly affect how the x-ray image looks: *density, contrast, distortion*, and *spatial resolution*. Density and contrast are considered photographic properties. Distortion and recorded detail are considered geometric properties. An understanding of these factors is essential to the discussion and evaluation of x-ray image. Each factor is influenced and controlled differently. Knowledge about these concepts enables the radiographer to identify the nature of problems that relate to film quality and to solve these problems effectively.

Density

Density is a photographic property that refers to the overall blackness or darkness of the radiographic image. An image that is neither too dark nor too light when seen on the viewing monitor is said to have the correct radiographic density. Fig. 7-2 provides examples of varying radiographic density. Note that density affects the *visibility of detail*. Some detail in the image is lost when the image is either too dark or too light.

Radiographic density is the result of setting the prime factors of exposure. Therefore the quantity of exposure to the IR determines the radiographic density. The greater the quantity of exposure, the darker the image will be. An image that is too dark is said to be **overexposed,** and one that is too light is **underexposed.** *Density is primarily controlled by varying the mAs*, usually by increasing or decreasing the exposure time.

Although kVp and SID also affect radiographic density, they are not used to control it. SID is usually kept constant, and kVp is used to control contrast and to penetrate the body part.

Do not confuse tissue density with radiographic density. **Tissue density** refers to the mass density, or atomic number, of the body part. Increased tissue density—as in bone, for example—causes a lighter area on the radiograph because it absorbs more of the primary radiation, leaving less exposure on the IR. On the other hand, fat has a much lower tissue density than bone. It will absorb less primary radiation and will produce a darker area on the image. Increased radiographic density means that the image is darker, whereas increased tissue density results in a lighter area on the image. In other words, radiographic density and tissue density are *inversely* related to each other. This can be quite confusing if the term *density* is used without qualification.

Digital imaging is used predominantly today. Using digital imaging, the x-ray exposure is processed in a computer and all x-ray images are looked at on a viewing monitor. In this digital environment in which there are no longer "films," the term **brightness** is used in place of density. The brightness (density) on the viewing monitor is adjusted by a control called the **window level.** Because of the newness of the digital environment, density continues to be used to evaluate the blackening level of the image.

Contrast

Contrast is a photographic property defined as the difference in radiographic density between adjacent portions of the image. Fig. 7-3 illustrates differences in **radiographic contrast.** Adequate contrast is also a key factor in the *visibility of detail*. Contrast is what makes the anatomy more visible. Images with contrast that is too low have little density difference between the anatomical structures. They have a flat, gray appearance, and details

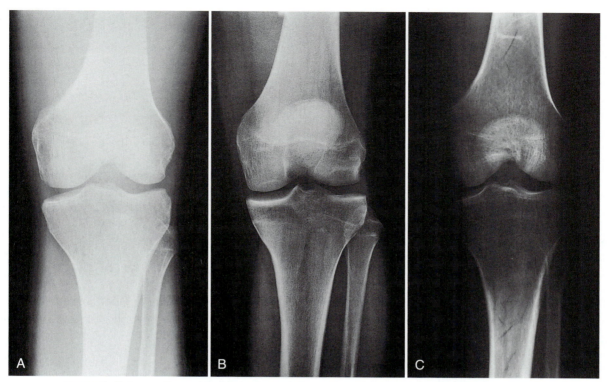

Fig. 7-2 Sufficient radiographic density is needed to make a diagnosis. **A,** Radiograph of the knee with insufficient density, 10 mAs, 80 kVp. It is too light to make a diagnosis and a repeat radiograph is needed. **B,** Radiograph of the knee with proper density, 20 mAs, 80 kVp. All bony aspects of the knee are seen, including soft tissue detail around the bone. **C,** Radiograph of the knee with too much density, 40 mAs, 80 kVp. Diagnosis cannot be made and a repeat radiograph is needed.

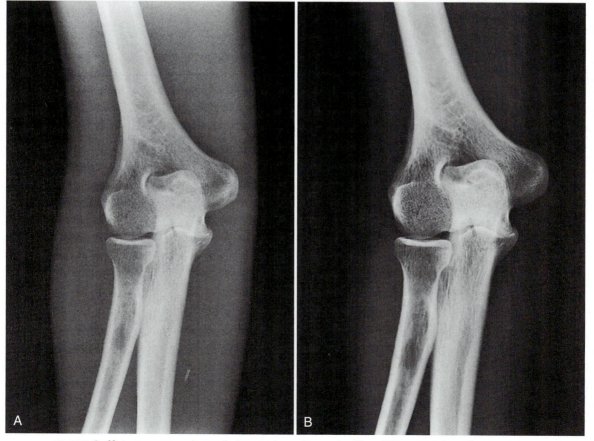

Fig. 7-3 Sufficient contrast is needed to make a diagnosis. Two different scales of contrast are shown on the elbow. **A,** Long scale (low contrast). **B,** Short scale (high contrast).

may be so similar in radiographic density that they are difficult to differentiate from each other. Images with too much contrast have a "black-and-white" appearance. They contain some areas that are very dark and others that are very light. These images have a great difference between the anatomical structures. It is difficult to see detail in areas with extremes of density. Optimum contrast provides sufficient differences in density to easily make out details in all portions of the image.

Optimal contrast can be either high or low depending on the body part. For example, an image of a hand requires a high contrast in order to be optimal, whereas an image of a chest requires a low contrast in order to be optimal. Sometimes the radiologist may request that an additional image be done on a body part at a different contrast level to visualize different anatomy.

Contrast is primarily controlled by kVp. A decrease in kVp produces increased contrast; increased kVp reduces contrast.

Fig. 7-4 illustrates a tool called a **penetrometer.** It is a solid piece of aluminum with steps of varying thickness. A penetrometer is often referred to as *step-wedge* because of its shape. A radiographic image of a penetrometer is a gray scale that shows the amount of penetration of each step. It simulates the different densities that would be seen on a patient's radiograph. Fig. 7-5 illustrates the gray scales produced by radiography of a penetrometer at different kVp settings. At 40 kVp, the number of gray tones between black and white is five. Note that there is considerable difference in radiographic density between each of these steps. This would be considered high contrast. High contrast is also called **short-scale contrast** because the range of densities is short. At 100 kVp, there are more than 15 gray tones between black and white, but the difference in radiographic density between these steps is slight. This would be considered low contrast. Low contrast is called **long-scale contrast** because the range of densities is long.

Contrast is significantly influenced by the tissue densities within the patient, referred to as **subject contrast.** Subject contrast is the range of differences in the intensity of the x-ray beam after it has been attenuated by the patient. It is affected by the kVp and the tissue density.

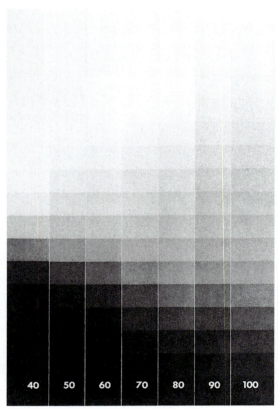

Fig. 7-5 Radiographs of a penetrometer at seven kVp levels demonstrate changes in contrast with varying kilovoltage (kVp). High contrast is produced at 40 kVp and low contrast is produced at 100 kVp. As kVp is increased, more steps are seen.

For example, the abdomen has many structures with similar tissue density and therefore displays low subject contrast. Abdominal structures, such as the liver and the kidneys, will appear similar, so abdominal radiographs tend to have a gray appearance (Fig. 7-6). On the other hand, the chest organs display a high degree of subject contrast. The tissues are very dense in the center, where the x-ray beam must penetrate the sternum, the spine, and the heart, but the lungs are air-filled and easily penetrated. The contrast in tissue density between these structures produces a "black-and-white" appearance (Fig. 7-7). A long scale of contrast is desirable for structures such as the chest that have a high degree of subject contrast. To achieve this, a high kVp (100 to 120) typically is used. Conversely, when the subject contrast is low, such as in the abdomen, a short scale of contrast produces a better image. To achieve this, a lower kVp (75 to 90) typically is used.

Contrast is directly influenced by the presence of fog and collimation. **Fog** is a general, unwanted exposure to the radiographic image. Fog produces an overall increase in density that causes all parts of the image to appear as though seen through a gray veil. It causes areas that would otherwise be bright or white to appear gray. Fog is primarily caused by scatter radiation. **Collimation** will also affect the contrast in the image. When the

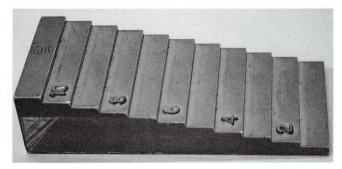

Fig. 7-4 Aluminum step-wedge–type penetrometer. Its radiographic image is a gray scale, as seen in Fig. 7-5.

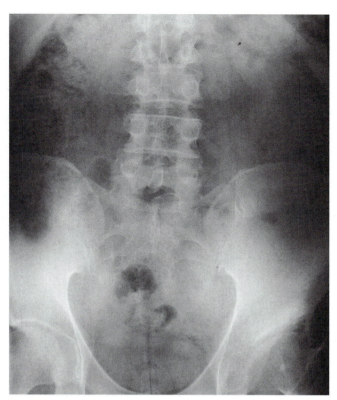

Fig. 7-6 Low subject contrast of the abdominal structures produces relatively low radiographic contrast.

collimator is opened too far, scattered x-rays will reach the IR and produce fog. These factors are discussed in Chapter 9. Fog and collimation that is too wide decreases contrast.

In the new digital environment, the term contrast continues to be used. The contrast on the viewing monitor is adjusted by a control called the **window width.**

Radiographic Distortion

Distortion is a geometric property and refers to differences between the actual subject and its radiographic image. Because the subject is three-dimensional and the image is flat (two-dimensional), all radiographic images have some degree of distortion. Distortion is unequal magnification of different portions of the same object. Radiographic distortion may be categorized by whether it affects primarily the size of the object or its shape. **Size distortion** is always in the form of magnification enlargement. **Shape distortion** is the result of unequal magnification of the actual shape of the structure.

Size Distortion

Size distortion occurs when the part is magnified. **Magnification** is a result of the geometry of the imaging setup. It is a function of the relationship between the SID and the distance between the subject and the IR. This distance is called the **object–image receptor distance (OID).** As you can see in Fig. 7-8, when the SID is great and the OID is minimal, there is little magnification distortion. The object and its image are almost the same size.

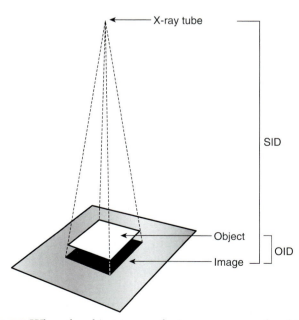

Fig. 7-8 When the object is near the image receptor, the object and its image are nearly the same size. *OID,* Object–image receptor distance; *SID,* source–image receptor distance.

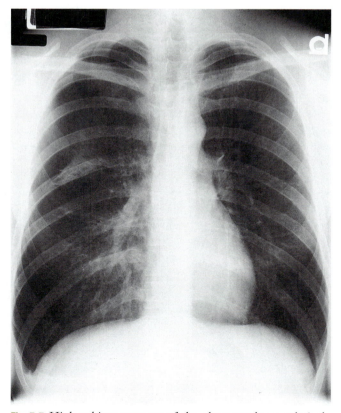

Fig. 7-7 High subject contrast of the chest produces relatively high radiographic contrast.

As the OID is increased, the magnification increases and distortion of the part occurs (Fig. 7-9). You can demonstrate this principle by using a flashlight to project a shadow of your hand on a flat surface. The farther your hand is from the surface, the greater is the size of its shadow. Fig. 7-10 illustrates the increased magnification caused by a decrease in SID.

Radiographic images can never be smaller than their actual size in the body. All images are magnified slightly because the body part is always above the IR. For the great majority of images, the goal is to keep magnification as low as possible to prevent size distortion. The limited operator should recognize, from study of Figs. 7-9 and 7-10, that size distortion will occur when either the OID increases or the SID decreases from the normal positioning. Size distortion therefore is controlled by positioning the body part as close to the IR as possible and using the longest SID practical.

Although magnification of body parts is not desirable in radiographic imaging, there are times when magnification is used to see a part better. For example, the odontoid process is often magnified (see page 276). Reducing the SID from the usual 40 inches to 30 inches to magnify the part enables the surrounding bony area to be spread outward and the field of view of the odontoid to increase.

Shape Distortion

Shape distortion, as stated before, is the result of unequal magnification. The least shape distortion occurs when the plane of the subject is parallel to the plane of the IR and the central ray is perpendicular to both (Fig. 7-11). Angulation of the part in relation to the IR, or angulation of the x-ray beam, produces shape distortion (Figs. 7-12 and 7-13). For these reasons, effort is made to position the patient so that the object of clinical interest is as parallel to the IR as possible and to minimize the need for tube angulation. Even when the x-ray beam is directed perpendicular to the IR, only the central ray is truly perpendicular. Therefore the least distortion occurs at the center of the image. Structures at the outer edges of the radiograph will exhibit some degree of distortion, especially when the IR is large. For this reason, the object of primary clinical interest is usually placed in the center of the field.

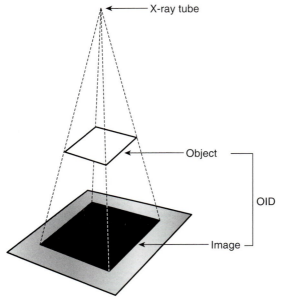

Fig. 7-9 With increased distance between the object and the image receptor (OID), the image is magnified.

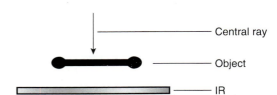

Fig. 7-11 The least distortion occurs when the object is parallel to the image receptor (IR) and the central ray is perpendicular to both.

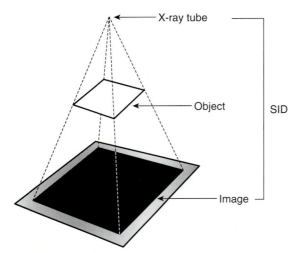

Fig. 7-10 With decreased distance between the radiation source and the image receptor (SID), magnification increases.

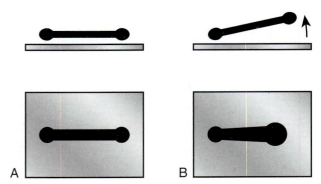

Fig. 7-12 A, Object and image receptor (IR) are parallel. **B,** When the object is not parallel to the image receptor, unequal magnification creates shape distortion. Note also that the object is foreshortened.

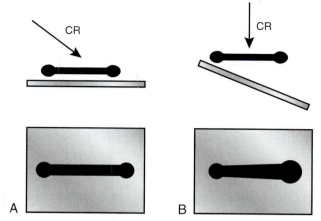

Fig. 7-13 Shape distortion occurs when the x-ray tube and image receptor (IR) are not aligned **(A),** or the object and IR are not aligned **(B).** Note elongation in both of the images. In **B,** there is both elongation and magnification. *CR,* Central ray.

Shape distortion displaces the projected image of an object from its actual position. It can be projected either shorter or longer. Two terms are used to describe shape distortion: *foreshortening* and *elongation*. **Foreshortening** projects the part so it appears *shorter* than it really is. This

usually occurs when the body part is not correctly aligned (see Fig. 7-12). **Elongation** projects the object so it appears *longer* than it really is. This distortion occurs when either the IR or the x-ray tube is not correctly aligned with the part (see Fig. 7-13).

When considering shape distortion, one must also keep in mind that many body parts are distorted by virtue of their position in the body and not because of misalignment of the central ray (CR), IR, or body part. For example, the scaphoid bone in the wrist is naturally foreshortened in the standard posteroanterior projection (Fig. 7-14, *A* and *B*). To better visualize the scaphoid, the operator often angles the CR 20 degrees to reduce the foreshortening. Angling the CR to this bone aligns it to be more parallel with the x-ray tube and displays it with less distortion (Fig. 7-14, *C* and *D*). See Box 7-2 for a summary of the factors that affect distortion.

Tube angulation, or positioning that causes distortion, is sometimes used to prevent structures from being superimposed, that is, projected on top of one another. Because superimposition may obscure details in the primary subject, distortion is sometimes tolerated.

Distortion is primarily controlled by the OID, SID, CR angle, part position, and IR position.

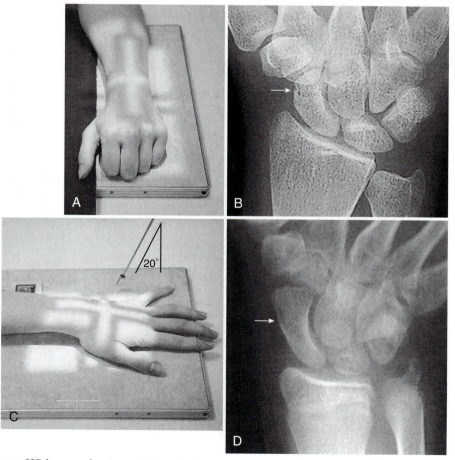

Fig. 7-14 With normal wrist position **(A),** the scaphoid bone *(arrow)* is somewhat foreshortened **(B)** because it does not lie parallel to the image receptor. Angulation of the central ray aligns it more perpendicularly with the scaphoid *(arrow)* **(C)** and improves visualization **(D).**

Box 7-2

Factors Affecting Distortion

Distortion

Size
- Object–image receptor distance
- Source–image receptor distance

Shape
- Alignment
  - Central ray (CR)
  - Part
  - Image receptor
- CR angulation
  - Direction
  - Degree

Spatial Resolution

Spatial resolution is also a geometric property. Before digital imaging, it was referred to as *recorded detail*. Spatial resolution refers to the sharpness of the image. It is more casually referred to as *resolution, sharpness, definition,* or simply *detail*. It is the edge sharpness of all portions of the image that determines whether the image appears sharp or blurred. When resolution is optimum, the edge sharpness of structures in the image is crisp and accurately rendered. Poor resolution tends to appear "fuzzy" or unclear. Several key factors that affect spatial resolution include patient motion, OID, SID, and the focal spot.

Geometric Factors

The geometric factors that control the formation of the image are *SID, OID,* and *focal spot size*. If these three factors are controlled properly, maximum spatial resolution will be seen in the image.

To promote understanding of how spatial resolution is maintained or improved, several terms are used. The **umbra** is the actual anatomic area, body part, or structure shown in the radiographic image. The **penumbra** describes the "unsharp edges" of the umbra, or body part (Fig. 7-15). All body parts will have some unsharpness at the edges in the radiographic image. The goal in radiographic imaging is to reduce the penumbra as much as possible. Penumbra is referred to as *blur* or *geometric unsharpness* in some texts.

X-rays are not emitted from a point source in the target of the x-ray tube. The rectangular area of the target where the electrons strike is called the *focal spot* (Fig. 7-16). The x-ray photons are emitted from this area. Conventional x-ray tubes will have two focal spots, generally termed a *small focal spot*, which is usually about 0.6 mm, and a *large focal spot*, which is usually about 1.2 mm. When the small focal spot is activated, the x-rays are emitted from an area half the size of the large focal spot.

Fig. 7-17 demonstrates that focal spot size affects the size of the penumbra. The smaller the effective focal

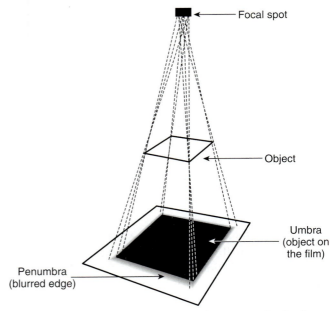

Fig. 7-15 X-rays are emitted from several points on the focal spot of the x-ray tube. This creates unsharp edges of objects called *penumbra*.

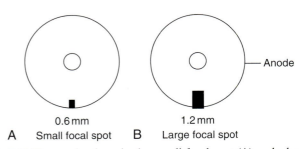

Fig. 7-16 X-ray tubes have both a small focal spot (**A**) and a large focal spot (**B**). The small focal spot creates less penumbra and greater spatial resolution.

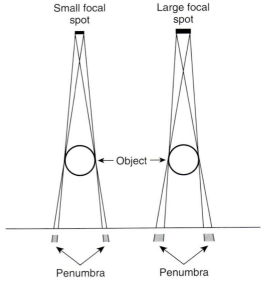

Fig. 7-17 A small focal spot produces less penumbra than a large focal spot. The small focal spot produces greater spatial resolution.

spot, the less the penumbra and the greater the spatial resolution. When the OID decreases, the penumbra decreases, prompting greater spatial resolution (Fig. 7-18). When the SID increases, the magnification and penumbra decrease, also prompting greater recorded detail (Fig. 7-19). Thus, whenever there is magnification of the image, there is also magnification of the penumbra. For this reason, *magnification results in image unsharpness.* These relationships are summarized in Table 7-1. The limited operator should always use the smallest focal spot possible. Because only the OID and SID affect magnification, the shortest OID and the longest SID possible should be used.

When there is a significant OID that cannot be minimized by positioning, increasing the SID and using the small focal spot will improve image quality. A good example is the lateral (side) projection of the cervical spine (see page 277). The location of the shoulder prevents

Table 7-1

Effects of Image Geometry on Spatial Resolution

Factor	Direction of Change	Effect on Resolution
Focal spot size	Decrease	Increase
Object–image receptor distance	Decrease	Increase
Source–image receptor distance	Increase	Increase

placement of the neck close to the IR. To avoid undue loss of detail, the projection is done at a 72-inch SID using the small focal spot.

It is important to remember that the distance between the patient's skin and the IR does not necessarily represent the OID. It is the distance between the IR and the object of clinical interest within the patient that matters. For this reason, an effort is made to perform radiography with the object of clinical interest as close to the IR as possible.

It is also important to note that all radiographic images have less resolution than the anatomic part itself. The challenge in radiography is to control the degree of unsharpness so that it does not interfere with image diagnosis.

Motion

Any movement during radiography will cause blurring of the radiographic image (Fig. 7-20), reducing spatial resolution. This applies to patient motion, of course, but also to movement of the IR or the x-ray tube. To prevent motion, the IR is placed in a firm, stable location and the tube is locked in position. The discussion that follows is intended to assist you in avoiding patient motion.

Patient motion may be categorized as either voluntary or involuntary. **Involuntary motion** involves movements over which the patient has no control, such as tremors, peristalsis, and heartbeats. **Voluntary motion** is normally controllable, although certain patients may be unable to control them (e.g., unconscious patients or small babies cannot hold their breath for a few seconds; patients who are in severe pain; or those who are unable to cooperate).

The first step in avoiding motion is to make every effort to ensure that the patient understands what is expected and is willing to cooperate. *Effective communications with both adults and children are key in avoiding motion.* Try to place the patient in a position that is as stable and comfortable as possible. When patients are standing for radiography, have them space their feet shoulder-width apart for a broad base of support and position them firmly against the film holder for stability. Minimize the time that a patient must maintain an awkward or

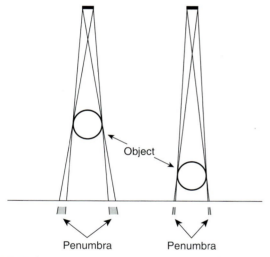

Fig. 7-18 Reducing the object–image receptor distance reduces penumbra and creates greater spatial resolution.

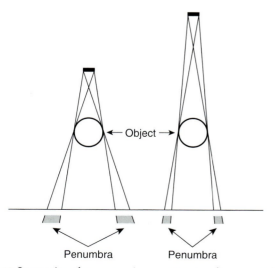

Fig. 7-19 Increasing the source–image receptor distance reduces penumbra and creates greater spatial resolution.

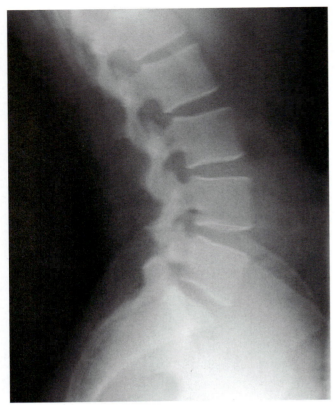

Fig. 7-20 Movement of the patient, tube, or image receptor during exposure causes image unsharpness called *motion blur.*

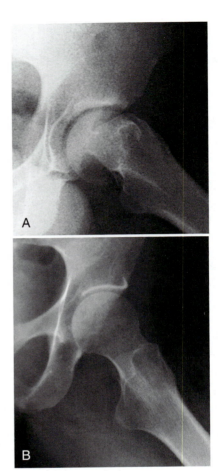

Fig. 7-21 A, Radiographic image of a hip showing quantum mottle. Note the noise and graininess in the image. **B,** Same image showing excellent spatial resolution.

uncomfortable position. Instructions should be clear and complete, with time allowed for the patient to comply.

Immobilization devices are used to minimize motion in certain cases. For example, a sandbag placed strategically over the arm may aid in immobilization of the hand. Devices and methods for pediatric immobilization are discussed in Chapter 18.

The principal means of controlling involuntary motion is to use a short exposure time. This is especially important for chest radiography, in which heart motion tends to blur the lung image, and for radiography of children. If motion is anticipated, or if motion is seen on the image and it has to be repeated, the standard mA and exposure time must be changed. A reduction in exposure time, with a corresponding increase in mA to maintain mAs and density, will reduce motion. For example, if 200 mA and 0.20 second (40 mAs) was used for a projection and motion was seen, adjusting the technique to 800 mA and 0.05 second (40 mAs) would significantly reduce motion in the image.

Two important points must be made regarding motion in radiographic imaging. First, the limited operator should learn to anticipate motion (especially when working with small children and infants) and adjust the exposure technique to avoid repeating the radiograph and to prevent giving a second radiation dose to the patient. Second, the great majority of patients will be able to cooperate and hold their breath. Therefore the standard

exposure technique should not be adjusted to a high mA and short exposure time for every patient. Use of a high mA (usually more than 200 mA) will reduce recorded detail because a high mA requires that the large focal spot be used.

Quantum Mottle

Quantum mottle is a term used to describe the situation in which a grainy or mottled (spotty) image is created. It occurs when the imaging system does not record the anatomic densities, usually because of lack of photons. Quantum mottle will occur when either the mAs or the kVp is set too low. This results in a blotchy, grainy, or noisy image (Fig. 7-21). The result is decreased spatial resolution.

Spatial resolution is primarily controlled by the OID, SID, focal spot, motion, and quantum mottle.

SUMMARY

The four prime factors of exposure are mA, time, kVp, and SID. The quantity of exposure is proportional to both the mA and the time. The mAs is the product of mA and time and indicates the total quantity of exposure. The kVp affects the quantity of exposure by determining how much of the primary beam will penetrate the subject and expose the film. The quantity of exposure in a given area of the IR is influenced by the SID according to the inverse square law, which states that radiation intensity is inversely proportional to the square of the distance.

Radiographic density refers to the overall blackness of a radiograph. It is influenced by all factors that affect exposure and is primarily controlled by mAs. An increase in exposure produces a darker image.

Radiographic contrast. The kVp is used to control the penetration of the x-ray beam and the contrast on the radiograph. High kVp produces a long scale of contrast, providing the latitude needed to make radiographs of subjects with a wide range of tissue densities. A short scale of contrast, produced by low kVp, results in greater density differences between portions of the subject that are similar in tissue density.

Distortion refers to both magnification and changes in the shape of the image as compared with the object. Magnification is enlargement of the image as a result of the relationship between the OID and the SID. Shape distortion is caused by unequal magnification. Shape distortion is controlled by alignment of the object to the IR and by the alignment of the x-ray beam.

Spatial resolution refers to the sharpness of the radiographic image. It is affected by geometric factors (SID, OID, and focal spot size), motion, and quantum mottle.

Digital Imaging

At the conclusion of this chapter, you will be able to:

- Define the key terms used in digital imaging
- List the equipment needed to perform digital imaging
- Explain the computed radiography (CR) digital system
- Explain the digital radiography (DR) system
- Compare CR and DR digital systems
- Describe terms used in image processing
- Recognize the importance of using exposure technique charts with digital imaging
- Describe the processing and postprocessing of a digital image
- Explain the functions of the digital processing system
- Explain what a picture archival and communications system (PACS) is and how it is used
- Recognize the common artifacts seen in digital images
- Explain the technical considerations for everyday use of digital systems

Key Terms

analog-to-digital converter (ADC)
artifacts
backscatter radiation
brightness
complementary metal oxide semiconductor (CMOS)
computed radiography (CR)
contrast resolution
conventional radiography
CR reader
dead pixels
DICOM
DICOM gray-scale function
digital imaging
digital radiography (DR)
direct conversion
dynamic range
edge enhancement
exposure index (EI)
exposure indicator number
flat-panel detector (FPD)

health level-7 (HL-7)
image annotation
image stitching
imaging plate (IP)
indirect conversion
matrix
photostimulable phosphor (PSP)
picture archival and communication system (PACS)
pixel
postprocessing
quantum mottle
radiolucent
rescaling
smoothing
shuttering
signal-to-noise ratio (SNR)
spatial resolution
window level
window width

This chapter presents an overview of the new digital imaging processing systems, computed radiography and digital radiography. The basic definitions associated with this new area of radiology are presented.

Today, well over 90% of radiology departments are using digital systems. Therefore, it is important for the limited operator to understand the basic terminology and concepts so that these systems can be used effectively with patients.

DIGITAL IMAGING

With the old conventional processing, the image of the body part appeared on the sheet of film. The film was taken to the radiologist and placed on the illuminator for interpretation (Fig. 8-1). After interpretation, the film was stored in a paper envelope and sent to the physician or filed in a radiology file room. From this description it can be noted that there is a lot of manual work involved in the process of creating the x-ray image.

Digital imaging, by definition, is the process of acquiring images of the body using x-rays, displaying them digitally, and viewing and storing them on a computer and in computer files. Digital imaging in radiology was first used in the early 1970s with the introduction of the computed tomography (CT) scanner by Godfrey Hounsfield of England. Since then, other areas of radiology, such as conventional radiology and ultrasound, have converted to digital imaging. Most medical imaging modalities (CT, magnetic resonance imaging [MRI], ultrasound, nuclear medicine, and **conventional radiography**) produce digital images that can be sent through a computer network to numerous computers inside and outside the medical facility (Fig. 8-2). In the near future,

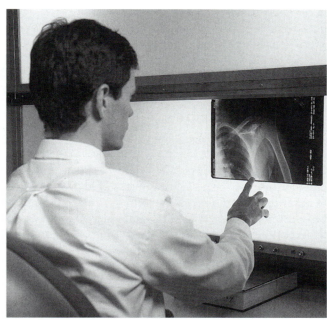

Fig. 8-1 A radiologist interpreting a shoulder x-ray image on a sheet of film using an illuminator in conventional radiology.

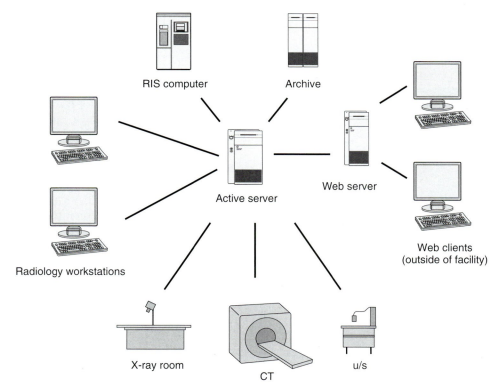

Fig. 8-2 A typical digital computer network showing the modalities feeding images to the workstations, viewing stations, servers, and archives. *CT,* Computed tomography; *RIS,* radiology information system; *u/s,* ultrasound.

all radiography departments will have converted to digital methods, whereas conventional screens and film, and darkrooms with mechanical processors to process films, will be obsolete. It should be noted that *digital imaging* is a general term also used outside of the radiology department. For example, nearly everyone has a digital camera, and pictures (images) are stored in a computer or flash drive. Digital imaging is what allows word files, photos, and videos to appear on the World Wide Web. YouTube and Facebook are fully digital systems.

The terms *digital imaging* and *digital radiography* have generated much confusion over the past years as the digital world evolved in the x-ray department. Both terms are used, and very often, interchanged.

Computed Radiography

Computed radiography (CR) is one of the two types of digital imaging systems. CR was introduced in the United States in 1983 by Fuji Medical Systems of Japan. CR can be referred to as *cassette-based* digital imaging because the image of the body part is obtained using a cassette that contains a storage phosphor plate (Fig. 8-3, *A*). These CR cassettes are often referred to simply as **imaging plates (IPs)**. The plate contains a **photostimulable phosphor (PSP)** that stores the latent image of the body part until it is processed. The phosphor absorbs the energy of the x-rays and, with it, the image of the body part. Most IP phosphors are made of barium fluorohalide with europium. Essentially, there are two types of IPs: a *standard-resolution IP,* which has a thick phosphor layer, and a *high-resolution IP,* which has a thin phosphor layer. High-resolution IPs have greater resolution and sharpness

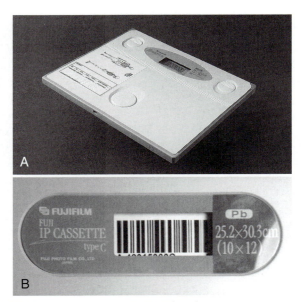

Fig. 8-3 A, Conventional CR IP. The plate contains a storage phosphor that stores the x-ray energy. **B,** Barcode label on the CR cassette allows matching of the image with the correct patient.

Table 8-1	
Most Common Computed Radiography (CR) Plate Sizes	
Inches	**Centimeters**
8 × 10	18 × 24
10 × 12	24 × 30
14 × 14	35 × 35
14 × 17	35 × 43
14 × 36	35 × 91

because of the thinner phosphor layer. The front of the cassette containing the IP is made of a **radiolucent** material that does not absorb primary x-rays. This allows the maximum number of x-rays to reach the IP. The back side of the cassette has a lead lining to prevent **backscatter radiation** from reaching the IP. Backscatter can cause image artifacts.

CR cassettes come in the same sizes and shapes as traditional film cassettes (Table 8-1). The plates also contain a barcode label or barcode sticker that allows the limited operator to match the image information with the patient-identifying barcode on the examination request (Fig. 8-3, *B*). To process and view the image, five additional equipment components are required: a **CR reader** unit, a limited operator computer workstation, a computer system with monitors for the radiologist to view the images, a printer if images need to be printed on film, and a computer server to store the images (Fig. 8-4).

After an IP is exposed, it is inserted into the CR reader (see Fig. 8-4, *A*). Once the plate is inside the reader, the phosphor is scanned with a laser beam. This releases the stored energy in the form of visible light (Fig. 8-5). Special electronics convert the light into an electric signal to produce the digital image of the body part on a computer screen (see Fig. 8-4, *B*). After the plate is scanned inside the reader, it is exposed to an intense white light to erase it. This ensures that any residual image on the IP is erased. Photostimulable phosphor plates can be reused at least 10,000 times before they need to be replaced.

A very important aspect of the IP is that it will absorb more low-energy scatter compared with the old film/screen cassettes. This means that appropriate collimation and kilovoltage peak (kVp) must be used to achieve optimal images. *This also makes the IP more sensitive to scatter radiation both before and after exposure to the x-ray beam.* The IP is also sensitive to background radiation and should be erased if it is not used in 48 hours; otherwise there will be fog on the image.

Digital Radiography

Digital radiography (DR) is a second type of digital imaging system. DR systems are often referred to as *cassetteless* because they do not use a cassette with an IP. Instead there

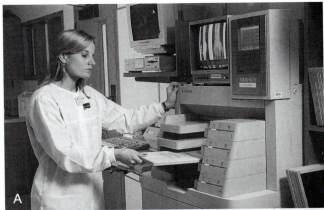

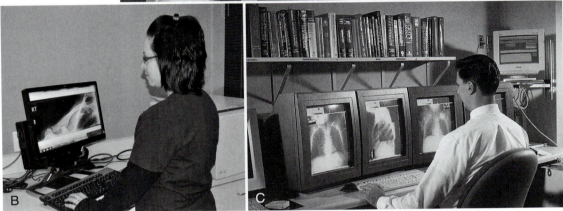

Fig. 8-4 A, Limited operator inserting an IP into the CR reader for processing of the image and plate erasure. **B,** The operator's computer workstation. Here the operator checks the image for quality control, adjusts the image as needed, and sends it electronically to the radiologist for interpretation. **C,** The radiologist at the reading station. Note that several images can be viewed at one time. Images are retrieved from the department server for reading.

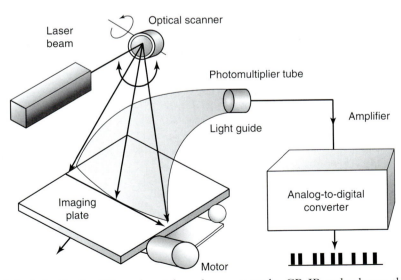

Fig. 8-5 A look inside the CR reader. A laser beam scans the CR IP and releases the stored energy as visible light. A photomultiplier tube converts the light to an electric signal. A converter creates the digital image, which is then sent to the computer system.

is a detector unit built into the table and upright wall unit. **Flat-panel detectors** (FPDs) consist of either a scintillation screen or a photoconductor, which converts the x-ray photons directly into electrical signals. With DR, the FPD is hard wired into the x-ray table and upright unit and a CR reader device is not needed. For protection it is permanently sealed inside a rigid protective housing. The FPD in the table or upright unit is 17 × 17 inches to accommodate horizontal and transverse body part projections. DR systems can be divided into two categories: indirect conversion and direct conversion systems.

Indirect conversion DR is a two-step process in which the x-ray energy is first converted into light and then converted into an electric signal. This method uses a scintillator to convert the x-ray energy into light. A scintillator is a device that glows when hit by the high-energy x-ray photons, and often it is made of cesium iodide. A photodiode made of amorphous silicon then converts the light into an electric signal. Adjacent to the photodiode layer is a thin-film transistor (TFT) array that allows readout of the x-ray image (Fig. 8-6, *A*). This occurs with the use of an **analog-to-digital converter (ADC).** The ADC takes the stored charge and converts it into digital values. From there, it is sent to the computer for processing and viewing.

The charged coupled device (CCD) is a type of indirect conversion detector. In this system, there is no photodiode and instead the CCD converts the light from the scintillator to the electric signal. The CCD device uses optics and light and therefore is often referred to as a CCD camera. The flat panel detector or CCD is built into the x-ray table (Fig. 8-7, *A*) or upright wall unit (Fig. 8-8). It is important to note that, unlike CR, DR requires installation of a new radiography room of equipment because the FPD system is integrated into the table, generator, and other electronics.

Another type of indirect conversion detector is the complementary metal oxide semiconductor (CMOS). CMOS detectors convert light into electrons very similar to CCD technology. With CMOS, the electrons are stored in capacitors. The semiconductor is a solid chemical element or a compound that allows excellent control of electrical current. The most common CMOS semiconductor is silicon. An ADC is use with this detector to convert the image into digital format.

Direct conversion is a one-step process. Detectors convert the x-ray energy directly to an electric signal through an amorphous selenium detector without the light conversion (Fig. 8-6, *B*). A TFT array is used also to collect and store the image for readout. DR images,

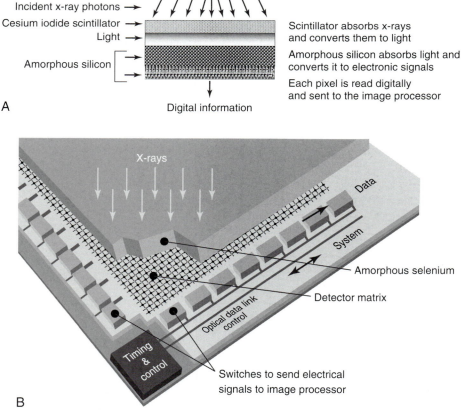

Fig. 8-6 A, Cross-sectional drawing of an indirect conversion detector showing the scintillator, the light given off, and the amorphous silicon layer that converts the light into the electric signal. **B,** Flat panel detector in a direct conversion system in which the x-ray energy is converted directly to an electric signal. Amorphous selenium layer is shown.

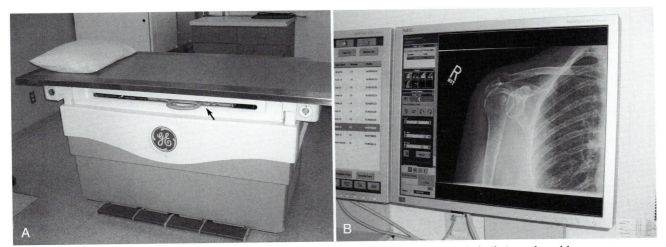

Fig. 8-7 A, Digital radiography x-ray table. The flat panel detector unit is built into the table *(arrow).* There is no Bucky tray for either a conventional film cassette or a CR IP. **B,** The image is displayed on the monitor in the x-ray room in 3 to 5 seconds for viewing.

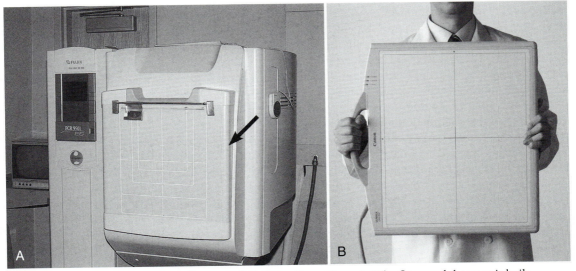

Fig. 8-8 A, An upright or wall-mounted digital radiography unit. The flat-panel detector is built into the front of the unit *(arrow).* This unit is used for radiography of upright chests and abdomens primarily but can be used for any x-ray projection that is done in the upright position. **B,** A DR cassette containing a flat-panel detector. These plates can be carried anywhere for obtaining fast images.

especially those from direct conversion detectors, are available within seconds of making the exposure, whereas with CR the plate has to be manually inserted into the reader unit for processing before it can be viewed. *The ability to see x-ray images very fast is one of several major advantages of CR and DR systems.* With DR, images can be processed and seen in 3 to 5 seconds (Fig. 8-7, *B*). The best systems on the market can process an image in as little as 1 second.

DR technology is now available in cassette form. Many manufacturers now build DR "plates" that have the flat-panel detector built into the cassette (see Fig. 8-8, *B*). These DR plates can be used to take x-rays on patients in

wheelchairs, on carts, and outside the department using a mobile x-ray machine. Some DR plates are connected to the processor via a cord (tethering), and some plates are "wireless" and can transmit the image information to the processor using a radio signal.

Regardless of the type of digital imaging system, CR or DR, the x-ray generator, the overhead tube crane and tube, and the patient table and upright wall unit remain. Digital imaging starts when the x-rays exit the patient's body. With digital imaging, the x-ray image is produced, processed, viewed, and stored within a computer-based system, which provides many efficiencies for the radiology department.

Digital Images

Images created by digital means require a much different terminology than the old film and screen technology. Limited operators should become familiar with this new terminology because it is used every day in the production of digital images.

Matrix and **pixel** are digital terms used to describe the viewing monitor and the image. The digital image as seen on the monitor is described as having a matrix, very similar to a regular computer monitor. The actual matrix is a series of thousands of very small boxes or squares. Placing a magnifying glass on a monitor will show the matrix squares. The individual matrix squares are known as picture elements or pixels (Fig. 8-9). Each of these pixels presents a visual brightness or density level. The matrix is laid out in a rectangular or square box. The matrix is the computer monitor's active area. For example, a typical digital monitor might have a matrix of 2000×2500 pixels. Multiplying these two numbers presents a monitor with 5,000,000 total pixels that form the image.

Dead pixels are defects in the components, which is a possibility in any imaging system. This may cause a loss of patient information. The manufacture of the pixels is so complex, it is inevitable that the detector array will suffer some damage. Dust, scratches, and interactions between materials can occur, resulting in some defective pixels. These pixels may be malfunctioning or dead, that is, not functioning at all. As the detector ages, the number of dead pixels increases but may not be detected if they are located on the edges of the panel. Manufacturers make efforts to maintain a standard of less than approximately 0.1% to 0.2% defective pixels and build software programs into their systems to identify and isolate dead pixels. The software uses a method to "fill in" the dead pixels with information using the surrounding pixels as a guide.

Spatial resolution is a critical image quality factor. A basic definition of spatial resolution is the amount of detail or sharpness of an image as seen on the monitor. The matrix size has a direct effect on spatial resolution. *The larger the matrix and the smaller the pixels, the greater the spatial resolution.* Thus a 1000×1000 matrix (1,000,000 pixels) in a 20-inch monitor will present greater resolution than a 512×512 matrix (262,144 pixels) in that same 20-inch monitor. Fig. 8-10 illustrates that smaller size pixels, or a greater number of pixels, will produce images with better resolution than larger pixels. Monitors can be purchased with different resolution capabilities. Very high–resolution monitors are used by the radiologist to read the images. These monitors can have a matrix as large as 4096×4096.

Contrast resolution and **dynamic range** are two other image quality factors that work together. Contrast resolution is the ability to distinguish anatomical structures of similar subject contrast, such as liver–spleen and gray matter–white matter. If contrast resolution is not adequate, it is very difficult to see the difference between the organs described and other body structures, especially very small structures. Dynamic range is the response of the detector to different levels of radiation exposure. A digital image can be produced with a wider range of exposures. Because of this response, overexposures and underexposures may not need to be repeated. However, a technique chart should still be used to determine the correct exposure and not just set a "range" exposure for a given body part. Both CR and DR detectors are capable of producing a much wider gray scale in the image. Digital imaging systems are capable of producing better contrast resolution and a wider dynamic range than the old film/screen systems. Contrast resolution and gray scale of any image are manipulated by adjusting the window described in the next section.

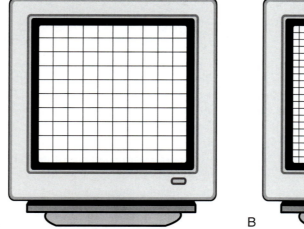 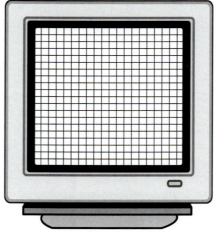

A   B

Fig. 8-9 A computer monitor's matrix and pixels shown. **A,** Monitor with a 10×10 matrix and 100 pixels. **B,** Monitor with a 20×20 matrix and 400 pixels. An image on the B monitor would display greater spatial resolution because of the larger matrix and smaller size of the pixels.

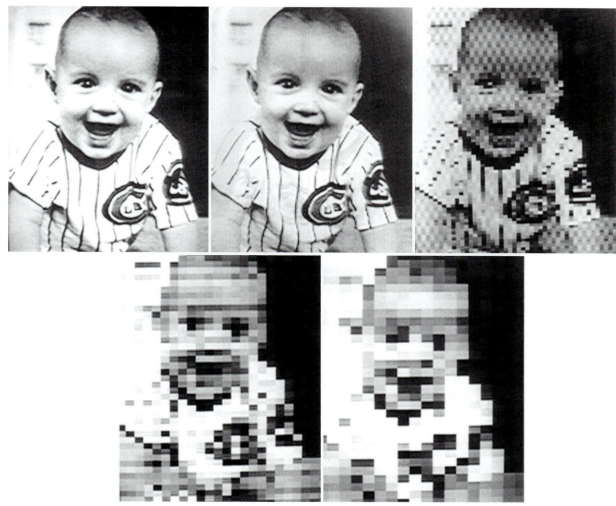

Fig. 8-10 Top image of child made with a large matrix and very small pixels. Bottom image made with smaller matrix and larger pixels resulting in poorer spatial resolution.

Signal-to-noise ratio (SNR) describes the ability of the digital system to convert the x-ray input electric signal into a useful radiographic image. *Signal* refers to the useful information in the image. *Noise* refers to the amount of information that is not useful. Noise can be caused by **quantum mottle** or inherent electrical noise. Quantum mottle occurs when there are not enough photons in the detectors to provide a high-quality image. This is usually the result of mA or kVp set to low. The goal in digital imaging is to reduce the amount of noise. The more signal that is present, the less noise, and the higher the quality of the image. When there is a high SNR, or low system noise, the greatest amount of information is captured. When the SNR is poor, contrast resolution is directly affected.

FUNCTIONS OF THE PROCESSING SYSTEM

Image Manipulation

The most common image processing parameters are those for brightness and contrast. **Window level** controls the density in the image. In digital imaging the word **brightness** is used in place of density. **Window width** controls the contrast in the image. The limited operator or physician can manipulate both of the controls, width and level, by simply clicking on the mouse (see Fig. 8-4, *B* and *C*).

Shuttering

When proper collimation is used there is a clear area around the collimated image. This clear or white area presents excess white light, which can interfere with viewing and interpretation (Fig. 8-11). Automatic **shuttering** is used to blacken out the white collimation borders. This eliminates the glare to the eyes. Shuttering is aesthetic and is a viewing technique only. It should never be used to mask poor collimation practices. For example, if there was wide, or open, collimation of the body part, scatter is introduced and contrast decreased. The image quality will be reduced even though the shuttering did not show the larger collimated area. All body parts should be collimated in the usual way when using digital systems. For DR, in which there is no cassette to

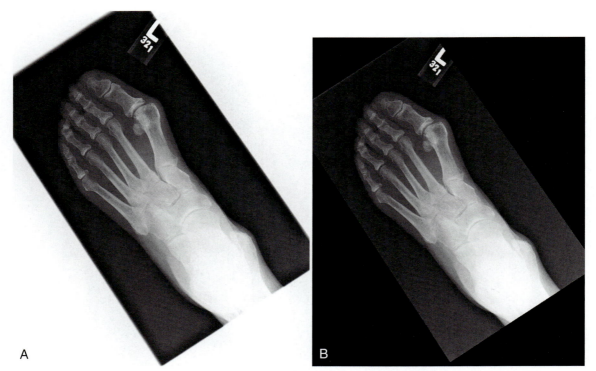

Fig. 8-11 Shuttering. **A,** Anteroposterior (AP) foot with proper collimation. **B,** Same foot with collimation and shuttering. Note shuttering surrounded the image with black area preventing bright light from showing around the image.

automatically set the collimator via a microswitch, standardized collimation settings are now stated in positioning textbooks.[b,c]

Image Stitching

When anatomy or the area of interest is too large to fit on one IR, multiple images can be "stitched" together using a special computer program, a technique called **image stitching.** This is used most often when doing full-spine posteroanterior (PA) projection images for scoliosis. Imaging the full spine requires a long IR plate. In digital imaging, a special plate consisting of two interlocked 14- × 17-inch cassettes in a 14- × 34-inch plate is used. Image stitching software automatically merges the two, or with some systems three, images together. One image will appear on the viewing monitor (Fig. 8-12).

Image Annotation

Many times, information other than standard identification must be added to the image. **Image annotation** allows the limited operator to add text that is useful to

have on the image. This can include information such as time, exposure technique, or patient position. In many digital software systems there is a preset selection of annotation items to choose from, or else the operator can manually insert these into the image. *Annotation should never be used to place a right (R) or left (L) marker on the image.* Identification markers should be placed directly on the IR or tabletop. This is a medicolegal issue. Right or left side errors can easily be made when annotation is used in place of lead markers.

Edge Enhancement

Edge enhancement is a processing technique in which images can be made sharper and have greatly increased contrast; however, it does introduce some noise. This is done by the computer software using various algorithms. A high-pass filter can scan the image's digital file and remove information that is not useful in the image. Edge enhancement can aid the radiologist when interpreting an x-ray examination; however, it can result in the loss of small detail. It is important for the operator to realize that the information content of a digital image is still totally dependent on the correct exposure technical factors. The appropriate exposure technique of kVp and mAs must still be set on the generator, the body part properly penetrated, and appropriate collimation used. Although enough radiation dose should be used to obtain an optimal image, the

---

[b]Long BW, Hall-Rollins J, Smith BJ: *Merrill's atlas of radiographic positioning and procedures,* St. Louis, 2015, Elsevier.
[c]Long BW, Hall-Rollins J, Smith BJ: *Merrill's pocket guide to radiography,* St. Louis, 2015, Elsevier.

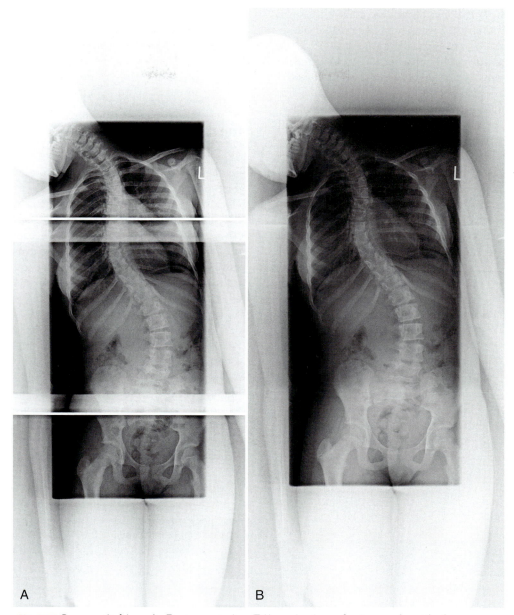

Fig. 8-12 Image stitching. **A,** Posteroanterior (PA) projection of spine made with three exposures. **B,** All three images joined together by image stitching.

dose should be as low as possible without compromising the image quality. Postprocessing techniques with software algorithms should not be the factor used to improve image quality.

Smoothing

Smoothing is another type of processing technique. With this technique each pixel's frequency is averaged with the surrounding tissue's pixel values. This is done to remove noise, which can be bothersome to the radiologist. Less contrast is also seen in the image. This technique is useful in viewing very small structures and the fine details of bone.

EXPOSURE TECHNIQUE CHARTS

Exposure technique charts must be used with digital imaging systems. Technique charts are described in Chapter 10. The milliamperage (mA), kilovoltage peak (kVp), exposure time, and automatic exposure control selections that were used for each body part in conventional imaging must be used with digital imaging. The IR systems in digital imaging prompt a much wider dynamic range. This means that the computer can correct for exposure technique errors within a limited range. If an image is too dark, it can be lightened, and if an image is too light, it can be darkened. Contrast can also be corrected. Although the computer can make these corrections, it is still the responsibility of the limited operator to set the correct exposure techniques. This allows optimal image quality and keeps the radiation exposure to the patient "as low as reasonably achievable" (ALARA). In recent years, the profession has seen "dose creep," an increase in doses to patients and operators, because of inappropriately increasing the exposure technique in an effort to avoid a repeat examination. In addition, state laws and the Joint Commission require that exposure technique charts be available in the x-ray room for reference to each x-ray projection performed. Thus, although the computer and software systems may be able to correct for overexposure and underexposure, this should not be seen as a reason to set broad exposure factors. Use of an exposure technique chart is more critical with digital systems. An exact kVp and mAs must be set for each body part.

One of the most important aspects of setting the exposure technique using digital imaging is correctness of the kVp chosen to penetrate the body part. If the kVp is too low and underpenetration occurs, a poor-quality image will be produced, as shown in Fig. 8-13, and a repeat will have to be done. This will result in additional exposure to the patient and to the limited operator. Quantum mottle, described previously, will occur in digital imaging also if there are too few photons reaching the IR. If exposure factors are set too high, the patient can receive excessive and unnecessary radiation. In addition, if the exposure is too high, image contrast is decreased because of excessive scatter radiation and other factors. *It is unethical for the limited operator to intentionally set the exposure technique too high to avoid having to obtain a repeat image.* As great as computers are, they cannot make excessive overexposure or underexposure produce an optimal image.

Rescaling

When the x-ray exposure is greater or less than what is needed to produce an image, automatic rescaling occurs. This processing system is designed to display all the pixels for the area of interest. Automatic **rescaling** means that images are produced with *uniform density and contrast*, regardless of the amount of exposure. Problems occur with rescaling when too little exposure is used, resulting in quantum mottle, or when too much exposure is used, resulting in loss of contrast and loss of distinct edges because of increased scatter radiation. Rescaling is no substitute for appropriate technical factors. There is a danger in relying on the system to "fix" an image through rescaling and in the process using higher milliamperage seconds (mAs) values than necessary to avoid quantum mottle. The term *dose creep* is widely used to explain this phenomenon. It refers to the use of automatic rescaling without regard to appropriate exposure amount. What may be appropriate for one patient may be too much exposure for another; however, the same factors are used. Therefore the dose creeps up over time.

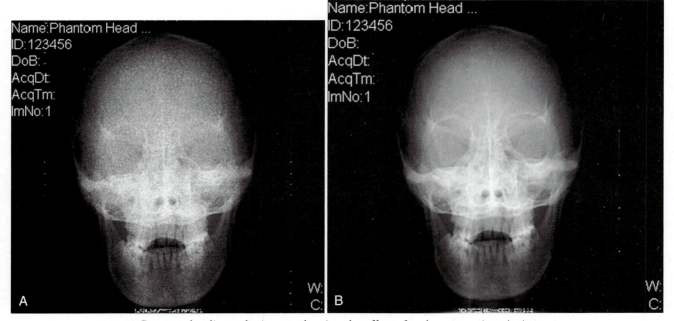

Fig. 8-13 Computed radiography images showing the effect of underpenetration. **A,** Anteroposterior projection of the skull underpenetrated at 58 kVp. The computer was unable to create a diagnostic image because not enough x-rays reached the detector. Quantum mottle, or noise, is evident. **B,** Same projection correctly penetrated at 85 kVp. Use of the correct kilovoltage is critical when using digital systems.

Table 8-2

Recommended Exposure Indicator Values

Company	Overexposure	Underexposure	Adult: Nongrid/Grid	Distal Limbs Nongrid
Carestream	>2500	<1600 tabletop; <1800 Bucky	1800–2100	2200–2400
Agfa	>2.9	<2.1	2.1–2.3	2.4–2.6
Fuji	<100	>250 tabletop; >400 Bucky	200–300	75–125

EXPOSURE INDICATORS

The amount of light given off by the phosphors in the IP is a result of the radiation exposure the plate has received. The light is converted into a signal that is used to calculate the **exposure indicator number.** Some refer to this as the *exposure index*. The total signal is not a measure of the dose to the patient but indicates how much radiation was absorbed in the phosphors, which gives only an idea of what the patient received. *The base exposure indicator number for all manufacturers' systems designates the middle of the detector operating range.* Unfortunately, the exposure indicator numbers are not standardized among the different manufacturers of digital systems and in fact they can vary widely (Table 8-2). The exposure indicator should be checked on every image. Fortunately, most departments have only one manufacturer's system, so understanding these numbers is made easier for the operator.

Because manufacturers differ in the way exposure is numerically represented, it can be difficult to calculate exposure amounts. The radiography profession has been calling for exposure indicator standardization for several years. Standardization will give the limited operator more confidence in adjusting technical factors while following the ALARA principle. Limited operators should use their vendor's proprietary exposure indices for reference to the correct exposure.

POSTPROCESSING

Another important component of digital imaging is **postprocessing** because a repeat exposure may not be necessary. With postprocessing, any image of a body part can be further adjusted with the computer software to visualize areas of interest better. Two common postprocessing techniques are subtraction and contrast enhancement. With the subtraction technique (Fig. 8-14), the computer can remove anatomy such as the bones or organs. With the contrast enhancement technique (Fig. 8-15), contrast can be changed from very high to very low. However, the more an image is postprocessed, the less information is transferred to the physician. Therefore manipulation of the image should be kept to a minimum.

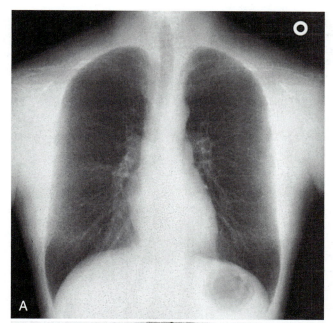
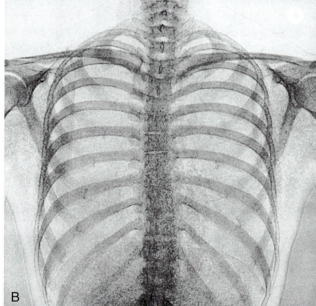

Fig. 8-14 Postprocessing subtraction technique. **A,** Ribs are removed to only show the lungs. **B,** Lungs and soft tissue are removed to show only the bony areas.

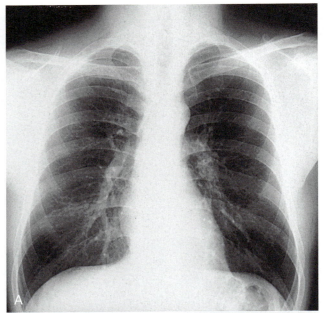

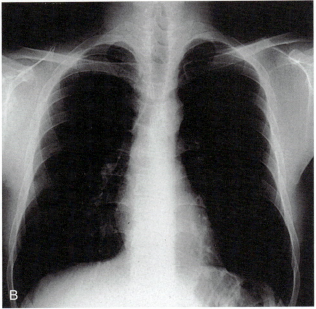

Fig. 8-15 Postprocessing contrast enhancement technique. **A,** This chest image shows the standard long scale of contrast for the lungs. Note that the trachea and bones of the shoulder do not show. **B,** Contrast adjusted to display a short scale of contrast. Note how the trachea and bones of the shoulder are now displayed.

Digital Imaging and Communications in Medicine and Health Level-7

Digital imaging and communications in medicine **(DICOM)** is a universally accepted standard for exchanging medical radiographic images within the institution and in the many areas where the images are viewed. In addition, the DICOM system allows physicians and others to view x-ray images made on different manufacturers' systems in a "cooperative" computer environment. For example, images made with a Fuji system can be read with an Agfa or Carestream system. Changes are made annually to the DICOM software, and limited operators should watch for bulletins with these updates.

One of the more important functions of the DICOM software is that it specifies a standardized display function for consistent display of gray-scale images. This is important because the scale of densities shown on an image in the original system, and a diagnosis made on that system, must be able to be duplicated exactly in a competitor's system. The **DICOM gray-scale function** provides methods for calibrating a particular viewing monitor display system for the purpose of presenting images consistently on different display monitors and printers.

Health level-7 (HL-7) is a communication standard for all of the hospital or clinic's information systems. For example, this standard allows the institution's patient demographics system, admissions and discharge system, and nursing information systems, along with the radiology department's patient information and image storage systems, to be integrated. This standard also allows the different manufacturers' software systems for the above to communicate effectively.

ARTIFACTS

CR and DR systems produce unique artifact patterns in digital imaging. Generally, an artifact is considered an *error* on the image. Some of the more common artifacts are described below.

- *Quantum mottle* is caused by an inadequate exposure technique. This can be because of either low mAs or low kVp (Fig. 8-16).
- *Moiré pattern.* This artifact occurs when the grid lines are not aligned with the laser scanning frequency of the CR reader (Fig. 8-17).
- *Light spots* are usually caused by dust or other foreign material on the IP. *CR phosphor* plates can be cleaned, but this must be done carefully according to the manufacturer's recommendations to avoid permanent damage.
- *Phantom or ghost images* may appear as a result of incomplete IP erasure. This artifact requires troubleshooting of both the CR plate preparation system and the display systems. Extreme overexposure may require two erasure cycles to completely remove the image (Fig. 8-18).
- *Scratches or tears* are permanent artifacts caused by damage to CR plates. Replacement of CR plates is expensive, but it is the only solution because these artifacts cannot be repaired (Fig. 8-19).
- *Extraneous line patterns* are linear lines caused by noise in the image reader electronics. They can run lengthwise or crosswise (Fig. 8-20).
- *Fogging* from background or scatter radiation is because of the CR plates being much more sensitive than the former film.

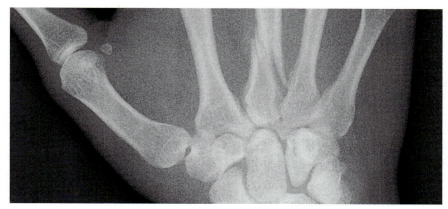

Fig. 8-16 Grainy appearance artifact of the bones. Quantum mottle appeared because of insufficient exposure to the IP.

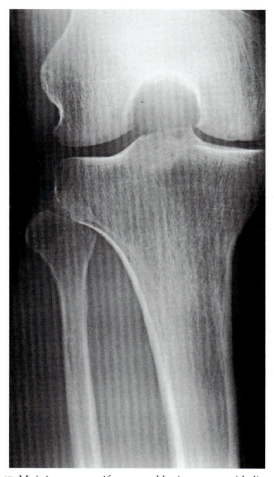

Fig. 8-17 Moiré pattern artifact caused by incorrect grid alignment with laser scan direction.

PICTURE ARCHIVAL AND COMMUNICATION SYSTEMS

In a typical radiology department, thousands of x-ray images can be processed in a given day. Before digital imaging, these images were on film and stored in envelopes in

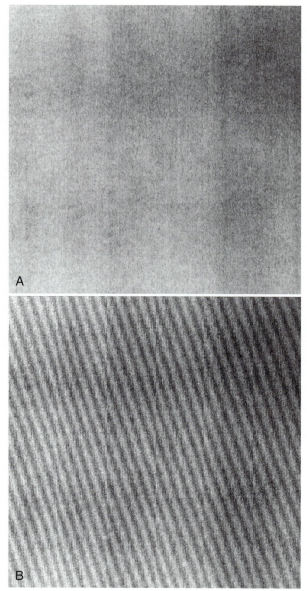

Fig. 8-18 A and **B,** Phantom or ghost image artifacts. These can occur from many sources including double-exposed IPs and scatter radiation. The actual artifact can appear as though it is in the patient's body, leading to incorrect diagnosis.

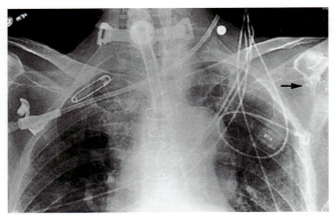

Fig. 8-19 Scratch artifacts are typically permanent because they occur inside the IR plate and in the phosphor.

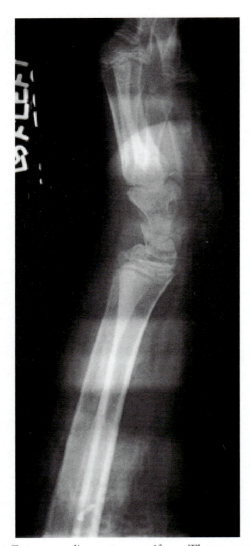

Fig. 8-20 Extraneous line pattern artifacts. These are typically caused by the CR reader device and malfunctioning electronics.

large file rooms. With digital imaging, the images are totally contained within computer systems; therefore a system is needed to view and file them. The image management system used in radiology departments is called a *PACS. PACS* is short for **picture archival and communication system.** The system consists of an extensive networked group of computers, servers, and archives (Fig. 8-21). A PACS will contain all the digital images that are produced in the department, including CT, MRI, ultrasound, and nuclear medicine images. This extensive computer system allows multiple users inside and outside the department to view images. A PACS typically is specially designed for the hospital or clinic depending on factors such as the volume of patients, the number of radiologist reading stations, the number of outside department physician viewing stations, and so on. The software with the PACS system must conform to DICOM standards.

TECHNICAL CONSIDERATIONS FOR EVERYDAY USE

Attention to detail is very important when using digital imaging systems. This section addresses the technical considerations that are different from those in conventional radiography.

Patient ID

Every image, including digital images, must include four items of information: the patient's name or institution ID for a given patient, a birth date or institution ID specific for a given patient, the date of the examination, and the name and location of the x-ray facility.

Kilovoltage

Because of the wider dynamic range of digital systems, a higher kVp setting may be acceptable for radiography projections that are done using the Bucky and a grid. The kVp may be increased as much as 10 kVp with little effect on contrast. This will help reduce radiation exposure to the patient because a higher kVp will penetrate better and reduce the exposure time. However, this can only work using automatic exposure control (AEC) or systems that have anatomically programmed radiography (APR). Limited operators need to be cautious with kVp. Using a kVp that is too low and will not penetrate the part adequately can create a poor-quality image as described earlier (see Fig. 8-13). Slightly overpenetrating the body part is better than underpenetrating it. An optimum kVp range should be posted on the technique chart for all projections using digital systems. In addition, for body parts that have widely different thicknesses of structures and densities but must be imaged on one projection (e.g., a chest, lateral hip, femur, foot), the thickest part must be

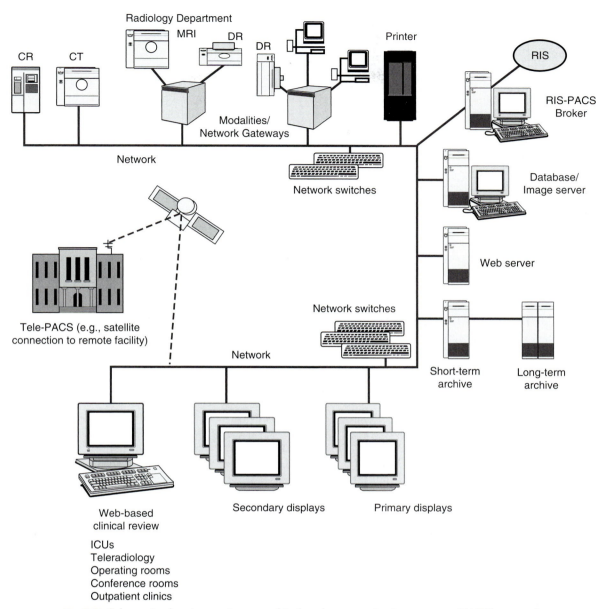

Fig. 8-21 Schematic showing a picture archival and communications system (PACS) network. *CR,* Computed radiography; *CT,* computed tomography; *DR,* digital radiography; *ICU,* intensive care unit; *MRI,* magnetic resonance imaging; *RIS,* radiology information system.

penetrated. Compensating filters should be used for body parts that have extreme differences in tissue density (see Chapter 10).

Part Centering

The body part that is being radiographed must always be placed in or near the center area of the CR plate or DR detector. If the central ray is directed to a body part that is positioned at the periphery of the IR (e.g., a finger placed near the edge), the computer may not be able to process the image properly. This also depends on whether the computer is in the autoprocessing or manual-processing mode. CR plates can be split in half and used

for two separate exposures because the image reader will note the two areas of exposure. However, this practice is not encouraged by the digital manufacturers.

Split Cassettes

If a CR cassette is divided in half and used for two separate exposures, the side not receiving the exposure *must always be covered with a lead shield.* Storage phosphors in the CR plate are hypersensitive to small levels of exposure, and these may show on the image as artifacts if the plate is not properly shielded. Covering the unused half prevents scatter radiation from reaching the unexposed side of the CR plate. Although this technique was practiced in conventional radiography, it is more critical with CR. Depending on the specific technical factors used, if shielding is inadequate, the images may not appear at all, may contain artifacts, or may display other image-processing failures. In addition, technical factors and body part thickness for the two exposures must be relatively close to each other.

Overexposure and Underexposure

A light or dark image on the display monitor may not indicate that the body part was underexposed or overexposed with x-rays as in conventional radiography. A wide array of computer-related factors can cause a light or dark image when digital processing is used. Digital images are often processed with unique numbers, described earlier as *exposure indicator numbers*, which indicate the amount of the exposure reaching the plate. The determination of overexposure or underexposure is made by evaluating this number and not the lightness or darkness of the initial image on the monitor. The manufacturer usually provides a range of numbers that indicate appropriate exposure. Using techniques that yield a number in the center of that range will result in low patient dose and good images.

Collimation

As with conventional radiology, the x-ray beam must be collimated carefully to the body part being radiographed. In addition to the usual image quality issues associated with excessive scattered or off-focus radiation, poor collimation practices with digital systems can result in digital processing errors. These errors are frequently related to inability of the system to identify and separate image information from primary beam exposure at the collimated edges of the image field, which results in images with inappropriate brightness or contrast. The collimation sizes indicated in this text for each projection should be used for all projections. The body part and collimated field should always be centered with regard to the IR when possible. If possible, *the collimated field should be placed so that all four margins are seen on the IR, or at least two sides of collimation should appear on the image.* When multiple exposures are produced on a CR IR, the collimated fields should be spaced and oriented to prevent overlap of adjacent collimated edges.

Open Cassettes

Once an exposure is made on a plate, the cassette can be opened momentarily and exposed to light without compromising the image—a 15-second exposure will begin the erasure process. Exposing the phosphor to ambient light starts the erasure process, but the process is slow. With CR plates, the latent image remains stored in the phosphor. The latent image will lose about 25% of its energy in 8 hours. All exposures on CR plates should be processed immediately. The cassette is not designed to be light-tight but is designed to protect the IP from dust, scratches, and other damage. This is different from conventional radiography, in which the film inside the cassette is ruined even if momentarily exposed to light.

Grids

The IRs used in digital radiography systems are much more sensitive to scatter radiation. Controlling scatter is a critical consideration in optimizing image quality when using digital imaging systems. Some projections may require a grid if the kVp is above a certain level. For example, one manufacturer requires that a grid be used for any exposure above 90 kVp. This consideration is particularly important in mobile radiography, in which many projections are done without a grid. The common problems associated with grids will occur with digital systems—grid cutoff and moiré artifacts. With digital systems, examination routines may need to be reevaluated to determine the need for a grid.

Display Monitor Quality Assurance

The viewing monitor is often the weakest link in the digital imaging chain. The monitor has a direct effect on the quality of the image that is viewed. The American College of Radiology (ACR) suggests that the monitor be checked for quality at daily, monthly, and quarterly time frames. The main quality control tools are the Society of Motion Pictures and Television Engineers (SMPTE) and American Association of Physicists in Medicine (AAPM) test patterns (Fig. 8-22). These patterns are in the computer software and can be retrieved to perform the tests. The most important monitor tests include:
- Viewing surface and airflow
- Image quality and appearance using a test pattern
- Geometric distortion
- Luminance, reflection, noise, and glare
- Resolution

In most instances these QC tests of the viewing monitor will be performed by trained QC radiologic technologists or a physicist.

Markers

ID markers, such as right (R) or left (L), should be placed on the CR cassette or the DR table, similar to using conventional screen/film combinations. *As mentioned earlier, although the R and L markers can be placed on the image using the computer software after the image is processed, this is not recommended because of the great potential for error and legal implications.* This is especially true when patients are examined in the prone position.

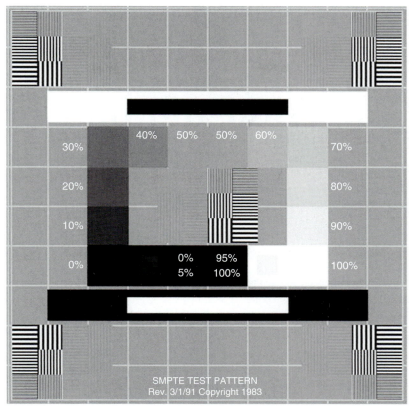

Fig. 8-22 SMPTE test pattern, as seen on a monitor, used to check viewing monitor performance including distortion, luminance, noise, contrast, and resolution.

SUMMARY

The new radiography systems—computed radiography and digital radiography—were introduced in this chapter. New terminology associated with these systems was also presented. The differences between these new digital processing systems and conventional radiography screens and film are important to understand and are brought out in the discussions. The unique differences between the IR used in computed radiography and in digital radiography are presented. The importance of using exposure technique charts and practicing the ALARA concept is discussed because there can be a greater likelihood of overexposing patients when using digital systems. Because film is not used in digital systems, and the storage of x-ray images is in computer servers, the picture archival and communication systems used in digital radiography are discussed. When using digital systems, the limited operator has to change many of his or her daily technical considerations. This chapter presented all of the technical considerations that are different when using digital systems. Technical items such as the kVp, part centering, splitting cassettes, overexposure and underexposure, collimation, grid use, and ID markers were all discussed.

Chapter 9

Scatter Radiation and Its Control

Learning Objectives

At the conclusion of this chapter, you will be able to:

- List and explain three types of interactions between radiation and matter that produce scatter radiation
- Explain the problems caused by scatter radiation in radiography
- List factors that affect the quantity of scatter radiation fog on a radiograph
- Identify scatter radiation fog on a radiograph
- List four measures that can be taken to reduce the quantity of scatter radiation fog on radiographs
- Define grid ratio, grid frequency, and grid radius
- List common grid ratios and state the appropriate application of each
- Define what is meant by "grid cutoff" and list four causes of this phenomenon
- Explain the difference between a Bucky and a stationary grid
- State the criteria for determining whether grid use is appropriate

Key Terms

backscatter
Bucky
coherent scattering
Compton effect
coned-down image
crosshatch grid
focal range
focused grids
fog
grid
grid cassette

grid cutoff
grid frequency
grid lines
grid radius
grid ratio
parallel grid
photoelectric effect
scatter radiation
secondary radiation
stationary grid

Scatter radiation is produced as a result of the attenuation of the x-ray beam by matter. This chapter explores the production of scatter radiation and the factors that influence its formation. In addition, this chapter covers methods used to minimize the fog that this radiation causes on radiographs.

RADIATION INTERACTIONS WITH MATTER

When x-rays completely *penetrate* the body, there is no interaction with matter, and no scatter or scattered radiation is formed as a result. When x-rays are *absorbed* in the body, however, their energy is "scattered," or converted into new scatter x-rays. Three types of interactions occur when radiation is absorbed by matter: *coherent scattering, Compton effect,* and *photoelectric effect.*

The result of either coherent scattering or the Compton effect is termed **scatter radiation** or simply *scatter.* Radiation produced by the photoelectric effect is correctly referred to as **secondary radiation.** Because more than one type of interaction takes place during radiography and the resulting radiation is so similar, the terms are often used interchangeably. When referring to both scatter and secondary radiation, this text uses the term *scatter radiation.*

The interactions that produce scatter radiation in radiography occur primarily within the patient. Some scattering also occurs as a result of interactions between the x-ray beam and the tabletop and image receptor (IR), and any other matter that happens to be within the radiation field.

Coherent Scattering

Coherent scattering is also known as *Thompson scatter.* This type of interaction takes place at relatively low energy levels (below 10 keV). Fig. 9-1 shows the path of the x-ray photon during this interaction. Because coherent scattering occurs in the very low energy ranges, and outside the usual range for diagnostic imaging, this interaction has no significance to our daily work. It is mentioned here only to demonstrate that at very low kilovolts peak (kVp) levels there is an interaction in the body.

Compton Effect

The **Compton effect** occurs at energy levels throughout the diagnostic x-ray range of 40 to 125 kVp. The incoming x-ray photon interacts with an *outer* orbital electron of an atom, removing it from the atom (ionization), and then proceeds in a different direction. The majority of the photon's energy is converted into a new photon of scatter radiation (Fig. 9-2). This new photon has less energy than the incoming primary beam photon and therefore a longer wavelength. It also travels in a new direction. Compton scatter travels in all directions. If it is directed back toward the x-ray tube, it is termed **backscatter.** Most of the photons that are scattered will scatter in a more forward direction. *As the kVp is increased, Compton interactions are increased.*

Photoelectric Effect

The **photoelectric effect** is similar to that which forms characteristic radiation in the x-ray tube (see Chapter 5). In this case, however, the incoming energy is an x-ray photon interacting with an atom in the body rather than an electron interacting with the tungsten anode.

In a photoelectric interaction, the incoming photon from the primary beam collides with an *inner* orbital electron of an atom. The photon is totally absorbed in the process and creates an absorbed dose in the patient. The electron's departure leaves a "hole" in the orbit, which is filled by an electron from an outer shell. The difference in binding energy between the two shells is emitted as a new x-ray photon (Fig. 9-3). This photon is referred to as a *characteristic photon* and is considered *secondary* radiation because it is radiation actually produced in the body. The photon will have a new direction. Its energy will be less than that of the primary photon. Photoelectric interactions are less prevalent in the

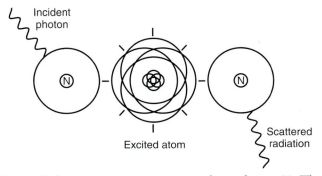

Fig. 9-1 Coherent scattering occurs in three phases. (1) The x-ray photon enters the atom. (2) The photon's energy is momentarily transferred to the atom, causing an excited state. (3) The energy is given up by the atom as a photon of the same energy but with an altered direction. *N,* Nucleus.

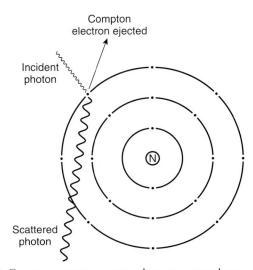

Fig. 9-2 Compton scatter occurs when an x-ray photon collides with an outer orbital electron of an atom. The electron is ejected from its orbit. The photon is deflected from its path and continues with decreased energy as a scattered photon. *N,* Nucleus.

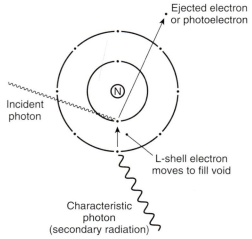

Fig. 9-3 Photoelectric effect occurs when an x-ray photon collides with an inner-shell orbital electron of an atom. The photon's energy is absorbed in the process of ejecting the electron. When an outer orbital electron moves to the inner orbit to fill the space vacated by the departing electron, the difference in binding energy between the two electron shells is emitted in the form of a new characteristic photon and secondary radiation. *N*, Nucleus.

diagnostic energy range than Compton interactions. The likelihood of a photoelectric interaction is determined by both the kVp level and the electron-binding energy of the atom in which the interaction occurs.

Because no part of the energy of the incoming photon exits the atom, photoelectric interactions are sometimes referred to as *true absorption*. In this text, references to scatter also apply to secondary radiation formed by the photoelectric effect. *As kVp is increased, photoelectric effect is decreased.* Note that this is the opposite of the Compton effect. In the diagnostic range of kVp used (50 to 100 kVp), the majority of radiation interactions with the body are Compton interactions.

RADIOGRAPHIC EFFECT OF SCATTER RADIATION

The production of scatter radiation during an exposure results in **fog** on the radiograph. Fog is unwanted exposure to the image. It does not strike the IR in a pattern that represents the subject, and it contributes nothing of value to the image. This fog produces an overall increase in radiographic density. The result is also a reduction in radiographic contrast, as stated in Chapter 7. Although increased density in the darker areas of the image is scarcely noticeable, areas that would otherwise be bright or white will instead be gray because of the fog. The intermediate gray tones will appear more similar to each other, which makes it difficult to distinguish recorded detail within those portions of the image that have similar tissue densities. In other words, *scatter radiation creates fog that reduces both contrast and the visibility of detail* (Fig. 9-4).

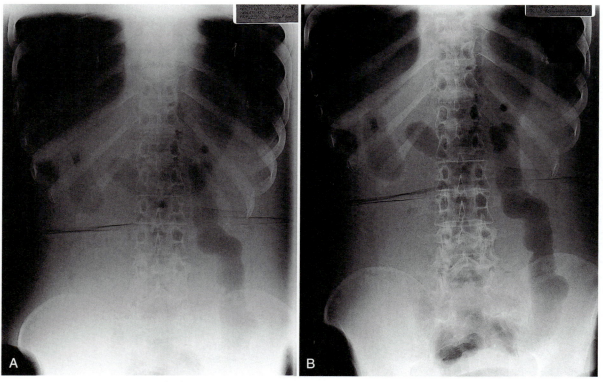

Fig. 9-4 A, Uncontrolled scatter radiation causes decreased contrast on this radiograph of a phantom abdomen. **B,** When the Bucky is used to control scatter radiation, contrast improves significantly.

FACTORS AFFECTING QUANTITY OF SCATTER RADIATION FOG

Four primary factors directly affect the quantity of scatter radiation fog on the radiograph (Box 9-1): *volume of tissue, kilovoltage, density of the matter,* and *field size.*

Volume of Tissue

The primary scatter consideration is the volume of tissue irradiated. *The thicker or larger the body part is, the greater are the scatter and the fog.* When there is a greater quantity of tissue in the path of the x-ray beam, there will be greater absorption of the x-ray beam and more interactions that produce scatter radiation. The volume of tissue irradiated is determined by the thickness of the subject and the size of the radiation field. When the subject is more than 10 to 12 cm in thickness, the amount of fog becomes objectionable unless the field size is very small.

Because a thicker subject requires a greater quantity of exposure, there will be more primary x-ray photons and more interactions. This is another reason why there will be more scatter radiation when the thickness of the subject is increased.

Kilovoltage

Kilovoltage also affects the quantity of scatter radiation that reaches the IR. *Higher kVp results in more scatter radiation fog.* When high-energy photons interact with matter, the scatter radiation that is produced is also of a higher energy. This high-energy radiation is better able to escape the subject without being reabsorbed and so is more likely to cause fog on the radiograph.

Density of Absorbing Matter

The density or atomic number of the absorbing matter also influences the quantity of scatter radiation fog. *The denser the body part, the less the scatter.* This is because there is more photoelectric effect. A very dense body part (higher atomic number), such as a bone, will absorb a large quantity of primary radiation. The prevalence of scatter radiation in radiography indicates that there must be some matter that produces scatter radiation and permits it to escape. In fact,

this is the case with all matter that is similar in density to water. Because the human body is largely made up of water, *the patient is the principal source of scatter radiation in radiography.*

Field Size

Maintaining the correct field size through collimation is one of the most important things a limited operator can do to control scatter radiation. *As collimation is increased, or made larger, scatter radiation fog increases.* Collimation should be restricted to only the body part being radiographed. This is also important because the smaller the field size, the fewer body parts are subjected to x-rays and the smaller the dose is to the patient.

CONTROLLING SCATTER RADIATION FOG

From this discussion, it is clear that scatter radiation fog becomes increasingly objectionable as the thickness of the subject increases. To obtain diagnostic quality radiographs of the trunk of the body, it is absolutely essential to employ some means of limiting the fog effect on the IR. The principal method for reducing scatter radiation fog is the use of a radiographic **grid**. A grid is used when the body part becomes greater than 10 to 12 cm in thickness or kVp settings are greater than 60. Additional strategies include beam restriction and reduction of kVp.

Grids

A grid is a device placed under the table between the patient and the IR (Fig. 9-5). It has the appearance of a thin metal plate (Fig. 9-6) and is constructed of tiny,

Box 9-1

Factors Affecting Scatter Radiation Fog

↑ Volume of Tissue	= ↑ scatter	= ↑ fog
↑ Kilovoltage	= ↑ scatter	= ↑ fog
↑ Field Size	= ↑ scatter	= ↑ fog
↑ Density of Matter	= ↓ scatter	= ↓ fog

↑, Increased; ↓, decreased.

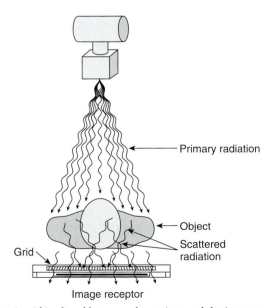

Fig. 9-5 A grid is placed between the patient and the image receptor to absorb scatter radiation. Scattered x-rays not moving in the same direction as the primary x-ray beam are absorbed by the grid.

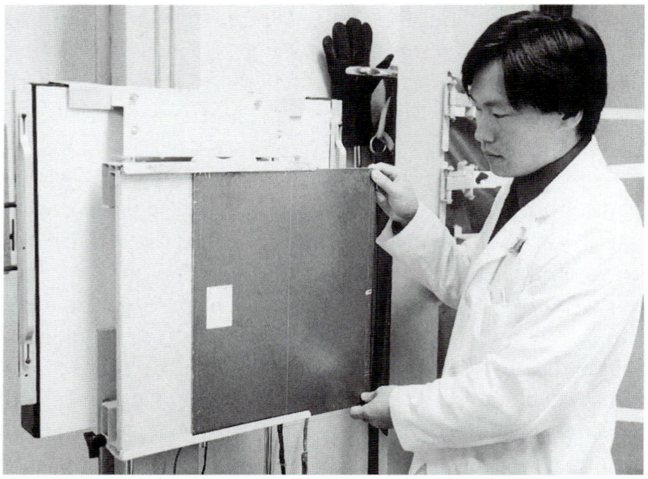

Fig. 9-6 A grid has the form of a thin plate and is covered by a protective aluminum coating.

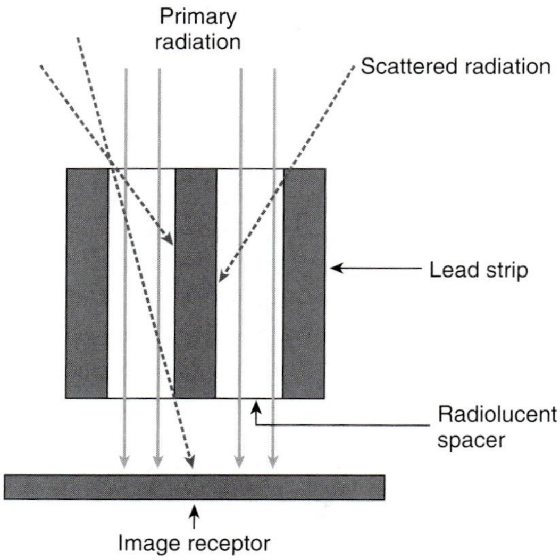

Fig. 9-7 Cross section of a grid demonstrating its function. The grid consists of lead strips on edge, separated by radiolucent interspacing material.

tissue-thin lead strips, placed on edge. The lead strips are held in place by a radiolucent interspacing material, usually aluminum. Because they are aligned to the x-ray beam, the lead strips tend to absorb scatter radiation while permitting remnant radiation to pass through (Fig. 9-7).

The effectiveness of a grid is determined by the **grid ratio,** that is, the relationship between the height of the lead strips and the width of the spaces between them (Fig. 9-8). This ratio determines how much variation in the direction of the incoming photon is allowed without the photon being absorbed by the grid. The higher the ratio, the less variation is permitted and the greater is the efficiency of the grid in absorbing the unwanted photons. Typical grid ratios range from 5:1 to 16:1. Table 9-1 lists common grid ratios and their usual applications. The x-ray table and upright unit will have a built-in grid that cannot be changed. Different grids are used for mobile x-ray projections. Limited operators may use a grid IR when taking an x-ray on a patient in a wheelchair or on a cart.

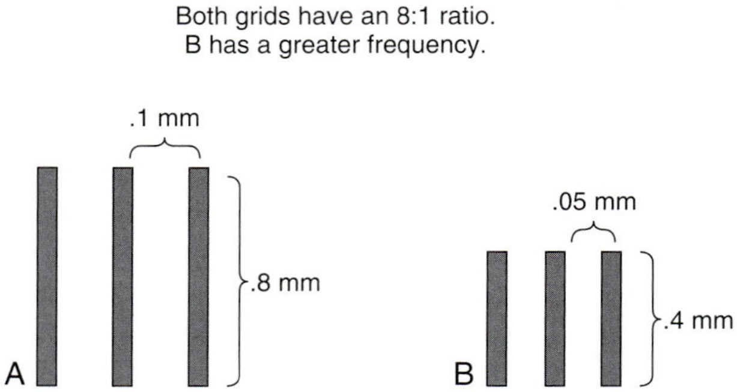

Fig. 9-8 The grid ratio is the relationship between the height of the lead strips and the width of the interspacing material. These two grids are different but have the same ratio. Note that the same degree of variation in direction of the x-rays is permitted by both.

Table 9-1
Grid Applications

Ratio	Application
5:1 and 6:1	Grid cassettes, mobile radiography
8:1	General purpose
12:1	General purpose, chest radiography
16:1	High-kilovoltage radiography

As seen in Fig. 9-8, grids with the same ratio may have many strips close together or fewer strips farther apart. The number of lead strips per inch is called the **grid frequency.** Grid frequencies range from 60 to 196 lines/inch.

Grids for general-purpose use are called **focused grids** because the lead strips are aligned in the direction of the diverging primary x-ray beam (Fig. 9-9). The lead

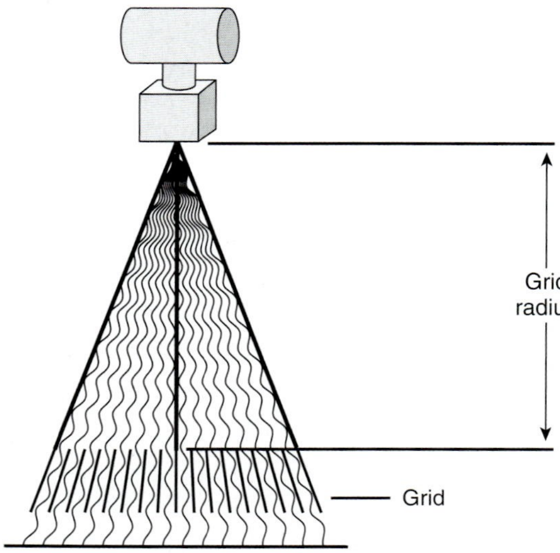

Fig. 9-9 The grid radius is the distance at which the primary x-ray beam is parallel to the focused lead strips of the grid.

strips of a focused grid are precisely aligned with the x-ray beam at a specific source–image receptor distance (SID), which is called the **grid radius.** Because the alignment does not need to be exact for the useful photons to pass through the grid, there is a range of distances within which the grid will not absorb an undue amount of useful radiation. This is referred to as the **focal range** of the grid. The SID employed with a grid should always be within the grid's focal range. The most commonly used SIDs are 40, 48, and 72 inches. Each usually requires a different grid with a suitable focal range. Grids with extra-long focal ranges are now available, however. Some have a focal range of 40 to 72 inches.

Grid Focal Range

The range of source–image receptor distances at which the grid will not absorb significant amounts of primary radiation.
Example: A grid with a 40-inch radius may have a focal range of 36 to 48 inches.

Each grid has a label indicating its ratio, its frequency, and its radius or focal range. This label is placed on the

side of the grid that faces the x-ray tube when the grid is in use. There is usually also a line down the middle that indicates the long axis of the lead strips and the grid's focal center.

Because the grid absorbs some useful radiation, the radiographic image includes an image of the grid itself. This grid image is called **grid lines** or *grid striping* (Fig. 9-10). Grid lines that appear on the image are objectionable and can reduce recorded detail. Two methods are employed to prevent objectionable grid lines: the grid may be moved during the exposure or the grid may have a very high frequency (i.e., many fine lines very close together).

Moving Grid

A moving grid is called a **Bucky.**
Moving the grid during the exposure blurs the image of the grid lines so that the grid image is not visible on the film.

A moving grid is called a **Bucky,** so named after Dr. Gustav Bucky, who invented it in 1913. A Bucky is a part of a radiographic table (Fig. 9-11) or an upright

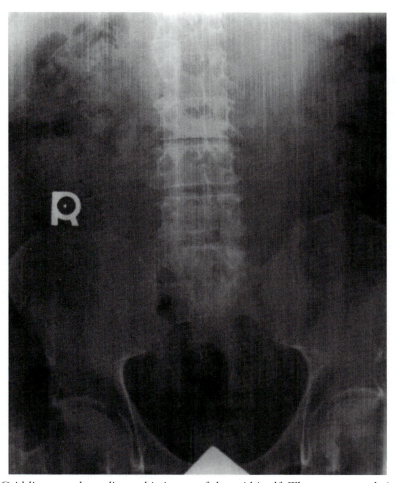

Fig. 9-10 Grid lines are the radiographic image of the grid itself. They are most obvious when the grid is stationary and the grid frequency is low.

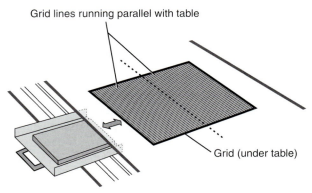

Grid lines running parallel with table

Grid (under table)

Fig. 9-11 A Bucky is a moving grid installed under the tabletop or in an upright cabinet.

cassette holder. The Bucky grid is mounted in a frame that incorporates a small motor. The motor causes the grid to oscillate back and forth rapidly during an exposure. This movement blurs the image of the grid lines, making them invisible on the radiograph. The Bucky device also includes the IR tray that holds the cassette in place when making Bucky exposures. A table Bucky has rollers that allow it to be moved along a track under the tabletop. This permits placement of the Bucky and the film at any location along the length of the table. Bucky grids typically have a ratio of 12:1 to 16:1 and a frequency of 85 to 103 lines/inch.

Stationary Grids

- Do not move during the exposure
- Should have many very fine lines (high frequency) to avoid objectionable grid lines on images
- Commonly used today in upright cassette holders

A high-frequency grid that does not move during the exposure is called a **stationary grid.** Such a grid produces grid lines, but the lines are very tiny and close together and are not readily seen at a normal viewing distance. Their appearance is acceptable because they are almost invisible and do not adversely affect the diagnostic quality of the image. Stationary grids may be part of a Bucky-like device in the radiographic table, and they are often used in upright cassette holders called *grid cabinets*. Stationary grids for permanent installations typically have a ratio of 8:1 or 12:1 and a frequency of at least 103 lines/inch.

Portable stationary grids come in various sizes and may be attached to a cassette when needed in locations other than the permanent installations. A **grid cassette** is a special cassette with a grid built into the front side. Both portable grids and grid cassettes are used for mobile and surgical radiography and for special applications when the patient cannot be positioned on the table or at

the upright grid cabinet. Grid cassettes typically have lower ratios than the grids used in permanent installations. Ratios of 5:1, 6:1, and 8:1 are common. Grid cassettes should be clearly marked and kept in a separate place from the regular cassettes. They must never be used in the Bucky.

Grids are precision instruments and are very expensive to replace. Special care must be taken to ensure that they are not damaged by dropping, striking, or bending. Such damage causes the lead strips to become misaligned, which makes the grid useless.

Grid Cutoff

Focused grids are designed to allow the passage of radiation that is aligned with the lead strips. Any misalignment of the primary x-ray beam will result in undesirable absorption of useful radiation by the grid. Excessive absorption of useful radiation by the grid is called **grid cutoff.** Grid cutoff appears as *decreased* radiographic density on the side of the image (Fig. 9-12).

No grid cutoff occurs when the x-ray beam is correctly aligned with the grid (Fig. 9-13). Grid cutoff occurs when the x-ray tube is centered to one side of the grid rather than to the focal center line (Fig. 9-14). Cutoff also occurs when the x-ray tube is angled toward one side

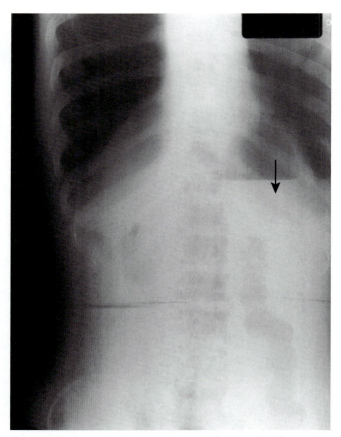

Fig. 9-12 Grid cutoff appears as areas of decreased radiographic density *(arrow)* on one side of the image. It occurs when the x-ray tube and the grid are not correctly aligned with each other.

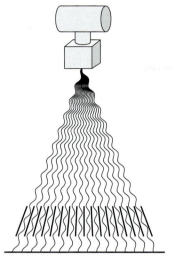

Fig. 9-13 When the x-ray beam is correctly aligned with a focused grid, no cutoff occurs.

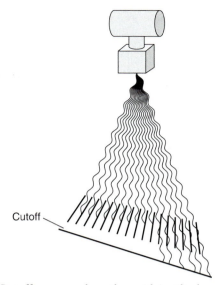

Fig. 9-15 Cutoff occurs when the grid is tilted or when the x-ray beam is angled across the grid.

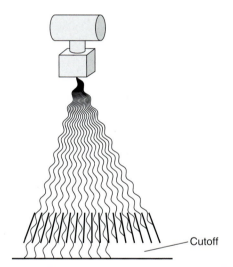

Fig. 9-14 Grid cutoff occurs when the x-ray beam is off center to one side of the grid.

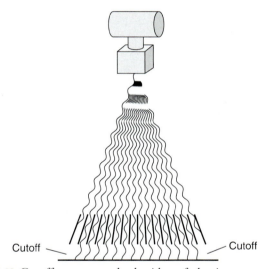

Fig. 9-16 Cutoff occurs on both sides of the image receptor when the source–image receptor distance is outside the focal range of the grid.

of the grid, rather than perpendicular to its center. The same effect is encountered if the grid is tipped side to side in relation to the primary beam (Fig. 9-15). Both of these problems involve only centering and angulation with respect to the *sides* of the grid. Cutoff does *not* result when the x-ray tube is off center lengthwise or angled along the length of the lead strips.

When a grid is used at a distance outside its focal range, cutoff will occur on both sides of the film (Fig. 9-16).

When the grid is reversed—that is, the wrong side is facing the x-ray tube—grid cutoff prevents most of the primary radiation from reaching the film (Fig. 9-17). A film taken with the grid reversed will show exposure only in a line down the center. The remainder of the film will be very light and streaked with grid lines.

Grid cutoff is prevented by ensuring that the x-ray beam is always properly aligned with the center of the grid at the appropriate distance. The precision required when aligning the x-ray beam to the grid is determined by the grid ratio. The higher the grid ratio, the more precise the alignment must be. This is why relatively high-ratio grids are used only in permanent installations where alignment is easily maintained. Lower-ratio grids are used for bedside radiography and other portable applications where it is more difficult to ensure precise alignment.

Specialty Grids

Specialty grids are available for special situations but are not suitable for general-purpose use. A grid with strips that are parallel to each other, rather than focused, is called a **parallel grid** (Fig. 9-18). The radius

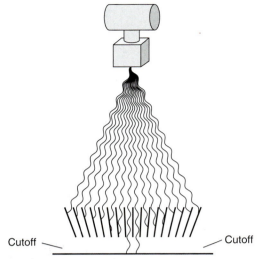

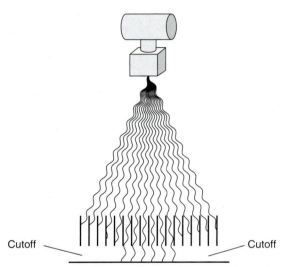

Fig. 9-17 Severe cutoff occurs when the grid is reversed. The image is visible only in the center, and grid lines are apparent.

Fig. 9-18 Lead strips of a parallel grid are not focused. This grid is practical for use only with very small fields and long source–image receptor distances (SIDs). The x-ray beam may be centered to the grid at any point. A short SID as shown will create cutoff at both sides.

of a parallel grid is infinity. Parallel grids can be used for radiography at very long SIDs because the useful portion of the x-ray beam is nearly perpendicular to the grid when the distance is great. They are available only in lower ratios. Parallel grids are also used in fluoroscopic spot film devices.

Another type of specialty grid is the **crosshatch grid,** sometimes called a *crossed grid.* This is actually a composite of two grids with the lead strips at right angles to each other (Fig. 9-19). A crosshatch grid is desirable because it has an effective ratio that is greater than the ratios of the two grids combined. For example, a crosshatch grid made of two 8:1 grids would be more efficient at preventing scatter radiation fog than a regular 16:1 grid, but would

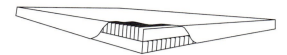

Fig. 9-19 A crosshatch grid consists of two grids laminated together with their lead strips perpendicular to each other. The x-ray tube cannot be angled when using a crosshatch grid.

have the alignment flexibility of an 8:1 grid. The limitation of the crosshatch grid is that it produces unacceptable grid cutoff when the x-ray tube is angled. It is useful only for procedures done with the central ray perpendicular to the grid and the film. This consideration makes it unsuitable for general use.

> ### Methods of Scatter Radiation Fog Control
>
> - Use grid device—grid placed between patient and film to absorb scatter
> - Use air gap—increased object–image receptor distance decreases scatter intensity at film
> - Minimize field size—decreases volume of scattering tissue
> - Decrease kilovoltage—decreases energy of scatter and increases contrast

Field Size and Collimation

Because field size and collimation significantly affect the volume of tissue irradiated, a reduction in field size will decrease the scatter radiation fog on the radiograph. For this reason, the radiation field is collimated to expose only the area of clinical interest. Decreasing the collimation improves contrast even when a grid or Bucky is used because it decreases the quantity of scatter that penetrates the grid (Fig. 9-20). When fog compromises the ability to see specific details in a large body part, it is common to take a **coned-down image** (Fig. 9-21). This term refers to a radiograph of a very small area of the subject. Most coned-down images are taken using an 8- × 10-inch IR and a 5- or 6-inch square field. They are centered precisely to the area of interest. Coned-down images demonstrate increased contrast compared with images of the same anatomy seen within a larger field. When a specific area of interest is centered to the field, as in a coned-down image, the decreased distortion also improves image quality.

Collimator and Central Ray Alignment

A quality control (QC) check is regularly performed on the collimator to ensure accuracy and to meet state and federal regulations. At the same time the collimator is tested, the x-ray beam alignment, or central ray alignment, is checked because in many instances it is the alignment of the tube that needs adjustment and not the collimator itself. This check is easily done

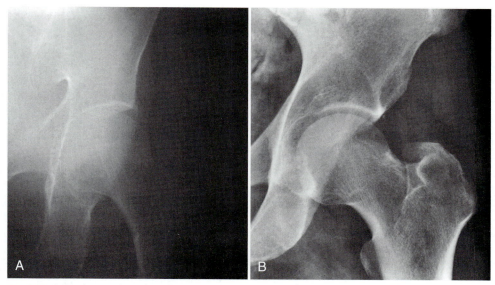

Fig. 9-20 A, Radiograph with collimator inadvertently opened to size 14 × 17 inches. Scattered radiation reduces contrast, and a poor-quality image results. **B,** Radiograph with collimator set correctly to 8 × 10 inches, which improves contrast and the visibility of detail.

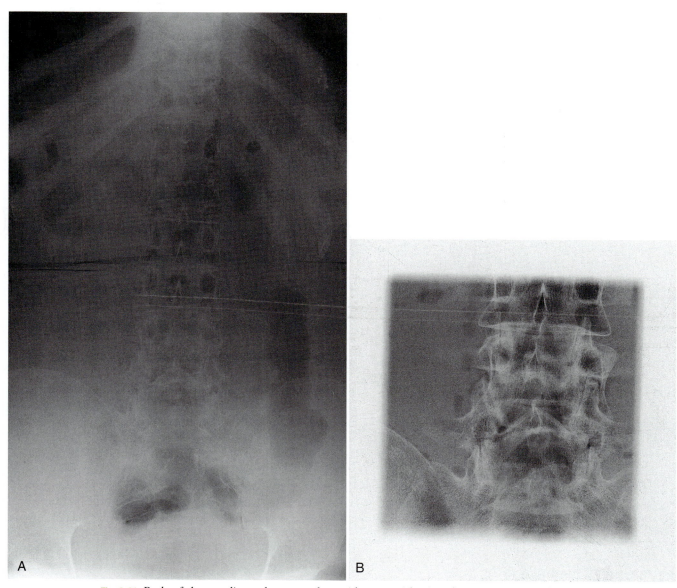

Fig. 9-21 Both of these radiographs were taken without a grid using the same exposure factors. **A,** A 35- × 43-cm image receptor results in excessive scatter radiation fog. **B,** A 5- × 5-inch coned-down radiation field significantly reduces scatter, improving visibility of detail on the image.

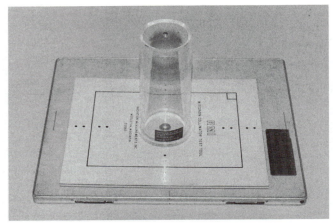

Fig. 9-22 Setup for the collimator and beam alignment quality control test. The template is placed on a cassette to check the collimator. The alignment cylinder is placed in the center of the template to check the beam alignment. Note the black square that the field light is collimated to.

with a *collimator template* and a *beam alignment cylinder* (Fig. 9-22). With the collimator test tool, an exposure is made with the template placed on the IR, and the light field is collimated to the indicated square. The standard control limit for the collimator is that the x-ray light field and the radiation field must be within ±2% of the SID. This means that at a 40-inch SID, the light field must be within 0.8 inch of the radiation field (Fig. 9-23).

An efficient quality control check can be done when the collimator template and a beam alignment cylinder are used together. Both the collimator and the alignment can be checked at the same time. The beam alignment cylinder (see Fig. 9-22) is placed directly on the collimator template, and the alignment is checked with the same exposure. A small lead bead at the top of the cylinder should be aligned with the small bead at the bottom of the cylinder if the alignment is correct. The standard control limit for the tube's CR beam alignment is that the tube must be mounted so that the x-ray beam is within *1 degree of perpendicular*. Fig. 9-23 shows two radiographs from the collimator and beam alignment test.

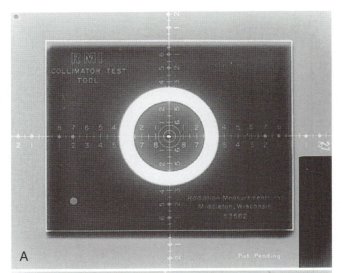

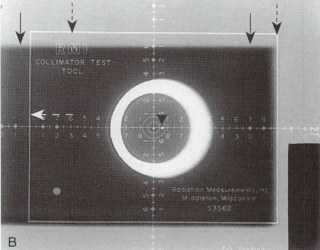

Fig. 9-23 Radiograph of the collimator and beam alignment test. **A,** Note that the radiation field falls almost directly on the square, indicating acceptable x-ray field and radiation field alignment. The beam alignment cylinder is sharp, and the two beads are directly on top of one another, indicating acceptable beam alignment. **B,** Unacceptable collimation and beam alignment. The radiation beam does not align with the collimator field light. Note that the collimator is clipping on one side *(black arrows)* and extending too far on another side *(white arrow)*. The beam alignment cylinder shows a blurred cylinder edge, and note that the two lead beads are not aligned *(arrowhead)*. Both the collimator and the beam alignment must be brought back into standard on this machine.

Grid Cutoff

Caused by misalignment between grid and x-ray beam.
- Lateral decentering
- Source–image receptor distance outside focal range
- Lateral angulation or grid off level
- Grid reversed

Decreasing Kilovoltage

When other methods fail to provide sufficient contrast, a decrease in kVp should be considered. Decreasing kVp increases contrast in two ways. First, this narrows the scale of contrast, as explained in Chapter 7. Second, lower kVp levels decrease the energy of the scatter radiation and decrease the fog, as explained earlier in this chapter. Of course, when kVp is decreased, radiographic density will also decrease. This requires an increase in milliampere-seconds to compensate. The mathematical calculations for maintaining radiographic density when changing kVp are discussed in Chapter 10. This change in exposure factors results in increased radiation dose to the patient, and so it should be used only when necessary. *Caution should also be used when lowering the kVp because the body part may not be penetrated if the kVp is lowered too much.*

SUMMARY

When diagnostic x-rays are absorbed by matter, they are "scattered," forming scatter and secondary radiation by means of coherent scattering, the Compton effect, or the photoelectric effect. The greatest quantity of scatter formed during routine radiography is caused by the Compton effect, which scatters photons in all directions.

This scattered radiation causes fog on the radiograph, decreasing radiographic contrast and decreasing the visibility of detail. The fog level becomes objectionable when the thickness of the subject is greater than 10 to 12 cm.

Scatter radiation fog is controlled primarily by using either a stationary grid or a moving grid device called a *Bucky*. The grid ratio indicates the efficiency of the grid in cleaning up scatter radiation and the precision with which the x-ray beam must be aligned with the grid. When the x-ray beam and the grid are not properly aligned with each other, grid cutoff results. Other means for reducing scatter radiation fog include reducing the field size and decreasing kVp.

Chapter 10

Formulating X-ray Techniques

At the conclusion of this chapter, you will be able to:

- Read and use an x-ray technique chart
- List methods for obtaining and/or creating an x-ray technique chart
- Accurately measure a body part using an x-ray caliper
- Compare fixed kilovolts peak (kVp) technique charts with variable kVp technique charts and state which is preferable
- Explain what is meant by "optimum kVp" and how this value is determined
- Select an appropriate milliamperage station for a given set of circumstances
- Take appropriate steps when the technique chart fails to provide an appropriate exposure
- Calculate exposure adjustments for changes in patient part size
- Determine the technique change required when radiographs are too dark or too light
- Suggest appropriate technique changes for increasing or decreasing the scale of contrast
- Calculate technique changes for variations in source–image receptor distance
- Explain the use of compensating filters for certain body structures
- Select the appropriate compensating filter for given body parts

Key Terms

caliper
compensating filter
fixed kVp chart
latitude
optimum kVp

radiographic phantom
technique chart
The Joint Commission
variable kVp chart

Most radiography departments have a functional technique chart that provides appropriate exposures for most circumstances. This chapter explores the components of technique charts and explains their limitations. When there is no chart or when the existing chart is inadequate, the limited operator must obtain or create a suitable chart. It is important to remember that no chart meets the requirements for every circumstance. When the planned procedure differs from the chart, the operator must make appropriate changes in the exposure settings. These radiographic examinations might include those involving patients who are larger or smaller than the measurements provided on the chart or patients whose conditions affect the amount of exposure required. Permanent changes in the type of grid, kilovoltage (kVp), milliamperage (mA), or source–image receptor distance (SID) will require a change in technique.

There is no one perfect set of factors that must be used for each exposure. A number of possible combinations may produce a diagnostic radiograph. The limited operator is responsible for ensuring that the technique chart is available, complete, and consistent. It must meet the requirements of the equipment and the preferences of the physician who will interpret the radiographs.

This chapter contains some formulas and mathematical calculations that all limited operators must master. The basic mathematical skills needed to perform these calculations are reviewed in Chapter 3, which also includes additional examples and practice problems to increase your proficiency.

TECHNIQUE CHARTS

A **technique chart** is a listing of the various radiographic examinations performed in the facility. It provides exposure factors for each body part according to its thickness. Table 10-1 is an example of a portion of a manual exposure technique chart. It is called *manual* because each technical factor is set "manually" by the x-ray operator. It includes the following information: type of examination, projection, SID, patient/part measurement (in centimeters), kVp, mA, exposure time, and a grid (Bucky) notation.

X-ray machines that use automatic exposure control (AEC) or anatomically programmed radiography (APR) systems must also have a technique chart. The chart should indicate all the items that a manual technique chart does, except the exposure time (which is automatic). The AEC chart will also have to indicate which of the three detectors to use for each projection. Most of these charts will have a combination of both AEC and manual techniques (Table 10-2).

Some limited operators become so familiar with the operation of their equipment over time that they tend to memorize or estimate exposures and do not feel the need for a technique chart. This practice may result in outdated or unavailable charts and may cause unnecessary exposure errors. Radiation control regulations may require posting of a current technique chart and may also specify the information to be included. In Oregon, for example, regulations require that technique charts include a notation that gonad shielding is required for specific examinations. **The Joint Commission,** the official organization that accredits hospitals and clinics, establishes standards for institutions that receive Medicare payments, and these standards include requirements for x-ray technique charts in radiography departments. Limited operators must be aware of requirements for technique charts and ensure that their charts conform to the regulatory standards.

Table 10-1

Example of Portion of a Manual Exposure Radiographic Technique Chart

	Lumbar Spine					
	AP and Oblique 40-inch SID Bucky			Lateral 40-inch SID Bucky		
cm	mA	sec	kVp	mA	sec	kVp
18–19	200	.04	86			
20–21	200	.05	86			
22–23	200	.06	86			
24–25	200	.08	86	200		96
26–27	200	.1	90	200	.15	96
28–29	200	.15	90	200	.2	96
30–31	200	.2	90	200	.25	96
32–33	200	.25	90	200	.37	96
34–35	200	.37	95	200	.5	102
36–37	200	.5	95	200	.65	102
38–39	200	.65	95	200	.85	102
40–41	200	.85	95	200	1.2	102

NOTE: Measure at level of anterior superior iliac spine. Use gonad shielding.
AP, Anteroposterior; *SID,* source–image receptor distance.

Table 10-2

Exposure Technique Chart for Shoulder Girdle Projections

				Shoulder Girdle				
Part	**cm**	**kVp***	**sec**	**mA**	**mAs**	**AEC†**	**SID**	**IR**
Shoulder— *AP‡*	18	75		200s		□□■	48 in	24 × 30 cm
Shoulder— *transthoracic lateral‡*	40	80		200s		□□■	48 in	24 × 30 cm
Shoulder— *axillary§*	18	75	.08	200s	16		48 in	10 × 12 inch
Shoulder— *PA oblique scapular Y‡*	24	85	.08	200s	16		48 in	24 × 30 cm
Intertubercular *groove§*—	3	55	.01	200s	2		48 in	8 × 10 inch
A-C articulation— *AP‡*	14	70	.15	200s	30		72 in	18 × 43 cm
Clavicle— *AP, PA‡*	16	70	.06	200s	12		48 in	24 × 30 cm
Scapula— *AP‡*	18	75		200s		□□■	48 in	24 × 30 cm
Scapula— *lateral‡*	24	85	.08	200s	16		48 in	24 × 30 cm

From Frank ED, Long BW, Smith BJ: *Merrill's atlas of radiographic positions and radiologic procedures*, ed 11, vol 1, St Louis, 2007, Mosby. Note that both manual and AEC techniques are shown.

*Kilovoltage values are for a three-phase 12-pulse generator.

†Each of these squares represents one of the three detectors in the AEC device.

‡Bucky, 16:1 grid.

§Tabletop, 8:1 grid.

A-C, Acromioclavicular; *AEC*, automatic exposure control; *AP*, anteroposterior; *IR*, image receptor; *PA*, posteroanterior; *s*, small focal spot; *SID*, source–image receptor distance.

Technique charts are unique to each x-ray machine and each facility. The x-ray machine manufacturer cannot supply a definitive chart with the machine because the exposures will vary considerably depending on the types of grids, tabletops, and SID. When a new chart is necessary, there are several possible sources.

Some of the major x-ray vendors will supply computer-generated charts for their customers. The local technical representative of your x-ray supply company may come to your department on request and do some testing to obtain the necessary data. These data are submitted to the company, and the chart is sent to your facility.

In some communities, experienced radiologic technologists will prepare a technique chart for a fee. This option is often advantageous because the chart can be made specifically for your facility and equipment, using only settings available on your control panel. Exposures may be provided for any procedures unique to your facility. Such a chart is also more likely to conform to local radiation control regulations.

A chart that needs to be changed because *all* of the exposures are too light or too dark can probably be modified easily. When the chart is consistent throughout—that is, all of the exposures are too light or too dark to about the same degree—it is a simple matter of increasing or decreasing all of the exposure times by a specific percentage to correct the radiographic density for all exposures. If your existing chart is not consistent, the use of a consistent chart borrowed from another facility with the identical equipment or from Appendix D may provide a starting point.

An exposure technique chart should be prepared with a calibrated x-ray machine and the specific type of image receptor (IR) used. After this, a technique chart that is not working will require checking the calibration of the x-ray machine, the digital processor system, or both. Sometimes the problem is an x-ray operator who is not following the techniques posted on the chart. *Technically, a well-prepared exposure technique chart should never be changed.* Also a chart should not be changed because of temporary changes in the calibration of the x-ray machine. Before a chart that has been working well is changed, all potential factors that could affect the techniques should be evaluated. A radiologic technologist with experience in using quality control test tools can easily determine if the x-ray machine is calibrated before calling the service personnel to invasively check the machine.

Finally, if you decide to prepare a chart yourself, products are available to assist you. Supertech Inc.[d] offers both computer software and a handheld slide rule to calculate exposures. Both products are supplied with a small penetrometer and a master density chart (Fig. 10-1, *A*). These are used to test your system and gather the basic data needed to tailor the tool to your x-ray department. Complete instructions are included. The Supertech

[d]Supertech Inc., P.O. Box 186, Elkhart, IN 46515; www.supertechx-ray.com.

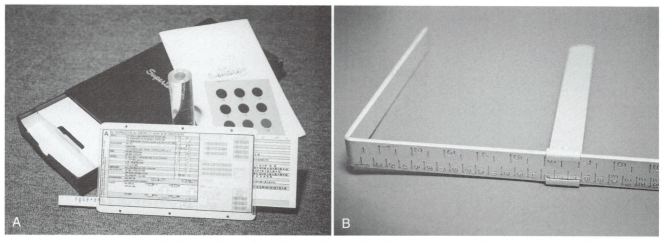

Fig. 10-1 A, Supertech calculator kit. **B,** X-ray caliper for measurement of body parts.

computer software generates technique charts that conform to The Joint Commission standards.

Regardless of whether you prepare the chart yourself or arrange for its preparation by someone else, some testing is needed to establish baseline data for your system. This testing should be done when the processor is functioning at optimal levels. The same IRs that will be used with the chart should be used for testing. It is helpful to have a record of exposures kept over a period of time that lists the examination, measurement, exposure factors, and an assessment of the images produced.

Before using your technique chart to take radiographs of patients, it is helpful to test some of your exposures using a **radiographic phantom.** A radiographic phantom is a human skeleton, or portion of a skeleton, encased in a plastic material that is similar in density to human tissue. You may already be familiar with phantoms through experience in your radiography education program. A good phantom provides an excellent simulation of radiography of a human patient. It may be possible to borrow one from your film company's technical representative, from your x-ray supply dealer, or from a radiography education program.

Computerized control units with programmed exposure settings or "anatomic programming" such as APR will automatically select the kVp, milliampere-seconds (mAs), and AEC detectors for an examination when the radiographer selects the body part and enters the measurement. To function accurately, these units must first be programmed with exposures that meet the requirements of the facility. In other words, a technique chart must be created and entered into the control's computer. Even with this type of equipment, radiation control agencies may require posting of a printed technique chart.

PATIENT MEASUREMENT

Technique charts are based on the measurement of the body part to be radiographed. The radiographer must measure the body part accurately to select the correct exposure from the technique chart or to obtain the correct exposure with a programmable computerized control.

The tool for body part measurement is called a **caliper** (Fig. 10-1, *B*). The main shaft of the caliper is a flat strip of metal, calibrated in both inches and centimeters. There are two perpendicular extensions from the shaft: one is permanently affixed to one end of the shaft and the other slides up and down the shaft. These two extensions form "jaws" between which the body part is measured.

It is usual for technique charts and computerized controls to specify the part measurement in centimeters. The dimension to be measured is the thickness through which the x-ray beam will pass. Measurements of the trunk of the body should always be made in the same general position as for radiography because measurements may change significantly when the patient changes position. For example, upright measurements of the abdomen are often 4 to 6 cm greater than measurements of the same region when the patient is lying down.

When a body part is measured, the fixed jaw of the caliper is placed under or against the part and the movable jaw is brought snugly and firmly against the patient on the opposite side (Fig. 10-2). You must take care that the jaws of the caliper remain parallel to each other. Pressing the jaws too tightly against the patient may cause them to spread apart at the open end, resulting in an inaccurate measurement. You must also take care that you do not measure air space. For instance, if the patient is lying on the table and you are measuring the thickness of the patient at the waist, the arch of the patient's back may leave a space between the back and the tabletop. Measuring from the tabletop to the surface of the patient's abdomen will give an inaccurate measurement. *Both jaws of the caliper must be firmly in contact with the body part.*

Body parts are usually measured through the path of the central ray. Some parts, however, may be measured through their thickest portion, or another method may

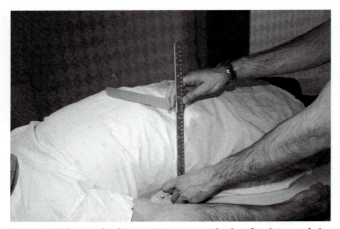

Fig. 10-2 When a body part is measured, the fixed jaw of the caliper is placed under or against the part and the movable jaw is brought snugly and firmly against the patient on the opposite side. Take care that the jaws of the caliper remain parallel to each other.

be used. For example, exposures for the anteroposterior (AP) open-mouth projection of the upper cervical spine are usually based on the cervical spine measurement taken in the midcervical region. When there is variation in measurement method, it should be stated in the technique chart. The technique chart is designed for a specific measurement method and will not produce accurate results unless the measurement is consistent with the method intended by the chart.

FIXED KILOVOLTAGE VERSUS VARIABLE KILOVOLTAGE

Years ago, it was common to construct technique charts based on a specific mAs value for each projection and to vary the kVp by 2 to 3 kVp/cm for changes in patient/part size. This type of chart is called a **variable kVp chart.** One of the advantages of a variable kVp chart is that overall image contrast is higher, which may provide greater visibility of detail. Also, variable kVp enables small incremental changes in exposure techniques that mA and exposure time cannot. Another type of chart is a **fixed kVp chart.** For this method, an optimum kVp value is established for each projection and the mAs is varied according to the patient/part thickness. The advantages of a fixed kVp chart are as follows. When the kVp levels are kept to the high end of the optimum range, exposures will have more **latitude** for exposure error. Latitude means that a wider range of densities, especially grays, are shown on the image. Exposures may be designated for small, medium, large, and extra-large patients, rather than having a separate listing for each centimeter measurement. When this is the case, each size category should state the size range in centimeters. Radiation exposure to patients may be somewhat lower with fixed kVp technique charts. In most departments, there

are some charts that are set up as variable kVp and some that are fixed kVp.

An experienced radiologic technologist and a radiologist will usually, together, determine the best type of chart for a particular facility. In most instances, a combination of both is used.

Some control panels do not have a sufficiently wide range of possible mAs combinations to provide ideal exposures at fixed kVp for all patient/part sizes. Small kVp changes can be used to "fine tune" exposures between mAs settings to obtain a proper exposure for each measurement. This results in a modified fixed kVp chart in which mAs is the primary variable but kVp fluctuates within a range of ±4 kVp from the optimum level.

OPTIMUM KILOVOLTAGE

The kVp setting for any examination must first provide sufficient penetration of the body part to create an image. Kilovoltage settings that are too low will result in a high-contrast image that may not show all the anatomic parts and a higher dose to the patient. The best policy is to use the highest kVp setting that will produce sufficient contrast for acceptable image quality. This setting is referred to as **optimum kVp.** This approach will result in the least patient exposure and the greatest exposure latitude.

The optimum kVp for a specific examination may be determined by taking a series of images with a radiographic phantom. Fig. 10-3 illustrates such a series, taken at 15% rule (exposure doubled) increments. In each case, the mAs was reduced 50% to maintain approximately the same radiographic density on all of the radiographs. It is not possible to evaluate the contrast of a radiograph that is too dark or too light. The radiographic density must be in an acceptable range for contrast to be apparent. The mAs must be adjusted to maintain the desired radiographic density when changing kVp. These adjustments are explained later in this chapter. The ideal kVp levels for your facility will depend on the grid ratio and phase of generator and should also correspond with the preferences of the radiologist who will read the radiographs. Useful ranges have been well established by the experience of others. Appendix E provides a listing of suggested optimum kVp ranges that will assist you by providing a starting point.

The kVp for a body part is established for a given room and for each projection in that room. Once established on the technique chart, the kVp should never be changed unless the contrast in the image needs to be adjusted.

CRITERIA FOR MILLIAMPERAGE SELECTION

Many of the exposure changes in this chapter involve changes in the mAs value. Most computerized control

55 kVp, 12 mAs

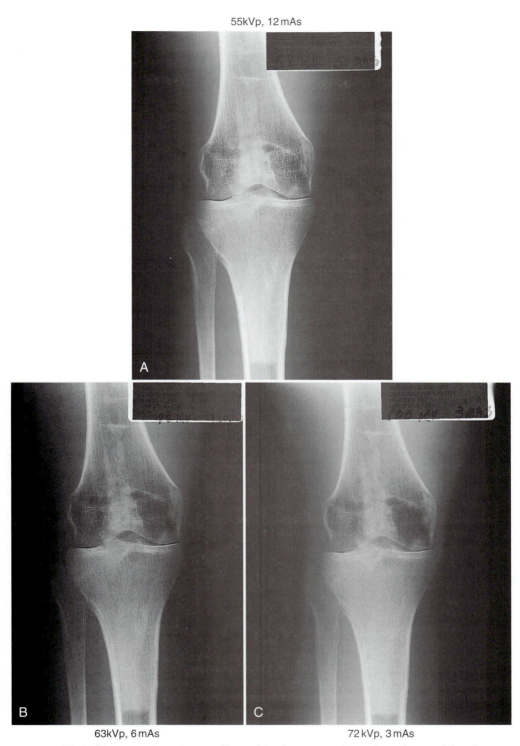

A

63 kVp, 6 mAs

72 kVp, 3 mAs

Fig. 10-3 Typical image series using a radiographic phantom to determine adequate kilovoltage. Note that **A** has high contrast, **B** has moderate contrast, and **C** has low contrast. The correct contrast level will be determined by the radiologist. Note the kVp doubled (using the 15% rule) and the mAs was reduced by 50% to keep image density the same.

panels provide the option of setting the mAs directly. Older units, however, will require you to decide how a given quantity of mAs will be obtained. As explained in Chapters 5 and 7, mAs is the product of mA and time, and several possible combinations of mA and time may be used to achieve the desired quantity of exposure. For

example, 10 mAs may be obtained using any of the following combinations:

$$50 \text{ mA}, 0.2 \text{ sec} = 10 \text{ mAs}$$
$$100 \text{ mA}, 0.1 \text{ sec} = 10 \text{ mAs}$$
$$200 \text{ mA}, 0.05 \text{ sec} = 10 \text{ mAs}$$

When a technique chart is being created or mAs values are being adjusted, the question then arises as to which of several possible combinations is best. In choosing an mA setting, the limited operator should consider the tube rating, focal spot size, exposure time requirements, and available mA and time settings.

CALCULATING EXPOSURE TIME

When the desired mAs is known and you have selected an mA setting according to the criteria discussed earlier, the next step is to determine the exposure time. To determine the exposure time, divide the desired mAs by the selected mA. This is a variation of the mAs formula:

$$\frac{mAs}{mA} = \text{Time (sec)}$$

Example: Suppose the desired mAs is 50, and you have decided to use 200 mA.

Using the formula:

$$\frac{50 \text{ mAs}}{200 \text{ mAs}} = 0.25 \text{ sec}$$

It is helpful to make an mAs chart for your machine. Create a column for each mA station and label the rows with the exposure time settings available on your control panel. Then calculate the mAs for all possible combinations and enter them on the chart. An example of such a chart is included in Appendix F. An mAs chart is a helpful reference when creating a technique chart or when departing from the usual exposure for a particular case, such as a patient who is unable to hold still.

TECHNIQUE CHART "FAILURE"

When a technique chart produces inconsistent results, it is often because the kVp levels are not optimal. Too low a kVp range will tend to produce too much contrast for smaller part measurements. For larger part measurements, insufficient penetration will result in films that are too light. When the fixed kVp is too high, radiographs will lack contrast, especially when the part measurement is at the upper end of the size range. These problems are solved by adjusting the level of the fixed kVp for those categories that are causing problems. Changes in kVp will require adjustments in mAs. The calculation of these adjustments is discussed later in this chapter.

Even the best technique charts do not always produce ideal radiographs. One possible cause is variation in generator x-ray output and calibration. When x-ray images are too dark or too light, it is wise to perform a quality control check of the digital system or the generator, or an experienced radiologic technologist can check the kVp, mA, and exposure time using quality control tools before modifying the technique chart. Another possible cause is inconsistency

in patient/part measurement, which will produce inconsistent results. It is important that the measurement method conform to the technique chart. Some radiographers always measure body parts through the path of the central ray. Others may measure at the thickest portion of the part for some or all examinations. It is helpful to include measurement instructions on the technique chart. Accurate body part measurement is explained earlier in this chapter.

Technique charts are constructed to meet the requirements of average or normal tissue densities for each body part. Tissue density may vary significantly because of disease, age, or muscle tone. An athlete or laborer may have muscle tissue that is much greater in density than average, requiring more exposure. Elderly patients usually have diminished bone density and muscle tone, requiring less exposure. As you gain experience you will learn to recognize patients whose tissue density requires adjustments to the exposures provided in the technique chart. Box 10-1 lists conditions that require an increase

 Box 10-1

Conditions Requiring an Exposure Increase (Hard to Penetrate)

Chest Conditions
Atelectasis
Bronchiectasis
Cardiomegaly
Congestive heart failure
Edema, pulmonary
Empyema
Hemothorax
Hydropneumothorax
Metastases (blastic)
Pleural effusion
Pneumoconiosis diseases
Pneumonia
Tuberculosis (calcific, miliary)

Conditions of Bone
Acromegaly
Arthritis, rheumatoid
Osteochondroma
Osteomyelitis, healed
Osteopetrosis (marble bone)
Paget disease

Abdomen
Ascites
Cirrhosis of liver

Soft Tissue
Edema

Generalized Conditions
Heavy musculature
Large bones

For each of the conditions listed above, increase body part measurement by 2 to 4 cm, depending on severity.

 Box 10-2

Conditions Requiring an Exposure Decrease (Easy to Penetrate)

Chest Conditions
Chronic obstructive pulmonary disease (emphysema)
Pneumothorax
Tuberculosis, active

Conditions of Bone
Arthritis, degenerative
Gout
Hyperparathyroidism
Metastasis, lytic
Multiple myeloma
Necrosis
Osteomyelitis, active
Osteoporosis
Sarcoma

Abdomen
Bowel obstruction
Pneumoperitoneum

Generalized Conditions
Advanced age
Atrophy
Emaciation

For each of the conditions listed above, decrease body part measurement by 2 to 4 cm, depending on severity of condition.

in exposure; Box 10-2 lists conditions that require a decrease in exposure. Some lists of this type suggest a specific amount of exposure change for each condition. The proper adjustment will depend on the severity of the condition. An increase or decrease of 2 to 4 cm from the patient measurement is a convenient method for arriving at a suitable technique.

ADJUSTMENT OF TECHNIQUES

Variations in Patient/Part Size

As the thickness of the subject increases, radiographic density will decrease unless adjustments are made in exposure. This adjustment is usually in the form of a change in mAs. A 30% mAs increase will compensate for a 2-cm increase in part size. This change compounds, like compound interest, and adjustment may require multiple steps. When decreasing technique to compensate for a smaller part size, the mAs is reduced by 20% for each 2 cm of part size reduction.

Example: Your routine technique for a lumbar spine measuring 20 cm is 200 mA, 0.15 second, 80 kVp, 40-inch SID. What technique would you use for a patient whose lumbar spine measured 24 cm?

Adjust for part size by increasing mAs 30% for each 2 cm of additional size.
First, determine the mAs:

$$200 \text{ mA} \times 0.15 \text{ sec} = 30 \text{ mAs}$$

To increase to 22 cm, multiply the mAs by 1.3 (100% + 30%):

$$30 \text{ mAs} \times 1.3 = 39 \text{ mAs}$$

To increase to 24 cm, multiply the new mAs (39) by 1.3:

$$39 \text{ mAs} \times 1.3 = 50.7 \text{ mAs (round off to 50 mAs)}$$

In this case, as with others in this chapter, the "ideal" mAs value may be one that is not available on the control panel. Because mAs variations of up to 20% are scarcely noticeable on the radiograph, the ideal mAs can usually be rounded up or down to the nearest available mAs value without any significant effect on radiographic density. If in doubt about which of the available mAs values to select, always select the highest. Now you must select appropriate mA and time settings to produce the calculated mAs, as explained earlier in this chapter.

It is also possible to compensate for part size variations using kVp, but this method should be used only when the size variation is relatively small because a large change in kVp will also alter contrast and may have negative effects on radiographic quality. A change of 2 kVp/cm is sufficient below 85 kVp; above 85 kVp, a 3-kVp change is necessary.

Example: A satisfactory lateral cervical spine radiograph is made on a patient measuring 12 cm using 100 mA, 0.05 second, and 76 kVp at 72-inch SID. Vary the kVp to alter this exposure for a patient measuring 10 cm.

Because the size variation is small, kVp may be used in this instance. Since the original kVp is less than 85, the compensation will be a reduction of 2 kVp/cm. The size difference is 2 cm (12 cm − 10 cm).

$$2 \text{ cm} \times 2 \text{ kVp/cm} = 4 \text{ kVp}$$
$$76 \text{ kVp} - 4 \text{ kVp} = 72 \text{ kVp}$$

Therefore, the new exposure will be 100 mA, 0.05 second, 72 kVp, 72-inch SID. Chapter 3 contains further discussion of these methods of technique adjustment with additional examples and practice problems.

Pediatric Techniques

If babies, small children, youngsters, and small teenagers are having x-ray examinations in your department, a special technique chart will have to be established. In Chapter 11 you will learn that *the rapidly developing tissues of children are much more sensitive to radiation damage than adults.* Therefore careful attention to providing accurate exposure techniques for x-ray of children is crucial. Repeats on children should be kept to a minimum. Also, your department should provide special training in positioning, restraining, and setting exposure techniques in children. Chapter 18 provides additional information on working with pediatrics.

Obese Patient Techniques

Modified x-ray exposure techniques need to be used on obese patients. The main factors have to be increased, including the mA, kVp, and exposure time. The *major limitation* in obtaining images of obese patients is inadequate penetration of the body part. This situation results in increased quantum mottle (noise) and very low image contrast. The increased exposure time required in these patients can also contribute to motion artifacts in the image. The single most important adjustment that should be made is an increase in the kVp. Increasing the kVp increases the penetration of the x-ray beam. The mA and exposure time (mAs) have to be increased; however, caution should be used in increasing the mA. Greater exposures can be obtained safely by using low mA settings and longer exposure times. (See tube rating chart in Chapter 6.)

Motion is not a major problem in imaging obese patients because the weight of the patient prevents most body parts from moving, and mA settings of about 320 can be used. This setting may increase the exposure time; however, with an explanation of the importance of holding the breath, most obese patients can do so. With repeated use of high exposure factors, the x-ray tube can become very hot. Limited operators should ensure that adequate cooling of the anode and tube as a whole occurs; this can be accomplished by simply taking more time between exposures. It is also important to point out that obese patients often are not able to have an x-ray done, in particular in the abdominal and pelvic areas. The maximum weight of the x-ray table is 450 lb but many manufacturers are increasing this to about 700 lb. Ensure that your table can handle the weight of these patients.

Alteration of Radiographic Density

When an image is too light, the best solution is usually an increase in mAs. *The minimum change necessary to cause a visible change in image density is 30% of mAs.* Likewise, when the image is too dark, mAs may be decreased. There are very few instances in which the kVp is changed when images are too light or too dark. Changing mAs by a specific quantity does not always produce the same result. It is the *percentage change* that is significant. Fig. 10-4 illustrates changes in radiographic density produced by various percentages of mAs increase. If an image is so light that it must be repeated to obtain diagnostic quality, at least a *doubling* (100% increase) is usually necessary. When decreasing density, a smaller percentage change is required. That is, a 50% mAs reduction produces the same amount of change as a 100% increase (see Fig. 10-4). *The general rule of thumb for mAs changes is to make adjustments in increments of doubles or halves.*

Although these changes will become much easier for you to estimate with experience, the main lesson here is

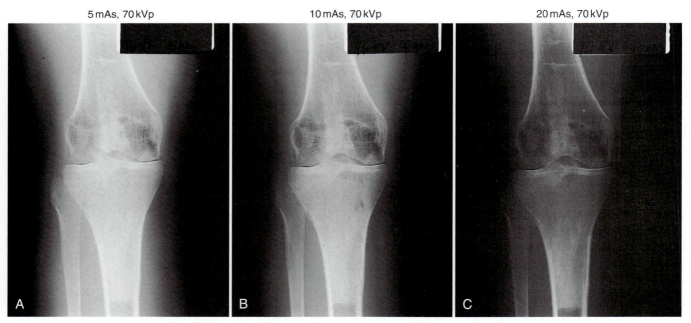

| 5 mAs, 70 kVp | 10 mAs, 70 kVp | 20 mAs, 70 kVp |

Fig. 10-4 Adjusting milliampere-seconds (mAs) to correct an image that is too light or too dark. Note that the knee in **A** is too light, and doubling the mAs will produce an acceptable density as in **B**. Image **C** is too dark, and reducing its mAs by 50% will produce an acceptable density as in **B**. Doubling the mAs or cutting the mAs by 50% will have a visible effect on density as shown.

that you must be bold when making changes. Trying to correct improper density with very small increments of change is ineffective.

Alteration of Contrast Levels

A change in kVp is often used to alter contrast. Because kVp affects the quantity of exposure to the IR, changing kVp will also affect radiographic density. For this reason, when an image of appropriate density requires a change in contrast, it is necessary to change both the kVp and the mAs. Whether working with an entire technique chart or a single exposure, the 15% rule can be used to change the level of contrast while keeping the density constant.

The 15% Rule

The 15% rule is based on the fact that a 15% change in kVp will produce approximately the same change in radiographic density as a doubling or halving of the mAs.

To decrease contrast, increase kVp by 15% and divide the mAs by 2. This application of the 15% rule increases latitude and creates a longer scale of contrast.

Example: A radiograph is made using 20 mAs and 68 kVp. The radiographic density is acceptable, but a longer scale of contrast is desired. To calculate the new exposure, first increase kVp by 15% (100% + 15% = 115%, or 1.15):

$$68 \text{ kVp} \times 1.15 = 78.2 \text{ kVp (round off to 78 kVp)}$$

Next, divide the mAs by 2:

$$20 \text{ mAs} \div 2 = 10 \text{ mAs}$$

Therefore the new exposure is 10 mAs at 78 kVp (Fig. 10-5).

To increase contrast, decrease kVp by 15% and multiply the mAs by 2. This application of the 15% rule decreases latitude and creates a shorter scale of contrast.

Example: A radiograph is made using 10 mAs and 65 kVp. The radiographic density is acceptable, but a shorter scale of contrast (high contrast) is desired. To calculate the new exposure, first decrease kVp by 15%.

$$65 \text{ kVp} \times 0.15 = 9.75 \text{ kVp (round off to 10 kVp)}$$
$$65 \text{ kVp} - 10 = 55 \text{ kVp}$$

Next, multiply the mAs by 2:

$$10 \text{ mAs} \times 2 = 20 \text{ mAs}$$

Therefore the new exposure is 20 mAs at 55 kVp.

Fig. 10-6 illustrates application of the 15% rule for increasing radiographic contrast. See also Chapter 3.

Variations in Source–image Receptor Distance

Changes in SID are not routine. A standard distance is established for each procedure, and the technique chart provides the correct exposure for the standard distance. Sometimes it will be necessary to modify exposures for changes in distance. For example, bedside and surgical radiography with mobile equipment may not permit use of the usual distance.

As explained in Chapter 7, variations in SID result in changes in radiation intensity. If the SID is to be changed without altering radiographic density, the mAs must be modified accordingly. The formula for this change is shown. The mAs is directly proportional to SID. If the SID is increased, the mAs is increased and vice versa. The

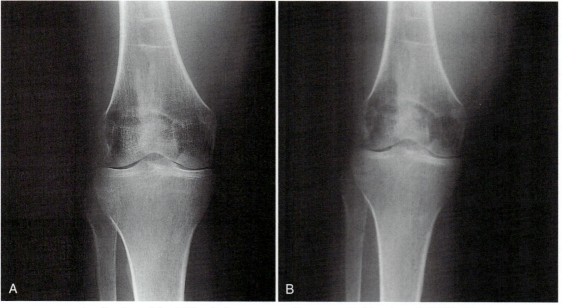

Fig. 10-5 Application of the 15% rule for contrast adjustment. **A,** 20 mAs and 68 kVp. **B,** 10 mAs and 78 kVp. Note less contrast in **B** because of a higher kilovoltage (kVp).

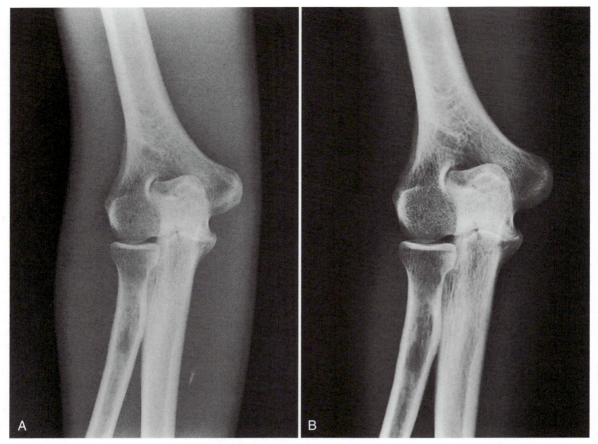

Fig. 10-6 Application of the 15% rule for contrast adjustment. **A,** 10 mAs and 65 kVp. **B,** 20 mAs and 55 kVp. Note higher contrast in **B** because of lower kilovoltage (kVp).

SIDs are always in this formula. The SIDs are always squared in this formula.

$$\frac{mAs_1}{mAs_2} = \frac{D_1^2}{D_2^2}$$

Example: Suppose that the usual technique for chest radiography of a patient measuring 20 cm is 4 mAs, 110 kVp, at 72-inch SID. In this case it is necessary to perform the examination at a 60-inch SID. How should the technique factors be changed? The solution to this distance problem involves a change in the mAs according to the formula given earlier. To solve it, substitute known values in the equation:

$$\frac{4\ mAs}{X} = \frac{72^2}{60^2}$$

Square the distances:

$$\frac{4\ mAs}{X} = \frac{5184}{3600}$$

Cross multiply and divide:

$$4 \times 3600 = 14,400$$

and

$$14,400 \div 5184 = 2.78$$

Table 10-3

Approximate Calculations for Changes in Source–image Receptor Distance (SID)

From 40-inch SID to	60 inch	72 inch	80 inch
Multiply mAs by	2	3	4

mAs, Milliampere-seconds.

Round the mAs:

$$X = 3\ mAs$$

Table 10-3 provides guidelines for approximate exposure changes for common variations in SID. See also Chapter 3.

COMPENSATING FILTERS

Radiography is usually accomplished using a single exposure technique for a given body structure. However, some structures contain areas of significantly varied tissue density that must be shown on one image. These structures present special challenges in demonstrating the anatomic structures with an acceptable range of densities. Often,

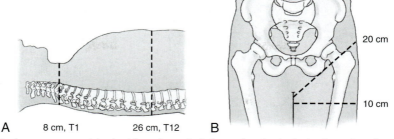

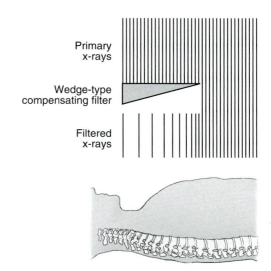

Fig. 10-7 Body structures with significantly varied tissue density include thoracic spine (antero-posterior) **(A)** and hip (lateral) **(B)**.

two exposures must be made on these body structures, which doubles the radiation exposure to the patient. Typically, if one exposure is used, a technique is selected to adequately penetrate the densest area of anatomy. In this case, the radiologist will highlight the dark anatomic area on the image with a "hot light." However, these images often have to be viewed by other physicians who do not have such a light available. With digital radiography systems, the image can be adjusted with the computer to lighten the dark area of anatomy; however, the large difference in transmitted x-rays often exceeds the dynamic range of the software. This can result in images that appear low in contrast, contain high noise, or show processing artifacts.

Examples of x-ray projections that have to demonstrate significantly varied tissue density include the *AP projection of the thoracic spine and the axiolateral projection (Danelius-Miller method) of the hip* (Fig. 10-7), *AP shoulder, lateral C7-T1 cervicothoracic area, AP foot, and AP and lateral scoliosis spine.* Exposure of these structures with a uniformly intense x-ray beam results in the production of an image with areas of underexposed or overexposed anatomy. To compensate for these variations in tissue density, specially designed attenuating devices called **compensating filters** can be placed between the radiographic tube and the IR. The resulting attenuated beam more appropriately exposes the various tissue densities of the anatomy and reveals more anatomic detail. Equally important, the filter will somewhat reduce the entrance skin exposure and therefore the dose to some of the organs in the body (Fig. 10-8).

Fig. 10-9 includes some of the most common filters in use today. These filters can be used with both screen/film and digital imaging systems to improve the image quality of a variety of anatomic areas. With most digital systems, filters are necessary to obtain a diagnostic image of an extreme density-different body part. In addition, radiation exposure to the patient is lowered through elimination of the extra exposures needed to demonstrate all of the anatomy and through the absorption of x-rays in some areas of the filter itself.

The appropriate use of radiographic compensating filters is an important aspect of the work of the limited

Fig. 10-8 Wedge-type compensating filter in position for an anteroposterior projection of the thoracic spine. Note how the thick portion of the wedge partially attenuates the x-ray beam over the upper thoracic area while the nonfilter area receives the full exposure to penetrate the thick portion of the spine. An even image density results.

operator. The operator determines whether or not to use a filter based on an assessment of the patient and then determines the type and exact position of the filter. This is accomplished while positioning the patient. Radiographic projections of the lateral hip and the lateral C7 to T1 cervicothoracic region in most instances will require a filter to demonstrate all the anatomy on one image. Projections such as the AP shoulder and AP thoracic spine may not need a filter on patients with hyposthenic physiques; however, on patients with hypersthenic physiques and patients who are barrel-chested or obese, a filter is necessary. Pediatric patients seldom require a filter, except when AP lateral projections of the full spine are done in cases of spinal curvatures such as scoliosis. The use of compensating filters for full-spine radiography not only allows the entire spine to be imaged with one exposure, it also significantly reduces the radiation exposure to the young age group that requires these images.

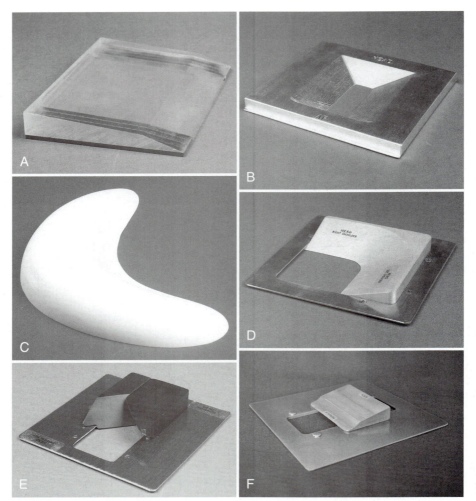

Fig. 10-9 Examples of compensating filters in use today. **A,** Supertech wedge, collimator-mounted Clear-Pb filter used for the anteroposterior (AP) projection of the hips, knees, and ankles on long (51-inch) film. **B,** Trough, collimator-mounted aluminum filter with a double wedge used for AP projections of the thoracic spine. **C,** Boomerang contact filter used for AP projections of the shoulder and facial bones. **D,** Ferlic collimator-mounted filter used for AP and posteroanterior oblique (scapular Y) projections of the shoulders. **E,** Ferlic collimator-mounted filter used for lateral projections of the cervicothoracic region (swimmer's technique) and axiolateral projections (Danelius-Miller method) of the hip. **F,** Ferlic collimator-mounted filter for AP projections of the foot.

Placement

Compensating filters are most often placed in the x-ray beam between the x-ray tube and patient. Broadly, filters fall into two categories based on their location during use: *collimator-mounted* filters and *contact* filters. The collimator-mounted filters are the most common and are mounted on the collimator, either using rails installed on both sides of the window on the collimator housing (Fig. 10-10) or using magnets. Generally, those filters placed between the primary beam and the body will have the added benefit of a reduction in radiation exposure to the patient because of the beam-hardening effect of the filter, whereas those placed between the anatomic part and the IR will have no effect on patient exposure. Measurements provided with the Ferlic filters[e]

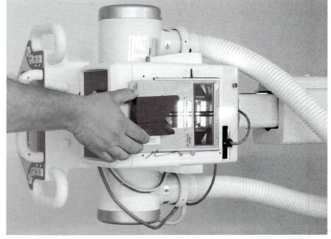

Fig. 10-10 The Ferlic collimator-mounted filter being positioned on the underside collimator for an anteroposterior projection of the shoulder.

[e]Ferlic Filter Company LLC, White Bear Lake, Minn.

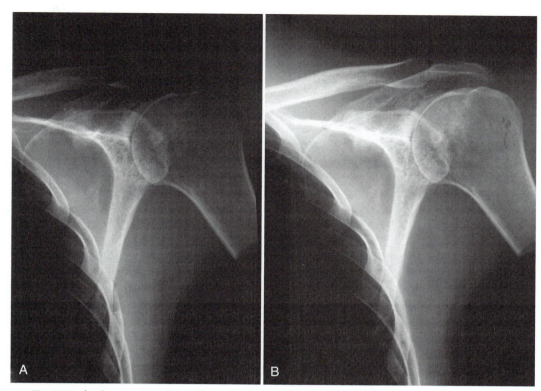

Fig. 10-11 A, Anteroposterior (AP) projection of the shoulder without a compensating filter. **B,** Same projection using the Ferlic shoulder filter, collimator mounted. Note greater visualization of the acromion, acromioclavicular (AC) joint, and humeral head.

show radiation exposure reductions of between 50% and 80%, depending on the kVp, in the anatomic area covered by the filter. Measurements by Frank, Stears, Gray, et al[f] and Gray, Stears, and Frank[g] show exposure reductions of between 20% and 69% to the thyroid, sternum, and breasts for scoliosis radiography. Both types of filters have the same effect on the finished image, which is a more uniform radiographic density, even though the tissue density varies greatly. Filters can be improvised as well, with radiographers creating their own versions of attenuation control devices such as filled bags of saline solution. Bags of solution, however, will increase radiation scattering. Use of improvised filters is not recommended because there is potential for creating unknown artifacts in the image. An example of the improvement in image quality using a compensating filter can be seen in the AP projection of the shoulder in Fig. 10-11.

Limited operators must use caution when mounting and removing compensating filters on the collimator while the x-ray tube is over the patient. There have been instances in which filters did not attach properly, did not get positioned into the filter track, or were forgotten and fell onto the patient when the tube was moved. All compensating filters, especially the aluminum ones, are moderately heavy with sharp edges; therefore they can cause injury to the patient if dropped. When the filter is positioned to the underside of the collimator and when it is removed, two hands must be used (Fig. 10-12). One hand should attach the filter while the other is positioned to catch the filter if it does not attach properly.

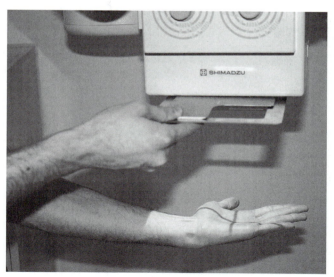

Fig. 10-12 Two hands must be used to attach and remove collimator-mounted filters. Note that one hand is used to catch the filter in case it is dropped.

[f]Frank ED, Stears JG, Gray JE, et al: Use of the posterior-anterior projection as a method of reducing x-ray exposure to specific radiosensitive organs, *Radiol Technol* 54:343, 1983.

[g]Gray JE, Stears JG, Frank ED: Shaped, lead-loaded acrylic filters for patient exposure reduction and image quality improvement, *Radiology* 146:3, 1983.

When using compensating filters, the exposure factors on the technique chart may have to be changed, depending specifically on the projection and patient. If compensating filters are new in your department, you may want to refer to a radiographer for appropriate use of the filter and also for accurate exposure techniques.

SUMMARY

A good variable or fixed kVp technique chart is required to produce consistent exposure results. Technique charts are based on body part measurements in centimeters taken using a caliper. Proper measurement according to the method specified by the technique chart is essential. Optimum kVp ranges are established for each body part, and the mAs is varied to adjust the exposure for changes in patient/part thickness. The mA is selected to conform to the requirements of the tube rating chart and to provide the desired focal spot size. The highest mA settings are used when short exposure times are required. Exposure times are determined by calculation, based on the required mAs and the desired mA.

Technique charts are necessary to program computerized controls and may be required by radiation control regulations and The Joint Commission standards. They should be updated when there is a change in the system that affects exposure requirements. Technique charts are designed for normal tissue density and usual radiographic procedures. They must be adjusted for patients whose tissue density is outside the normal range and for procedures that depart from the usual SID, grid, or IR system speed.

The mAs is used to adjust radiographic density. Bold changes are needed when images must be repeated because they are too dark or too light. Contrast levels may be adjusted without affecting density by using the 15% rule.

Some parts of the body contain areas of significantly varying tissue density that must be shown on one image. To compensate for these variations in tissue density, compensating filters should be used and exposure techniques adjusted accordingly.

Chapter 11

Radiobiology and Radiation Safety

At the conclusion of this chapter, you will be able to:

- State the units used to measure radiation exposure, absorbed dose, and dose equivalent using the Système International
- Discuss the potential effects of radiation injury to cells
- Define and compare radiation risks according to type: somatic vs. genetic and short-term vs. long-term
- Discuss the risks of exposure to low doses of ionizing radiation and compare these with other familiar health risks
- Explain the significance of the ALARA (as low as reasonably achievable) principle
- List and explain methods for minimizing patient dose during radiography
- Explain what is meant by "low-dose techniques"
- List and explain precautions for the safety of limited operators
- List potential risks of radiation exposure during pregnancy and explain ways to reduce these risks

Key Terms

absorbed dose (D)
air kerma
ALARA (as low as reasonably achievable) principle
biologic damage
chromosomes
cumulative effective dose (CumEfD)
deoxyribonucleic acid (DNA)
dominant genes
dose equivalent
effective dose (EfD)
entrance skin exposure (ESE)
enzymes
erythema

free radicals
genes
gonad shields
gonads
Gray (Gy)
ionizing radiation
mutations
optically stimulated luminescence (OSL)
radiation protection
radiation weighting factor
recessive genes
Sievert (Sv)
Système International (SI)

The health risks involved in radiation use are not well understood by the general public. Diagnostic radiography involves low doses of radiation, and the risks to both patients and limited operators are extremely small. It is important to understand the risks associated with radiography and to commit to the practice of radiation safety in all aspects of radiography work. When used properly, radiation from x-ray examinations also has benefits. The diagnostic information that the patient's physician receives from the x-ray examinations far outweighs the risks.

Ionizing radiation is radiation that, when passing through the body, produces positively and negatively charged particles. **Radiation protection** is the measures taken to safeguard patients, personnel, and the public from unnecessary exposure to ionizing radiation.

This chapter is about the measurement of radiation, the effects of radiation exposure, and the ways in which limited operators can minimize the potential hazards to their patients, their co-workers, themselves, and future generations.

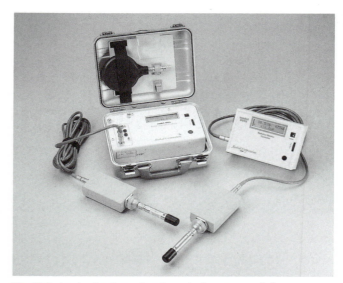

Fig. 11-1 An ionization chamber dosimeter used for accurate measurement of diagnostic x-rays.

RADIATION MEASUREMENT

Two systems were used for many years to measure radiation and radiation dose: the units of the conventional (British) system and the **Système International (SI)** units established by the International Commission on Radiation Units in 1980. The conventional system is now gone, and the SI system is the predominant system used by the scientific community, the government, and all foreign countries. Table 11-1 lists the three key radiation measurements used today and their associated units in the SI system. *All units in this chapter will be stated in the new SI units.* Should you encounter an old conventional value in a reading, you can simply multiply that value by 0.01 to obtain the value in the SI system.

Unit of Exposure

Air kerma is the SI unit term for radiation exposure. It represents a measurement of the radiation intensity *in the air*. This is determined by the ionization of air resulting from interaction with the x-ray beam. Air kerma is measured with an ionization chamber (Fig. 11-1). A simple way to describe "exposure" is to think of the amount of

x-rays that are in the air between the x-ray tube and the patient. It is also the volume of x-rays that strike the surface of the body.

The measuring unit of exposure in the SI system is the **Gray,** abbreviated Gy-$_a$. The subscript "a" is used with the unit Gy to indicate "air."[1,2] Many exposures in radiology are very low and therefore the prefix "milli," which is 1/100 of the unit it precedes, is very often used with the Gy to make numbers easier to relate to. For example, the very small exposure value 0.012 Gy would be stated as 12 mGy. *To convert Gy to mGy, multiply Gy × 1000.*

Unit of Absorbed Dose

Absorbed dose (D) is the amount of energy (x-ray) absorbed by the irradiated tissue. It is an important value because it measures the amount of energy that is absorbed by the patient. To measure specific tissue doses received in diagnostic applications, the SI unit is also the Gray. The subscript "t" is used with the unit Gy to indicate "tissue."[1,2] Dose values are indicated as Gy-$_t$. Therefore Gy-$_a$ is the exposure in *air* value and Gy-$_t$ is the absorbed dose in *tissue* value. Similar to exposure, dose values can be quite low and the prefix "milli" is used with the Gy to make the numbers easier to relate to. For example, if a patient received an absorbed dose of 0.150 Gy, this could be stated as 150 mGy.

It is important for the limited operator to understand that for every x-ray projection taken, the patient receives both an exposure and an absorbed dose. For example, for an abdomen x-ray series, the patient may receive an

Table 11-1	
SI Units of Exposure and Dose	
SI Unit of:	**SI Term**
Exposure	Air Kerma (Gy-$_a$)
Absorbed dose	Gray (Gy-$_t$)
Dose equivalent	Sievert (Sv)

SI, Système International.

[1]Wagner LK, Archer, BR: *Minimizing risk from fluoroscopic x-rays,* PRM, 2007.
[2]Bushong SC: *Radiologic science for technologists,* ed 10, St. Louis, 2013, Mosby.

exposure of 16 mGy-$_a$ and from that exposure an *absorbed dose* of 1.2 mGy-$_t$. The absorbed dose will always be less than the initial air exposure. The differences between the units, *exposure*, and *absorbed dose* are also determined by their very words. Whenever "exposure" is used, it means radiation in air. Whenever "absorbed dose" or "dose" is used, it means absorbed dose in the body.

Unit of Dose Equivalent

The biologic effect of radiation exposure varies according to the type of radiation involved and its energy. Equal doses of various types of radiation will not necessarily result in equal biologic effects. Some radiation workers, such as engineers in nuclear power plants or technologists in nuclear medicine laboratories, may be exposed to several types of radiation with unequal levels of biologic effect. Neither the Gray-$_a$ nor the Gray-$_t$ is a useful unit for measuring the occupational dose of combined radiations with different levels of effects. **Dose equivalent** is the term used to describe or clarify the absorbed dose in the body based on the *type* and *energy* of the radiation the person was exposed to. For example, a nuclear power plant worker receives a much different type of radiation and energy than a limited operator in a clinic. The **Sievert (Sv)** is the SI system's unit of dose equivalent. Similar to exposure and absorbed dose described earlier, many dose equivalent values are small, and therefore the prefix "milli" is used with Sv to make the numbers easier to relate to. For example, a dose equivalent of 0.200 Sv could more easily be stated as 200 mSv.

To simplify the process of measuring occupational dose, a **radiation weighting factor** is assigned to each type of radiation, based on the variation in biologic damage that is produced when an individual receives exposure from different types of radiation. Table 11-2 lists the radiation weighting factors for the different types of radiation. For example, if a worker received an absorbed dose of 10 Gy-$_t$ of protons, the total dose equivalent would be 20 Sv. The dose equivalent is obtained by multiplying the absorbed dose by the weighting factor.

Understanding the dose equivalent is made easy for limited operators and others who work in diagnostic radiology. Because the weighting factor for x-ray photons

is "1" (see Table 11-2), the *absorbed dose* and the *dose equivalent* are always identical numbers.

In our everyday work, the dose equivalent is primarily used for radiation protection purposes. Specifically, occupational doses such as the readings from radiation dosimeters and the doses patients receive from radiation, as well as the occupational doses published in journals, are stated as dose equivalent. Limited operators will receive regular dose-related communications in the radiology department from state and federal entities. Depending on the nature of the material, the radiation values could be stated in exposure, absorbed dose, or dose equivalent values. Some communications may have all three values stated.

The conversion of any of the units of exposure, absorbed dose, and dose equivalent from the stated value to a milli-value, or from a milli-value to its stated value, can be better understood by reviewing a series of common radiation dose values side by side. Table 11-3 shows a scale of Gy-$_t$ values converted to mGy-$_t$. It should be evident why most values in radiology are stated as "milli" values. Note that by changing to mGy-$_t$ the stated numbers become easier to relate to than numbers with many zeros and decimal points. Conversion of Gy-$_a$ and Sv to "milli" values will demonstrate the same effect. When large exposures are discussed, the value is typically not converted to milli. For example, an exposure of 20 Gy-$_a$ would not be converted to 20,000 mGy-$_a$.

Estimation of Dose from X-ray Exposure Factors

Radiographers and limited operators usually think of radiation dose in terms of the prime factors of milliampere-seconds (mAs), kilovolts peak (kVp), and source–image receptor distance (SID). These values for a given x-ray exposure will determine the absorbed dose a patient receives. On a daily basis, limited operators never have to calculate dose for x-ray examinations. Also, dose is not tracked in patient histories. Knowing how dose can be affected with changes in the prime factors can help in understanding radiation. A special graph is necessary to

Table 11-2

Radiation Weighting Factors for Different Types of Ionizing Radiations

Type of Radiation	Radiation Weighting Factor
X-ray photons	1
Gamma photons	1
Low-energy internal protons	2
Fast neutrons	20
Alpha particles	20

Table 11-3

Conversion of Gy-$_t$ to mGy-$_t$

Gy-$_t$	mGy-$_t$
0.005	5
0.010	10
0.050	50
0.100	100
0.250	250
0.500	500
1.00	1000
2.50	2500

Table 11-4

Typical Exposures and Doses for Radiographic Examinations

Examination	Entrance Skin Exposure (mGy-$_a$)*	Mean Bone Marrow Dose (mGy-$_t$)	Gonad Dose (mGy-$_t$)
Skull	2.00	0.10	<1
Chest	0.1	0.02	<1
Cervical spine	1.5	0.20	<1
Abdomen	4.0	0.30	1.25
Pelvis	1.5	0.20	1.50
Limb	0.5	0.02	<1

*Note how much higher the exposure (in air) is compared with the absorbed dose (in tissues).

Modified from Statkiewicz Sherer MA, et al.: *Radiation protection in medical radiography,* ed 7, St Louis, 2014, Mosby.

convert technical factors into units of dose. Appendix G contains the dose curve for exposures. Use this chart only to see how the dose changes when mAs, kVp, or SID changes.

Patient dose in radiography is usually calculated according to the exposure level at the skin. This is called the **entrance skin exposure (ESE).** Some typical doses for radiographic exposures are listed in Table 11-4. Note the differences in exposure for various examinations and compare the ESE with the dose to bone marrow and gonads (reproductive organs). It is apparent that the highest ESE exposures are received with examinations of the skull, abdomen, and lumbar spine, although the greatest bone marrow and gonad doses are associated with examinations of the abdomen, lumbar spine, and pelvis.

BIOLOGIC EFFECTS OF RADIATION EXPOSURE

Cellular Response

To understand how cells are affected by radiation exposure, it is helpful to understand something of the composition of a typical cell. Fig. 11-2 is a simplified diagram of a cell. The cell is surrounded by the plasma membrane. At its center is the nucleus, which contains the nucleoli.

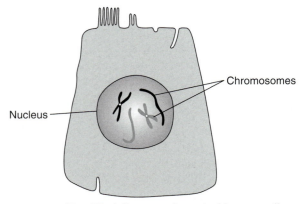

Fig. 11-2 Simplified diagram of a typical human cell.

Inside the nucleoli are 23 pairs of **chromosomes,** microscopic bodies that contain the **genes.** Genes are the determiners of heredity and are made of a unique protein called **DNA** (deoxyribonucleic acid). The chromosomes contain the coded "information" that the cell needs to function.

As discussed in Chapter 4, x-rays can ionize substances, removing electrons from their orbits. This process results in a free, negatively charged electron and leaves the remainder of the atom with a positive charge. When cells are irradiated, ionization may occur to any part of the cell, such as the material that makes up its membrane, the water within the membrane, or the DNA. The initial ionization may produce a "domino effect," causing ionization in the surrounding area.

Most of these effects are extremely short-lived. Electrons quickly find new homes in the orbits of other atoms, and the balance of charges returns to normal. **Free radicals** combine to form more stable compounds. Some cells may sustain damage that requires several days for the body to repair. Biologic chemicals called **enzymes** repair damage to cell membranes and DNA, correcting an additional 5% to 9% of the damage within a period of about 3 days. Occasionally, however, the damage is not resolved. A cell may be so injured that it cannot sustain itself and will die. Cell death is not serious unless it involves large numbers of cells. A cell may be damaged in such a way that its DNA "programming" is changed and the cell no longer behaves normally. This type of injury may cause malfunction of the cell or may affect its ability to divide and multiply. Another possible result is the runaway production of new, abnormal cells, causing cancer or a malignant blood disease such as leukemia.

Law of Bergonié and Tribondeau

The relative sensitivity of different types of cells is summarized in the Bergonié-Tribondeau law, which states that cell sensitivity to radiation exposure depends on four characteristics of the cell:

1. *Age.* Younger patient cells are more sensitive than older ones.

2. *Differentiation.* Simple cells are more sensitive than highly complex ones.
3. *Metabolic rate.* Cells that use energy rapidly are more sensitive than those that have a slower metabolism.
4. *Mitotic rate.* Cells that divide and multiply rapidly are more sensitive than those that replicate slowly.

According to this law, blood cells and blood-producing cells have characteristics that cause them to be very sensitive. Cells that are in contact with the environment are quite simple, have relatively short lives, and are quite sensitive. These include the cells of the skin and the mucous membranes that line the mouth, nose, stomach, and bowel. Some glandular tissue is also particularly sensitive, especially that of the thyroid gland and the female breast. The tissues of embryos, fetuses, infants, children, and adolescents tend to be more sensitive than those of adults both because of their age and because of their higher metabolic and mitotic rates. Nerve and muscle cells, which have a long life and are quite complex, are much less vulnerable to radiation injury. Cortical bone cells are also relatively insensitive.

Ionizing radiation produces **biologic damage** as it interacts with the body tissue. The destructive interactions occur at the atomic level, leading to cellular damage. Table 11-5 provides the known biologic effects of different radiation dose equivalents.

Classification of Radiation Effects

Radiation effects are classified in various ways. The most common are *short-term*, *long-term*, *somatic*, and *genetic*. The likelihood of these effects occurring after radiation exposure to x-rays is proportional to the dose received.

Table 11-5

Radiation Dose Equivalent and Subsequent Biologic Effects Resulting from Acute Whole Body Exposures

Radiation Dose Equivalent	Subsequent Biologic Effect
250 mSv	Blood changes (e.g., measurable hematologic depression, decreases in the number of lymphocytes present in the circulating blood)
1500 mSv	Nausea, diarrhea
2000 mSv	Erythema (diffuse redness over an area of skin after irradiation)
2500 mSv	If dose is to gonads, temporary sterility
3000 mSv	50% chance of death; lethal dose for 50% of population over 30 days (LD 50/30)
6000 mSv	Death

Note: Radiation exposures are delivered to the entire body over a time period of less than a few hours.
Adapted from Statkiewicz Sherer MA, et al.: *Radiation protection in medical radiography*, ed 7, St Louis, 2014, Mosby.

Short-term effects are those observed within 3 months of the exposure. They are associated with high radiation absorbed doses, typically greater than 500 mGy-$_t$. Short-term effects may be further categorized according to the body system affected: *hematologic system* (blood), *gastrointestinal system* (digestive tract), and *central nervous system* or *CNS* (brain and spinal cord). Today, there are very few short-term effects seen from diagnostic x-ray procedures.

Long-term effects, sometimes referred to as *latent effects*, are not observed until several years after exposure; in fact, they may not be apparent for as long as 30 years. In general, it is the long-term effects that we are most concerned about in diagnostic radiology. These would be the effects shown after a patient has undergone many years of average to high radiation exposure.

Somatic effects are those that affect the body and tissues of the individual who is irradiated. There are both short-term and long-term somatic effects. We should always be concerned about the somatic effects and think of this effect every time we set a technical exposure value on the generator and repeat an x-ray.

Genetic effects occur as a result of damage to the reproductive cells of the irradiated person and are observed as defects in the children or grandchildren of the irradiated individual.

Short-term Somatic Effects

Short-term somatic effects occur with high doses of radiation and they are predictable. One observable short-term effect is reddening of the skin, called **erythema.** This phenomenon is sometimes called a *radiation burn.* This burn can be observed with a dose to the skin of 2,000 mSv. In the very early days of radiation use, the amount of radiation necessary to produce reddening of the skin was called the *erythema dose* and was the first unit used to measure radiation.

Other short-term effects have been observed and studied in radiation therapy patients and in the victims of nuclear accidents and atomic bomb blasts. This type of radiation involves vastly more exposure than is delivered by diagnostic x-ray machines. Extremely high doses produce CNS effects, causing seizures and coma and resulting in death in a short period of time. Lesser doses result in "radiation sickness," a gastrointestinal effect in which the mucosal lining of the digestive tract is damaged, breaks down, and becomes infected by the bacteria that normally inhabit the bowel. These victims also have a compromised immune system, caused by the death of white blood cells, and are unable to fight the infection. Radiation sickness is usually fatal, but suffering may be prolonged. A lesser dose, affecting primarily the blood and blood-forming cells of the bone marrow, results in hematologic effects: anemia and compromise of the immune system. These victims are prone to infectious diseases that may or may not be fatal, depending on the radiation dose and the severity of the disease process.

Human beings who receive whole-body doses of radiation in excess of 5,000 mGy-$_t$ may die within 30 to 60 days because of the effects related to depletion of the stem cells and of the hematopoietic system. The whole body radiation dose that is fatal to 50% of the irradiated human population within 30 days is stated as a "lethal dose" (LD). We therefore use "LD 50/30" to describe this situation. The lethal dose for human beings is generally estimated to be 3,000 to 4,000 mGy-$_t$ without treatment.

Long-term Somatic Effects

The time required for long-term effects to become apparent is generally considered to be 5 to 30 years, with the greatest percentage of effects occurring between 10 and 15 years.

Short-term radiation effects are predictable, and the quantity of exposure required to produce them is well documented. Long-term effects, on the other hand, are random. They may involve repeated small doses, such as those used in radiography.

Long-term radiation effects are not predictable because they occur so long after exposure and because these same effects also occur in the absence of radiation exposure. Only extensive research with large populations using computer analysis can demonstrate the role of radiation in causing these effects. The incidence of certain conditions is shown to be increased when results for irradiated groups are compared with those for nonirradiated control groups. The documented latent effects of low doses of ionizing radiation include the following:

- *Cataractogenesis:* the formation of *cataracts*, clouding of the lens of the eye. This effect is of concern to radiologists and radiographers who work extensively in fluoroscopy and who perform other work that involves repeated exposure to the eyes.
- *Carcinogenesis:* increased risk of malignant disease, particularly cancer of the skin, thyroid, and breast, and leukemia, a malignant disease of the blood that has been clearly demonstrated to be associated with radiation exposure.
- *Life span shortening: shorter life span than without having been exposed to ionizing radiation.* A study of the life span of radiologists who died during a 3-year period before 1945 showed that they had shorter life spans than physicians who did not use radiation in their practices. This group of radiologists included those who had been using radiation since the early days of x-ray science. More recent studies show that the decreased occupational exposure typical today has no measurable effect on the life span of radiologists. Radiation exposure is still definitely linked to life span shortening, however. This is a public health concern and another reason to practice a high level of radiation safety.
- *Leukemia: cancer of the blood or bone marrow.* In the early 1900s when x-ray was in its infancy, this was one of the earliest effects seen in people who worked in radiology and in people who received x-rays.

Genetic Effects

Genetic effects are changes or **mutations** to the genes of the reproductive cells. They occur as a result of radiation exposure to the reproductive organs called **gonads,** the female ovaries or the male testes. In the female, all the ova (egg cells) that the individual will ever produce are present in the ovaries in an immature state at birth. Because no new egg cells are produced as the individual ages, the effect of radiation exposure to the ovaries is cumulative. Radiation to the testes also has longer-term genetic effects than might at first be presumed because damage to the stem cells that produce the sperm may result in the continued production of sperm that carry the genetic mutation. The vast majority of genetic mutations are considered to be negative, or to make cells less well suited to survival than nonmutated cells.

Reproductive cells have only half the number of chromosomes of other cells. Each parent contributes one chromosome to each pair in the new individual, and nature makes the choice as to which gene of each pair will determine the characteristics of the offspring. Those genes that are "chosen" are said to be **dominant genes** and those that are not selected are called **recessive genes.** Genes that have mutated are usually recessive and so do not affect the characteristics of the child. Both dominant and recessive genes, however, occur in the reproductive cells of the child and may be passed on to future generations.

Because the population is exposed to radiation from natural, occupational, and health care sources, there is likelihood that individuals will be conceived with mutation of both genes in a strategic pair, resulting in some type of deformity, defect, or characteristic that is less well suited to survival. Mutations may appear as cleft palates, spina bifida, and polydactyly. Public health officials and governments are very concerned about preserving the integrity of the population's gene pool by minimizing radiation that may cause defects in future generations. This concern should motivate those who use ionizing radiation to minimize gonad doses in every way possible. Gonad shielding for this purpose is addressed later in this chapter.

Genetic effects from mutations caused by x-ray exposure have long been demonstrated in animal research. Interestingly, very little genetic effect has so far been confirmed by continuing research involving the Japanese populations exposed to radiation when the atomic bombs were dropped on Hiroshima and Nagasaki during World War II. Individuals who were children at that time are now becoming grandparents. Studies of this new generation and those that follow will be necessary before the genetic effects on bomb survivors can be evaluated completely.

Comparative Risks

The average American was, in earlier times, exposed to an annual dose of 3.6 mSv of radiation from all sources—natural and man-made. The natural sources of radiation remain the same today but unfortunately the man-made radiation (from x-ray examinations) has soared. Today the average American is exposed to 6.3 mSv, a 75% increase. The increase is primarily because of increases in dose from computed tomography (CT) and interventional procedures. Naturally occurring radiation from space, from the earth, and from radon gas accounts for 82% of this exposure (Fig. 11-3). Today, a greater percentage of the dose Americans receive is from medical x-ray examinations, and this dose equals 3.2 mSv. The remaining dose, 3 mSv, comes from natural sources.

The increase in patient radiation dose requires that radiographers and limited operators exercise more control over medical imaging. We must be more aware of the appropriateness of performing x-ray examinations and gain control over unnecessary examinations.

Certainly the percentage of observable effects from the radiation involved in typical x-ray examinations is extremely low, and the risk to any one patient is minimal. Most of us take greater risks daily when we drive a car or cross a busy street.

Many people may be outdoors during a thunderstorm. Few, if any, will be struck by lightning. People struck by lightning may be killed or only slightly injured. The chance of being struck by lightning is extremely remote, but it is greater if you make it a habit of standing in high places during thunderstorms. Scientists can predict fairly accurately the annual rate at which lightning will strike human beings, but it is impossible to predict who will be struck and who will not.

Similarly, radiation causes increased *risk* of the effects outlined, but the effects cannot be predicted with respect to any one individual. Table 11-6 provides some interesting

Table 11-6

Decrease in Life Expectancy from Various Causes

Cause	Days
Unmarried male	3500
Cigarette-smoking male	2250 (20 cigarettes/day)
Heart disease	2100
Unmarried female	1600
Overweight 30%	1300
Coal miner	1100
Overweight 20%	900
Less than eighth-grade education	850
Cigarette-smoking female	800 (20 cigarettes/day)
Low socioeconomic status	700
Stroke	520
Pipe smoking	220
Increasing food intake 100 cal/day	210
Job with radiation exposure (1 rem/yr for 40 yr)	40
Natural radiation (BEIR)	8
Medical x-ray films	6
Coffee consumption	6
Oral contraceptive use	5
5 rem/yr (occupational exposure)	5
Diet drink consumption	2
Reactor accidents	0.02*
Radiation from nuclear industry	0.02*
Papanicolaou test	−4
Smoke alarm in home	−10
Airbags in car	−50
Mobile coronary care unit	−125

*These items assume that all U.S. power is nuclear.
BEIR, Biologic effects of ionizing radiation.

comparisons between the risks involved in radiography and other more familiar risks.

Scientists agree that any one individual's risk from radiography is *extremely small*, but exposure to the entire population does pose public health risks. The increase in the average dose, however, is a growing discussion in the radiography and governmental communities. Even when the chance of serious effects is one in a million, that adds up to 250 serious problems in a nation of 250 million people. Although the risk from a chest x-ray is frequently quoted as typical, the dose for a lumbar spine examination may be 50 times greater, increasing the risk. All who are involved in applying ionizing radiation to human beings share the responsibility for ensuring that everything possible is done to keep these risks as low as possible.

RADIATION SAFETY

Clearly, exposure to x-rays creates some risk for patients, limited operators, radiographers, and radiologists. It is

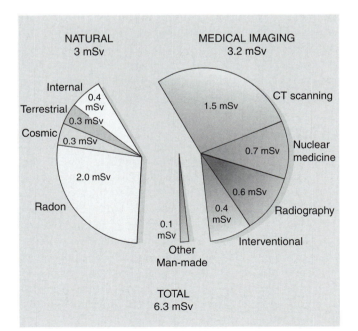

Fig. 11-3 Current estimated levels of human radiation exposure. For the first time, medical imaging exposure values have exceeded natural background exposures.

therefore an essential part of your education and your ethical responsibility to be knowledgeable about radiation safety and to use this knowledge to prevent all unnecessary radiation exposure to your patients, your co-workers, and yourself.

The federal government issues regulations and recommendations to ensure the safety of patients and radiation workers. State agencies incorporate federal guidelines into the state regulations. Additional laws and regulations may apply in individual states. The state radiation control agencies are responsible for the administration of both state and federal regulations. Your state may have a regulation that requires the posting of a summary of the regulations that apply to your facility. Limited operators are responsible for knowing and following the laws and regulations that apply to their work.

Patient Protection

There is no arbitrary limit on the amount of radiation exposure a patient may receive. The guiding philosophy is called the **ALARA principle.** The ALARA principle states that all radiation exposure to humans should be limited to levels that are as low as reasonably achievable. Radiation control agencies use this guideline to compare the quantities of radiation used for specific procedures within the community. If the average ESE for a specific examination in your community is 0.20 mGy, this provides evidence of what is reasonably achievable. If the dose in your facility for the same examination is much greater than the average, the level is unacceptable and must be reduced to meet regulatory requirements. The limited level can reduce radiation to patients by reducing repeat exposures, avoiding mistakes, using the smallest radiation field, using the highest kVp, and maintaining the SID at 40 inches.

The greatest cause of unnecessary radiation to patients that can be controlled by limited operators is repeat exposures. Repeat exposures are undesirable for many reasons. They require extra time and materials that increase health care costs, in addition to increasing patient dose, so it is important to avoid the need for repeats. On the other hand, exposures *must* be repeated when image quality is inadequate. Reduction of patient dose is not a valid reason for failing to repeat an image that is not diagnostic.

To minimize the need for repeat exposures, limited operators must take care to avoid mistakes. Double-check requisitions and patient identification so that the right patient gets the right examination. Establish good routine procedures and follow them strictly so that careless errors do not necessitate repeat exposures. Provide clear instructions to patients so that they will cooperate in obtaining a successful examination.

Another cause of unnecessary exposure that limited operators control is the size of the radiation field. Radiation exposure can be substantially controlled by the proper use of collimation. *Use the smallest radiation field that will cover the area of clinical interest.* In no case should the size of the radiation field be greater than the size of the film. Whenever possible, collimate to exclude sensitive tissue, such as the eyes, the thyroid gland, the female breasts, and the gonads. As you practice positioning and centering with precision, you will gain confidence that the essential anatomy can be visualized successfully without using an excessive field size.

In addition to developing good habits of procedure and collimation, the limited operator can reduce patient exposure by using "low-dose techniques." Low-dose techniques involve using optimum kVp and a minimum SID of 40 inches (with 48 inches preferred).

The highest kVp that will produce acceptable contrast results in less exposure to the patient than a low-kVp technique. An increase in kVp with no other change will increase the patient dose rate slightly. However, when the mAs is adjusted down to compensate for the kVp increase, the net result is a reduction in dose. The use of the 15% rule to increase kVp and decrease mAs (see Chapter 10) results in a dose reduction of approximately 34%.

Routine radiography should never be performed at less than a 40-inch SID. The tube housing permits leakage of some radiation that increases patient dose without being useful in image formation. In addition, interaction between the primary x-ray beam and the parts of the collimator produces scatter radiation. Patient dose from these sources is relatively insignificant at a 40-inch SID but increases dramatically, according to the inverse square law, when the tube is closer to the patient. A 48-inch SID is now becoming commonplace. This results in greater recorded detail and less dose to the patient.

As stated in Chapter 9, the use of a grid requires a significant increase in exposure compared with the same examination performed without a grid. For this reason, grids and Buckys should be used only when necessary to control scatter radiation. Small body parts that do not generate large quantities of scatter should be radiographed on the tabletop. The exposure technique chart should indicate whether a grid is used or not.

Gonad Shielding

Lead shields that prevent unnecessary radiation to the reproductive organs are required by regulation in most jurisdictions. **Gonad shields** are used to reduce the likelihood of genetic radiation effects. Gonad shields must be used when the patient is of reproductive age or younger, whenever the gonads are within the primary x-ray beam, and when the shield will not interfere with the purpose of the examination. Generally, this applies to most patients under the age of 55. A shield device consisting of at least 0.5 mm lead equivalent is placed between the x-ray tube and the patient. Shields attached to the collimator are called *shadow shields.* The limited operator positions them by viewing their shadows within the collimator light field (Fig. 11-4). Shields placed on or near the patient's body

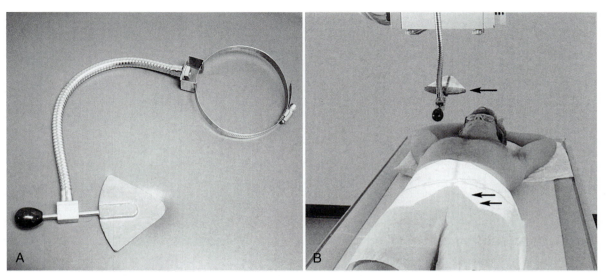

Fig. 11-4 Shadow shield is attached to the collimator or tube housing **(A)** and placed by observing the location of its shadow *(arrows)* in the collimator light field **(B).**

are called *contact shields* and are somewhat more effective than shadow shields (Fig. 11-5). Both types meet the legal requirements for gonad shielding. Fig. 11-6 demonstrates shield placement for both males and females. It is helpful to note that the pubic symphysis (the center of the pubic bone) is at the same level as the greater trochanter of the femur, which avoids the necessity of palpating the pubic bone for proper shield placement.

Gonad shields should also be used when the primary radiation field is *near* the gonads, even though this may not be required by regulation. *Whenever the gonads are within 5 cm of the margin of the radiation field, gonad dose will be significantly reduced by shielding.* When the field is more than 5 cm from the gonads, shielding has little effect with respect to protection from primary radiation. On the other hand, scatter radiation may provide some level of gonad dose for *any* examination when the gonads are not shielded. Little extra effort is required to provide a lead apron or lead shield. Most limited operators feel better about their work when they shield conscientiously, and patients also appreciate this level of concern.

Shields may be purchased that provide precise shielding of the gonads when doing radiography of adjacent structures. It is almost always possible to shield the male gonads, regardless of the examination. A female gonad shield may sometimes interfere with the purpose of the examination. The abdomen, sacrum (pelvic portion of the spine), and coccyx (tailbone), for example, cannot be well visualized with an ovary shield in place. When the ovaries cannot be shielded, the ovarian dose is greatly reduced if the patient can be radiographed prone (face down) or facing away from the x-ray tube. In this position, the tissue of the buttocks and the bones of the pelvis absorb a significant quantity of radiation that would otherwise increase the gonad dose. Variations from standard positioning should first be approved by the radiologist.

Personnel Safety

Limited operators may potentially be exposed to radiation either from the primary x-ray beam or from scatter radiation. Because limited operators are considered to be "occupationally exposed individuals," they are prohibited from activities that would result in direct exposure to the primary x-ray beam. This means that *limited operators are not allowed to hold patients or image receptors during x-ray exposures.* Nonoccupationally exposed personnel, who are not pregnant and who are wearing protective apparel, should hold patients whenever possible.

The procedures with greatest risk for occupational exposure are those involving fluoroscopy and mobile radiography. These procedures are not commonly performed by limited operators. Fluoroscopy involves direct observation of the x-ray image in motion during procedures commonly used to visualize the digestive tract or the circulatory system. Special fluoroscopic x-ray equipment is required. Limited operators assisting with fluoroscopy may have to be in the room to change cassettes and to assist with patient positioning and the administration of contrast media during these procedures. Mobile radiographic examinations are sometimes referred to as *portable radiography.* These examinations are performed in the surgical suite or at the patient's bedside where there is no protective control booth. Scattered radiation from the patient and other objects poses the greatest hazard for radiography personnel.

Time, Distance, Shielding

The three principal methods used to protect limited operators from unnecessary radiation exposure are *time,* *distance,* and *shielding.* Time and distance apply principally to radiographers who are involved in fluoroscopy and mobile radiography. Shielding is employed to protect all radiographers.

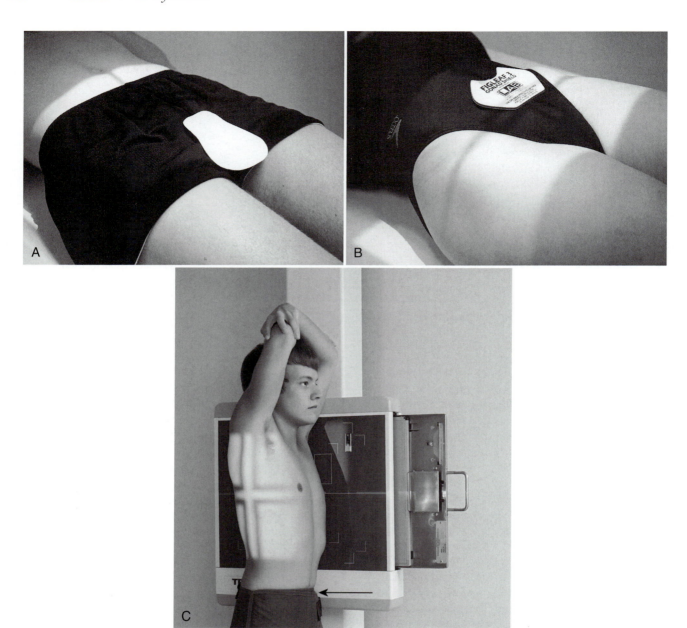

Fig. 11-5 Contact shields are placed on the patient's body during exposure. **A,** Male shielding. **B,** Female shielding. **C,** Wrap-around shield *(arrow)* is placed on the waist for a chest x-ray.

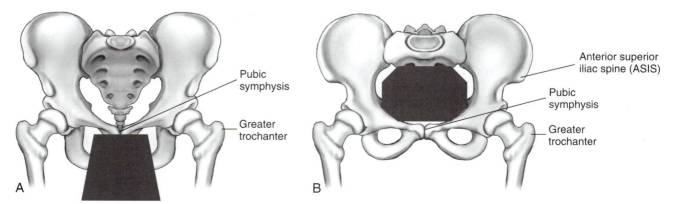

Fig. 11-6 Shield placement. **A,** The top of the male shield is 1 inch inferior to the top of the pubic symphysis, which is at the level of the greater trochanter. **B,** The female shield is placed in the midline, midway between the level of the anterior superior iliac spine and the pubic symphysis.

The amount of exposure received is directly proportional to the time spent in a radiation field, so occupational dose is decreased when this time is minimized. For example, a limited operator might shorten the time of exposure by stepping into the control booth during fluoroscopic procedures when not required to be near the patient.

The second method involves using distance. Increasing the distance between yourself and a radiation source decreases your exposure in proportion to the square of the distance, so small increases in distance have a relatively large effect. Mobile x-ray units have long cords on the exposure switches, which enables the radiographer to get at least 6 feet away from the patient and machine while making an exposure.

The third method is shielding, and this is by far the most common method of protection. The lead wall of the control booth provides protective shielding and is the limited operator's primary defense. Limited operators are unlikely to be exposed to any significant amount of radiation when standing well within the protection of the control booth. Other types of shielding include lead aprons, gloves, and thyroid shields (Fig. 11-7). These types of shields are worn during fluoroscopic procedures and mobile radiographic examinations. They are also worn by personnel who have to hold patients.

The preexposure safety check introduced in Chapter 2 is an essential safety practice. It is the principal method used to ensure that you do not accidentally expose your co-workers. When you perform the safety check, you make certain that no one is in the x-ray room unnecessarily, that everyone in the control booth is completely behind the lead barrier, and that the x-ray room door is closed. Doors are usually open or ajar except during exposures. A closed door indicates that it is not safe to enter.

Quality Control: Aprons and Gloves

A *quality control check* is regularly performed on the lead aprons and gloves used in the department to meet state and federal regulations. The minimum standard lead equivalency for the aprons should be 0.5 mm and for the lead gloves should be 0.25 mm. Radiographers perform this quality control check every 6 months. The check is performed simply by placing the apron or glove on a fluoroscopic x-ray table and checking the entire area of lead using the fluoroscopic beam. If any cracks are seen, the apron or glove must be taken out of service. The check of these protective devices must be documented in the department's quality control logs.

Personnel Monitoring

Devices for monitoring radiation exposure of radiation workers are called *personal dosimeters*. Monitoring is required whenever radiation workers are likely to risk receiving 10% or more of the annual occupational effective dose limit of 50 mSv. Thermoluminescent dosimeters (TLD) were used until recently but are now becoming obsolete.

Optically stimulated luminescence (OSL) refers to a recently developed monitoring dosimeter (Fig. 11-8) that uses aluminum oxide as a radiation detector. This dosimeter is processed using laser light. OSL dosimeters are similar to TLDs and have several additional advantages. They can measure small doses more precisely and can be reanalyzed to confirm results. They are accurate over a wide dose range and have excellent long-term stability.

Personal dosimeter laboratories provide badges, processing service, and reports, and they keep permanent records of the radiation exposure of each person monitored. Service may be arranged on a weekly, monthly, or quarterly basis (Fig. 11-9). Personnel who

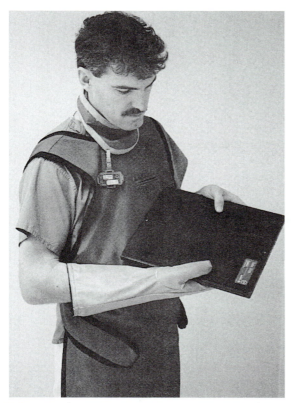

Fig. 11-7 Limited operator wears protective apparel while holding a patient or during mobile radiographic examinations. Note radiation badge worn outside the apron at the collar.

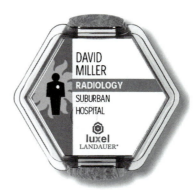

Fig. 11-8 Example of optically stimulated luminescence (OSL)–type personal dosimeter.

SAMPLE ORGANIZATION
RADIATION SAFETY OFFICER
1000 HIGH TECH AVENUE
GLENWOOD, IL 60425

LANDAUER®

Landauer, Inc. 2 Science Road Glenwood, Illinois 60425-1586
Telephone: (708) 755-7000 Facsimile: (708) 755-7016
www.landauerinc.com

RADIATION DOSIMETRY REPORT

ACCOUNT NO.	SERIES CODE	ANALYTICAL WORK ORDER	REPORT DATE	DOSIMETER RECEIVED	REPORT TIME IN WORK DAYS	PAGE NO.
103702	RAD	9920800151	06/11/04	06/07/04	4	1

luxel®

PARTICIPANT NUMBER	NAME (ID NUMBER / BIRTH DATE)	SEX	DOSIMETER	USE	RADIATION QUALITY	DOSE EQUIVALENT (MREM) FOR PERIODS SHOWN BELOW: DEEP DDE	EYE LDE	SHALLOW SDE	QUARTERLY ACCUMULATED DOSE EQUIVALENT (MREM): DEEP DDE	EYE LDE	SHALLOW SDE	YEAR TO DATE DOSE EQUIVALENT (MREM): DEEP DDE	EYE LDE	SHALLOW SDE	LIFETIME DOSE EQUIVALENT (MREM): DEEP DDE	EYE LDE	SHALLOW SDE	RECORDS FOR YEAR	INCEPTION DATE (MM/YY)
FOR MONITORING PERIOD:						05/01/04 - 05/31/04			QTR 2			2004							
0000H	CONTROL CONTROL CONTROL		Ja Pa U	CNTRL CNTRL CNTRL		M M	M M	M M M										5	07/97 07/97 07/97
00191	ADDISON, JOHN	M	Ja	WHBODY	PN P NF	90 60 30	90 60 30	90 60 30	90 60 30	90 60 30	90 60 30	100 70 30	100 70 30	100 70 30	200 170 30	200 170 30	200 170 30	5	07/97
00192	JORGENSON, MIKE	M	Pa U	WHBODY RFINGR		M	M	M M	M	M	M M	M	M	M 70	M	M	M 100	5	07/97 07/97
00193	THOMAS, LEE	M	Pa U	WHBODY RFINGR		ABSENT ABSENT			M	M	M M	M	M	M M	M	M	M M	5	07/97 07/97
00196	WALKER, JANE	F	Pa	WHBODY		3	3	3	12	11	11	12	11	11	22	21	21	5	11/97
00197	EDWARD, CHRIS	M	Pa	WHBODY		M	M	M	M	M	M	M	M	M	M	M	M	5	01/98
00198	ZERR, ROBERT	M	Pa	WHBODY NOTE		40 CALCULATED	40	40	160	160	160	200	200	200	240	240	240	5	07/98
00199	ADAMS, JANE	F	Pa	WHBODY		M	M	M	M	M	M	9	10	12	9	10	12	5	07/98
00200	MEYER, STEVE	M	Pa Pa U	COLLAR WAIST ASSIGN NOTE RFINGR	PL	105 M 4 ASSIGNED DOSE BASED ON EDE 1 CALCULATION	105 M 105	105 M 105 140	6	162	165 400	11	327	334 690	51	1247	1284 2180	5	08/98 08/98 08/98
00202	HARRIS, KATHY	F	Pa U	WHBODY RFINGR		M	M	M M	M	M	M M	M	M	M 30	M	M	M 30	4	02/99 02/99

QUALITY CONTROL RELEASE: VS   20 - PR 6774 - RPT130 - N1   - 02013

M: MINIMAL REPORTING SERVICE OF 1 MREM
ELECTRONIC MEDIA TO FOLLOW THIS REPORT

NVLAP®
NVLAP LAB CODE 100518-0**

Fig. 11-9 Personnel monitoring report for a radiology department. The quarterly, year-to-date, and lifetime radiation levels are shown for each individual.

receive relatively high doses of occupational exposure change their badges most frequently. Because these dosimeters cannot accurately measure total exposures of less than 0.05 mSv, personnel who receive very small amounts of exposure will get more accurate measurements with less frequent badge changes. Personnel involved in diagnostic radiography who are always, or nearly always, in a control booth during exposures get the most accurate reports with quarterly service. Those who work in fluoroscopy and do mobile radiography are usually best monitored with monthly service.

Service companies provide an extra personal dosimeter in every batch that is marked "Control." The purpose of this dosimeter is to measure any radiation exposure that might occur to the entire batch while in transit. Any amount of exposure measured from the control dosimeter will be subtracted from the amounts measured from the other dosimeters in the batch. The control dosimeter should be kept in a safe place, away from any possibility of x-ray exposure. *It should never be used to measure occupational dose or for any other purpose.*

Radiation dosimeter service companies will want to know the name, birth date, and Social Security number of all persons to be monitored so that all records will be accurately identified. If there has been a history of previous occupational radiation exposure and the dose is known, this information should also be provided so that the record will be complete and accurate. Dosimeter reports are sent to the subscriber for each batch, and an annual summary of personnel exposure also is provided. Personnel should be advised of the radiation exposure reported from their badges and should be provided with copies of the annual reports for their own records. Occupationally exposed personnel should not leave their employment without a complete record of their radiation exposure history. Employers are required to provide this information.

Personal dosimeters should be worn in the region of the collar on the anterior surface of the body and should be outside the lead apron when a lead apron is worn (see Fig. 11-7). These dosimeters should never be clipped to straps worn around the neck, hanging near the center abdomen. Additionally, they should never be taken from the clinic or hospital to go shopping, home, or to other nonmedical areas.

Effective Dose Limits

Federal government standards must be met with regard to the amount of radiation an occupationally exposed person receives annually and in his or her lifetime. The National Council on Radiation Protection and Measurements (NCRP) prepares the standards and makes the recommendations to the government.

The **effective dose (EfD)** system is a limiting system used to calculate the upper limit of occupational exposure permissible. *For occupationally exposed personnel, the upper EfD limit is 50 mSv.* This applies to workers over the age of 18 who are not pregnant, and it is assumed to be a whole body dose. This limit applies to occupational exposure only, not to exposure that workers may receive from x-ray examinations related to their own health care or from natural background exposure. The effective dose is measured by the personal dosimeter readings.

To ensure that the lifetime risk of occupationally exposed persons remains within acceptable limits, an additional recommendation indicates that the *lifetime effective dose* in mSv should not exceed 10 times the occupationally exposed person's age in years. This is referred to as the **cumulative effective dose (CumEfD)**. *The CumEfD limits a radiation worker's lifetime effective dose to his or her age in years times 10 mSv.* For example, a 30-year-old worker with no previous occupational exposure would have a CumEfD limit of 300 mSv.

The established EfD limits ensure that the safety of radiation workers is comparable to that of workers in other occupations. The risk from the allowable exposures indicated earlier is considered to be low. The occupational dose received by limited operators is usually well below the established limits.

The ALARA principle is the guiding philosophy associated with the use of EfD limits. It is important that limited operators not be complacent simply because their dose is below the limit. It is required by radiation control agencies that employers and employees make every effort to ensure that occupational dose is kept to the lowest levels that are reasonably achievable.

Radiation and Pregnancy

It has long been recognized that radiation exposure poses risks to the developing embryo or fetus. In general, we now know that radiation exposure during pregnancy may result in spontaneous abortion, congenital defects in the child, increased risk of malignant disease in childhood, and an increase in significant genetic abnormalities in the children of parents who were exposed before birth.

Animal studies first alerted scientists to the fact that radiation could cause spontaneous abortion of the developing embryo and could increase the rate of congenital abnormalities seen in those who survived to birth. These findings have been confirmed in humans by studying the pregnancies of women who survived the atomic bomb blasts of Hiroshima and Nagasaki and the nuclear accident at Chernobyl, Russia. In the 1950s, Alice Stewart, an English researcher, demonstrated a fourteenfold increase in the incidence of childhood leukemia among children who had been exposed to radiation in utero as a result of maternal x-ray pelvimetry examinations in the third trimester of pregnancy.

According to the NCRP, studies of groups of women exposed to radiation as a result of diagnostic and therapeutic procedures confirm that radiation *in excess of 150 mGy-t* to the uterus is cause for concern. Table 11-7

Table 11-7
Estimation of Fetal Radiation Dose

Maternal X-ray Examination	ESE (Gy-$_a$)	Fetal Dose (mGy-$_t$)
Skull	0.70	0
Cervical spine	1.10	0
Chest (posteroanterior)	0.10	0
Lumbar spine	2.50	0.80
Pelvis	2.95	0.50
Wrist or foot	0.05	0

Modified from Bushong SC: *Radiologic science for technologists,* ed 10, St Louis, 2013, Mosby.
ESE, Entrance skin exposure.

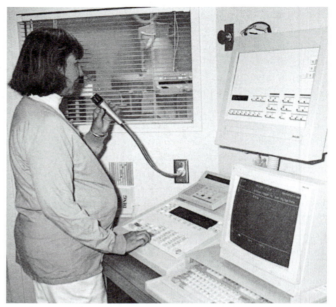
Fig. 11-10 Lead barrier of control booth protects pregnant limited operator and her unborn child.

lists the average fetal doses associated with various radiographic examinations.

The greatest risks for spontaneous abortion, fetal death, and birth defects exist when significant levels of exposure occur during the first trimester of pregnancy, that is, the first 3 months. The embryo is most vulnerable to radiation while tissues are in the process of differentiation. Unfortunately, this creates the greatest hazard at a time when a woman may not yet be aware that she is pregnant.

Radiation control agencies address the issue of radiation exposure of pregnant radiation workers. Regulations regarding pregnant workers use the term *declared pregnant woman.* When a worker voluntarily notifies her employer, in writing, that she is pregnant, the employer is responsible for ensuring that her dose equivalent remains below the established limit for pregnancy. *The NCRP-recommended EqD limit to the embryo/fetus for a pregnant worker is 0.5 mSv.* The radiation safety officer should provide essential counseling, and the worker should be given a second dosimeter, which is worn at the waist level for all radiation procedures. If a protective lead apron is worn, the second dosimeter is worn under the apron. *There is also a limit for the 9 months of the pregnancy. This limit is set at 5.0 mSv.* Table 11-8 shows the dose limits that are important to occupational radiation workers. The work assignment should be evaluated to minimize exposure. For a pregnant limited operator, the safest work assignment would be one in which a permanent lead barrier (control booth) always shields the worker during exposures (Fig. 11-10). Here again, the ALARA

principle is important. Every effort should be made to minimize exposure, keeping the dose received as far below the established limit as possible. Pregnant workers, or those of childbearing age who *may* be pregnant, should pay particular attention to personal safety measures when assisting with fluoroscopy or using mobile x-ray equipment.

The public is generally aware that radiation is to be avoided during pregnancy, and this may lead to irrational fears on the part of pregnant women or their families. The chance is extremely remote that a routine x-ray examination of the chest or an extremity would result in harm to the developing child. The risk of abnormality in the child as a result of a diagnostic x-ray examination in the first trimester of pregnancy is considered to be 1 in 1000 or less, depending on the examination. On the other hand, examinations requiring direct radiation to the pelvis, especially relatively high-dose fluoroscopic studies or CT scans of the abdomen or lumbar spine, may be cause for concern.

Radiation control regulations require that women of childbearing age be advised of potential radiation hazards before an x-ray examination. This requirement is usually met by posting signs in the radiology department advising women to tell the limited operator before the examination if there is any possibility that they may be pregnant (Fig. 11-11). Such signs should be written in all languages commonly used in the community.

The patient's physician is in the best position to be aware of an early pregnancy. The patient's history may indicate the possibility of pregnancy, and specific questions to rule out pregnancy should be a part of any medical history that precedes the ordering of pelvic or abdominal x-ray examinations. If pregnancy is a possibility, an early pregnancy test, easily and quickly performed in the physician's office, may clarify the situation. If the

Table 11-8
Effective Dose Limits for Occupational Workers

	mSv
Annual	50
Cumulative	age × 10 mSv
Embryo/fetus (mo)	0.5
Entire gestation	5.0

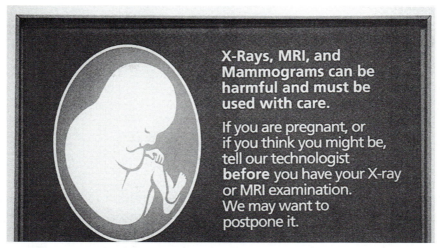

X-Rays, MRI, and Mammograms can be harmful and must be used with care.

If you are pregnant, or if you think you might be, tell our technologist **before** you have your X-ray or MRI examination. We may want to postpone it.

Fig. 11-11 Signs in dressing rooms, waiting areas, and imaging suites alert patients to the potential hazard of examination when pregnant.

patient is pregnant and the proposed x-ray examination involves direct pelvic radiation, the physician must weigh the potential risks and benefits of the examination and discuss them with the patient before proceeding with the study. In the case of minor or chronic complaints, it is common to delay the examination until after the birth of the child.

In practice, however, the possibility of pregnancy may not even be considered. This is especially true in the case of accident or injury, for which the emergency room or office visit is brief and the history is limited to the injury complaint. For this reason, *it is essential that the limited operator be mindful of the possibility of pregnancy whenever the patient is a female of childbearing age.* Specific questions should be asked to determine that the patient's physician has addressed the issue of pregnancy before ordering the examination. When the radiographic examination does not involve the abdomen and pelvis, it is good practice to provide a lead apron for women of childbearing age, whether pregnant or not (usually for those aged 10 to 55).

If x-ray examinations of a pregnant patient must be done, modifications in procedure can help to minimize dose to the embryo or fetus. If the part to be examined is *not* the abdomen or pelvis, this area can be shielded with a lead apron. If the abdomen or pelvis is to be examined, the number of projections and the size of the radiation field may be minimized, and a high-kVp technique will result in less radiation exposure than that from a routine procedure. The decision to do a limited study and the determination of the exact limitations to be imposed are up to the patient's physician or the radiologist.

SUMMARY

SI units are used to measure radiation exposure and dose. *ESE* stands for *entrance skin exposure,* the most common dose measurement in diagnostic radiography.

Cellular response to radiation exposure is the result of ionization that may involve a direct hit to the DNA of a cell's chromosome or may damage the cell indirectly as a result of the ionization of water and the formation of free radicals. Most cellular damage is repaired within a very short period of time. Cellular sensitivity is greatest for cells that are young, simple, rapidly dividing and multiplying, and have a rapid metabolism. Blood cells and blood-forming cells are very sensitive, as are skin cells, mucosal cells, and the cells of the thyroid gland and female breast; brain cells and cortical bone cells are relatively insensitive.

Low doses of radiation, typical of those received in diagnostic radiography, produce effects that are long term. They include the formation of cataracts, cancer, and leukemia and the possibility of birth defects in children irradiated during early gestation. Genetic effects are the result of mutations in genes caused when the reproductive organs are exposed. They may result in malformations or other defects in future generations.

Limited operators can reduce radiation risk to their patients by minimizing the need for repeat exposures, collimating well, and using low-dose techniques. Gonad shielding is required in some cases to reduce the likelihood of genetic effects.

Personnel safety is ensured by the proper use of time, distance, and shielding. Preexposure safety checks help prevent accidental exposure to co-workers. Limited operators' occupational dose is monitored using an OSL-type dosimeter. It is worn on the collar and evaluated monthly or quarterly by a qualified laboratory. Reports should be available to limited operators on either a monthly or a quarterly basis. The occupational dose for limited operators is typically well below the established EfD limit of 50 mSv per year.

Warning signs, early pregnancy tests, interviews, and double-checks by the limited operator are used to prevent the possibility of inadvertent exposure of a developing embryo or fetus that would increase the risk of spontaneous abortion, birth defects, or childhood cancer.

Radiographic Anatomy, Positioning, and Pathology

PART III

Radiographic Anatomy, Positioning, and Pathology

Chapter 12

Introduction to Anatomy, Positioning, and Pathology

Learning Objectives

At the conclusion of this chapter, you will be able to:

- Explain the differences between cells, tissues, organs, and systems
- List the systems of the human body and state the basic components and function of each
- Describe the structure of bone
- List the three classifications of joints and give an example of each
- Use correct terminology to describe joint motions
- Demonstrate anatomic position
- List and define the planes of the body
- Use correct terminology to describe anatomic locations and relationships
- Use correct terminology when referring to radiographic positions and projections
- Given a position/projection description from one of the following chapters, select, mark, and place the image receptor correctly
- Modify standard procedures to produce quality radiographic images of obese patients
- Define common terms used to describe or classify disease processes
- Explain the differences between acute and chronic conditions and between benign and malignant conditions
- Define inflammation and describe its possible consequences

Key Terms

abrasions
acute
anatomic position
anomalies
articulations
atrophy
benign
cartilage
central nervous system (CNS)
chronic
congenital
contusions
degeneration
diagnosis
dislocation
edema
fracture
gastrointestinal (GI) tract
hormones
iatrogenic
idiopathic
infections
inflammation
ischemia

lacerations
lesion
ligaments
lymph
malignant
metastasis
microorganisms
neoplasms
nosocomial
obese
pathology
peripheral
prognosis
projections
signs
sprain
strain
symptoms
syndrome
tendons
trauma
ulcer
vascular insufficiency

This chapter, the first in Part III, introduces the subjects of anatomy, radiographic positioning, and pathology to familiarize the reader with general concepts and terminology. This will improve understanding of the material included in the chapters to follow. Each of the other chapters in Part III discusses the anatomy, radiographic positioning, and common pathology of a particular body part. The term *anatomy* refers to the *structure* of the body. A comprehensive knowledge of the anatomy to be radiographed is essential for accurate radiographic positioning and for correct evaluation of finished radiographs. Physiology, on the other hand, refers to the function of the body. Although the primary emphasis in this text is on anatomy, function is included in the discussion of tissue and of organ systems.

In preparation for the study of radiographic positioning, this chapter includes the terms used to describe body positions and radiographic projections. Also included are details of common tasks performed during radiographic procedures. These include image receptor (IR) selection and use; alignment of radiographic tube, body part, and IR; placement of radiographic markers; and patient instructions.

Pathology is the study of disease that causes abnormal changes in the structure or function of body tissue and organs. A general knowledge of pathology will improve understanding of why many radiographic procedures are performed. This awareness may improve the diagnostic results of the procedure. The performance of radiography is more interesting and rewarding when the results make a positive contribution to the diagnosis and treatment of the patient.

ANATOMY

There are six levels of structural organization of the human body (Fig. 12-1). The body, like all matter, is made up of atoms and molecules. This is referred to as the *chemical level* of organization. The next level is the *cellular level*. Cells are the smallest units of living things. Groups of similar cells that work together to perform a common function are called *tissues*. An *organ* is a group of tissues that act together to perform a special function. A *system* is a group of organs that work together to perform complex functions. The sixth and highest level of structural organization is the *body as a whole*.

Cells

Cells are the smallest units of all living things. The human body is made up of many trillions of living cells. Cells are too small to be seen with the naked eye but can be examined using a microscope. There is great variation among cells with respect to size, shape, and function. For example, the ovum (female sex cell) is more than 100 times the size of a red blood cell. Some

cells are flat, some are brick-shaped, some are threadlike, some have irregular shapes, and some are capable of changing shape. Cells function as parts of tissue, so their function is explained under that heading.

The three main parts of a cell are the plasma membrane, the cytoplasm, and the nucleus. The plasma membrane encloses the cytoplasm and forms the outer boundary of the cell. The membrane also serves to provide communication between the cell and the rest of the body. Hormones or other chemical compounds can attach to the cell membrane and affect the activities within the cell. The cytoplasm is a highly specialized living material inside the plasma membrane and surrounding the nucleus. The cytoplasm consists of fluid and a variety of tiny structures called *organelles* that perform the work of the cell. The nucleus of the cell contains the chromosomes, the hereditary structures that contain the "blueprint" for cell structure and function. They are made up of the complex protein, DNA.

Tissues

Four main types of tissue compose the body's many organs: epithelial, connective, muscle, and nervous.

There are a number of types of epithelial tissue, but all perform the basic function of protecting underlying tissues. The skin is made up of epithelial tissue, as are the linings of the stomach and the air passages of the lungs. Some epithelial tissues also absorb and/or secrete substances. For example, the lining of the stomach absorbs nutrients from food and secretes chemicals that aid in digestion.

Connective tissue is the most widely distributed of all tissue and has the greatest variety of form and function. Connective tissue is found between tissues and between organs and serves to hold them together. It also makes up the structure of bone, cartilage, and fat.

Muscle tissue is capable of stretching and contracting. Its function is to produce movement. Different types of muscle tissue serve to move the bones, cause the heart to beat, and provide the movements required by other body organs.

Nervous tissue consists of the nerve cells, called *neurons*, and support cells. Neurons conduct electric impulses, providing rapid communication between body structures and control of body functions.

Organ Systems

Organ systems are the largest and most complex units of the body. The 11 major organ systems that compose the human body are the integumentary, muscular, nervous, endocrine, circulatory, lymphatic, respiratory, digestive, urinary, reproductive, and skeletal systems.

A brief overview is provided for the majority of the organ systems. The skeletal system is discussed in greatest detail because this is the most common organ system radiographed by the limited operator. The majority of

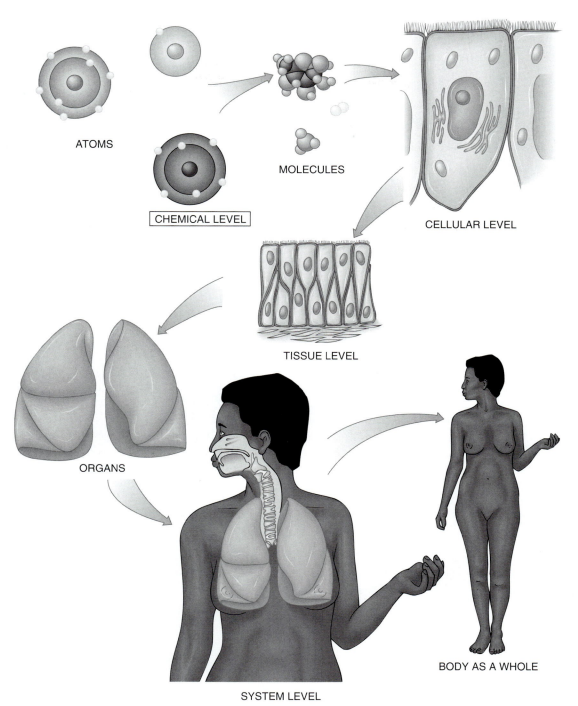

Fig. 12-1 Levels of structural organization.

chapters in Part III are concerned with radiography of a particular portion of the bony skeleton. Part III also covers radiography of the chest, which contains the major portion of the respiratory system, and radiography of the abdomen, which contains the major parts of the digestive and urinary systems.

Integumentary

The integumentary system (Fig. 12-2) consists principally of the skin. It also includes the hair and the

nails. The glands within the skin that secrete oil and sweat are parts of the integumentary system as well. Special microscopic organs in the skin sense contact with the outside world, enabling the body to respond to pain, pressure, touch, and changes in temperature.

Muscular

The muscular system (Fig. 12-3) consists of the voluntary muscles, which control the movements of the skeleton

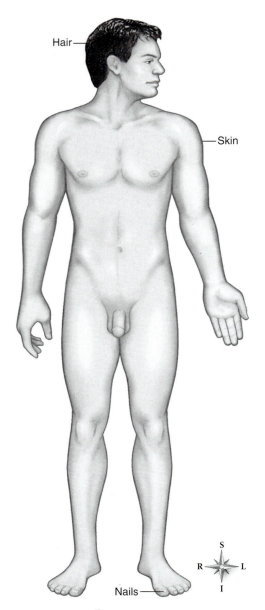

Hair

Skin

Nails

Fig. 12-2 Integumentary system.

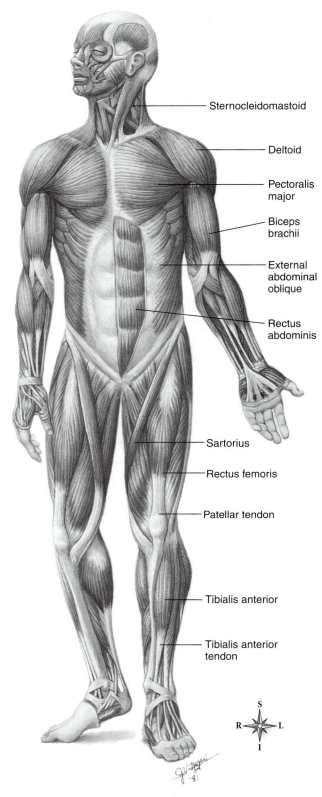

Sternocleidomastoid

Deltoid

Pectoralis major

Biceps brachii

External abdominal oblique

Rectus abdominis

Sartorius

Rectus femoris

Patellar tendon

Tibialis anterior

Tibialis anterior tendon

Fig. 12-3 Muscular system.

and are under conscious control, and the involuntary muscles, which function to produce the movements of organs. Muscles produce heat, maintaining a constant body temperature. Some specific muscles will be introduced in Chapter 23 in the discussion on intramuscular injections.

Nervous

The nervous system (Fig. 12-4) consists of the brain, the spinal cord, and the nerves. The brain and the spinal cord are referred to as the **central nervous system (CNS).** The nerves that carry information between the CNS and all parts of the body comprise the **peripheral** nervous system. Nervous system functions include communication, integration and control of body functions, and recognition of stimuli. Stimuli are agents, such as light, heat, pressure, and sound, that evoke sensations and perceptions. The functions of the nervous system are accomplished by the transmission of tiny electric impulses along the nerve pathways.

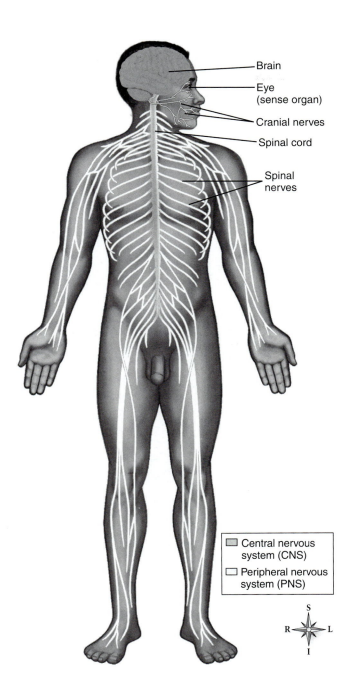

Fig. 12-4 Nervous system.

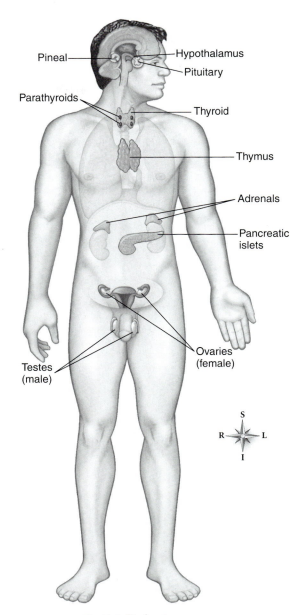

Fig. 12-5 Endocrine system.

Endocrine

The endocrine system (Fig. 12-5) consists of glands that secrete special chemicals called **hormones.** Endocrine glands are sometimes referred to as *ductless glands* because their secretions are released directly into the bloodstream, rather than being transported by a draining duct. They serve some functions similar to those of the nervous system in that they communicate, integrate, and regulate body functions. The hormones of the endocrine system provide slower, longer-lasting control of body function than the rapid electric impulses of the nervous system.

Circulatory

The circulatory system (Fig. 12-6) is also referred to as the *cardiovascular system.* It consists of the heart and the blood vessels. There are three types of blood vessels: *arteries,* which carry blood away from the heart; *veins,* which carry blood back to the heart; and *capillaries,* tiny vessels between the arteries and the veins that provide oxygen and nutrients to the cells. The heart provides a pumping action to keep blood flowing throughout the circulatory system. The major portions of the circulatory system will be addressed in more detail with the anatomy of the chest and abdomen in Chapter 16. Specific arteries and veins will be introduced when learning the procedures for taking a pulse in Chapter 22 and for drawing blood samples in Chapter 24.

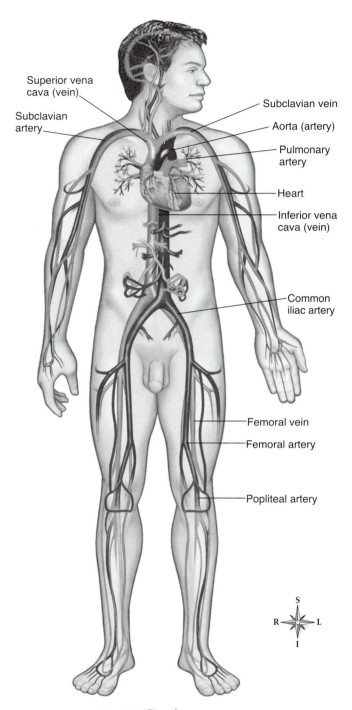

Fig. 12-6 Circulatory system.

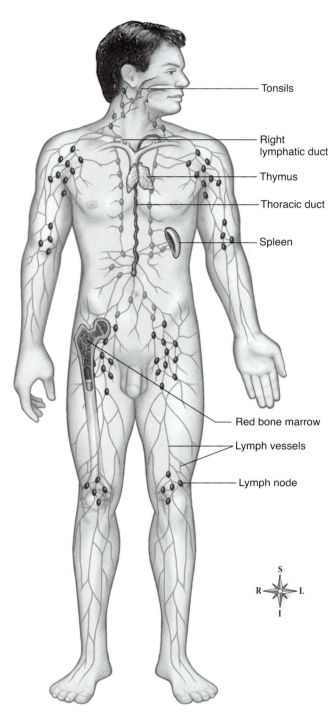

Fig. 12-7 Lymphatic system.

Lymphatic

The lymphatic system (Fig. 12-7) consists of the lymph nodes and lymph vessels, plus the spleen, tonsils, and thymus gland. The lymphatic system provides the fluid called **lymph** that surrounds the cells and serves to move fluid and certain large molecules from the cells to the circulatory system. The lymphatic system communicates with the circulatory system by means of the thoracic duct in the chest. An important function of the lymphatic system is its role in the immune system, which protects the body from disease.

Respiratory

The respiratory system (Fig. 12-8) consists of the breathing passages of the body. Included are the nose and mouth, the *pharynx* (throat), the *trachea* (windpipe), the *bronchi* (singular, *bronchus*), and the lungs. The bronchi are branching tubes from the trachea to the tissues of the lungs. The small, peripheral branches of the bronchi are called the *bronchioles*. The bronchioles terminate in tiny sacs called *alveoli* that are surrounded by blood vessels. Oxygen from the air is transferred to the blood from the

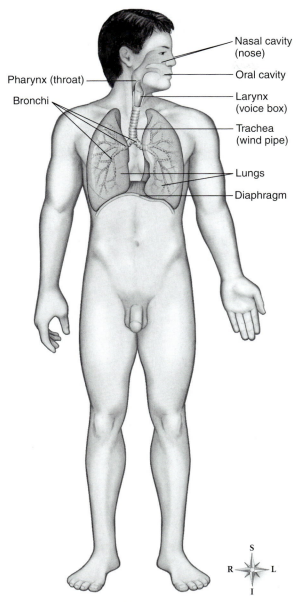

Fig. 12-8 Respiratory system.

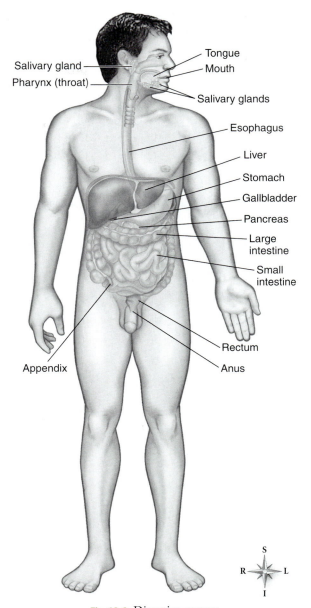

Fig. 12-9 Digestive system.

alveoli. Carbon dioxide, a gaseous waste produced when oxygen is used by the body, is transferred from the blood to the alveoli so that it can be exhaled from the lungs. More detailed anatomy of the respiratory system is covered in Chapter 16.

Digestive

The primary organs of the digestive system (Fig. 12-9) are the mouth, pharynx, esophagus, stomach, small intestine, large intestine, rectum, and anal canal. These organs constitute the **gastrointestinal (GI) tract,** also called the *alimentary canal,* a hollow tube that is open at both ends. The GI tract is the path of food from the time it enters the mouth until it is excreted as waste. It is lined with epithelial tissue called *mucous membrane.* Accessory organs of the digestive system, many of which aid in digestion, include the tongue, teeth, salivary glands, liver,

gallbladder, pancreas, and appendix. The major portion of the digestive system is contained within the abdominal cavity and is further discussed in Chapter 16.

Urinary

The urinary system (Fig. 12-10) consists of the kidneys, ureters, bladder, and urethra. The function of the urinary system is to eliminate excess fluid and the waste products of cellular activity from the body. The fluid and chemical waste are removed from the blood by the kidneys, forming *urine.* The urine flows through long tubes called *ureters* and into the bladder, where it is stored. Urine empties from the bladder through a tube called the *urethra.*

Reproductive

The reproductive system, unlike other organ systems, does not function for the survival of the individual. Its purpose

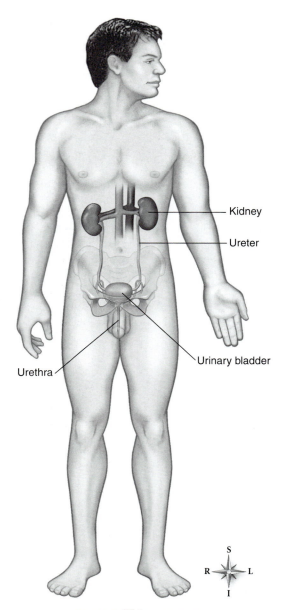

Fig. 12-10 Urinary system.

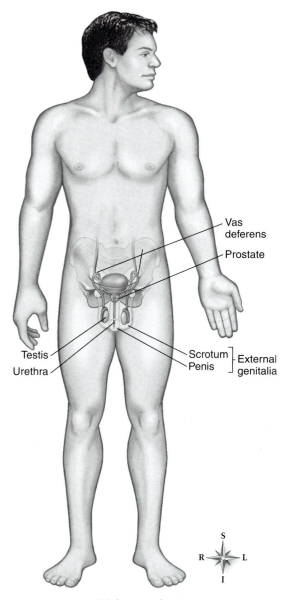

Fig. 12-11 Male reproductive system.

is the survival of the species; in our case the human race. Hormones produced by the reproductive organs promote the development of sexual characteristics. External organs or structures of the reproductive system are called *genitalia*. The organs that produce reproductive cells are called *gonads;* they were introduced in Chapter 11.

In the male reproductive system (Fig. 12-11), the external genitalia consist of the scrotum and the penis. The gonads are called *testes* (singular, *testis*). The testes are located within the scrotum. Sperm (male reproductive cells) from the testes travel through the vas deferens (a small, tubular structure) to the urethra, which opens to the outside. In the male, the urethra is a part of both the urinary system and the reproductive system. The prostate gland is an accessory organ of the male reproductive system. It surrounds the urethra at its junction with the bladder.

In the female reproductive system (Fig. 12-12), the external genitalia consist of the vulva, the soft tissues that surround the vaginal opening. The gonads are the ovaries, which are located within the pelvic portion of the abdomen. Fallopian tubes, which are also called *uterine tubes*, capture the ova when they are released by the ovaries and transmit them to the uterus. If the ovum is fertilized by a sperm, it attaches to the wall of the uterus, where the new life is nourished and protected as it grows until the fetus is mature enough to be born.

Skeletal

The skeletal system (Fig. 12-13) provides a rigid framework for the body. It consists of 206 bones with other associated tissues, such as cartilage and ligaments. **Cartilage** is a tough, fibrous connective tissue that is both stiff and flexible. The lay term for cartilage is *gristle*. **Ligaments** are

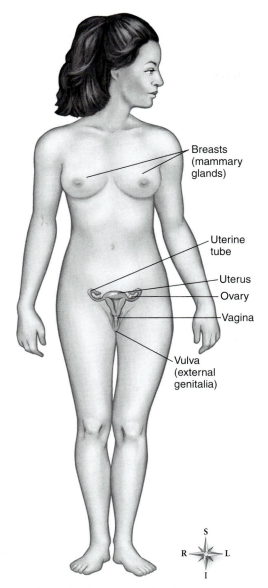

Fig. 12-12 Female reproductive system.

flexible bands of fibrous tissue that bind joints together and provide connections between bones and cartilage. **Tendons** are bands of fibrous tissue that attach muscles to bones.

The skeletal system is divided into the axial skeleton and the appendicular skeleton. The axial skeleton consists of the skull, spine, sternum (breast bone), and ribs. The appendicular skeleton includes the bones of the extremities (arms and legs), as well as those of the pelvis and shoulders. The remainder of this section discusses the physical characteristics of bone and the types of joints formed by the joining of particular bones.

Structure of Bone

The structure of bone varies considerably, depending on the specific type of bone. The four basic types are listed and described in Table 12-1.

The outer portion of most bones is a layer of hard, compact bone called the *cortex*. Inside the cortex is bone tissue that has a honeycomb, or *trabecular*, structure and is called cancellous or spongy bone. Long bones have a long cavity in the center called the *medullary canal*. The medullary canal and the spaces within spongy bone contain *marrow*, a fatty substance containing blood vessels and immature blood cells. The surfaces of bones that form moving joints are covered with *joint cartilage*. All other bone surfaces are covered by a tough, fibrous membrane called the *periosteum*.

The long bones are all found in the extremities. They include the major bones of the arms and legs and those that make up the fingers and toes. The parts of a long bone are illustrated in Fig. 12-14. The long shaft of the bone is called the *diaphysis*. At each end of the diaphysis is a flared portion called the *metaphysis*. The rounded ends that form joints are called the *epiphyses* (singular, *epiphysis*). Between the metaphysis and the epiphysis is the epiphyseal plate, or "growth plate." Early in life, this plate is made of cartilage and is the center for bone growth. When the bone is mature, the growth plate ossifies, meaning it turns to bone. The ossified growth plate is often seen on radiographs and is referred to as the *epiphyseal line*.

The features of bone shapes may be characterized as either **projections,** which grow out from the bone surface, or depressions, which are indentations or hollows in the surface. Specific terms are used to describe these features according to their characteristics.

Projections

Condyle—a rounded process that forms part of a joint (example: mandibular condyle of the temporomandibular joint)

Coracoid—a pointed projection (example: coracoid process of the scapula)

Coronoid—a beaklike projection (example: coronoid process of the ulna)

Crest—a bony ridge (example: crest of the ileum, a common positioning landmark)

Epicondyle—a projection above a condyle (example: medial epicondyle of the elbow)

Facet—a small, smooth process that forms part of a joint (example: articular surface of the superior articulating process of a vertebra)

Head—the rounded, wide end of a long bone (example: head of the humerus)

Malleolus—a club-shaped projection (example: medial malleolus of the distal tibia)

Process—a general term for a projection (example: coracoid process of the scapula)

Protuberance—a general term for a projection (example: external occipital protuberance of the skull)

Spine—a sharp process or a sharp ridge (example: scapular spine)

Styloid—a long, sharp process (example: ulnar styloid)

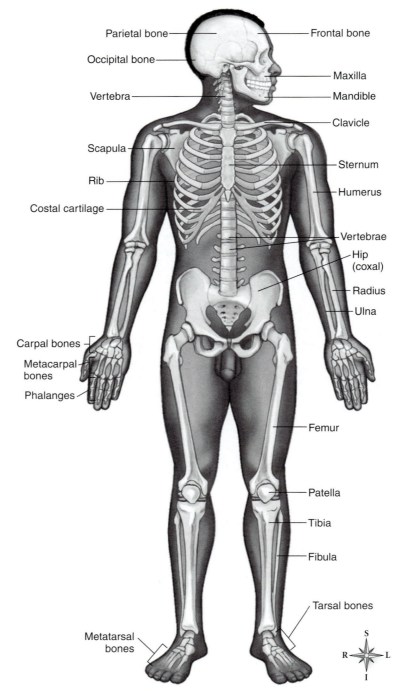

Parietal bone
Occipital bone
Vertebra
Scapula
Rib
Costal cartilage
Carpal bones
Metacarpal bones
Phalanges
Metatarsal bones

Frontal bone
Maxilla
Mandible
Clavicle
Sternum
Humerus
Vertebrae
Hip (coxal)
Radius
Ulna
Femur
Patella
Tibia
Fibula
Tarsal bones

Fig. 12-13 Skeletal system.

Trochanter—one of the large, rounded processes of the femur

Tubercle—a small, rounded process (example: greater tubercle of the proximal humerus)

Tuberosity—a rounded process larger than a tubercle, although the terms are sometimes used interchangeably (example: greater tuberosity of the proximal humerus)

Depressions

Fissure—a linear depression, a groove (example: orbital fissure)

Foramen (plural, *foramina*)—a hole in a bone for the passage of blood vessels and nerves (example: foramen magnum of the skull base)

Fossa (plural, *fossae*)—a pit or hollow (example: mandibular fossa of the temporal bone)

Groove—a shallow linear depression (example: bicipital groove of the proximal humerus)

Sinus—a cavity or hollow space (example: maxillary sinus)

Sulcus—a trenchlike depression, a deep fissure (example: carotid sulcus of the sphenoid bone)

Table 12-1

Bone Types

Bone Type	Description	Examples
Long	Long shaft with thick cortex and medullary canal; the two ends form joints	Humerus (upper arm), femur (thigh bone)
Short	Small bones made primarily of cancellous bone with a thin cortex	Bones of wrist and ankle
Flat	Two layers of compact bone with a thin cancellous layer between them	Cranium (outer skull), scapula (shoulder blade)
Irregular	Wide variety of shapes and structures	Vertebrae (spine), bones of the face

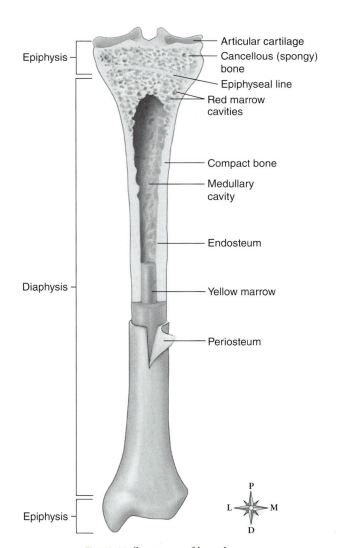

Epiphysis

Articular cartilage
Cancellous (spongy) bone
Epiphyseal line
Red marrow cavities

Compact bone
Medullary cavity

Endosteum

Diaphysis

Yellow marrow

Periosteum

Epiphysis

P
L — M
D

Fig. 12-14 Structure of long bones.

Joints

The places where bones are joined together are called *joints* or **articulations.** There are three classifications of joints based on their ability to move:

- *Synarthrosis* refers to a joint that does not move. With the exception of the mandible (jaw bone), the joints of the skull are all synarthrodial joints and are called *sutures.*
- *Amphiarthrosis* refers to a joint that has very limited motion. The articular surfaces that form these joints are covered by fibrous cartilage or cushioned by disks of fibrous cartilage. The joints between the bodies of the spinal vertebrae and the sacroiliac joints (between the spine and the pelvis) are examples of amphiarthrodial joints.
- *Diarthrosis* refers to a joint that can move freely. The bones that form these joints are shaped to fit together to accomplish the required movement, and their articular surfaces are covered by articular cartilage. A fibrous capsule that is lined with synovial membrane surrounds the joint. This membrane secretes *synovial fluid*, providing moisture to lubricate the joint.

Some diarthrodial joints have sacs filled with synovial fluid. These are called *bursae* (singular, *bursa*). They serve to cushion the movements of tendons or muscles. Important bursae are located at the shoulder, elbow, hip, and knee.

Joint Movements

Joints allow a number of body movements. The following terms are used to describe these movements. Many are used in the radiographic positioning instructions in this book.

Four types of movement are found in diarthrodial joints:

Circular movement is the arclike rotation of a structure around an axis. Circular movements include rotation, circumduction, supination, and pronation.

- *Rotation* is the pivoting of a bone on its axis. Moving the head from side to side (indicating "no") requires pivoting the first cervical vertebra around the odontoid process of the second cervical vertebra.
- *Circumduction* moves the distal end of a bone in a circle, resulting in a conical-shaped motion. A baseball pitcher's throwing motion requires circumduction of the arm at the shoulder.
- *Supination* is lateral (or external) rotation of the bones of the forearm so the palm of the hand is facing up or anterior. This movement is illustrated in Fig. 12-15.
- *Pronation*, the opposite of supination, is medial (or internal) rotation of the bones of the forearm so the palm of the hand is facing down or posterior.

Angular movement is commonly referred to as bending, resulting in a change in angle between the long axis of the two bones making up the joint. These angular

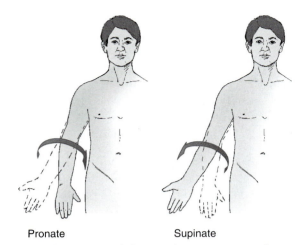

Pronate   Supinate

Fig. 12-15 Illustration of the circular movements of pronation and supination.

movements include flexion, extension, abduction, and adduction.

- *Flexion* is a bending motion that decreases the angle between two bones. An example would be to bend the arm at the elbow joint so the forearm moves closer to the humerus. This movement is illustrated in Fig. 12-16.
- A specific type of flexion, called *dorsiflexion*, occurs when the foot is moved so the toes are closer to the anterior surface of the lower leg. This decreases the angle between the top, or dorsal surface, of the foot and the anterior lower leg. *Plantar flexion*, the opposite of dorsiflexion, is movement of the foot away from the lower leg so the angle between them is increased.
- *Extension*, the opposite of flexion, is a bending motion that increases the angle between two bones. The arm is extended at the elbow joint when the flexed arm is returned to anatomic position. The term *hyperextension* is used when a joint is extended beyond its usual anatomic position. This is not considered a normal joint movement.

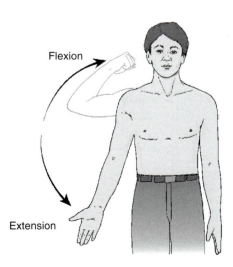

Flexion

Extension

Fig. 12-16 Illustration of angular movements of flexion and extension.

- *Abduction* is movement of a part away from the middle, or midline, of the body. An example would be movement of the arm or leg straight out to the side of the body, without moving it forward or back.
- *Adduction*, the opposite of abduction, is movement of a part toward the midline.

Gliding movement occurs when one bone slides over another. These simple motions occur without any circular or angular movements. Examples include the movement of the patella over the femur with knee flexion or extension and movement between the articular surfaces of the inferior and superior articular processes of adjacent vertebra.

The final types of diarthrodial joint movements are called *special movements*. They do not fit into the other types and occur in a limited number of joints. Special movements include inversion, eversion, protraction, retraction, elevation, and depression.

- *Inversion* is turning the sole, or plantar surface, of the foot inward (Fig. 12-17). This is a common movement when someone steps on something sharp in bare feet, then checks to see if damage has occurred. Unintentional inversion of the foot is a common cause of a sprained ankle.
- *Eversion*, the opposite of inversion, is turning the sole of the foot outward. Unintentional eversion can also result in a sprained ankle.
- *Protraction* is moving a part forward, or anterior. Holding an arm straight out in front of you requires protraction.
- *Retraction*, the opposite of protraction, is moving a part backwards, or posterior.
- *Elevation* moves a part up, or superior. Moving the top of your shoulder toward your ear requires an elevation movement.
- *Depression*, the opposite of elevation, moves a part down, or inferior.

Many of the body movements just described are performed by the patient during a radiographic procedure. The limited operator must frequently assist the patient, through either verbal instructions or physical manipulations, to achieve these movements. Care must be taken to assess the patient's physical abilities and response to pain during the positioning process to prevent injury.

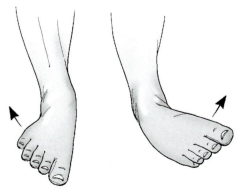

Fig. 12-17 Illustration of the special movements of eversion and inversion.

RADIOGRAPHIC POSITIONING

Radiographic positioning is the process of placing the body or a body part in proper position to create the desired radiograph. Chapters 13 through 17 contain descriptions and instructions for all common radiographic positions, projections, and methods. To properly perform a radiographic procedure, the limited operator must understand anatomic terms and terms for body position, radiographic position, and radiographic projection.

Radiographic positioning instructions frequently include terms that describe the relationship of body parts to each other and to the location or orientation of body surfaces or structures in space. Terms that indicate these anatomic relationships are based on **anatomic position** (Fig. 12-18).

The following terms are used to accurately describe anatomic locations, orientations, and relationships:

- *Anterior*—forward or front portion of the body or body part
- *Posterior*—backward or back portion of the body or body part; the opposite of anterior
- *Caudal/caudad*—away from the head
- *Cephalic/cephalad*—pertaining to the head; toward the head; the opposite of caudal
- *Central*—pertaining to the middle area or main part of an organ or body part
- *Peripheral*—away from the central mass of an organ, toward its outer limits; the opposite of central
- *Distal*—away from the source or point of origin; for example, the wrist is *distal* to the elbow, being farther from the point of origin of the arm, which is at the shoulder
- *Proximal*—toward the source or point of origin; the opposite of distal
- *Dorsal*—pertaining to the back part or surface of the body or part; the top surface of the foot; or the back of the hand
- *Ventral*—forward, front part; the opposite of dorsal
- *External*—to the outside, at or near the surface of the body or a body part
- *Internal*—deep, near the center of the body or a body part; the opposite of external
- *Inferior*—below, farther from the head
- *Superior*—above, toward the head; the opposite of inferior
- *Lateral*—referring to the side, away from the center to the left or right
- *Medial/mesial*—toward the center of the body or the center of a part; the opposite of lateral
- *Palmar*—referring to the palm (anterior surface) of the hand
- *Plantar*—referring to the sole of the foot
- *Parietal*—referring to the walls of a cavity
- *Visceral*—pertaining to organs

Procedures for radiographic positioning are also described using body planes (Fig. 12-19). The *sagittal plane* divides the body into right and left parts; the *midsagittal* or *median plane* divides the body into equal right and left parts. The *coronal plane* divides the body into anterior and posterior parts. The *midcoronal* or *midfrontal plane* divides the body into relatively equal parts; it passes through the external auditory meatus (the opening of the ear), the center of the shoulder, the greater trochanter (the bony prominence in the lateral hip area), and the lateral malleolus (the bony prominence on the lateral surface of the ankle). The *transverse* or *horizontal plane* divides the body into superior and inferior portions. It may be drawn at any level.

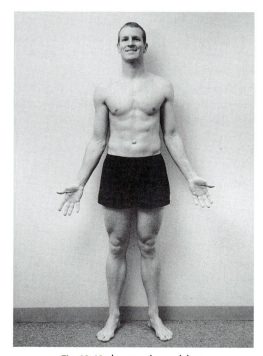

Fig. 12-18 Anatomic position.

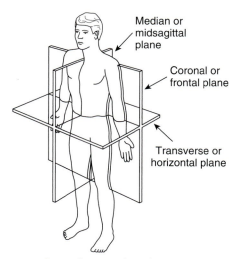

Median or midsagittal plane

Coronal or frontal plane

Transverse or horizontal plane

Fig. 12-19 Sagittal, coronal, and transverse planes.

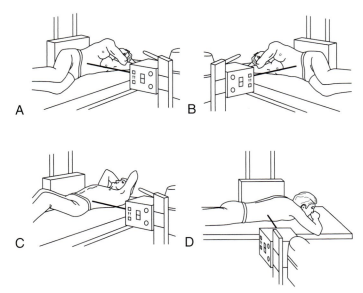

Fig. 12-20 Decubitus positions. Note horizontal orientation of the central ray. **A,** Left lateral decubitus position results in an anteroposterior (AP) projection. **B,** Right lateral decubitus position results in an AP projection. **C,** Dorsal decubitus position results in a lateral projection. **D,** Ventral decubitus position results in a lateral projection.

Body Positions

Radiographic positioning usually begins with proper placement of the patient's body. The following terms are used to describe body positions:
- *Prone*—lying face down
- *Recumbent*—lying down; the position is further described by adding the name of the body surface on which the patient is lying: *dorsal recumbent, lateral recumbent, ventral recumbent*
- *Supine*—lying on the back
- *Upright*—erect, standing or seated

Radiographic Positions

Radiographic positions describe the placement of the body part in relation to the radiographic table or IR. The following terms are used to describe radiographic positions.

For a *decubitus* position, the patient is recumbent with the central ray (CR) horizontal, or parallel to the floor. This position is named according to the body surface on which the patient is lying: lateral decubitus (left or right), dorsal decubitus, or ventral decubitus. Fig. 12-20 illustrates the four decubitus positions.

A *lateral* position is achieved by placement of the body or body part with the sagittal plane parallel to the IR. It is named according to the side adjacent to the radiographic table or IR.

A *lordotic* position results in angulation of the coronal plane of the chest with the IR. It is achieved by having the upright patient lean back so that only the dorsal aspect of the shoulders is in contact with the IR.

An *oblique* position is achieved when the body part or entire body is placed so that the coronal plane is not parallel with the radiographic table or IR. The description is usually stated as a degree of rotation, either from a body plane or toward the affected side.

Radiographic Projections

A radiographic projection indicates the path of the CR from the radiographic tube and through the patient to the IR. Most are named, in anatomic terms, by the CR entrance and exit points in the body.

For *anteroposterior (AP)* projections, the CR enters the anterior surface and exits the posterior surface of the body or anatomic structure (Fig. 12-21).

For *posteroanterior (PA)* projections, the CR enters the posterior surface and exits the anterior surface of the body or anatomic structure (Fig. 12-22).

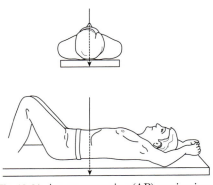

Fig. 12-21 Anteroposterior (AP) projection.

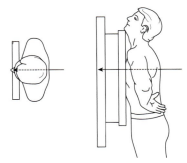

Fig. 12-22 Posteroanterior (PA) projection.

Lateral projections are those in which the sagittal plane of the body or body part is parallel to the IR. Lateral projections are always named for the side of the patient that is nearest the IR (Fig. 12-23). Lateral projections of the extremities are further described with the lateral

or medial entrance and exit of the CR: mediolateral or lateromedial.

Oblique projections are those in which the body is rotated so that the CR travels through the body on an oblique plane, rather than following an anatomic plane. Oblique projections are named by the entrance and exit points of the CR. For example, in an AP oblique projection, the CR enters the anterior aspect of the body and exits the opposite posterior aspect. Fig. 12-24 illustrates the AP and PA oblique projections

Axial projections are radiographs taken with a longitudinal angulation of the CR of 10 degrees or more. The angle may be either cephalad (toward the head) or caudad (away from the head) (Fig. 12-25).

Tangential projections are produced by directing the CR to "skim" the profile of the subject. Fig. 12-26 illustrates the tangential projection used to demonstrate the patella and patellofemoral joint space.

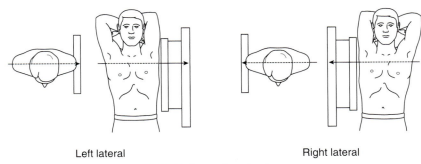

Left lateral   Right lateral

Fig. 12-23 Lateral projections.

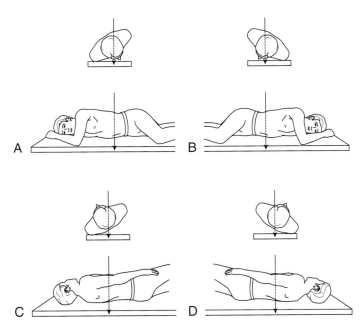

Fig. 12-24 Oblique projections. **A,** Posteroanterior (PA) oblique projection, right anterior oblique (RAO) position. **B,** PA oblique projection, left anterior oblique (LAO) position. **C,** Anteroposterior (AP) oblique projection, left posterior oblique (LPO) position. **D,** AP oblique projection, right posterior oblique (RPO) position.

Fig. 12-27 Lengthwise image receptor placement. Long dimension is parallel to long axis of the body.

provided with the position/projection descriptions in this text will work with both cassette-based CR IPs and DR IRs.

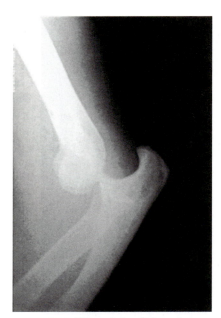

Fig. 12-43 Elbow joint dislocation.

force is called a **strain.** Other types of soft tissue trauma include **lacerations,** cuts or tears through the skin and underlying tissues; **abrasions,** scraping wounds to the skin; and **contusions,** closed wounds that cause bleeding under the skin and are commonly called *bruises.*

The principal chemical causes of disease are poisonings and drug reactions. Inhalation of toxic fumes or the absorption of toxic substances through the skin may also cause chemical injury to the body.

Exogenous diseases caused by microbiologic agents are called **infections.** Infections may occur in almost any part of the body but are most likely to affect structures that are in some way in contact with the outside world. The most common infections are those that occur in wounds and those that involve the respiratory system. Microbiologic agents are living organisms too small to be seen with the naked eye and are termed **microorganisms.** Many of these agents cause contagious diseases. Microorganisms are discussed in Chapter 21, which deals with infection control.

A crater-like sore on the skin or a mucous membrane is called an **ulcer.** There are many possible causes. Ulcers in the lining of the stomach, for example, may be caused by chemical injury from the acids produced by the body to aid in digestion.

When the cause of a disease is unknown, it is said to be **idiopathic.** Diseases that occur as the result of treatment by health professionals are termed **iatrogenic.** The term **nosocomial** refers to diseases that are acquired in hospitals.

Classification by Disease Process

Diseases are often classified according to the nature of the disease process itself. The disease process may involve inflammation, degeneration, or alterations in tissue growth.

Inflammation is the immune system's response to cellular injury. It is the initial part of the healing process. Inflammation is characterized by swelling, reddening, heat at the site, and pain. During this process, the blood supply to the injured area is increased. The term for swelling caused by vascular congestion is **edema.** White blood cells attack microorganisms and clean up dead tissue and other debris of injury. The terms used to define inflammatory conditions all end in *itis.* For example, *arthritis* refers to inflammation of a joint and *sinusitis* is the term for inflammation of the sinuses.

Chronic inflammation causes **degeneration,** further injury to cells and tissues. Degeneration may lead to **atrophy,** a decrease in the size or number of cells. Atrophy causes tissue to waste away and also causes impairment or loss of function. There are four types of atrophy: senile, disuse, pressure, and endocrine. Senile atrophy occurs as a result of age. Decreased muscle mass and strength in the elderly are manifestations of senile atrophy. Disuse atrophy occurs to any body part that is not used. For example, when a cast is used to treat a fracture of a limb, the muscles within the cast tend to shrink during the period that the cast is in place. An example of pressure atrophy is the deterioration of skin and underlying tissues that may occur in bedridden patients, causing bedsores, which are a form of ulcer. Endocrine atrophy is caused by a decrease in the supply of hormones. An example is the shrinkage of the ovaries and the uterus after menopause.

Hyperplasia and *hypertrophy* are both increases in the size of tissues or organs. *Hyperplasia* is defined as an increase in the number of cells, whereas *hypertrophy* refers to an increase in the size of the cells. These two conditions may exist together, and the two terms are often used interchangeably. These alterations in cell growth may be caused by inflammation or by an excess or deficiency of endocrine production.

Neoplasms are growths or tumors. They develop when changes in cells cause failure of the mechanisms that control normal cell growth. The names of neoplasms usually end with *oma.* Some examples include *carcinoma, sarcoma, melanoma, lipoma, lymphoma,* and *adenoma.* Most neoplasms can be classified as either benign or malignant. **Benign** neoplasms are single masses of cells that remain at one location and are limited in their growth. **Malignant** neoplasms are cancers. They tend to invade surrounding tissue and are capable of **metastasis,** that is, they may be transplanted to other locations in the body. Metastasis may occur through "seeding," the migration of cells through the cavities of the body, or the tumor may be spread through either the lymphatic system or the circulatory system.

SUMMARY

The human body is a highly organized and complex structure. Its fundamental units are cells. Groups of similar cells form tissues. Organs are combinations of tissues with a special function. Groups of organs form each of the 11 organ systems of the body. Each system has a unique structure that is suitable for its special functions. The limited operator should be familiar with the general structure and function of all body systems.

The limited operator requires a deeper understanding of the skeletal system because of its significance in radiography. An understanding of the structure of bones and joints and the names of their parts prepares the limited operator for a deeper study of each part of the skeletal system.

The terminology of body positions, radiographic positions, and radiographic projections is the essential language of radiographic positioning. Body positions include recumbent, prone, supine, and upright. Radiographic positions describe the placement of the body or body part in relation to the radiographic table. The radiographic positions are decubitus, lateral, lordotic, and oblique. Radiographic projections indicate the path of the CR from the radiographic tube through the patient to the IR. The CR entrance and exit points in the body most frequently name these projections. For example, the CR for the AP projection enters the body on the anterior surface and exits the posterior surface. All radiographic procedures consist of a set of steps designed to ensure patient safety and optimum diagnostic results. Each procedure has

patient care aspects, including assessment, communication, and both physical and radiation safety concerns. Technical aspects include selection and orientation of the IR; placement of exposure fields on the IR; alignment of the tube, body part, and IR; placement of radiographic markers; selection of appropriate exposure settings; and image evaluation.

Pathology is the study of disease. It includes many topics not usually thought of as diseases, such as injuries, birth defects, and anomalies. Diseases may be caused by circulatory system problems, by deficiencies or autoimmune conditions within the body, or by trauma, chemical injury, or infection from outside the body. Fractures, dislocations, and sprains are injuries caused by trauma to the skeletal system. Strains, lacerations, abrasions, and contusions are soft tissue injuries.

The response of the immune system to cellular injury is called *inflammation*. Chronic inflammation causes degeneration and atrophy of tissues, resulting in loss of function. Inflammation or endocrine imbalance may cause hyperplasia or hypertrophy, an increase in the size of an organ or structure. Neoplasms are tumors that may be benign or malignant. Benign neoplasms are self-limiting, but malignant neoplasms may invade surrounding tissue or spread to other parts of the body through a process called *metastasis*.

Chapter 13

Upper Limb and Shoulder Girdle

Learning Objectives

At the conclusion of this chapter, you will be able to:

- Name the bones that compose the upper limb and shoulder girdle and identify each on an anatomic diagram and on a radiograph
- Name and identify the significant bony prominences and depressions of the upper limb and shoulder girdle and identify significant positioning landmarks by palpation
- Demonstrate correct body and part positioning for routine projections and common special projections of the upper limb and shoulder girdle
- Correctly evaluate radiographs of the upper limb and shoulder girdle for positioning accuracy
- Describe and recognize on radiographs pathology common to the upper limb and shoulder girdle

Key Terms

acromion process
axilla
bursitis
carpal bones
carpus
clavicle
coracoid process
digits
fat pad sign
glenoid process
humerus
joint effusion
metacarpals
olecranon process
osteoarthritis

osteoblastic
osteolytic
osteomyelitis
osteophytes
phalanx (pl. phalanges)
radial deviation
radius
scapula
sesamoid bones
tendinitis
ulna
ulnar deviation

Although the focus of this chapter is on the upper limb and shoulder girdle, many of the principles introduced in this chapter apply equally well to the lower limb. For example, similar types of fractures and other pathologies occur in both the upper and the lower extremities.

ANATOMY

The upper limb, also called the upper extremity, includes the fingers, thumb, hand, wrist, forearm, elbow, humerus, and shoulder girdle (Fig. 13-1).

Fingers and Thumb

The fingers are called the **digits** and are considered to be part of the hand (Fig. 13-2). They are numbered from 1 to 5, beginning with the thumb. Digits 2 through 5 consist of three small long bones called **phalanges** (singular, **phalanx**). The phalanges are distinguished from one another as proximal (nearest the hand), middle, and distal. For example, the bone at the tip of the "ring finger" is called the *fourth distal phalanx*. The rounded tips of the distal phalanges are called *ungual tufts*. The hinge joints that connect the phalanges are called the *interphalangeal (IP) joints* and are distinguished as proximal and distal. The thumb has only two phalanges with one IP joint.

Hand

The bones of the hand are called **metacarpals.** They are numbered 1 through 5, starting on the lateral aspect. The numbers correspond to the digits with which they articulate. The distal end of a metacarpal is called its *head*, and the proximal end is referred to as the *base*. For example, the thumb is attached to the head of the first metacarpal. The hinge joints between the metacarpals and the proximal phalanges are called the *metacarpophalangeal (MCP) joints.*

There are usually one or more small bones in the region of the first MCP joint called **sesamoid bones.** These small, flat, oval bones within tendons are not counted among the bones of the body. They are called *sesamoid bones* because they resemble a sesame seed. They serve to protect the joint.

Wrist

The wrist consists of eight short bones called **carpal bones.** Together, they are referred to as the **carpus.** They are arranged in two rows. Beginning with the proximal row on the lateral aspect (thumb side), they are named *scaphoid, lunate, triquetrum,* and *pisiform.* The scaphoid is the most frequently fractured carpal bone. Continuing back toward the thumb, the distal row consists of the *trapezium, trapezoid, capitate,* and *hamate.* The capitate is the largest of the carpal bones. There is a small curved projection on the anterior aspect of the hamate called the *hook* or *hamulus.* As a whole, the wrist is capable of all joint motions except rotation. It moves in four directions: anterior, posterior, medial, and lateral. The greatest degree of movement is (anterior)

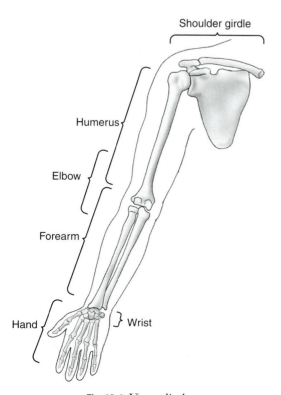

Fig. 13-1 Upper limb.

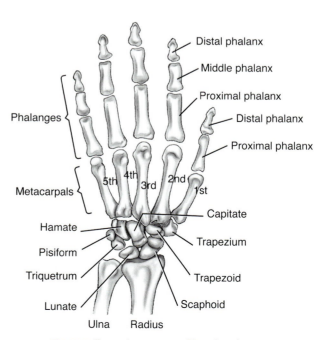

Fig. 13-2 Posterior aspect of hand and wrist.

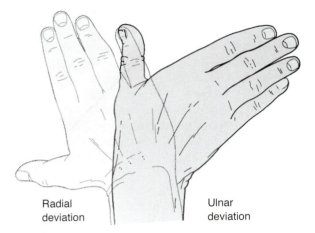

Radial
deviation

Ulnar
deviation

Fig. 13-3 Illustration of radial deviation and ulnar deviation at the wrist.

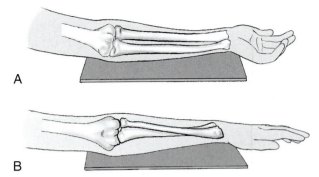

Fig. 13-5 Positions of forearm bones. **A,** Supination. **B,** Pronation.

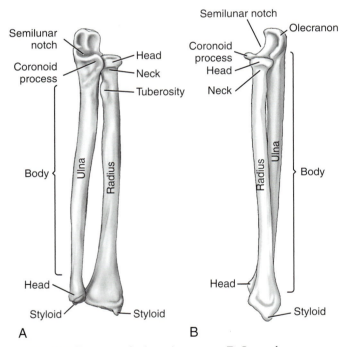

Fig. 13-4 Forearm. **A,** Anterior aspect. **B,** Lateral aspect.

flexion, followed by (posterior) extension, **ulnar deviation,** and **radial deviation** (Fig. 13-3). Ulnar deviation occurs when the hand is moved toward the medial (ulnar) side of the wrist. Movement of the hand toward the lateral (radial) side of the wrist is radial deviation.

Forearm

The forearm (Fig. 13-4) consists of two long bones, the **radius** and the **ulna.** The ulna is the longer, thinner bone on the medial aspect. The radius is thicker and

somewhat shorter and is located on the lateral aspect. The styloid process of the radius is a bony prominence that can be palpated on the lateral aspect of the wrist. The ulnar styloid can be felt on the posteromedial aspect of the wrist; it is most prominent when the hand is pronated. Pronation causes the radius to cross over the ulna (Fig. 13-5). The forearm is radiographed with the hand in supination to prevent this superimposition.

The proximal end of the radius is referred to as the *radial head.* The *radial tuberosity,* which is distal to the radial head, is a muscle attachment that is not normally palpable.

The proximal end of the ulna terminates in the posterior aspect of the olecranon process. In lay terms, the **olecranon process** is sometimes called the *funny bone* or *crazy bone.* Anterior to the olecranon process is the semilunar notch. The inferior lip of the semilunar notch is called the *coronoid process.*

Humerus

The single bone of the upper arm is called the **humerus** (Fig. 13-6). The distal end of the humerus is the humeral condyle. Just superior to the condyle are two palpable prominences, the medial and lateral epicondyles. Between the epicondyles on the posterior aspect is the olecranon fossa, a depression into which the olecranon process of the proximal ulna fits when the elbow joint is extended. There are two distal articular surfaces on the humerus: the rounded capitulum (also called the *capitellum*), which articulates with the head of the radius, and the trochlea, a spool-shaped process that articulates within the semilunar notch of the ulna. Just superior to the trochlea is the coronoid fossa, into which the coronoid process of the ulna fits when the elbow is flexed. Just superior to the capitulum is the radial fossa, a depression into which the radial head fits when the elbow joint is flexed.

The superior end of the humerus is called the *head.* The portion just inferior to the head is the *anatomic neck.*

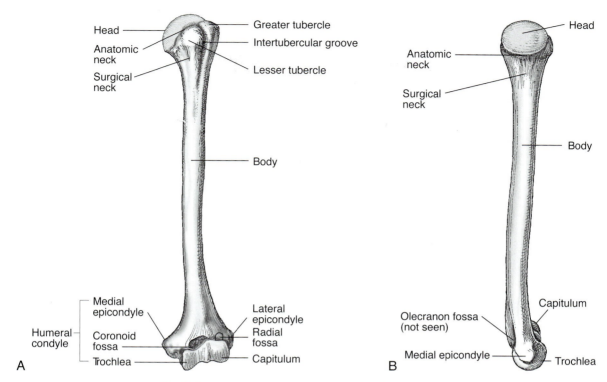

Fig. 13-6 Humerus. **A,** Anterior aspect. **B,** Medial aspect.

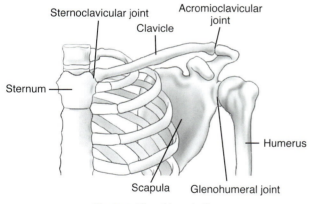

Fig. 13-7 Shoulder girdle.

Two prominences on the head of the humerus are significant: the greater tubercle, which is superior and lateral, and the lesser tubercle, which is medial and inferior. The greater tubercle can be felt on the upper outer aspect of the shoulder when the patient is in anatomic position. The constricted area just distal to the tubercles is called the *surgical neck*, which is a common site of fractures.

Shoulder Girdle

The bones of the shoulder are often referred to as the *shoulder girdle* (Fig. 13-7). They include the **scapula** (shoulder blade), the **clavicle** (collar bone), and the proximal portion of the humerus.

The scapula (Fig. 13-8) is a flat, triangular bone. Its three sides are called the *superior border*; the *lateral border*; and the *medial border*. The junction of the lateral and medial borders at the lower tip is called the *inferior angle*. The spine of the scapula is a bony ridge on the posterior surface that is inferior and somewhat parallel to the superior border. It serves as a muscle attachment. At the junction of the superior and lateral borders are three significant features: the acromion process, the coracoid process, and the glenoid process. The **acromion process** is a large, rounded projection that can be felt on the superior surface of the shoulder. The **coracoid process** is a muscle attachment on the anterior surface that is palpable just medial to the humeral head. The **glenoid process** is on the superior lateral aspect. It contains a cavity called the *glenoid fossa* that forms the socket of the shoulder joint. Its articulation with the humeral head is called the *glenohumeral joint.*

The clavicle (Fig. 13-9) is a long, narrow bone located anterior to the upper portion of the rib cage. Its medial end attaches to the sternum (breast bone), forming the *sternoclavicular (SC) joint*. Its lateral end forms a gliding joint with the acromion process of the scapula that is called the *acromioclavicular (AC) joint.*

Fig. 13-10 illustrates the palpable bony landmarks of the upper limb.

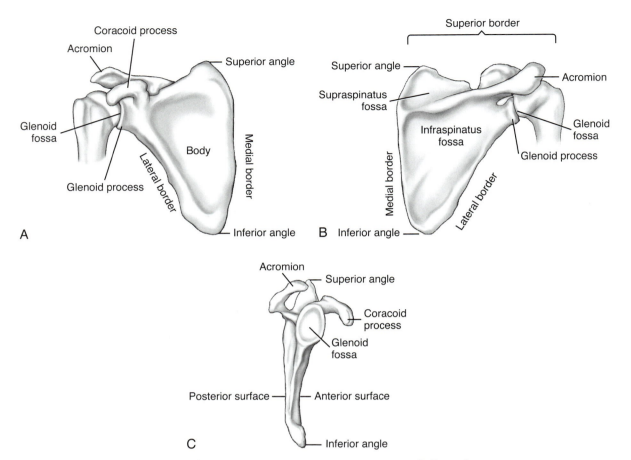

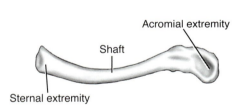

Fig. 13-8 Scapula. **A,** Anterior aspect. **B,** Posterior aspect. **C,** Lateral aspect.

Fig. 13-9 Anterior aspect of clavicle.

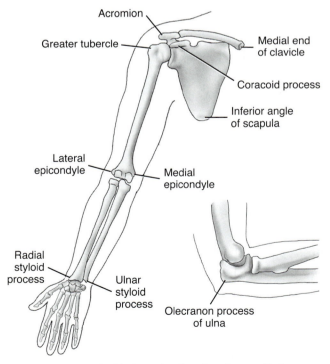

Fig. 13-10 Palpable bony landmarks of upper limb.

POSITIONING AND RADIOGRAPHIC EXAMINATIONS

Examinations of the upper limb from the fingertips through the elbow joint are usually done on the tabletop (the image receptor [IR] is placed on top of the radiographic table without a grid) with the patient seated at the end of the radiographic table (Fig. 13-11).

Each upper limb radiograph is created using a single IR. For example, a three-projection radiographic examination of the hand would require use of three computed

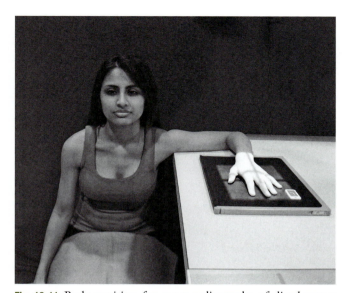

Fig. 13-11 Body position for most radiographs of distal upper limb. This position is comfortable for the patient and ensures that the gonads are not in close proximity to the x-ray exposure field.

radiography (CR) cassettes or three separate exposures on a digital radiography (DR) IR. The exception is radiography of a finger, when some institutions will allow multiple exposure fields (for all three projections) to be placed on a single CR imaging plate.

To prepare for these examinations, the patient removes any clothing or jewelry from the area that will be within the radiation field. This is usually a simple matter for examinations of the distal limb. Patients may need to remove outer clothing from the upper torso and don a gown for examinations of the shoulder region.

Although gonad shielding is not legally required for examinations of the upper limb, it is wise to shield whenever the patient requests or if the gonads are within or close to (about 5 cm) the primary x-ray beam. A lead shield placed in the lap is shown here for these examinations.

Hand

Routine Examination

The routine examination of the hand includes the posteroanterior (PA), PA oblique-lateral rotation, and lateral projections.

IR: 8 × 10 inches (18 × 24 cm) or 10 × 12 inches (24 × 30 cm)

Grid: No

Source–image receptor distance (SID): 40 inches minimum

Body position: Seated at end of table with elbow flexed 90 degrees and arm resting on the table.

Part position:

PA: Hand open, fingers extended, with palmar surface in contact with IR, fingers moderately separated (Fig. 13-12).

> **TIP:** If injury or deformity prevents full extension of the fingers, the hand cannot be placed flat, palm down on the IR. In such a case, a better result will be obtained with the anteroposterior (AP) projection, with the back of the hand placed on the IR. All other aspects of the radiograph are the same.

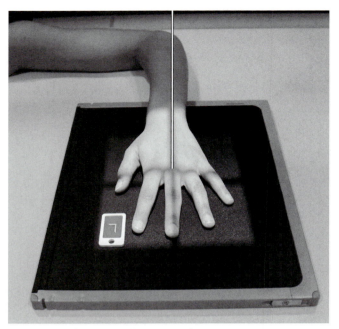

Fig. 13-12 Hand. Position for PA projection.

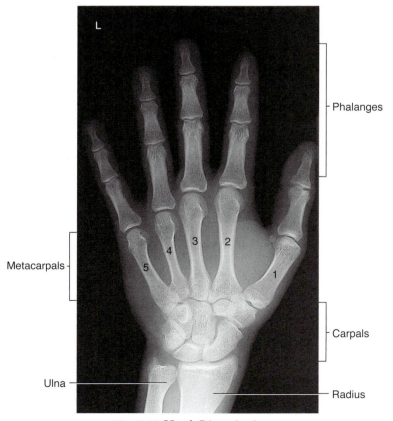

Fig. 13-13 Hand. PA projection.

PA oblique: From the PA, the hand is rotated laterally to place the anteromedial aspect in contact with IR. Coronal plane of hand forms a 45-degree angle with IR. Stair-step sponge is used to support and maintain position of fingers so that IP joints are clearly visualized (Fig. 13-14). Alternatively, without stair-step sponge, "modified teacup" position (named for position of hand when holding a teacup) is used when fingers are not of interest (Fig. 13-16).

Lateral: Medial aspect of hand is in contact with IR with coronal plane of hand perpendicular to IR. Thumb is positioned as for PA projection and is supported on a radiolucent sponge. Wrist will be slightly pronated (Fig. 13-18, *A*). Fingers may be separated (fanned) to prevent superimposition, if desired (Fig. 13-18, *B*).

Central ray:

PA and PA oblique: Perpendicular to third MCP joint.

Lateral: Perpendicular to second MCP joint.

Collimation: 1 inch (2.5 cm) on all sides of the hand, including 1 inch (2.5 cm) proximal to the ulnar styloid process.

Patient instruction: Do not move.

Structures seen: Entire hand (including fingertips), carpus, and most distal aspects of radius and ulna. PA: No overlap of metacarpals or digits (Fig. 13-13). PA oblique: No or minimal overlay of metacarpal shafts, with some overlap of metacarpal heads and bases. IP joint spaces open (stair-step sponge, Fig. 13-15) or not well demonstrated ("modified teacup," Fig. 13-17). Lateral: Superimposition of second through fifth metacarpals. Superimposition of second through fifth phalanges (extension, Fig. 13-19, *A*) or phalanges individually demonstrated (fanned, Fig. 13-19, *B*). Thumb is seen in PA projection.

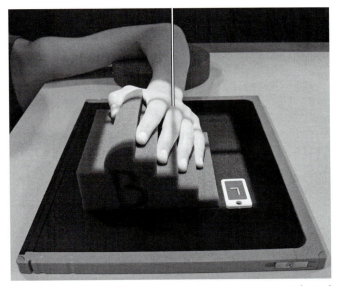

Fig. 13-14 Hand. Position for PA oblique projection—lateral rotation, using stair-step sponge.

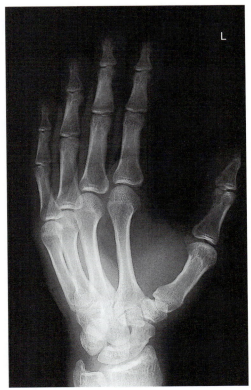

Fig. 13-15 Hand. PA oblique projection, using stair-step sponge.

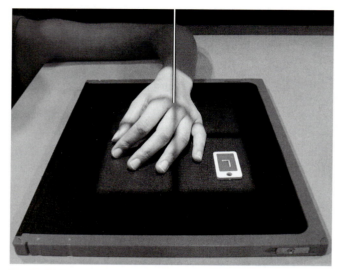

Fig. 13-16 Hand. Position for PA oblique projection—lateral rotation, "modified teacup" position.

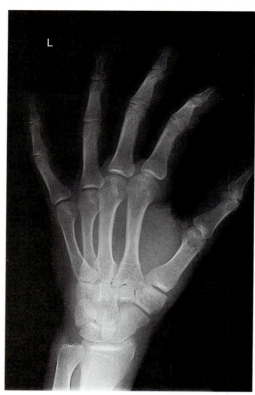

Fig. 13-17 Hand. PA oblique projection, "modified teacup" position.

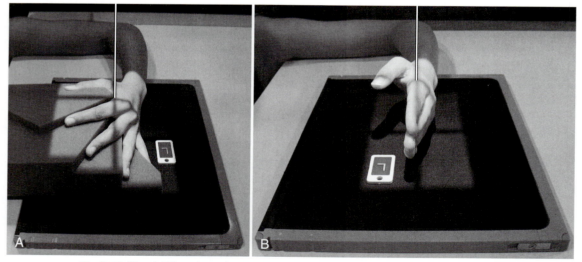

Fig. 13-18 Hand. Ulnar lateral position. **A,** Fingers in extension. **B,** Fingers fanned.

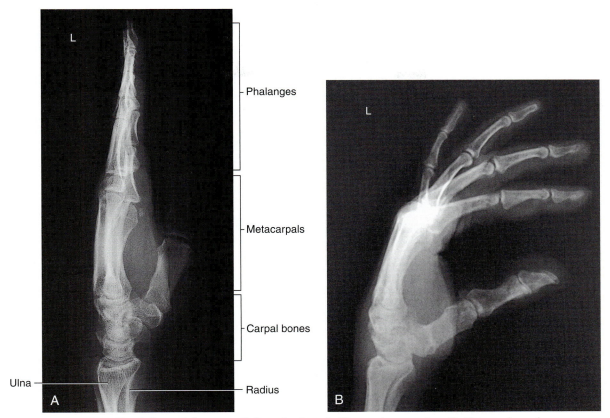

L

Phalanges

Metacarpals

Carpal bones

Ulna

A

Radius

L

B

Fig. 13-19 Hand. Lateral (lateromedial) projection. **A,** Fingers in extension. **B,** Fingers fanned.

Fingers

Although the fingers are included in the examination of the hand, separate finger studies are often performed when the area of clinical interest is limited to a specific finger. Depending on department protocol, the routine projections for the fingers may include a PA projection of the entire hand plus oblique and lateral projections of the affected finger, or the examination may be limited to the PA, oblique, and lateral projections of the affected finger only. Each projection of the finger should include at least the entire digit and the distal portion of the corresponding metacarpal. It is not uncommon that the digits on either side of the digit of interest are also included.

The hand position for lateral projections of the fingers will vary, depending on which finger is involved and what motions are possible for the patient.

Keep the finger as close to the IR as possible and maintain the finger in a position parallel to the IR. When the finger is angled in relation to the IR, visualization of the IP and MCP joint spaces is compromised (Fig. 13-20). A stair-step sponge is a desirable aid for oblique and lateral positioning because it supports the finger parallel to the IR. This position decreases distortion and improves visualization of the IP joints. A stair-step sponge or other radiolucent support also reduces the motion that is likely to occur if the finger trembles because it is not supported during the exposure.

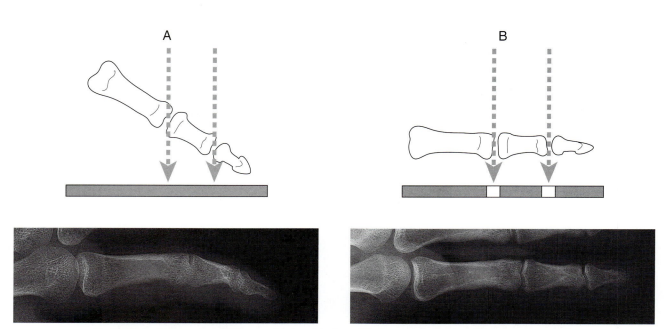

Fig. 13-20 A, Orientation of finger with hand in "modified teacup" position. Finger is not parallel to image receptor (IR). Articular surfaces are not parallel to central ray (CR), which obscures interphalangeal (IP) joint spaces. **B,** Orientation of finger when stair-step sponge is used. Finger is parallel to IR and articular surfaces are parallel to CR, so IP joint spaces are visible.

Routine Examination

The routine examination of the fingers includes the PA, PA oblique-lateral rotation, and lateral projections.

IR: 8 × 10 inches (18 × 24 cm) lengthwise

Grid: No

SID: 40 inches minimum

Body position:
Seated at end of table with elbow flexed and arm resting on table.

Part position:

PA: Hand is open with palmar surface in contact with IR. Fingers are moderately separated (Fig. 13-21).

PA oblique: From the PA, hand is rotated lateral to place anteromedial (palmar/ulnar) surface in contact with IR. Coronal plane of fingers is at a 45-degree angle to IR. Fingers are supported by stair-step sponge (Fig. 13-23). (The alternative to the use of a stair-step sponge is the "modified teacup" position, as shown for examination of the hand.)

Lateral: Medial or lateral surface of hand may be in contact with IR, depending on which brings finger of interest nearest to IR. Other fingers are flexed or extended as necessary to leave affected finger free of superimposition. Affected finger is supported parallel to IR (Figs. 13-25, 13-27, 13-28, and 13-29).

Central ray: Perpendicular to proximal IP joint.

Collimation: 1 inch (2.5 cm) on all sides of the digit, including 1 inch (2.5 cm) proximal to the MCP joint.

Patient instruction: Do not move.

Structures seen: Entire digit and distal portion of metacarpal with IP and MCP joint spaces open and clearly visualized (Figs. 13-22, 13-24, and 13-26). Department protocol may require including an adjacent digit in each image.

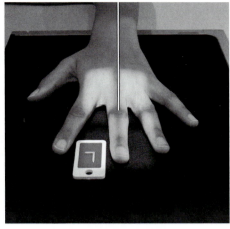

Fig. 13-21 Finger. Position for PA projection.

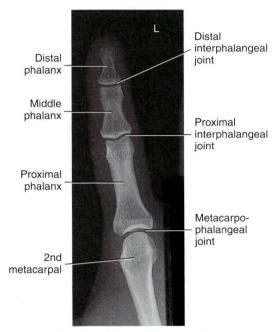

Distal phalanx

Middle phalanx

Proximal phalanx

2nd metacarpal

Distal interphalangeal joint

Proximal interphalangeal joint

Metacarpo-phalangeal joint

Fig. 13-22 Finger. PA projection.

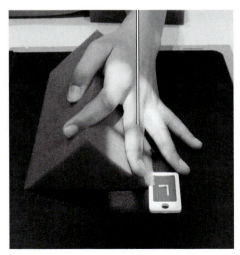

Fig. 13-23 Finger. Position for PA oblique projection—lateral rotation.

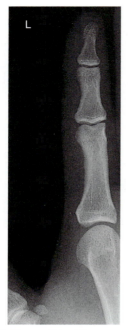

Fig. 13-24 Finger. PA oblique projection.

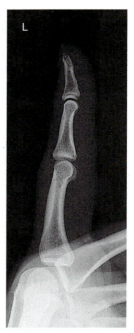

Fig. 13-26 Finger. Lateral projection.

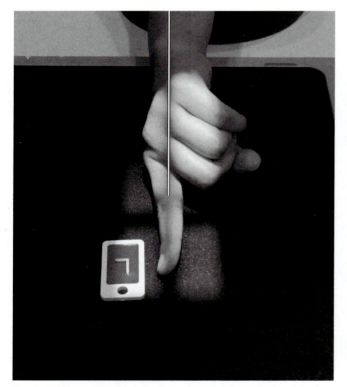

Fig. 13-25 Finger. Position for lateral projection of second (index) finger.

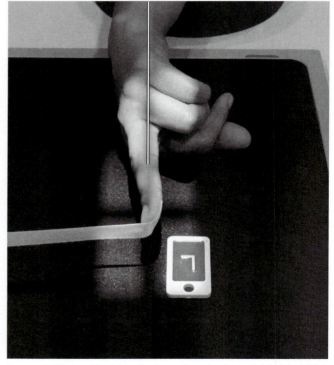

Fig. 13-27 Finger. Position for lateral projection of third (middle) finger.

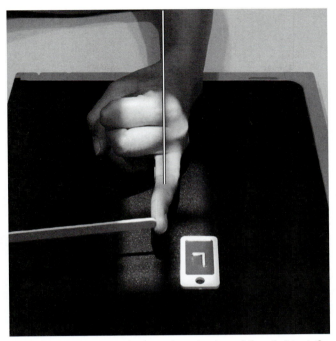

Fig. 13-28 Finger. Position for lateral projection of fourth (ring) finger.

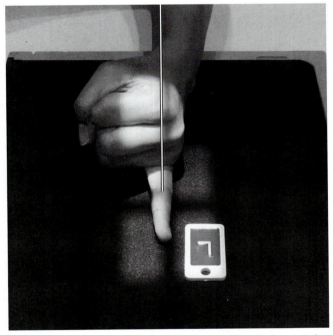

Fig. 13-29 Finger. Position for lateral projection of fifth (little or pinky) finger.

Thumb

Examination of the thumb differs from examinations of the other fingers because the thumb attaches to the hand at a different angle. In addition, examinations of the thumb must include the entire first metacarpal rather than only a portion of it. As with the finger, the thumb examination may include a PA projection of the entire hand. When this is the case, the PA hand position results in an oblique position of the thumb.

Routine Examination

The routine examination of the thumb includes the AP, PA oblique, and lateral projections.

IR: 8 × 10 inches (18 × 24 cm) lengthwise

Grid: No

SID: 40 inches minimum

Body position:

AP: Seated at end of table, leaning forward, arm abducted 90 degrees, with forearm rotated internally into exaggerated degree of pronation.

PA oblique and lateral: Seated at end of table with elbow flexed 90 degrees, arm fully supported, and palm resting on the IR.

Part position:

AP: Dorsal surface of thumb is in contact with IR. Coronal plane of thumb is parallel to IR. Plane of palm of hand is perpendicular to IR (Fig. 13-30).

> **TIPS:**
> - Place the fifth metacarpal and medial (ulnar) aspect of hand back far enough to avoid superimposition with the first metacarpal.
> - If patient is unable to assume a satisfactory position for this projection, substitute the PA projection.

PA oblique: Palmar surface of hand is in contact with IR as for PA projection of hand. Coronal plane of thumb will be 45 degrees to plane of IR (Fig. 13-32).

Lateral: Beginning with hand positioned for PA oblique thumb, patient flexes MCP joints 2 through 5 with the fingers extended, "tenting" hand until thumb is in lateral position (Fig. 13-34).

Central ray: Perpendicular to first MCP joint.

Collimation: 1 inch (2.5 cm) on all sides of the digit, including 1 inch (2.5 cm) proximal to the carpometacarpal (CMC) joint.

Patient instruction: Do not move.

Structures seen: Entire thumb and first metacarpal with all joint spaces open and clearly visualized (Figs. 13-31, 13-33, and 13-35).

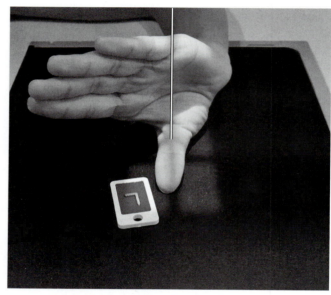

Fig. 13-30 Thumb. Position for AP projection.

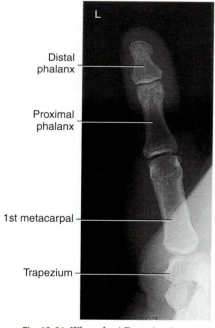

Fig. 13-31 Thumb. AP projection.

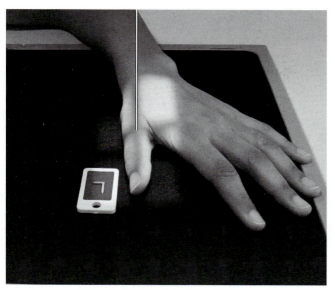

Fig. 13-32 Thumb. Position for PA oblique projection.

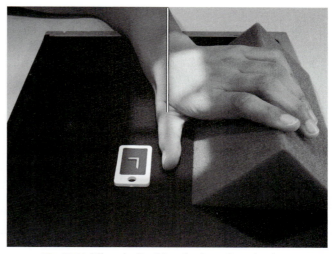

Fig. 13-34 Thumb. Position for lateral projection.

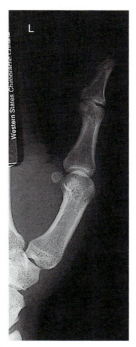

Fig. 13-33 Thumb. PA oblique projection.

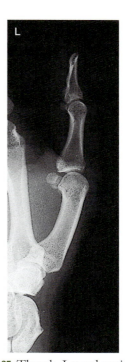

Fig. 13-35 Thumb. Lateral projection.

Alternative Thumb Projection: PA

When patients are unable to rotate the arm enough to assume the proper position for an AP projection, the PA projection is substituted. However, the resulting image will have less detail than the AP projection image because the increased object–image receptor distance (OID) results in greater magnification distortion (geometric unsharpness).

Body position: Same as for PA oblique and lateral thumb projections.

Part position: Medial (ulnar) aspect of hand is in contact with IR and palm of hand is perpendicular to IR. Thumb is supported with coronal plane parallel to IR (Fig. 13-36).

Central ray: Perpendicular to first MCP joint.

Collimation: 1 inch (2.5 cm) on all sides of the digit, including 1 inch (2.5 cm) proximal to the CMC joint.

Structures seen: Entire thumb and first metacarpal with all joint spaces open (Fig. 13-37).

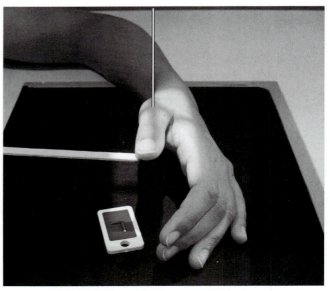

Fig. 13-36 Thumb. Position for PA projection.

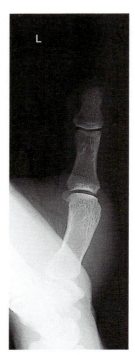

Fig. 13-37 Thumb. PA projection. (Note: Results in greater magnification and less detail than AP projection.)

Wrist

The wrist is a complex structure with many small bones and joints. Although the routine projections are usually sufficient, there are a number of supplemental projections and methods designed to demonstrate specific bones and joints of this region.

Routine Examination

The routine examination of the wrist includes the PA, PA oblique-lateral rotation, and lateral projections.

IR: 8 × 10 inches (18 × 24 cm) or 10 × 12 inches (24 × 30 cm) lengthwise

Grid: No

SID: 40 inches minimum

Body position: Seated at end of table with elbow flexed 90 degrees and forearm resting on table.

Part position:

PA: Anterior surface of wrist is in contact with IR. Fingers are flexed to form a loose fist, placing wrist in firmer contact with IR and opening intercarpal joints (Fig. 13-38).

PA oblique: Anteromedial surface of wrist is in contact with IR so that coronal plane of wrist forms a 45-degree angle with IR. Position may be supported by wedge sponge, stair-step sponge, or patient's thumb (Fig. 13-40).

Lateral: Medial surface of wrist is in contact with IR. Coronal plane of wrist is perpendicular to IR (Fig. 13-42).

Central ray: Perpendicular to the midcarpal area.

Collimation: 2.5 inches (6 cm) proximal and distal to the wrist joint and 1 inch (2.5 cm) on the sides.

Patient instruction: Do not move.

Structures seen: Distal portion of radius and ulna, carpal bones, and proximal halves of metacarpals (Figs. 13-39, 13-41, and 13-43).

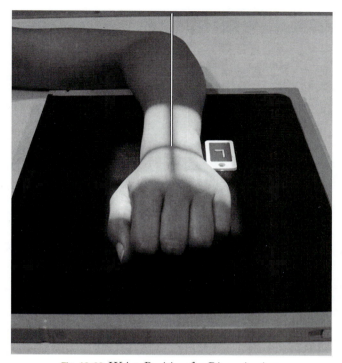

Fig. 13-38 Wrist. Position for PA projection.

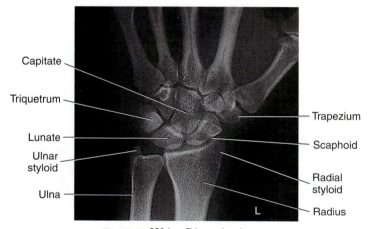

Fig. 13-39 Wrist. PA projection.

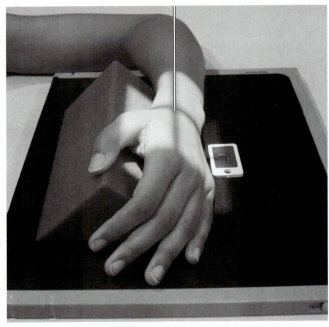

Fig. 13-40 Wrist. Position for PA oblique projection—lateral rotation.

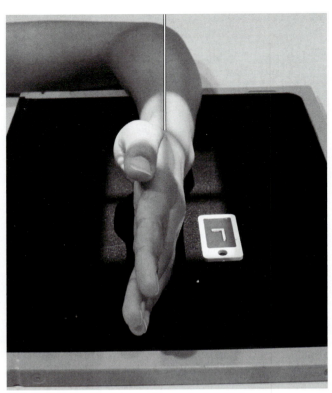

Fig. 13-42 Wrist. Position for lateral (lateromedial) projection.

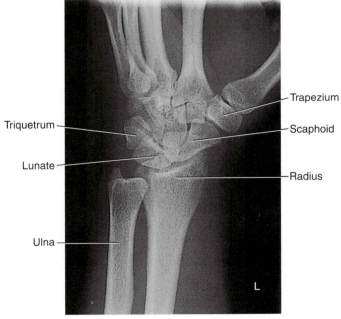

Triquetrum

Lunate

Ulna

Trapezium

Scaphoid

Radius

L

Fig. 13-41 Wrist. PA oblique projection.

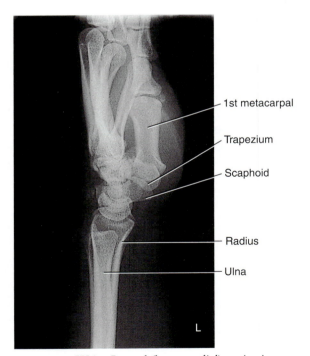

1st metacarpal

Trapezium

Scaphoid

Radius

Ulna

L

Fig. 13-43 Wrist. Lateral (lateromedial) projection.

Supplemental Projections

These supplemental projections and methods may be added individually to the routine examination according to the area of clinical interest and the instructions of the physician.

IR: 8 × 10 inches (18 × 24 cm) lengthwise

Grid and **SID** same as for routine examination.

AP Oblique Projection—Medial Rotation

The AP oblique projection with medial rotation is the opposite of the routine oblique. It is useful for demonstration of the medial aspect of the carpus, particularly the lunate and the pisiform.

Body position: Same as for other wrist projections.

Part position: Posteromedial surface of wrist is in contact with IR so that coronal plane forms a 45-degree angle with IR (Fig. 13-44).

Central ray: Perpendicular to midcarpal area.

Collimation: 2.5 inches (6 cm) proximal and distal to the wrist joint and 1 inch (2.5 cm) on the sides.

Structures seen: Distal portion of radius and ulna, carpal bones, and proximal halves of metacarpals (Fig. 13-45).

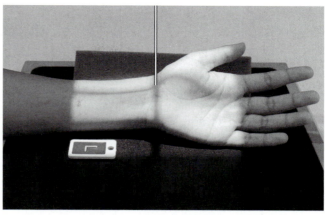

Fig. 13-44 Wrist. Position for AP oblique projection—medial rotation.

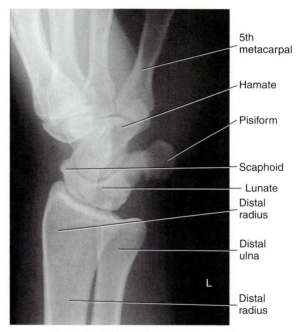

Fig. 13-45 Wrist. AP oblique projection.

PA Projection—Ulnar Deviation

The PA projection with ulnar deviation is performed when fracture of the scaphoid is suspected. It reduces foreshortening of the scaphoid.

Part position: Same as for PA wrist with fingers extended. Hand is then deviated outward, in the direction of ulna, to extent that patient can tolerate (Fig. 13-46).

Central ray: Perpendicular, centered to scaphoid (a point slightly proximal and medial to first metacarpal base).

Collimation: 2.5 inches (6 cm) proximal and distal to the wrist joint and 1 inch (2.5 cm) on the sides.

Structures seen: Distal portion of radius and ulna, carpal bones, and metacarpals deviated toward ulna. Scaphoid seen with minimal foreshortening (Fig. 13-47).

PA Axial Projection (Stecher Method)

The Stecher method projection is performed when fracture of the scaphoid is suspected. It reduces foreshortening of the scaphoid. It is preferred when ulnar deviation is too painful for patient.

Part position: Arm is extended and parallel to long axis of table for correct alignment with angled x-ray beam. One end of the IR is elevated so the plane of the IR is 20 degrees with respect to tabletop. Wrist is positioned with anterior aspect on IR as for PA wrist, with the fingers oriented to the elevated end of the IR (Fig. 13-48).

Central ray: Perpendicular to table and directed to enter the scaphoid (a point slightly proximal and medial to first metacarpal base).

Collimation: 2.5 inches (6 cm) proximal and distal to the wrist joint and 1 inch (2.5 cm) on the sides.

Structures seen: Distal portion of radius and ulna, carpal bones, and proximal metacarpals. Scaphoid seen with minimal foreshortening (Fig. 13-49).

> **TIP:** A variation of the method is performed with a nonelevated IR and the CR angled 20 degrees in direction of elbow and centered to scaphoid (point slightly proximal and medial to first metacarpal base).

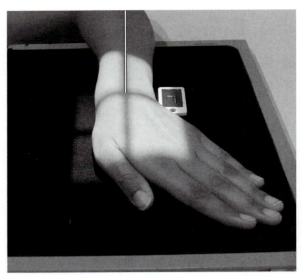

Fig. 13-46 Wrist. Position for PA projection—ulnar deviation.

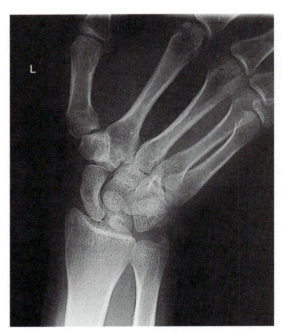

Fig. 13-47 Wrist. PA projection—ulnar deviation.

Tangential Projection (Gaynor-Hart Method)

The Gaynor-Hart method is used to demonstrate the carpal canal, usually in patients with symptoms of carpal tunnel syndrome or suspected fracture.

Part position: Arm is extended and parallel to long axis of table for correct alignment with angled x-ray beam. Wrist is extended to place the palm of hand perpendicular to IR, if possible (Fig. 13-50).

Central ray: Directed to the palm at a point approximately 1 inch (2.5 cm) distal to the base of the third metacarpal and at an angle of 25 to 30 degrees in direction of elbow. Greater angle may be required when the wrist cannot be extended as shown in Fig. 13-50.

Collimation: 1 inch (2.5 cm) on the three sides of the shadow of the wrist.

Structures seen: Carpal canal—anterior arch of carpal bones, including portions of the scaphoid, trapezium, pisiform, and hook of hamate (Fig. 13-51).

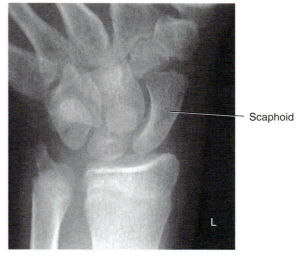

Fig. 13-49 Wrist. PA axial projection (Stecher method).

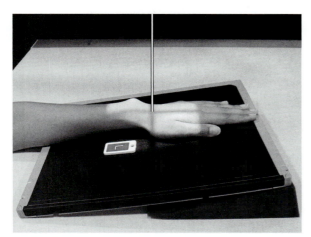

Fig. 13-48 Wrist. Position for PA axial projection (Stecher method).

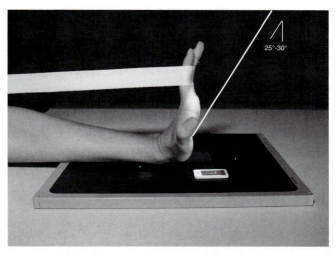

Fig. 13-50 Wrist. Position for tangential projection of carpal canal (Gaynor-Hart method).

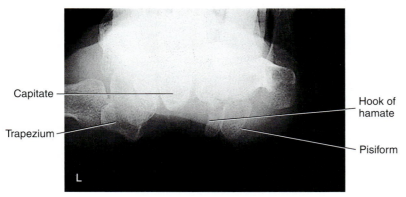

Fig. 13-51 Wrist. Tangential (inferosuperior) projection.

Forearm

Examination of the forearm is usually ordered when the area of clinical interest is in the shaft of the radius and/or the ulna. The examination should include the entirety of both bones and their articular surfaces.

Visualization of both joints is preferable. If only one joint is demonstrated, the *same* joint must be demonstrated on both projections. In this case, additional radiographs that include the other joint will be needed.

Routine Examination

The routine examination of the forearm includes the AP and lateral projections.

IR: 10 × 12 inches (24 × 30 cm) diagonal or 14 × 17 inches (35 × 43 cm) lengthwise

Grid: No

SID: 40 inches minimum

Body position: Seated at end of table with **axilla** (armpit) at table level; this may be achieved by lowering seat or by having patient lean toward table.

Part position:

AP: Arm is fully extended with hand supinated and posterior surface in contact with IR. Both wrist and elbow are supinated with coronal plane of arm parallel to IR (Fig. 13-52). This is achieved by adjusting the coronal plane of the humeral epicondyles parallel to the plane of the IR. A small sandbag in palm of hand can aid in maintaining position.

Lateral: Elbow is flexed 90 degrees with medial surface in contact with IR. Wrist is in lateral position (Fig. 13-54).

Central ray: Perpendicular to midpoint of the forearm.

Collimation: 2 inches (5 cm) distal to the wrist joint and proximal to the elbow joint and 1 inch (2.5 cm) on the sides

Patient instruction: Do not move.

Structures seen: Entire forearm, including both elbow and wrist joints (Figs. 13-53 and 13-55).

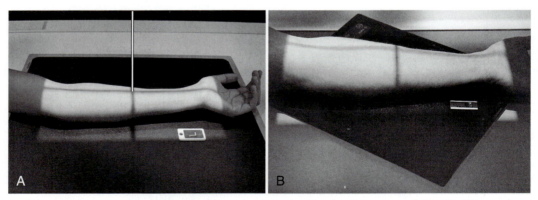

Fig. 13-52 Forearm. Position for AP projection. **A,** Usual orientation of IR. **B,** Diagonal placement of IR, when forearm is too long to fit within the long dimension of the IR. Exposure field must include entire corners of a computed radiography imaging plate to ensure good image quality.

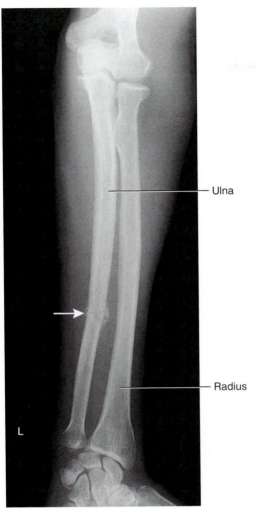

Fig. 13-53 Forearm. AP projection, with healing fracture of the ulnar shaft *(arrow)*.

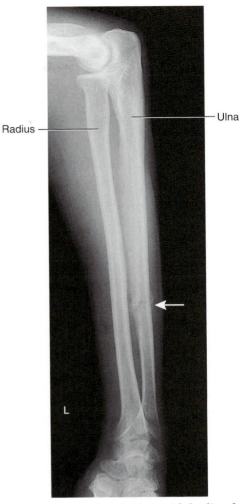

Fig. 13-55 Forearm. Lateral projection, with healing fracture of the ulnar shaft *(arrow)*.

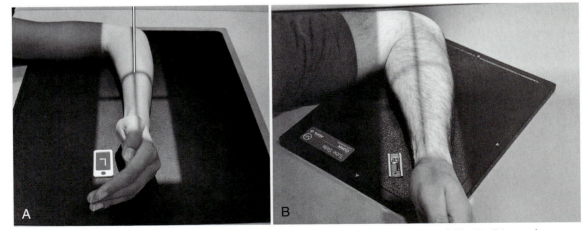

Fig. 13-54 Forearm. Position for lateral projection. **A,** Usual orientation of IR. **B,** Diagonal orientation of IR, when forearm is too long to fit within the long dimension of the IR.

Elbow

The positions for the routine examination of the elbow are the same as those for the forearm. Because it is often impossible for patients with an injured elbow to fully extend the elbow joint, alternatives are presented for the AP projection with the elbow partially flexed. Supplemental projections may be added to the basic examination for further visualization of specific aspects of the joint.

Routine Examination

The routine examination of the elbow includes the AP and lateral projections.

IR: 8 × 10 inches (18 × 24 cm) or 10 × 12 inches (24 × 30 cm) lengthwise

Grid: No

SID: 40 inches minimum

Body position:
Seated at end of table with axilla at level of table, as for AP forearm.

Part position:

AP: Arm is fully extended with hand supinated and posterior surface in contact with IR. Coronal plane of humeral epicondyles parallel to IR (Fig. 13-56). If patient is unable to fully extend arm, substitute alternate positions for AP projection with flexed elbow.

Lateral: Elbow is flexed 90 degrees with medial surface in contact with IR. Coronal plane of humeral epicondyles perpendicular to IR. Wrist is in lateral position to degree patient can achieve (Fig. 13-58).

Central ray: Perpendicular to elbow joint. For AP projection, joint is midway between humeral epicondyles. For lateral projection, it is at lateral epicondyle.

Collimation: 3 inches (8 cm) proximal and distal to the elbow joint and 1 inch (2.5 cm) on the sides.

Patient instruction: Do not move.

Structures seen: Elbow joint with portions of distal humerus and proximal forearm (Figs. 13-57 and 13-59).

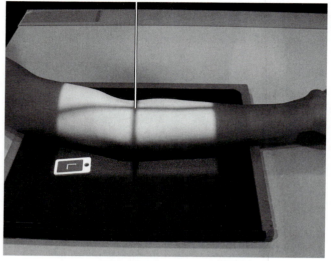

Fig. 13-56 Elbow. Position for AP projection.

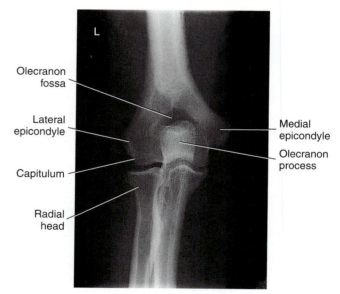

Olecranon fossa

Lateral epicondyle

Capitulum

Radial head

Medial epicondyle

Olecranon process

Fig. 13-57 Elbow. AP projection.

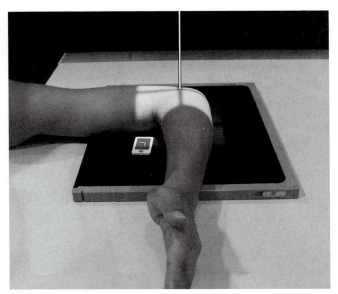

Fig. 13-58 Elbow. Position for lateral (lateromedial) projection.

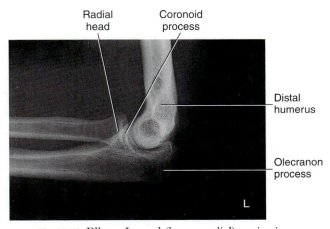

Fig. 13-59 Elbow. Lateral (lateromedial) projection.

Alternative Positions for AP Projections

When the patient is unable to fully extend the elbow joint for an AP projection, *both* of the following AP projections with flexed elbow are necessary to substitute for the routine AP projection.

IR: 8 × 10 inches (18 × 24 cm) lengthwise

AP Elbow, Proximal Forearm

Body position: Standing and leaning over table, if possible.

Part position: Posterior aspect of forearm rests on IR and elbow is extended as much as possible. Rotation of forearm adjusted so coronal plane of humeral epicondyles is parallel to IR (Fig. 13-60).

Central ray: Perpendicular to center of elbow. If the elbow is flexed 90 degrees or more, it is necessary to angle central ray 5 to 15 degrees in proximal direction to avoid superimposing distal humerus over proximal forearm.

> **TIP:** To ensure that the patient's head is not in the path of the x-ray beam, turn on the field light, look for the head shadow, and move the head out of the way, if needed.

Collimation: 3 inches (8 cm) proximal and distal to the elbow joint and 1 inch on the sides.

Structures seen: Proximal forearm portion of elbow joint. Distal humerus will be distorted (Fig. 13-62).

AP Elbow, Distal Humerus

Body position: With axilla at table level as for routine AP projection, elbow is extended as much as possible and forearm is supported. Arm is rotated to place coronal plane of humeral epicondyles parallel to IR (Fig. 13-61).

Central ray: Directed to center of joint. If elbow is flexed 90 degrees or more, it is necessary to angle central ray 5 to 15 degrees in distal direction to avoid superimposing proximal forearm over distal humerus.

Collimation: 3 inches (8 cm) proximal and distal to the elbow joint and 1 inch on the sides.

Structures seen: Distal humeral portion of elbow joint. Proximal forearm will be distorted (Fig. 13-63).

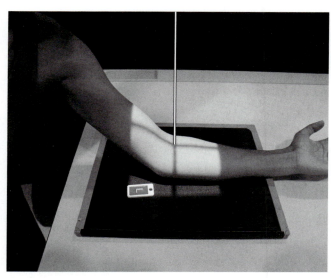

Fig. 13-60 Elbow. Position for AP projection of forearm portion with elbow flexed.

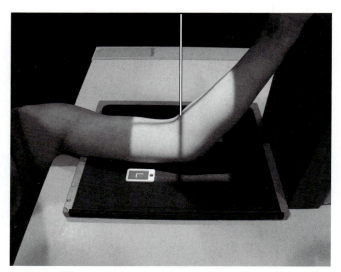

Fig. 13-61 Elbow. Position for AP projection of humeral portion with elbow flexed.

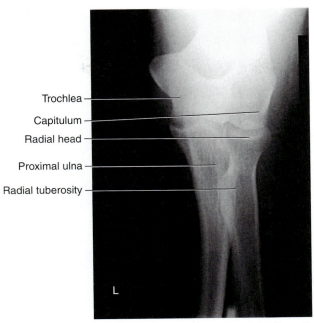

Fig. 13-62 Elbow. AP projection of forearm portion with elbow flexed.

Trochlea

Capitulum

Radial head

Proximal ulna

Radial tuberosity

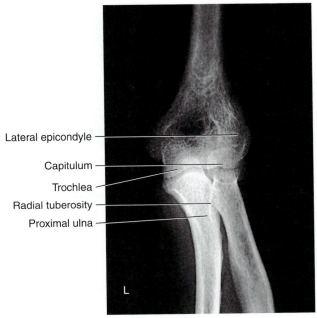

Fig. 13-63 Elbow. AP projection of humeral portion with elbow flexed.

Lateral epicondyle

Capitulum

Trochlea

Radial tuberosity

Proximal ulna

Supplemental Projections

IR: 8 × 10 inches (18 × 24 cm) lengthwise, for each.

Grid and **SID** same as for routine examination.

AP Oblique—Lateral Rotation

Performed when injury to the lateral portion of the elbow (radial head or capitulum) is suspected.

Body position: From AP position, leaning laterally and rotating shoulder externally so that posterior lateral aspect of elbow is in contact with IR.

Part position: Coronal plane of elbow forms angle of 45 degrees with IR (Fig. 13-64).

Central ray: Directed to center of elbow joint.

Collimation: 3 inches (8 cm) proximal and distal to the elbow joint and 1 inch on the sides.

Structures seen: Radial head and capitulum without superimposition of ulna (Fig. 13-65).

AP Oblique—Medial Rotation

Performed when injury to the medial portion of the elbow (coronoid process or trochlea) is suspected.

Body position: Same as for AP projection.

Part position: Hand pronated, which allows coronal plane of elbow to assume a 45-degree angle with IR (Fig. 13-66).

Central ray: Directed to center of elbow joint.

Collimation: 3 inches (8 cm) proximal and distal to the elbow joint and 1 inch on the sides.

Structures seen: Coronoid process and trochlea without superimposition (Fig. 13-67).

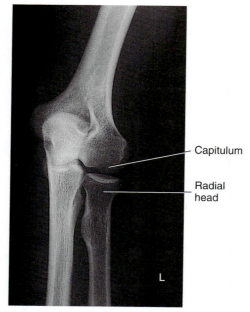

Fig. 13-65 Elbow. AP oblique projection with elbow in lateral rotation.

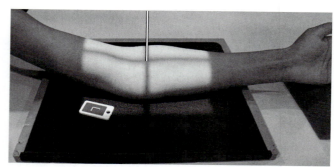

Fig. 13-66 Elbow. Position for AP oblique projection with medial rotation of elbow.

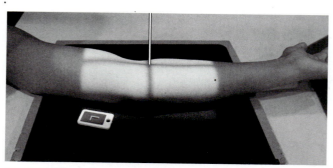

Fig. 13-64 Elbow. Position for AP oblique projection with lateral rotation of elbow.

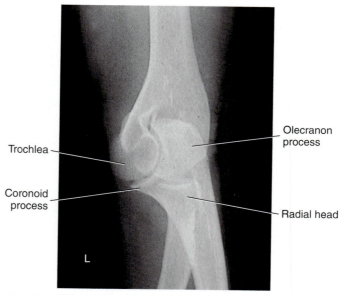

Fig. 13-67 Elbow. AP oblique projection with elbow in medial rotation.

Humerus

The humerus may be radiographed with the patient either upright or supine, depending on patient condition. Both methods are presented here. The thickness of the shoulder joint usually dictates that this study be done using a Bucky or grid. For relatively small patients, however, a grid is not necessarily required.

Routine Examination

Humerus (Upright Patient)

The routine examination of the humerus, with patient upright, includes AP and lateral projections.

IR: 14 × 17 inches (35 × 43 cm) lengthwise

Grid: Yes

SID: 40 inches minimum

Body position: Seated or standing with back to upright Bucky or grid cabinet. The body position, whether oblique or facing toward or away from the IR, is not critical as long as the epicondyles are oriented appropriately for the projection.

Part position: Adjust the height of the IR to place its upper margin about 1.5 inches (3.8 cm) above the head of the humerus.

AP: Arm slightly abducted with palm of hand supinated. Coronal plane of humeral epicondyles parallel to IR (Fig. 13-68).

Lateral: Elbow flexed approximately 45 degrees and palm of hand against hip so that fingertips point down and elbow is lateral with coronal plane of humeral epicondyles perpendicular to IR (Fig. 13-69).

Central ray: Perpendicular to midhumerus.

Collimation: 2 inches (5 cm) distal to the elbow joint and superior to the shoulder and 1 inch (2.5 cm) on the sides.

Patient instruction: Stop breathing. Do not move.

Structures seen: Entire humerus, shoulder joint, and elbow joint (Figs. 13-72 and 13-73).

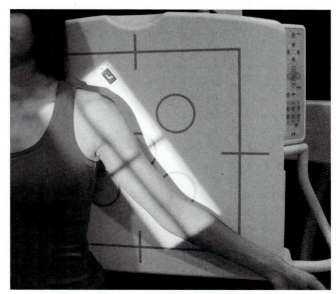

Fig. 13-68 Humerus. Position for AP projection, patient upright.

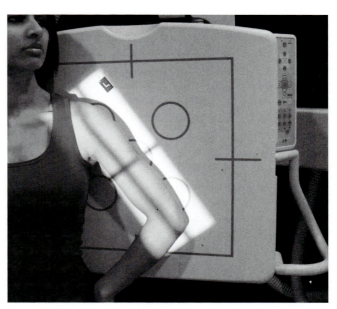

Fig. 13-69 Humerus. Position for lateral projection, patient upright.

Humerus (Recumbent Patient)

The routine examination of the humerus, with the patient recumbent, includes AP and lateral projections.

The procedure for radiography of the humerus in the recumbent position is similar to that used for upright studies. It varies somewhat because the width of the radiographic table may not allow room for the patient to lie safely when the arm is abducted and placed over the center of the grid. For this reason, the recumbent examination is done with the humerus nearer the trunk of the body, and the lateral projection is done without flexing the elbow.

IR: 14 × 17 inches (35 × 43 cm) lengthwise

Grid: Yes

SID: 40 inches minimum

Body position: Supine on radiographic table.

Part position: Adjust the height of the IR to place its upper margin about 1.5 inches (3.8 cm) above the head of the humerus.

AP: Arm extended and hand supinated. Arm rotated to place coronal plane of humeral epicondyles parallel to IR (Fig. 13-70).

Lateral: Arm medially rotated to exaggerated degree of pronation until coronal plane of humeral epicondyle is perpendicular to IR (Fig. 13-71). Posterior aspect of hand may be against the patient's side.

Central ray: Perpendicular to midhumerus.

Collimation: 2 inches (5 cm) distal to the elbow joint and superior to the shoulder and 1 inch (2.5 cm) on the sides.

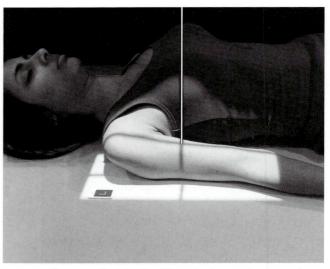

Fig. 13-70 Humerus. Position for AP projection, patient recumbent.

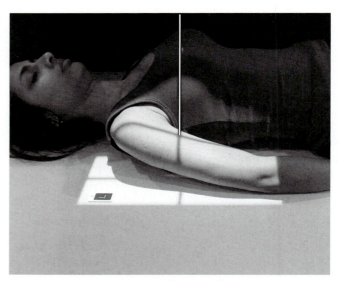

Fig. 13-71 Humerus. Position for lateral projection, patient recumbent.

Patient instruction: Stop breathing. Do not move.

Structures seen: Entire humerus, shoulder joint, and elbow joint (see Figs. 13-72 and 13-73).

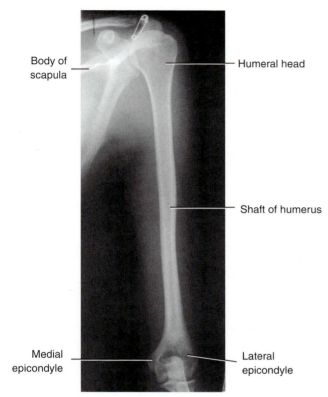

Body of scapula

Humeral head

Shaft of humerus

Medial epicondyle

Lateral epicondyle

Fig. 13-72 Humerus. AP projection.

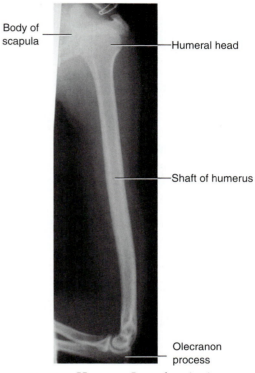

Body of scapula

Humeral head

Shaft of humerus

Olecranon process

Fig. 13-73 Humerus. Lateral projection.

Shoulder

Examinations of the shoulder girdle may be done with the patient recumbent on the radiographic table or upright using the upright Bucky or grid cabinet, depending on patient condition. In hospitals it is usual for patients who arrive in radiology on a stretcher to be kept in a recumbent position until their injuries have been evaluated. In outpatient facilities, ambulatory patients are frequently more comfortable in the upright position. Because a full lead apron may interfere with the examination, gonad shielding is shown here using a half-apron for examinations of the shoulder region.

The routine examination of the shoulder requires that the patient be able to rotate the humerus. This is usually possible for relatively mild or chronic complaints. In such cases, it is desirable to examine the entire shoulder girdle, so the routine study should include the scapula, clavicle, and proximal humerus. The IR is placed crosswise to accommodate the length of the clavicle.

Acute injuries to the shoulder may involve fractures of the proximal humerus or dislocation of the glenohumeral joint. In such cases, the patient cannot rotate the shoulder, and arm movement could cause additional injury. In cases of acute injury, the examination is performed without moving the arm. The IR is placed lengthwise to include a greater portion of the humerus. Both the routine procedure and the acute injury procedure are presented.

Routine Examination

The routine examination of the shoulder includes AP projections with both internal and external humerus rotation.

IR: 10 × 12 inches (24 × 30 cm) crosswise

Grid: Yes

SID: 40 inches minimum

Body position:
Standing or seated with back to upright Bucky or grid cabinet or supine on table; coronal plane of body parallel to IR.

Part position:

External rotation: Arm slightly abducted with palm of hand supinated. Arm adjusted to place coronal plane of humeral epicondyles parallel to IR (Figs. 13-74 and 13-76).

Internal rotation: Humerus and arm rotated internally until back of hand is against thigh. Arm adjusted to place coronal plane of humeral epicondyles perpendicular to IR (Figs. 13-75 and 13-77).

Patient instruction: Stop breathing. Do not move.

Central ray: Perpendicular to a point 1 inch inferior to coracoid process.

Collimation: Adjust to 10 × 12 inches (24 × 30 cm) on the collimator.

Structures seen: Entire clavicle and scapula and proximal third of humerus. External rotation demonstrates greater tubercle in profile (Fig. 13-78); internal rotation demonstrates lesser tubercle in profile (Fig. 13-79).

Compensating Filter: Use of a specially designed compensating filter for the shoulder improves the quality of the image. These filters are particularly useful when digital imaging (CR or DR) systems are used.

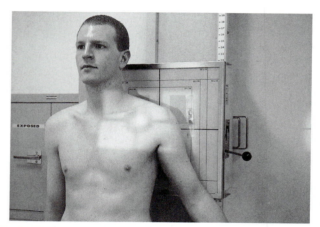

Fig. 13-74 Shoulder. Position for AP projection—external (arm) rotation, patient upright.

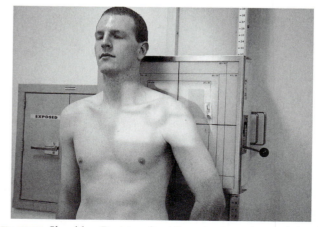

Fig. 13-75 Shoulder. Position for AP projection—internal (arm) rotation, patient upright.

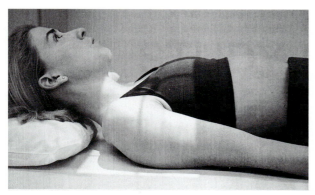

Fig. 13-76 Shoulder. Position for AP projection—external (arm) rotation, patient recumbent.

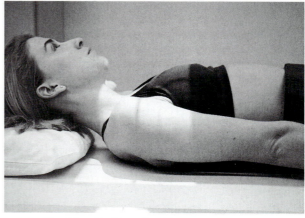

Fig. 13-77 Shoulder. Position for AP projection—internal (arm) rotation, patient recumbent.

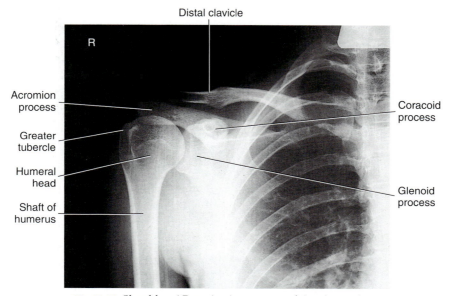

Distal clavicle

R

Acromion process

Greater tubercle

Humeral head

Shaft of humerus

Coracoid process

Glenoid process

Fig. 13-78 Shoulder. AP projection—external (arm) rotation.

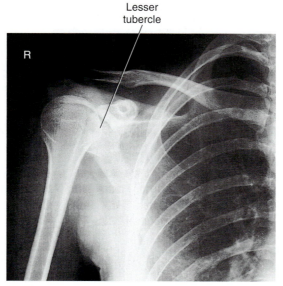

Lesser tubercle

R

Fig. 13-79 Shoulder. AP projection—internal (arm) rotation.

Additional Shoulder Projection

AP Oblique Projection (Grashey Method)

The AP oblique projection demonstrates the glenoid fossa in profile, allowing evaluation of glenohumeral joint integrity.

IR: 10 × 12 inches (24 × 30 cm) crosswise
Grid and **SID** same as for routine examination.

Body position: Patient upright or recumbent. Coronal plane of body aligned 35 to 45 degrees with respect to IR (Fig. 13-80).

Part position: Posterolateral aspect of shoulder in contact with upright Bucky or table; scapular body parallel to IR; arm in internal, external, or neutral rotation.

Central ray: Perpendicular through glenohumeral joint, at a point 2 inches (5 cm) medial and 2 inches (5 cm) inferior to superolateral border of shoulder.

Collimation: Adjust to 10 × 12 inches (24 × 30 cm) on the collimator.

Structures seen: Glenohumeral joint with open joint space and glenoid process in profile; coracoid process will usually obscure superior aspect of joint space (Fig. 13-81).

TIP: When patient is recumbent, body rotation of more than 45 degrees may be required to place the scapular body parallel to the IR and open joint space.

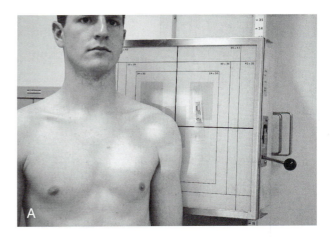

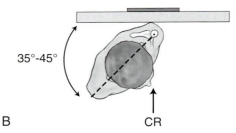

Fig. 13-80 Shoulder. **A,** Position for AP oblique projection (Grashey method). **B,** Top view of same position as in **A.**

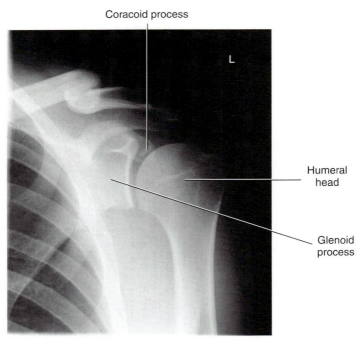

Fig. 13-81 Shoulder. AP oblique projection (Grashey method).

Alternate Examination for Acute Shoulder Injury

The routine examination for acute injury to the shoulder may include AP and transthoracic lateral or PA oblique (scapular Y) projections.

IR: 10 × 12 inches (24 × 30 cm) lengthwise

Grid: Yes

SID: 40 inches minimum

Body position: Standing or seated at upright Bucky or grid cabinet.

Part position: *AP:* With back to upright Bucky and without moving arm. Coronal plane of body is parallel to IR (Fig. 13-82).

Transthoracic lateral: Coronal plane of body is perpendicular to IR with affected side against upright Bucky. Unaffected arm is raised above head (Fig. 13-84).

PA oblique (scapular Y): Anterolateral aspect of shoulder against upright Bucky. Coronal plane of body 45 to 60 degrees to IR. Body rotation adjusted to place scapular body perpendicular to IR (Fig. 13-86).

Central ray: Perpendicular to center of IR, with top of IR 1.5 inches to 2 inches above top of shoulder.

Collimation: Adjust to 10 × 12 inches (24 × 30 cm) on the collimator.

Patient instruction: *AP and PA oblique:* Stop breathing. Do not move.

Transthoracic lateral: Use "breathing technique." (Exposure is made during slow, deep breathing. This technique effectively blurs superimposing rib and lung structures, improving visualization of humerus.)

Structures seen: Proximal half of humerus and portions of scapula and clavicle (Figs. 13-83, 13-85, and 13-87).

Demonstrates fractures of upper humerus and aids in evaluation of glenohumeral dislocation.

TIPS:

- For PA oblique (scapular Y), to ensure that the body of the scapula is perpendicular to the IR, grasp the lateral and medial border between the thumb and index finger. Rotate the patient's body until a line between the finger and the thumb is perpendicular to the IR.
- An AP oblique projection (Grashey method) may be added for suspected humeral dislocation.

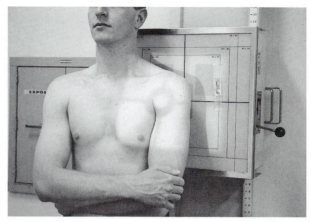

Fig. 13-82 Shoulder. Position for AP projection, when acute injury is suspected.

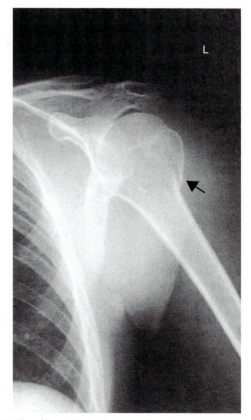

Fig. 13-83 Shoulder. AP projection, demonstrating surgical neck fracture of humerus (*arrow*).

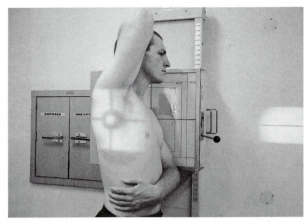

Fig. 13-84 Shoulder. Position for transthoracic lateral projection, used when acute injury is suspected.

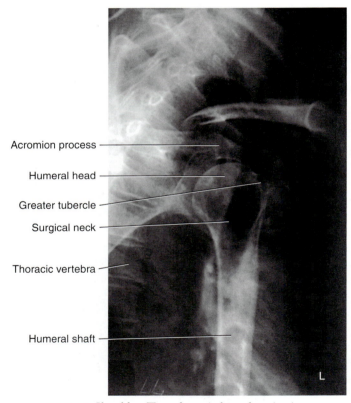

Acromion process

Humeral head

Greater tubercle

Surgical neck

Thoracic vertebra

Humeral shaft

Fig. 13-85 Shoulder. Transthoracic lateral projection.

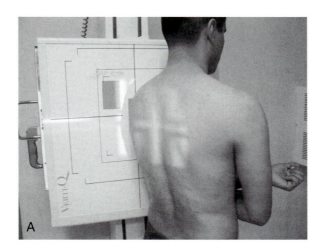

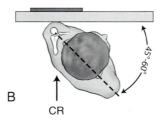

Fig. 13-86 Shoulder. **A,** Position for PA oblique projection (scapular Y). **B,** Top view of same position as in **A.**

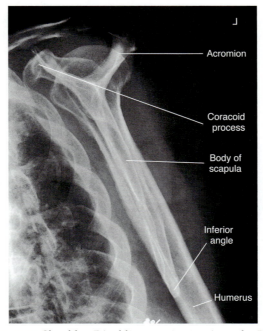

Acromion

Coracoid process

Body of scapula

Inferior angle

Humerus

Fig. 13-87 Shoulder. PA oblique projection (scapular Y).

Clavicle

Examination of the clavicle is routinely done in the PA and PA axial projections to keep the clavicle as close to the IR as possible. If the patient is recumbent, however, a supine position is more comfortable when the clavicle has been injured. Under these circumstances, AP and AP axial projections are performed.

Routine Examination

The routine examination of the clavicle includes the upright PA and PA axial projections, or recumbent AP and AP axial projections.

IR: 10 × 12 inches (24 × 30 cm) crosswise

Grid: Yes

SID: 40 inches minimum

Body position: Upright: Standing or seated facing Bucky with coronal plane parallel to IR. Head turned away from side of interest. Arm at side (Figs. 13-88 and 13-89).

Recumbent: Supine (Figs. 13-90 and 13-91).

Part position: See body position.

Central ray: PA or AP: Perpendicular to midclavicle.

PA axial: 15 to 30 degrees caudad to midclavicle.

AP axial: 15 to 30 degrees cephalad to midclavicle.

Collimation: Adjust to 8 × 12 inches (18 × 30 cm) on the collimator.

Patient instruction: Stop breathing. Do not move.

Structures seen: Entire clavicle and its articulations (Figs. 13-92 and 13-93).

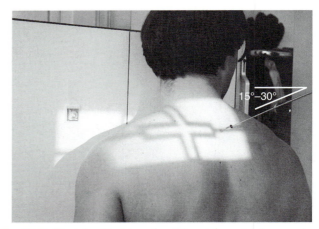

Fig. 13-89 Clavicle. Position for PA axial projection, patient upright.

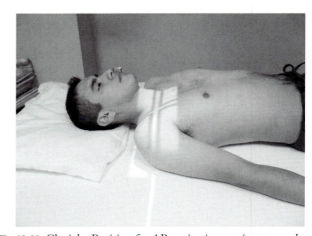

Fig. 13-90 Clavicle. Position for AP projection, patient recumbent.

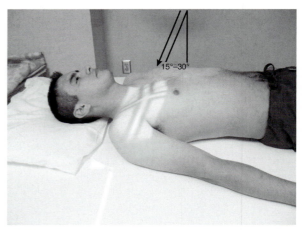

Fig. 13-91 Clavicle. Position for AP axial projection, patient recumbent.

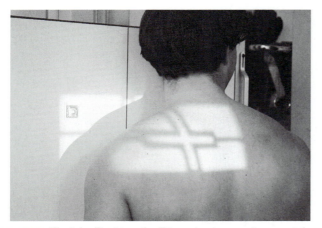

Fig. 13-88 Clavicle. Position for PA projection, patient upright.

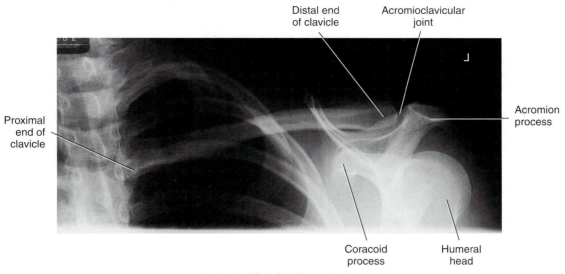

Distal end of clavicle

Acromioclavicular joint

Proximal end of clavicle

Acromion process

Coracoid process

Humeral head

FIG. 13-92 Clavicle. PA projection.

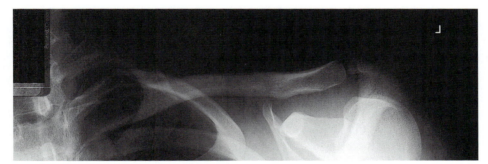

Fig. 13-93 Clavicle. PA axial projection.

Scapula

Routine Examination

The routine examination of the scapula includes the AP and lateral projections.

IR: 10 × 12 inches (24 × 30 cm) lengthwise

Grid: Yes

SID: 40 inches minimum

Body position: Standing or seated at upright Bucky or grid cabinet, or recumbent on table.

Part position:

AP: Arm abducted so that humerus is perpendicular to long axis of body. Elbow flexed 90 degrees. When patient is upright, patient may support position by grasping a pole (Figs. 13-94 and 13-97).

Upright lateral: Anterior oblique body position with affected side nearest IR. Adjust rotation of body (45 to 60 degrees) so that blade (body) of scapula is perpendicular to IR. Patient's forearm is positioned behind back with elbow flexed 90 degrees (Fig. 13-96). Alternatively, arm may be positioned over head or across chest, depending on structures of interest and patient's ability to comply (Fig. 13-95).

Recumbent lateral: Posterior oblique body position with unaffected side in contact with table. Rotation of body adjusted (45 to 60 degrees) so that blade (body) of scapula is perpendicular to IR. Patient's arm may be positioned across chest (Fig. 13-98).

> **TIP:** To ensure that the body of the scapula is perpendicular to the IR, grasp the lateral and medial border between the thumb and index finger. Rotate patient's body until a line between the finger and thumb is perpendicular to the IR.

Central ray: Perpendicular to midscapula. For the AP, this point is approximately 2 inches (5 cm) inferior to the coracoid process. For the lateral, this point is the middle of the medial border of the scapular body.

Collimation: Adjust to 10 × 12 inches (24 × 30 cm) on the collimator.

Patient instruction: Stop breathing. Do not move.

Structures seen: Entire scapula and its articulations with clavicle and humerus. AP projection demonstrates portions of scapula not obscured by ribs and clavicle (Fig. 13-99). Lateral projections demonstrate body of scapula free of superimposition by ribs, acromion, and coracoid process. Position of arm will determine portion of scapula obscured by proximal humerus (Fig. 13-100).

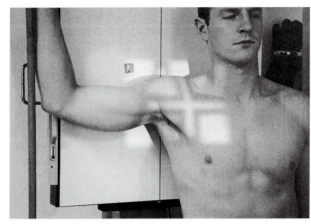

Fig. 13-94 Scapula. Position for AP projection, patient upright.

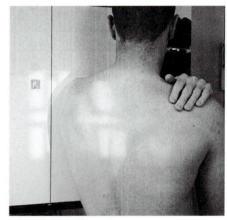

Fig. 13-95 Scapula. Position for lateral projection (anterior oblique position), arm across chest, patient upright.

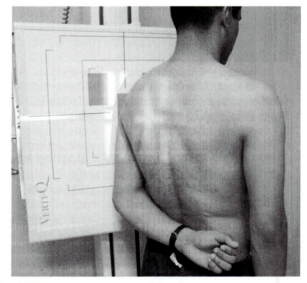

Fig. 13-96 Scapula. Position for lateral projection (anterior oblique position), forearm behind back, patient upright.

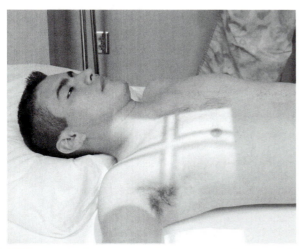

Fig. 13-97 Scapula. Position for AP projection, patient recumbent.

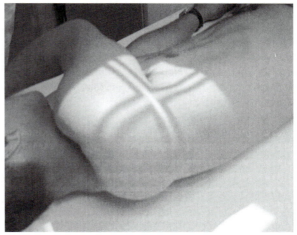

Fig. 13-98 Scapula. Position for lateral projection (posterior oblique position), patient recumbent.

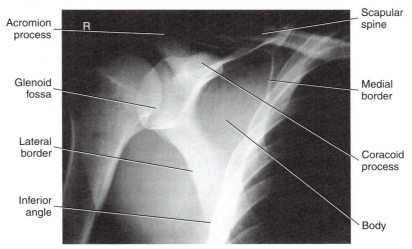

Acromion process

Glenoid fossa

Lateral border

Inferior angle

Scapular spine

Medial border

Coracoid process

Body

R

Fig. 13-99 Scapula. AP projection.

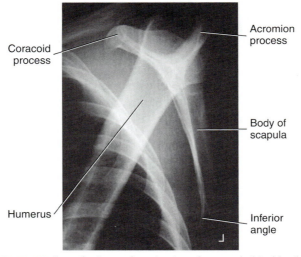

Coracoid process

Humerus

Acromion process

Body of scapula

Inferior angle

Fig. 13-100 Scapula. Lateral projection, forearm behind back.

Acromioclavicular Joints

Routine Examination

The routine examination of the acromioclavicular (AC) joints includes bilateral AP projections, both with and without weights. The purpose is to determine ligament integrity by demonstrating change in relative positions of the acromion and clavicle when under stress.

IR: 14 × 17 inches (35 × 43 cm) crosswise or two 10 × 12 inches (24 × 30 cm) lengthwise—one for each shoulder

Grid: Not required but may be used

SID: 40 inches minimum (or more as needed for wide shoulders)

Body position: Standing with back to IR(s).

Part position:

First exposure (no weights): Back of shoulders against lower half of IR(s). Arms relaxed at sides in neutral position (Fig. 13-101).

Second exposure (weights): Back of shoulders against upper half of IR(s). Arms at sides with 5- to 10-lb sandbag attached to each wrist (Figs. 13-102 and 13-104).

Central ray: Perpendicular to midline at level of acromion processes. Exposure field collimated to cover half of the IR (see Fig. 13-101).

TIPS:
- If the two sides are exposed separately, which is acceptable, patient must have sandbags on wrists for both weight-bearing radiographs.
- When the patient's shoulders are too wide to fit on a 35 × 43 cm IR, two 24 × 30 cm IRs can be placed side by side in the cassette holder (Fig. 13-103).
- Instruct the patient to stand tall but relax shoulders to allow weights to pull them down. This will result in best demonstration of AC joint separation.

Collimation: Adjust to 6 × 17 inches (15 × 43 cm) on collimator for large, single IR.
  Adjust to 6 × 8 inches (15 × 20 cm) for two smaller IRs.

Patient instruction: Stop breathing. Do not move.

Structures seen: Both AC joints for comparison to evaluate ligament integrity (Fig. 13-105).

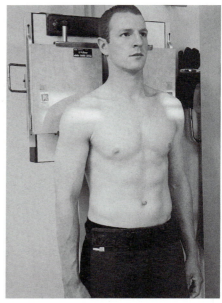

Fig. 13-101 Acromioclavicular joints. Position for bilateral AP projections, without weights.

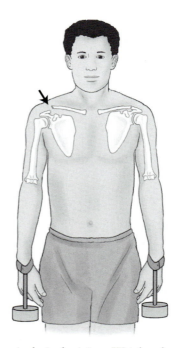

Fig. 13-102 Acromioclavicular joints. Weights should be attached to wrists as shown and not held in hands. Note how separation of the right AC joint is shown by pulling of weights *(arrow)*.

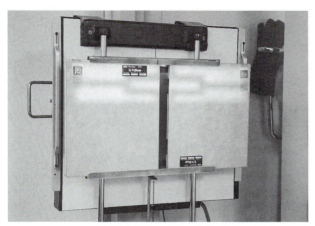

Fig. 13-103 Image receptor (IR) placement for acromioclavicular joint study using two IRs, no grid.

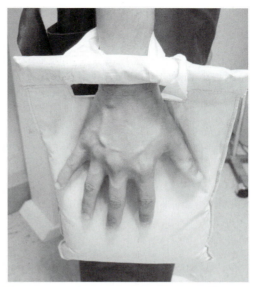

Fig. 13-104 Close-up of sandbag affixed to wrist. This is the ideal way to apply weight to the shoulders.

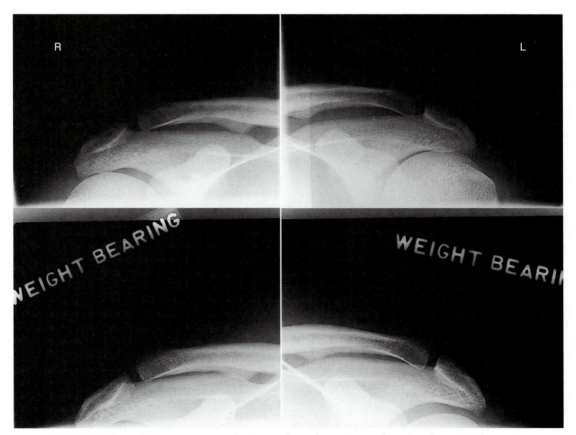

Fig. 13-105 Bilateral AP projections of acromioclavicular joints, with and without weights, using two IRs and nongrid holder.

PATHOLOGY

Probably the most significant pathology affecting the upper limb is trauma. Fractures and other injuries to this portion of the anatomy may vary greatly, and a sample of those seen with radiography is discussed here.

Common Fractures

The boxer's fracture is a common fracture of the fifth metacarpal, usually caused when the patient strikes a solid object with a closed fist (Fig. 13-106).

An important carpal bone injury is a fracture of the scaphoid (navicular), often caused by a fall on an outstretched arm. When they are new, scaphoid fractures may be occult, that is, very subtle or completely invisible on a radiograph. Special projections are often necessary to demonstrate this fracture, or it may be necessary to have the patient return for another radiographic examination after about 10 days (Fig. 13-107). It is especially important to identify these fractures because the scaphoid has a relatively inefficient blood supply, and there is a strong possibility of necrosis if the fracture is not identified early and treated correctly (Fig. 13-108). Necrosis of the scaphoid causes impairment of wrist function.

A Colles fracture (Fig. 13-109) is a common fracture of the distal radius, accompanied by posterior and medial displacement. A Monteggia fracture consists of a fracture of the ulna and dislocation of the radial head (Fig. 13-110).

The most common elbow fracture is a fracture of the radial head, which may occur as the result of a fall on an outstretched arm (Fig. 13-111). It is particularly important to demonstrate the soft tissue of the elbow joint in the lateral projection. When a fracture at the elbow causes **joint effusion** (increased fluid in the joint capsule), the fat pad in the joint region will be displaced. It moves upward from the joint area and can be seen radiographically as a dark shadow in the soft tissue anterior or sometimes posterior to the humerus. This **fat pad sign** (Fig. 13-112) may be the only radiographic indication of a fracture involving the elbow joint.

The humerus is most commonly fractured at its weak point, the surgical neck. An example is seen in the positioning section of this chapter (see Fig. 13-83).

Fig. 13-106 Boxer's fracture *(arrow)*.

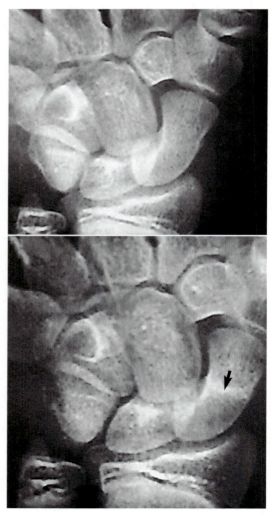

Fig. 13-107 Scaphoid fracture at injury and 3 weeks later *(arrow)*.

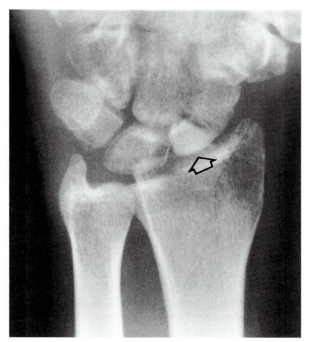

Fig. 13-108 Avascular necrosis of scaphoid *(open arrow)*.

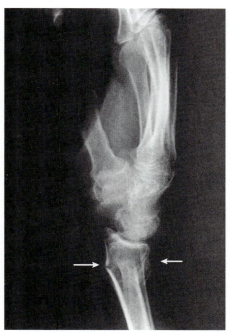

Fig. 13-109 Colles fracture *(arrows)*.

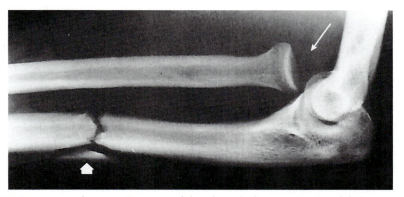

Fig. 13-110 Monteggia fracture. Fracture of the ulnar shaft *(arrowhead)* and dislocation of the radial head *(arrow)*.

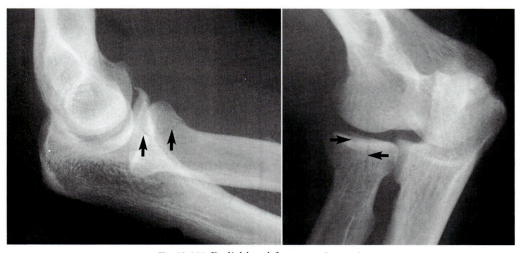

Fig. 13-111 Radial head fractures *(arrows)*.

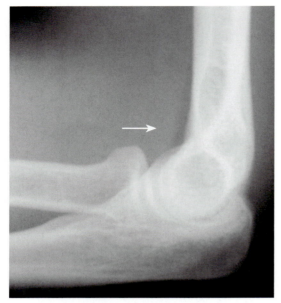

Fig. 13-112 Fat pad sign *(arrow)*.

Fractures of the clavicle are frequently seen, especially in children (Fig. 13-113).

Other Trauma Conditions

Dislocation of the shoulder (glenohumeral) joint is a fairly common injury. The humeral head may be displaced from the glenoid fossa either anteriorly or posteriorly (Fig. 13-114).

Injuries that introduce foreign bodies into the soft tissues may also be evaluated radiographically. In the upper limb, this is most commonly seen in the hand.

Nontraumatic Conditions

Chronic irritation to a bursa may lead to a condition called **bursitis,** inflammation of the bursa. Bursitis may cause calcific (calcium) deposits in the soft tissue of the joint region that are visible on radiographs. The shoulder is a very common site for calcific bursitis (Fig. 13-115). Inflammation of a tendon, called **tendinitis** or *tendonitis,* may occur at any tendon attachment in the body. It is

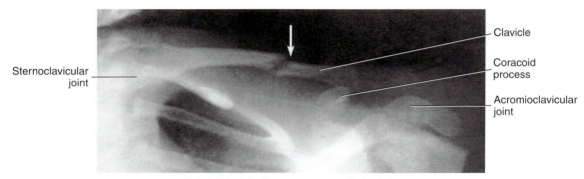

Fig. 13-113 Clavicle fracture in a small child *(arrow)*.

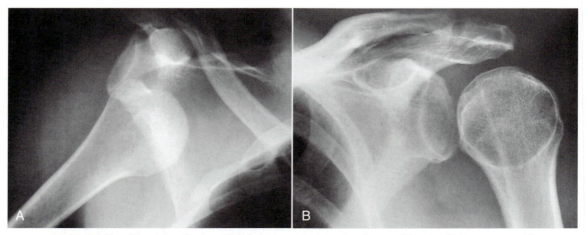

Fig. 13-114 Shoulder (glenohumeral) dislocations. **A,** Anterior: humeral head inferior to coracoid process. **B,** Posterior: humeral head trapped behind edge of glenoid process.

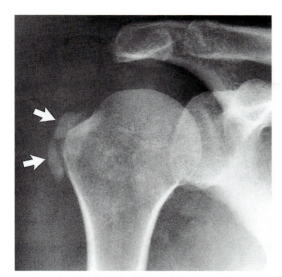

Fig. 13-115 Calcific bursitis *(arrows)*.

common at the shoulder and in the wrist. Tendinitis may also produce calcific deposits in the soft tissues.

Arthritis (joint inflammation) may affect any part of the body, and there are a number of different types. Rheumatoid arthritis (see Fig. 12-40) is a crippling disease that often involves the hands and is a common reason for radiography. The most common type of arthritis is a degenerative joint disease called **osteoarthritis** (Fig. 13-116). It is a chronic condition that causes hypertrophy of the bone. The enlarged, deformed portions of the bone are called **osteophytes.**

Osteomyelitis (Fig. 13-117) is inflammation of bone, especially the marrow, caused by a pathogenic organism. Bone infection may be caused by a number of different bacteria, including *Staphylococcus* and *Mycobacterium tuberculosis.*

Fig. 13-118 illustrates a bone cyst of the humerus. This fluid-filled cyst has a wall of fibrous tissue. Cysts of

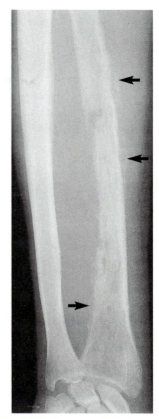

Fig. 13-117 Osteomyelitis *(arrows)*.

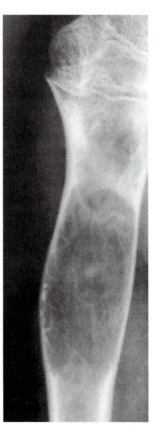

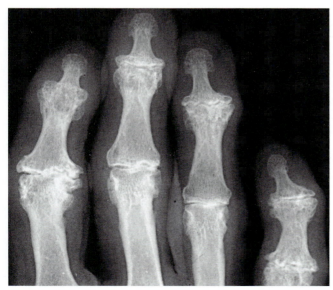

Fig. 13-116 Osteoarthritis of fingers, with obliteration of interphalangeal joint spaces and osteophyte formation.

Fig. 13-118 Bone cyst in humerus *(dark expanded area)*.

this type have no symptoms and are usually discovered only when they have weakened the bone sufficiently to cause a fracture. Fractures caused by underlying disease are called *pathologic fractures.* The cyst is actually a type of benign neoplasm. Other types of neoplasm and metastatic bone diseases may also affect the bones of the upper limb. They are called **osteoblastic** if they result in increased bone formation and **osteolytic** if they cause destruction of the bone.

SUMMARY

The bones of the hand and wrist include the phalanges, metacarpals, and carpals. The radius and ulna form the forearm, articulating at the wrist and the elbow. The humerus articulates with the forearm at the elbow and forms the shoulder joint where it articulates with the scapula. The scapula, clavicle, and upper humerus form the shoulder girdle. Important palpable bony prominences include the styloid processes of the distal radius and ulna, the olecranon process of the proximal ulna, the epicondyles and greater tuberosity of the humerus, and the acromion and coracoid processes of the scapula.

Radiography of the hand, fingers, thumb, wrist, forearm, and elbow is performed on the tabletop, without a grid. The patient is usually seated at the end of the table. Multiple projections may be included on a single IR. Examinations of the humerus and shoulder girdle, on the other hand, are done using a grid. The patient may be recumbent or upright. Examination of the AC joints requires a rather unusual combination of methods to produce bilateral projections taken with and without weights.

A variety of pathologies affect the upper limb, including trauma (fractures and dislocations) and nontraumatic conditions, such as arthritis, bursitis, tendinitis, infection, and neoplasia. Radiography has an important role in diagnosis of these conditions.

Chapter 14

Lower Limb and Pelvis

Learning Objectives

At the conclusion of this chapter, you will be able to:

- Name the bones that make up the lower limb and pelvis and identify each on an anatomic diagram and on a radiograph
- Name and identify the significant bony prominences and depressions of the lower limb and pelvis and identify significant positioning landmarks by palpation
- Demonstrate correct body and part positioning for routine projections and common special projections of the lower limb and pelvis
- Correctly evaluate radiographs of the lower limb and pelvis for positioning accuracy
- Describe and recognize on radiographs pathology that is common to the lower limb and pelvis

Key Terms

calcaneus
fabella
femur
fibula (pl. fibulae)
ilium (pl. ilia)
ischium (pl. ischia)
meniscus (pl. menisci)
metatarsals

patella (pl. patellae)
pedal digit
phalanges
prosthesis (pl. prostheses)
pubis (pl. pubes)
talus
tarsal bones
tibia

Many of the bones of the lower limb correspond to similar structures with similar functions in the upper limb. However, there are a number of significant differences, particularly in the ankle and knee joints. The understanding of both upper and lower extremities will be enhanced by comparing the two extremities.

ANATOMY

The lower limb includes the foot, toes, ankle, lower leg, knee, and femur (Fig. 14-1). The pelvis connects the lower limb to the axial skeleton, so it is included here.

Foot and Toes

The foot is commonly divided into three basic parts: the forefoot, the midfoot, and the hindfoot (Fig. 14-2). The bones of the forefoot include the **phalanges** and **metatarsals**. They correspond to the phalanges and metacarpals of the hand. The toes, sometimes called **pedal digits**, are numbered 1 through 5 from medial to lateral, just as are the fingers in the hand. The first pedal digit is called the *great toe* and has two phalanges. The rest of the toes have three phalanges. Just as in the hand, the hinge joints that connect the phalanges are called *interphalangeal (IP) joints* and are named *proximal* and *distal* in toes 2 through 5. The great toe has only one IP joint. The metatarsals are numbered 1 through 5, starting with the medial aspect. The numbers correspond to the digits with which they

articulate. The distal end of a metatarsal is called its *head*, and the proximal end is referred to as the *base*. The hinge joints between the metatarsals and the proximal phalanges are called *metatarsophalangeal (MTP) joints.*

There are usually two sesamoid bones in the region of the first MTP joint. These small, flat, oval bones were introduced in Chapter 13. They are located within tendons and are not counted among the bones of the body. They serve as a lever and to protect the joint.

The midfoot consists of five short bones called **tarsal bones.** The three cuneiform bones are named by location: medial, intermediate, and lateral. They articulate with the first, second, and third metatarsals, respectively. Lateral to the third cuneiform is the cuboid, which articulates with the fourth and fifth metatarsals. Proximal to the cuneiforms is the navicular bone.

The hindfoot includes the calcaneus and the talus. The **calcaneus** is commonly referred to as the *heel bone.* The **talus** is superior to the calcaneus and in addition articulates with the navicular, the tibia, and the fibula. The intertarsal (between the tarsal) joints are gliding joints with relatively small amounts of motion.

Ankle, Lower Leg, Knee, and Femur

The talus articulates with the tibia and fibula to form the ankle mortise. Weight is transferred from the shaft of the tibia through the talus, while the malleoli provide stability on either side. The entire joint is shaped like an

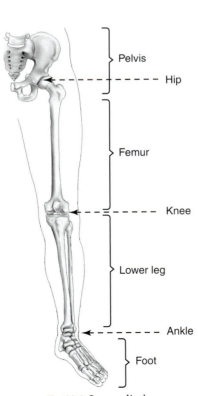

Fig. 14-1 Lower limb.

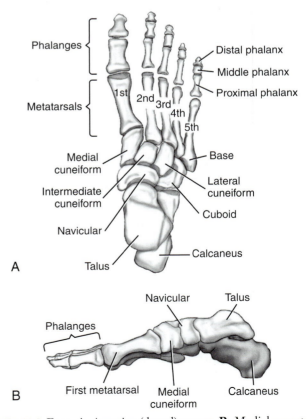

Fig. 14-2 Foot. **A,** Anterior (dorsal) aspect. **B,** Medial aspect.

inverted box (⊓) (Fig. 14-3). It is called a *mortise joint* because it resembles a carpenter's joint of the same name. The ankle is a hinge joint. When it flexes to raise the foot, the motion is called *dorsiflexion;* when it extends, pointing the toe downward, the motion is called *plantar flexion.* Lateral flexion of the ankle tends to roll the foot onto its medial aspect and is called *eversion.* Medial flexion causes the foot to roll onto its lateral aspect and is called *inversion.*

The lower leg (Fig. 14-4) consists of two long bones, the **tibia** and the **fibula.** The tibia is the longer, thicker bone on the medial side. The fibula is much thinner and somewhat shorter and is located laterally. The medial malleolus is a bony prominence that can be palpated at the ankle on the medial aspect of the distal tibia. The lateral malleolus is the rounded prominence on the distal aspect of the fibula and can be felt on the lateral aspect of the ankle.

A knoblike protuberance on the anterior surface of the tibia near the proximal end of the shaft is called the *tibial tuberosity.* The articular surface of the proximal tibia is a large, flat surface called the *tibial plateau.* The medial and lateral condyles are palpable projections on either side of the tibial plateau. Near the center of the tibial plateau are two superior projections called the *intercondylar eminences* or *tibial spines.*

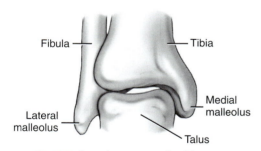

Fig. 14-3 Anterior aspect of ankle joint.

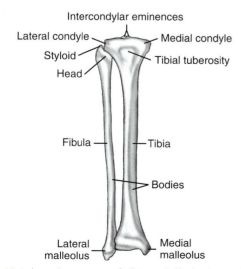

Fig. 14-4 Anterior aspect of tibia and fibula (lower leg).

The rounded proximal portion of the fibula is called the *head.* It terminates in a styloid process. The proximal fibula articulates with the metaphysis of the tibia at the inferior aspect of the lateral condyle. It is not a part of the knee joint.

The single long bone of the thigh is called the **femur** (Fig. 14-5). It is the largest, heaviest bone of the body. The distal end of the femur flares to form two palpable prominences, the medial and lateral condyles. Between the condyles on the posterior aspect of the leg is the intercondylar fossa. The distal articular surfaces of the condyles articulate with the tibial plateau to form the knee, which is a hinge-type joint. The articular surface of each condyle is cushioned by a C-shaped cartilage called a **meniscus.**

Anterior to the distal femur is the **patella,** commonly called the *kneecap.* It is a flat bone in the shape of a rounded triangle with its apex on the inferior margin. The patella is actually a large sesamoid bone, the only sesamoid bone numbered among the bones of the body. It is not unusual for there to be an additional small sesamoid bone posterior to the knee. This normal variation is called a **fabella.**

The rounded superior end of the femur is called the *head.* A small indentation on its posterior superior surface is called the *fovea capitis.* The narrow portion between the head and the shaft is the *neck.* The neck extends from the shaft at an angle, projecting superiorly and medially. Just inferior to the neck, the proximal shaft of the femur flares to form two prominences, the greater and lesser *trochanters.* The greater trochanter is a large projection on the lateral aspect that is palpable on the side of the upper thigh. The lesser trochanter is inferior to the greater trochanter and projects medially. It is not normally palpable. Between the two trochanters on the posterior aspect of the leg is a bony ridge called the *intertrochanteric crest.*

Fig. 14-6 illustrates the palpable bony landmarks of the lower limb.

Pelvis and Hip

The two bones that make up the halves of the pelvis are called the *hip bones,* also called the *os coxae* or *innominate bones* (Fig. 14-7). Each is a composite bone made up of three bones: the **ilium,** the **ischium,** and the **pubis.**

The ilium forms the upper portion of the pelvis. Its large, flat, superior portion is called the *ala,* or wing. It articulates with the sacral portion of the spine medially, forming the sacroiliac joint. Its rounded superior margin is palpable and is a common positioning landmark called the *iliac crest.* On the lateral aspect of the ilium is an anterior projection called the *anterior superior iliac spine (ASIS).* The ASIS is palpable on the anterior surface of the body in the hip region and is also a common positioning landmark.

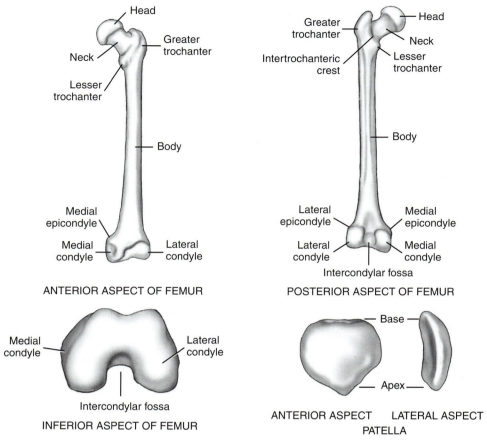

ANTERIOR ASPECT OF FEMUR

POSTERIOR ASPECT OF FEMUR

INFERIOR ASPECT OF FEMUR

ANTERIOR ASPECT   LATERAL ASPECT
PATELLA

Fig. 14-5 Femur and patella.

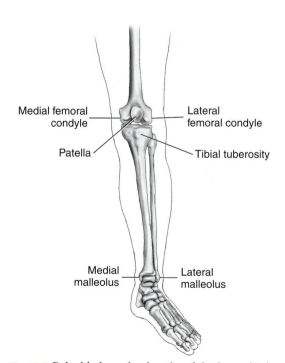

Fig. 14-6 Palpable bony landmarks of the lower limb.

The inferior portion of the pelvis is formed by the ischium, on the posterior aspect, and the pubis, on the anterior aspect. The most inferior portion of the ischium is a bony prominence called the *ischial tuberosity*. When one is sitting erect, the weight of the body is supported on the ischial tuberosities. They are palpable through the inferior portions of the buttocks. Together, the rami (branches) of the ischium and pubis form a bony ring. The hole within this ring is called the *obturator foramen*.

The ilium, ischium, and pubis join to form a synarthrodial joint at the acetabulum. The acetabulum is the rounded fossa that forms the socket of the hip joint. It articulates with the head of the femur. The right and left pubic bones join in the midline to form the pubic symphysis, an amphiarthrodial joint.

Fig. 14-8 illustrates the palpable bony landmarks of the pelvis and hip.

POSITIONING AND RADIOGRAPHIC EXAMINATIONS

Examinations of the lower limb from the toes up to the knee joint are usually done on the tabletop (nongrid),

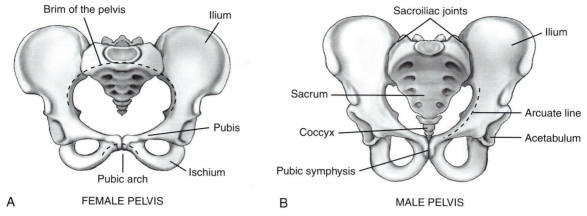

Fig. 14-7 Pelvis. **A,** Female. **B,** Male.

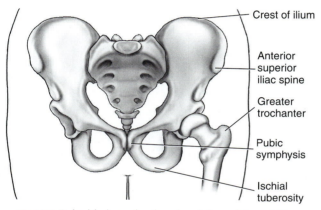

Fig. 14-8 Palpable bony landmarks of the pelvis and hip.

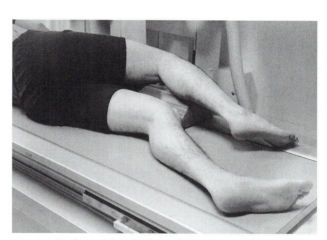

Fig. 14-9 Body position for lateral projections of lower limb.

with the patient sitting or lying on the radiographic table.

The shoe and stocking should be removed from the affected leg, as should any jewelry in the region. Trousers should be removed if they cannot be moved out of the radiation field, especially if the fabric is heavy, such as jeans. A rolled or bunched trouser leg will create an artifact on the image.

Although gonad shielding is legally required only for examinations of the femur, it is wise to shield whenever possible. A lead apron is shown for these examinations, when appropriate.

The body position illustrated in Fig. 14-9 places the entire lower limb in lateral position. This body position may be used for any lateral projection of the lower limb. Note that the coronal plane of the pelvis is perpendicular to the table, the knee is flexed approximately 45 degrees, and the ankle is dorsiflexed so that the foot forms an angle of 90 degrees with the lower leg. The unaffected leg is supported to prevent rotation of the pelvis. However, when the patient is unable to attain this position, the unaffected leg can be placed behind the affected leg as long as the lateral position is maintained.

Toes

Although the toes are included in the examination of the foot, separate studies of the toes may be performed when the area of clinical interest is limited to a specific toe. Each projection of the toe should include the entire digit and the distal portion of the corresponding metatarsal.

Toes 2 through 5 tend to curl downward. When the toes are angled in relation to the image receptor (IR), visualization of the joint spaces is compromised. When this is the case, an anteroposterior (AP) axial projection is recommended. For lateral projections of the toes, the foot may be positioned with either its medial or lateral aspect in contact with the IR, depending on which toe is involved. Keep the toe as close to the IR as possible and maintain the toe in a position parallel to the IR.

Routine Examination

The routine examination of the toe includes the AP or AP axial, AP oblique (medial rotation), and lateral projections.

IR: 8 × 10 inches (18 × 24 cm)

Grid: No

Source–image receptor distance (SID): 40 inches minimum

Body position: Seated or recumbent on table with knee flexed.

Part position:

AP axial: Plantar surface supported on a 15-degree wedge sponge (Fig. 14-10)

AP: Plantar surface is in contact with IR (Fig. 14-11).

AP oblique: Medial plantar surface of toe and forefoot is in contact with IR. Plantar surface of foot and toes forms a 30- to 45-degree angle with IR (Fig. 14-13).

Lateral: Medial or lateral surface of foot may be in contact with IR, depending on which brings toe of interest nearest to IR. Other toes are flexed or extended as needed to leave affected toe free of superimposition. Affected toe is supported parallel to IR. Toes may be held in position using tape or a bandage (Fig. 14-15) or a wooden tongue blade. Positioning a single toe apart from the others often demands some creativity on the part of the radiographer. Variations may be required depending on which toe is involved, configuration of toe, and movements tolerable for the patient.

Central ray:

AP axial: Angled 15 degrees posteriorly (toward heel) to MTP joints

AP, AP oblique, lateral: Perpendicular to MTP joints.

Collimation: 1 inch (2.5 cm) on all sides of the toes, including 1 inch (2.5 cm) proximal to the MTP joint.

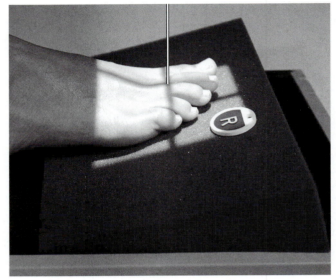

Fig. 14-10 Wedge sponge supports toes parallel to image receptor.

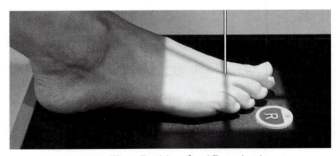

Fig. 14-11 Toes. Position for AP projection.

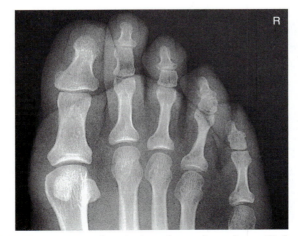

Fig. 14-12 Toes. AP axial projection of toes, elevated on a 15-degree wedge sponge.

Patient instruction: Do not move.

Structures seen: Entire digit and distal half of metatarsal with IP and MTP joint spaces open and clearly visualized (Figs. 14-12, 14-14, and 14-16).

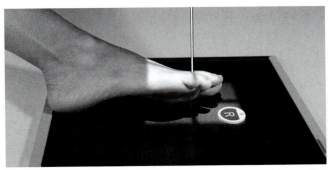

Fig. 14-13 Toes. Position for AP oblique projection—medial rotation.

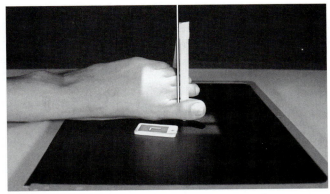

Fig. 14-15 Toes. Position for lateral projection of great toe.

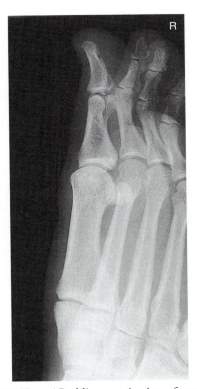

Fig. 14-14 Toes. AP oblique projection of great toe.

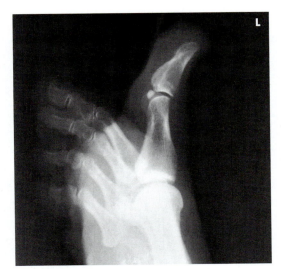

Fig. 14-16 Toes. Lateral projection of great toe.

Sesamoids

The sesamoid bones of the foot are located on the plantar aspect of the first MTP joint. These small bones are occasionally injured and are usually seen on foot radiographs. However, special positioning is required to demonstrate them without superimposition with other bones of the foot.

Routine Examination

The routine examination of the sesamoids includes the tangential projection.

IR: 8 × 10 inches (18 × 24 cm)

Grid: No

SID: 40 inches minimum

Body position: Standing, facing away from collimator, or prone.

Part position: Plantar surface of foot resting on IR in a position of dorsiflexion, and adjusted to place the ball of the foot perpendicular to the IR (Fig. 14-17*A*).

When the patient can't stand, the tangential projection can be performed with the patient seated, the foot pointing up, and the plantar surface at an angle of approximately 70 degrees with the plane of the IR (Fig. 14-17*B*).

Central ray: Perpendicular and tangential to the first MTP joint.

Collimation: Adjust to 3 × 3 inches on the collimator.

Patient instruction: Do not move.

Structures seen: Sesamoids and first metatarsal head in profile (Fig. 14-18).

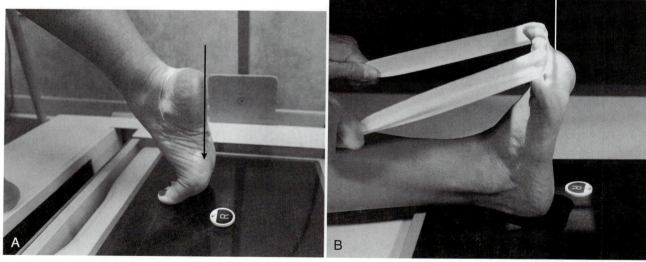

Fig. 14-17 Sesamoids. Position for tangential projection. **A,** Toes close to IR. **B,** Toes away from IR. This position is used when patient cannot stand.

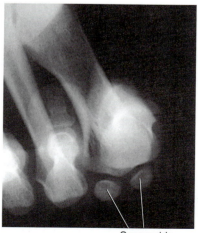

Sesamoids

Fig. 14-18 Sesamoids. Tangential projection.

Foot

The top of the foot is its dorsal aspect and the bottom its plantar surface, so the AP axial projection would more correctly be a dorsoplantar (DP) axial projection. However, this term is commonly used only in podiatric medicine. The central ray is angled posteriorly (toward the heel) for this projection to reduce foreshortening of the metatarsals and to better demonstrate the intertarsal articulations.

Routine Examination

The routine examination of the foot includes the AP axial, AP oblique (medial), and lateral projections.

IR: 10 × 12 inches (24 × 30 cm) lengthwise

Grid: No

SID: 40 inches minimum

Body position: Seated or recumbent on table with knee flexed. In podiatric practice, the AP (DP) and AP (DP) oblique projections are performed with the patient standing.

Part position: For all projections, foot is centered with regard to IR so that toes, heel, and both malleoli are within field.

AP axial: Plantar surface of foot is in contact with IR (Fig. 14-19).

AP oblique: Leg is rotated medially so that medial plantar aspect of foot is in contact with IR. Plantar surface of foot forms a 30-degree angle with IR (Fig. 14-21).

Lateral: Lateral aspect of foot is in contact with IR and foot is in true lateral position with plantar aspect of forefoot perpendicular to IR. Ankle is dorsiflexed so that long axis of foot is perpendicular to tibia (Fig. 14-23).

Central ray:

AP axial: Angled 10 degrees posteriorly (toward heel) and entering base of third metatarsal.

AP oblique and lateral: Perpendicular to base of third metatarsal.

Collimation:

AP axial and AP oblique: 1 inch (2.5 cm) on the sides and 1 inch (2.5 cm) beyond the calcaneus and distal tip of the toes.

Lateral: 1 inch (2.5 cm) on the sides of the shadow of the foot including 1 inch (2.5 cm) above the medial malleolus.

Patient instruction: Do not move.

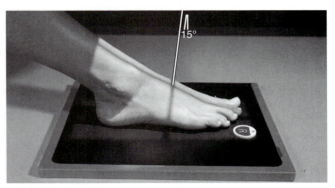

Fig. 14-19 Foot. Position for AP axial projection.

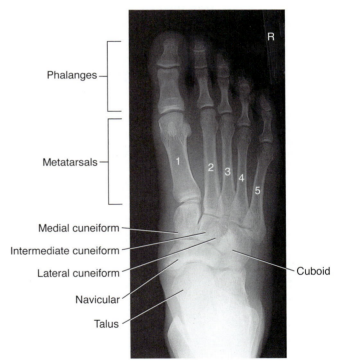

Fig. 14-20 Foot. AP axial projection.

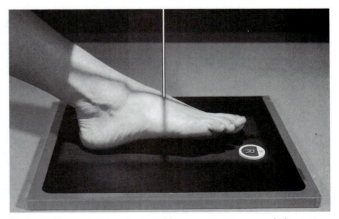

Fig. 14-21 Foot. Position for AP oblique projection—medial rotation.

Structures seen: Entire foot, including toes, metatarsals, and tarsal bones. On AP axial projection, calcaneus is obscured by superimposition of lower leg (Fig. 14-20). AP oblique projection with medial rotation should demonstrate the metatarsals and some tarsals (cuboid, navicular, lateral cuneiform) with minimal superimposition on one another (Fig. 14-22). Too much superimposition of these structures indicates that angle between plantar surface of foot and IR was too great; that is, foot was everted too much. Lateral projection shows superimposition of metatarsals, more proximal than distal. It should include the ankle joint (Fig. 14-24).

Compensating filter: A wedge-type compensating filter, attached to the collimator, may be used to produce a more even radiographic density on the AP axial projection, preventing overexposure of the toes and distal metatarsals. The filter is placed so that its thicker portion is projected over the toes and its thin edge is projected in the midmetatarsal region.

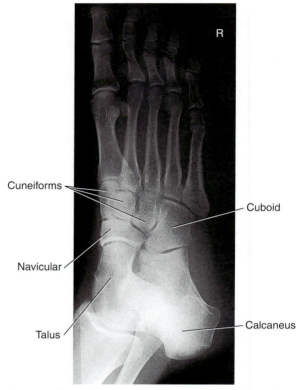

Fig. 14-22 Foot. AP oblique projection—medial rotation.

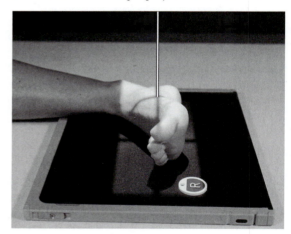

Fig. 14-23 Foot. Position for lateral projection.

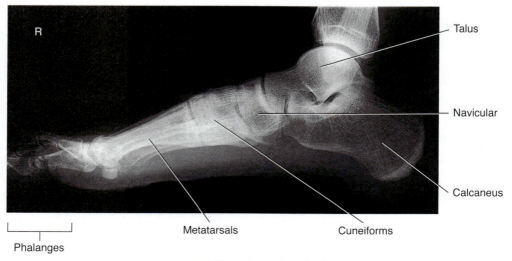

Fig. 14-24 Foot. Lateral projection.

Podiatry Examination

Radiographic examination of the foot in podiatric practice is usually performed with the patient standing to demonstrate the relationship of the bony structures during weight bearing. A podiatry examination includes AP axial, AP axial obliques (medial and lateral rotation), and lateral projections. The AP axial projection may include both feet taken with one exposure (bilateral) or a single foot (unilateral).

IR: 10 × 12 inches (24 × 30 cm) lengthwise

Grid: No

SID: 40 inches minimum

Body position: Standing.

Part position:

AP axial: Plantar surface of feet or foot in contact with IR or surface of IR tunnel (Fig. 14-25).

AP axial oblique (medial rotation):   Foot is rotated to place medial plantar aspect of foot in contact with IR or surface of IR tunnel. Plantar surface of foot forms a 30-degree angle with IR (Fig. 14-27).

AP axial oblique (lateral rotation):   Foot is rotated to place lateral plantar aspect of foot in contact with IR or surface of IR tunnel. Plantar surface of foot forms a 30-degree angle with IR (Fig. 14-29).

Lateral: Medial aspect of the foot in contact with IR. Long axis of foot is perpendicular to tibia (Fig. 14-31).

Central ray:

AP axial: Angled 10 to 15 degrees toward the heel. Directed between the feet at the level of the third metatarsal base for the bilateral exam. Directed to the third metatarsal base for a unilateral exam.

AP axial obliques: Angled 10 to 15 degrees toward the heel. Directed to the third metatarsal base.

Lateral: Horizontal and perpendicular to the third metatarsal base.

Collimation:

AP axial and AP axial obliques: 1 inch (2.5 cm) on the sides and 1 inch (2.5 cm) beyond the calcaneus and distal tip of the toes.

Lateral: 1 inch (2.5 cm) on the sides of the shadow of the foot including 1 inch (2.5 cm) above the medial malleolus.

> **NOTE:**   An AP oblique projection is sometimes performed with the foot flat on the IR or IR tunnel and the CR angled 30 degrees or 45 degrees from lateral to medial (Fig. 14-33).

Patient instructions: Do not move.

Structures seen: Entire foot, including toes, metatarsals, and tarsal bones. On AP axial projection, calcaneus is obscured by superimposition of lower leg (Fig. 14-26). AP oblique projection with medial rotation should demonstrate the metatarsals and some tarsals (cuboid, navicular, lateral cuneiform) with minimal superimposition on one another (Fig. 14-28). AP oblique projection with lateral rotation should demonstrate the medial and intermedial cuneiforms and the navicular (Fig. 14-30). Lateral projection shows superimposition of metatarsals, more proximal than distal. It should include the ankle joint (Fig. 14-32).

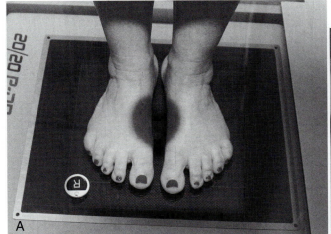
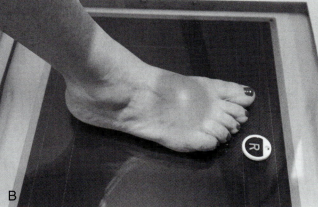

Fig. 14-25 Foot. **A,** Position for bilateral AP axial projection, patient standing. **B,** Position for AP axial projection, patient standing.

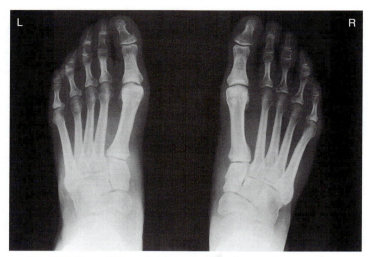

Fig. 14-26 Foot. Bilateral AP axial projection, patient standing.

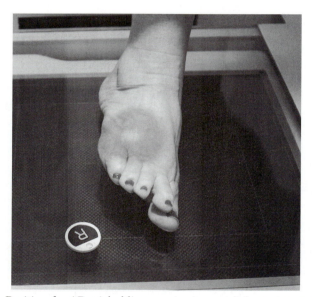

Fig. 14-27 Foot. Position for AP axial oblique projection–medial rotation, patient standing.

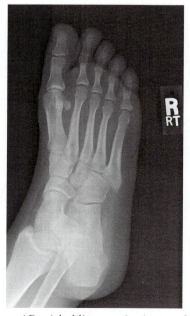

Fig. 14-28 Foot. AP axial oblique projection–medial rotation, patient standing.

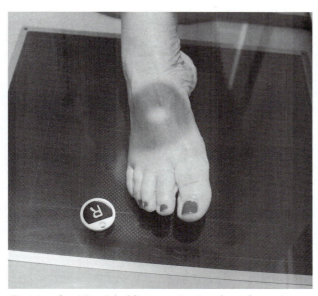

Fig. 14-29 Foot. Position for AP axial oblique projection–lateral rotation, patient standing.

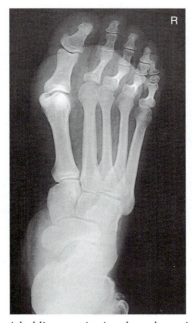

Fig. 14-30 Foot. AP axial oblique projection–lateral rotation, patient standing.

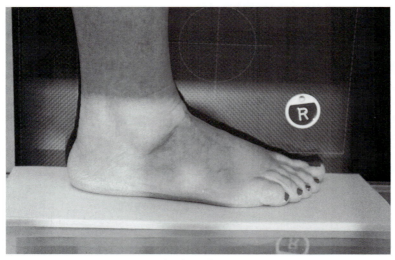

Fig. 14-31 Foot. Position for lateral projection, patient standing.

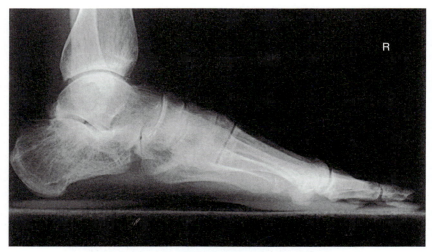

Fig. 14-32 Foot. Lateral projection, patient standing.

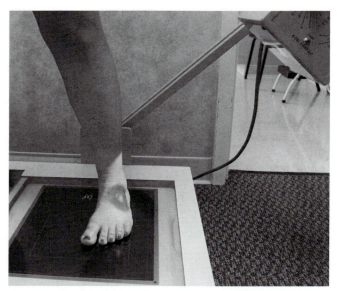

Fig. 14-33 Foot. Position for AP oblique projection (45-degree lateral to medial CR angle), patient standing. Note DR image receptor unit (dark rectangle) inside standing platform.

Calcaneus

Routine Examination

The routine examination of the calcaneus includes the axial (plantodorsal) and lateral projections.

IR: 8 × 10 inches (18 × 24 cm)

Grid: No

SID: 40 inches minimum

Body position:

Axial (plantodorsal): Seated or recumbent on table with leg extended.

Lateral: Seated or recumbent on table with knee flexed.

Part position:

Axial (plantodorsal): Posterior surface of ankle and heel is in contact with IR. Place foot so that malleoli are centered with regard to middle of IR. Sagittal plane of foot is perpendicular to IR. Foot is dorsiflexed as much as possible and held in position by patient using a strap or bandage (Fig. 14-34).

Lateral: Lateral surface of heel is in contact with IR. Part is positioned as for lateral projection of foot but with calcaneus centered to IR (Fig. 14-36).

Central ray:

Axial (plantodorsal): Angled 40 degrees cephalad to center of IR, entering at third metatarsal base.

Lateral: Perpendicular to center of IR, entering about 1 inch (2.5 cm) distal to medial malleolus.

> **NOTE:** In podiatric practices, an axial (dorsoplantar) projection may be taken with the patient standing on the IR. The central ray is angled 45 degrees anteriorly, entering the dorsal surface of the ankle joint and exiting the plantar surface of the heel at the level of the fifth metatarsal base (Fig. 14-38). This projection may be called the Harris-Beath method, Skier's position, or Coalition position.

Collimation:

Axial (plantodorsal): 1 inch (2.5 cm) on three sides of the shadow of the heel.

Lateral: 1 inch (2.5 cm) past the posterior and inferior shadow of the heel. Include the medial malleolus and base of the fifth metatarsal.

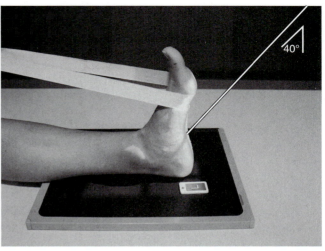

Fig. 14-34 Calcaneus. Position for axial (plantodorsal) projection.

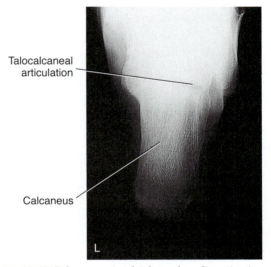

Talocalcaneal articulation

Calcaneus

L

Fig. 14-35 Calcaneus. Axial (plantodorsal) projection.

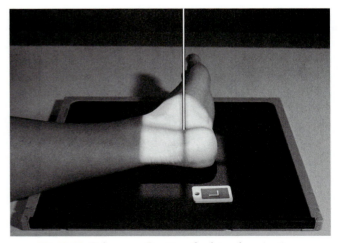

Fig. 14-36 Calcaneus. Position for lateral projection.

Patient instruction: Do not move.

Structures seen: Both projections demonstrate entire calcaneus and its articulation with talus (Fig. 14-35). Lateral projection also shows calcaneal articulations with cuboid and navicular anteriorly (Fig. 14-37).

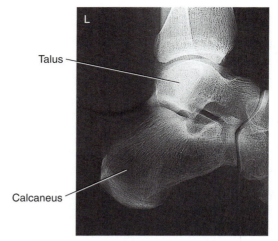

Fig. 14-37 Calcaneus. Lateral projection.

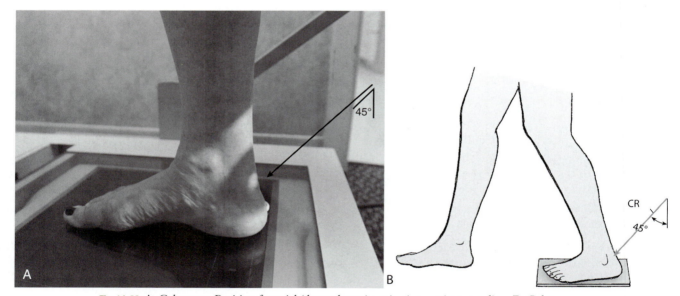

Fig. 14-38 A, Calcaneus. Position for axial (dorsoplantar) projection, patient standing. **B,** Calcaneus. Drawing demonstrating relationship between CR, calcaneus, and IR.

Ankle

There are two medial oblique ankle projections, one that best demonstrates the ankle mortise joint and one that best demonstrates the tibiofibular joint. The projections that constitute a routine examination must be determined by the physician who will interpret the images.

Routine Examination

The routine examination of the ankle includes the AP, AP oblique (medial rotation), AP oblique (medial rotation–mortise joint), and lateral projections.

IR: 10 × 12 inches (24 × 30 cm) lengthwise

Grid: No

SID: 40 inches minimum

Body position:

AP and AP obliques: Seated or recumbent on table with affected leg extended.

Lateral: Recumbent or semirecumbent on affected side with knee flexed 30 to 45 degrees.

Part position:

AP: Posterior surface of heel and lower leg is in contact with IR. Midpoint between malleoli is centered to IR. Foot is dorsiflexed so that plantar surface of foot forms a 90-degree angle with coronal plane of lower leg. Sagittal planes of leg and foot are perpendicular to IR (Fig. 14-39). Foot may be held in position by patient using a strap or bandage.

AP oblique (medial rotation): From position for AP projection, entire leg is rotated medially 45 degrees. Sagittal planes of foot and leg must remain aligned to each other (Fig. 14-41).

   NOTE: In podiatric practice, an AP oblique projection with a 45-degree lateral rotation may also be performed.

AP oblique (medial rotation—mortise joint): From position for AP projection, entire leg is rotated 15 to 20 degrees medially. Sagittal planes of foot and leg must remain aligned with each other (Fig. 14-43).

Lateral: Lateral surface (medial surface, if upright) of ankle is in contact with IR. Sagittal plane of foot and leg is parallel to IR. Foot is dorsiflexed so that plantar surface of foot forms a 90-degree angle with coronal plane of lower leg (Fig. 14-45).

   TIP: When pressure on the lateral malleolus is painful for the patient, a small sponge may be placed under the distal portion of the leg.

Central ray:

AP and AP obliques: Perpendicular to point midway between malleoli.

Lateral: Perpendicular to medial malleolus.

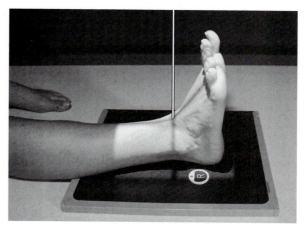

Fig. 14-39 Ankle. Position for AP projection.

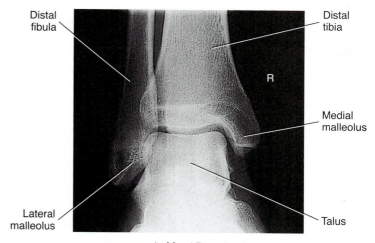

Fig. 14-40 Ankle. AP projection.

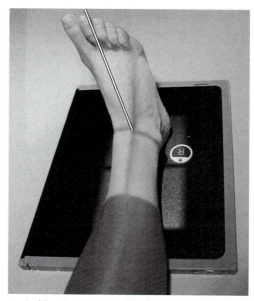

Fig. 14-41 Ankle. Position for AP oblique projection—45-degree medial rotation.

NOTE: In podiatric practice, all projections are performed with the patient standing. The IR will be vertical and the central ray horizontal. Part positions and central ray placement are as described for the AP (Fig. 14-47) and AP oblique (Fig. 14-48). However, the central ray enters at the lateral malleolus for the lateral (lateromedial) projection (Fig. 14-49).

Collimation:

AP and AP obliques: 1 inch (2.5 cm) on the sides of the ankle and 8 inches (18 cm) lengthwise to include the heel.

Lateral: 1 inch (2.5 cm) on the sides of the ankle and 8 inches (18 cm) lengthwise to include the heel and fifth metatarsal base.

Patient instruction: Do not move.

Structures seen: Superior portion of talus and distal portions of tibia and fibula (Fig. 14-40). AP oblique projection with a 45-degree medial rotation demonstrates tibiofibular joint without superimposition (Fig. 14-42). AP oblique projection with 15- to 20-degree medial rotation demonstrates mortise joint spaces without superimposition (Fig. 14-44). Lateral projection demonstrates tibiotalar and subtalar joints, and includes fifth metatarsal base (Fig. 14-46).

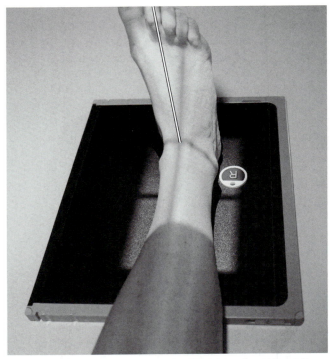

Fig. 14-43 Ankle (mortise joint). Position for AP oblique projection—15- to 20-degree medial rotation.

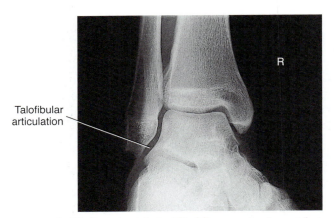

Talofibular articulation

Fig. 14-44 Ankle (mortise joint). AP oblique projection—15- to 20-degree medial rotation.

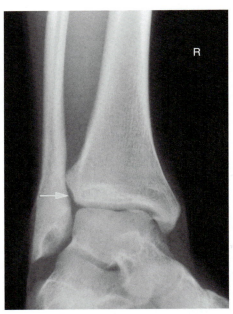

Fig. 14-42 Ankle. AP oblique projection—45-degree medial rotation. Note open tibiofibular joint *(arrow)*.

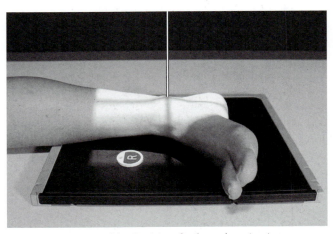

Fig. 14-45 Ankle. Position for lateral projection.

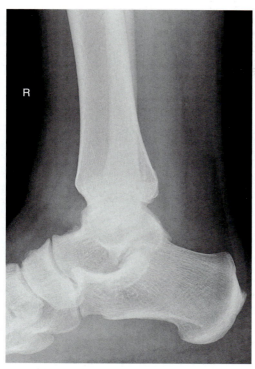

Fig. 14-46 Ankle. Lateral projection.

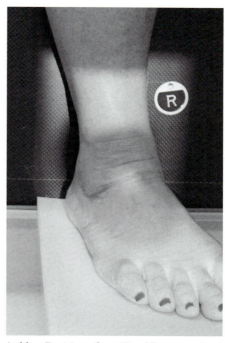

Fig. 14-48 Ankle. Position for AP oblique projection-medial rotation, patient standing.

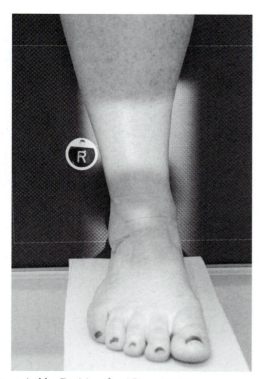

Fig. 14-47 Ankle. Position for AP projection, patient standing.

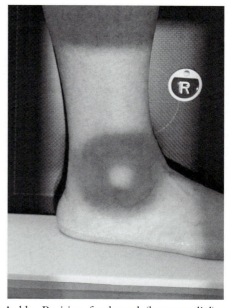

Fig. 14-49 Ankle. Position for lateral (lateromedial) projection, patient standing.

Lower Leg

The lower leg examination should include the entire tibia and the fibula and their articular surfaces. Visualization of both knee and ankle joints is preferable. If only one joint can be included on the largest IR available, the *same* joint must be demonstrated on both projections. In this case, additional radiographs will be needed to demonstrate the other joint. It is often necessary to use two 14 × 17 inch (35 × 43 cm) IRs diagonally to demonstrate both joints on adult patients.

Routine Examination

The routine examination of the lower leg includes the AP and lateral projections.

IR: 14 × 17 inches (35 × 43 cm) lengthwise or diagonal

Grid: No

SID: 40 inches minimum

Body position:

AP: Seated or recumbent on table.

Lateral: Recumbent on affected side with contralateral leg anterior or posterior to affected leg.

Part position:

AP: Leg is fully extended with posterior surface of lower leg in contact with IR. Margin of IR is placed 1 to 2 inches beyond joint of primary interest. Foot is dorsiflexed so that plantar surface of foot forms a 90-degree angle with coronal plane of lower leg. Sagittal planes of leg and foot are perpendicular to IR (Fig. 14-50). Foot may be held in position by patient using a strap or bandage.

Lateral: Knee may be flexed, if necessary, to ensure a true lateral position. Lateral surface of lower leg is in contact with IR. Leg is rotated to place sagittal plane of leg parallel to IR and coronal plane through patella perpendicular to IR. Margin of IR is placed 1 to 2 inches beyond joint of primary interest (Fig. 14-52).

Central ray: Perpendicular to center of IR entering midshaft of tibia.

Collimation: 1 inch (2.5 cm) on the sides and 1.5 inches (4 cm) beyond the ankle and knee joints.

Patient instruction: Do not move.

Structures seen: Entire lower leg and at least one joint (Figs. 14-51 and 14-53).

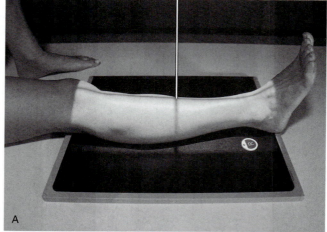

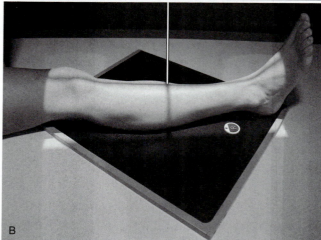

Fig. 14-50 Lower leg. Position for AP projection. **A,** Usual orientation of IR. **B,** Diagonal placement of IR, when lower leg is too long to fit within the long dimension of the IR. Exposure field must include entire corners of a computed radiography imaging plate to ensure good image quality.

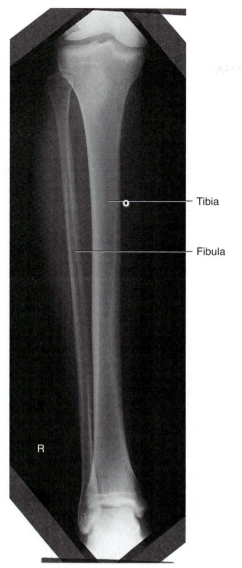

Tibia

Fibula

R

Fig. 14-51 Lower leg. AP projection.

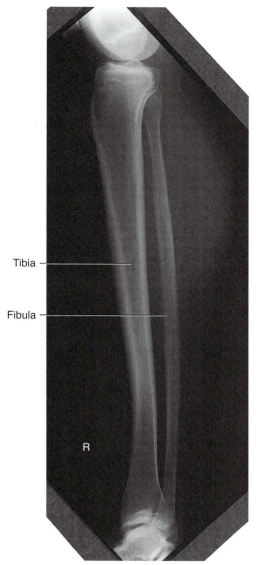

Tibia —

Fibula —

R

Fig. 14-53 Lower leg. Lateral projection.

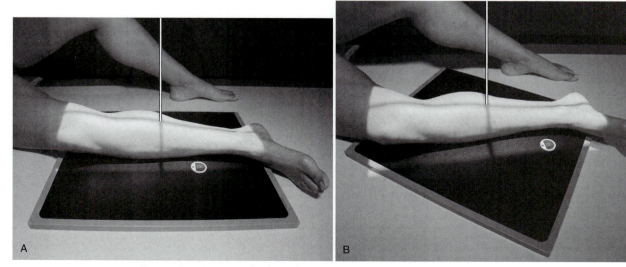

A   B

Fig. 14-52 Lower leg. Position for lateral projection. **A,** Usual orientation of IR. **B,** Diagonal placement of IR, when lower leg is too long to fit within the long dimension of the IR.

Knee

The routine examination of the knee consists of AP and lateral projections. However, an axial projection of the intercondylar fossa ("tunnel" or "notch") and a tangential projection of the patella are frequently requested for the evaluation of chronic knee complaints.

When the area of clinical interest is the patella, the routine examination includes posteroanterior (PA) and lateral projections. A tangential projection of the patella may be added for chronic conditions but should not be included when there is suspicion of patellar fracture. *Do not flex the knee more than 10 degrees when there is suspicion of fracture of the patella.* When this is the case, the lateral projection is taken with the knee extended.

Routine Examination

The routine examination of the knee includes the AP and lateral projections.

IR: 10 × 12 inches (24 × 30 cm) lengthwise

Grid: With or without is acceptable. For large knees, radiographic contrast is superior with a grid.

SID: 40 inches minimum

Body position:

AP: Seated or supine on table with leg extended.

Lateral: Recumbent on affected side with femur aligned with center of table. Unaffected leg is anterior or posterior to affected leg.

Part position:

AP: Leg is fully extended with sagittal plane of leg perpendicular to IR (Fig. 14-54).

Lateral: Knee is flexed 20 to 30 degrees. Sagittal plane of femur and lower leg is parallel to IR (Fig. 14-56).

Central ray:

AP: Entering 0.5 inch distal to apex of patella. Angle is variable, depending on the measurement between the ASIS and the tabletop, as follows:

<19 cm (thin patient)	3-5 degrees *caudad*
19 to 24 cm	0 degrees (perpendicular)
>24 cm (large pelvis)	3-5 degrees *cephalad*

Lateral: Angled 5 to 7 degrees cephalad entering 1 inch distal to medial epicondyle of femur.

Collimation: Adjust to 10 × 12 inch (24 × 30 cm) size on the collimator.

Patient instruction: Do not move.

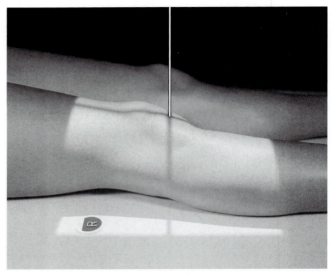

Fig. 14-54 Knee. Position for AP projection.

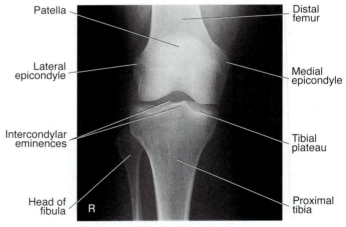

Fig. 14-55 Knee. AP projection.

Structures seen: Knee joint with portions of distal femur and proximal lower leg (Fig. 14-55). Lateral projection includes a profile of tibial tuberosity. It should demonstrate distal femur with condyles superimposed and joint space free of superimposition. Entire patella and retropatellar joint space should also be clearly visualized (Fig. 14-57).

Alternative Projection

The PA projection of the knee is sometimes substituted for the AP projection. This is especially desirable when the patella is of particular clinical interest.

IR size and orientation, **grid, SID,** and **collimation** are the same as for routine knee projections.

Body position: Patient prone.

Part position: Affected leg extended and sagittal plane of leg perpendicular to IR; foot on affected side is plantar flexed and rests on its dorsal aspect (Fig. 14-58).

Central ray: Directed 5 to 7 degrees caudad to exit 0.5 inch (1.3 cm) inferior to the patellar apex.

Structures seen: Knee joint with portions of distal femur and proximal lower leg. Greater visibility of the patella than on the AP projection (Fig. 14-59).

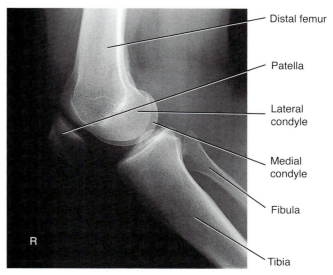

Distal femur
Patella
Lateral condyle
Medial condyle
Fibula
Tibia

R

Fig. 14-57 Knee. Lateral projection.

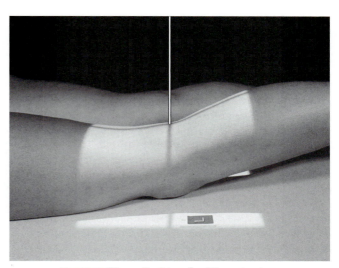

Fig. 14-58 Knee. Position for PA projection.

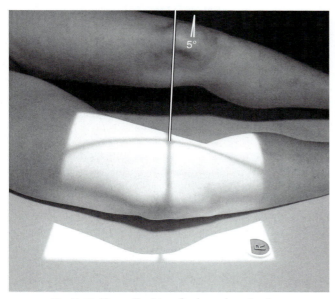

5°

Fig. 14-56 Knee. Position for lateral projection.

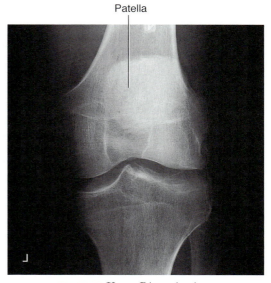

Patella

Fig. 14-59 Knee. PA projection.

Supplemental Projections

PA Axial Projections of the Intercondylar Fossa ("Tunnel")

Two methods are presented for demonstration of the intercondylar fossa. The Holmblad method, in which there is less distortion caused by tube angulation, is often preferred. The Camp-Coventry method may be desirable if the patient is unable to assume the correct position for the Holmblad method.

IR size and orientation, **grid, SID,** and **collimation** are the same as for routine knee projections.

PA Axial Projection—Holmblad Method

Body and part position: Patient is on hands and knees on radiographic table with affected knee flexed so that angle between femur and table is 70 degrees. Contralateral knee is flexed more and is forward to provide support (Fig. 14-60). Pelvis must remain level and sagittal plane of affected leg must remain perpendicular to the IR.

Central ray: Perpendicular to center of IR through center of knee joint.

Structures seen: Knee joint with portions of distal femur and proximal lower leg. Open intercondylar fossa (Fig. 14-61).

> **TIPS:**
> - Placing small level sponges under the knees helps provide patient comfort in this position.
> - An increase in milliampere-seconds (mAs) of 50% from that used for the AP or PA projection is needed to compensate for the increased tissue thickness at the distal femur.

PA Axial Projection—Camp-Coventry Method

Body and part position: Prone with affected knee flexed to form an angle of 40 or 50 degrees between tibia and table (Fig. 14-62).

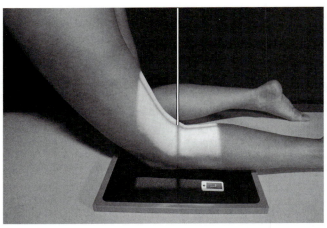

Fig. 14-60 Knee (intercondylar fossa). Position for PA axial ("tunnel") projection—Holmblad method.

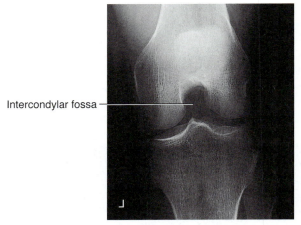

Intercondylar fossa

Fig. 14-61 Knee (intercondylar fossa). PA axial ("tunnel") projection—Holmblad method.

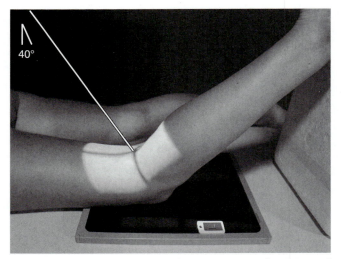

40°

Fig. 14-62 Knee (intercondylar fossa). Position for PA axial ("tunnel") projection—Camp-Coventry method.

Central ray: Angled 40 degrees caudad through knee joint to center of IR if leg is 40 degrees, and 50 degrees if leg is 50 degrees.

Structures seen: Knee joint with portions of distal femur and proximal lower leg. Open intercondylar fossa (Fig. 14-63).

> **TIP:** An increase in mAs of 50% from that used for the AP or PA projection is needed to compensate for increased tissue thickness caused by the angulation of the x-ray beam.

Tangential ("Sunrise") Projection of the Patella—Settegast Method

IR size and orientation, **grid**, **SID**, and **collimation** are the same as for routine knee projections.

Position: Prone with affected knee flexed as much as possible or until the patella is perpendicular to the IR. Sagittal plane of femur is perpendicular to IR. Position may be supported by a strap around the ankle that is extended over patient's shoulder and held by patient (Fig. 14-64). Alternatively, patient may be seated on the radiographic table (Fig. 14-65).

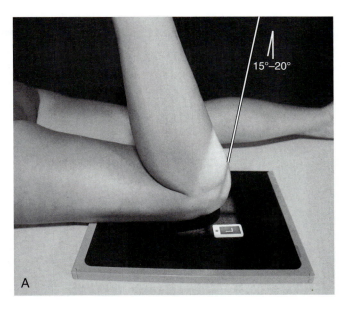
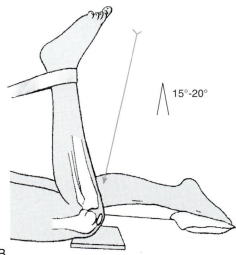

A

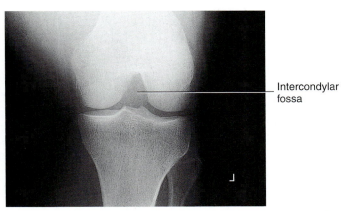

Fig. 14-63 Knee (intercondylar fossa). PA axial ("tunnel") projection—Camp-Coventry method.

Intercondylar fossa

B

Fig. 14-64 Patella. **A,** Position for tangential ("sunrise") projection—Settegast method (patient prone). **B,** Drawing demonstrating relationships between central ray, patellofemoral joint space, and image receptor.

Central ray: Angled 15 to 20 degrees cephalad and centered to inferior margin of patella. Angulation is adjusted so that central ray passes between patella and distal femur.

Structures seen: Patella in profile and open patellofemoral joint (Fig. 14-66).

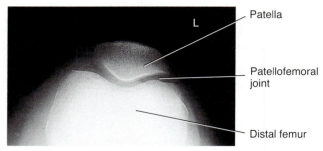

Fig. 14-66 Patella. Tangential projection.

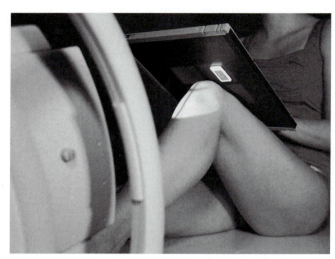

Fig. 14-65 Patella. Position for tangential ("sunrise") projection—Settegast method (patient seated).

Femur

For most adults, the entire femur is too long to be included on a 35 × 43 cm IR, so a choice must be made about which portion to include. Radiographs of the distal femur include the knee, whereas those of the proximal femur include the hip joint. When the entire femur is imaged, AP and lateral radiographs of both the proximal and distal femur are included.

Routine Examination

Distal Femur

The routine examination of the distal femur includes the AP and lateral projections.

IR: 14 × 17 inches (35 × 43 cm)

Grid: Yes

SID: 40 inches minimum

Body position:

AP: Supine with affected femur aligned with center of table.

Lateral: Recumbent on affected side with affected femur aligned with center of table. Knee and hip of unaffected limb are flexed, and leg is supported anterior to the body.

Part position:

AP: Leg is extended with sagittal plane perpendicular to IR. Ensure plane through epicondyles is parallel with IR. Inferior margin of IR is placed 1 to 2 inches below knee joint (Fig. 14-67).

Lateral: Knee of affected leg is flexed 30 to 45 degrees. Sagittal plane of femur is parallel to IR. Inferior margin of IR is placed 1 to 2 inches below knee joint (Fig. 14-69).

Central ray: Perpendicular to midpoint of IR.

Collimation: 1 inch (2.5 cm) on the sides of the shadow of the femur and 17 inches (43 cm) in length.

Patient instruction: Do not move.

Structures seen: Knee joint and distal three fourths of femur (Figs. 14-68 and 14-70).

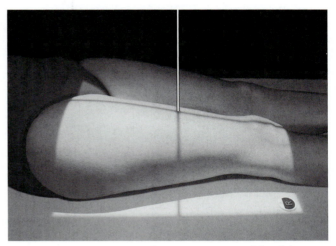

Fig. 14-67 Femur. Position for AP projection of distal femur.

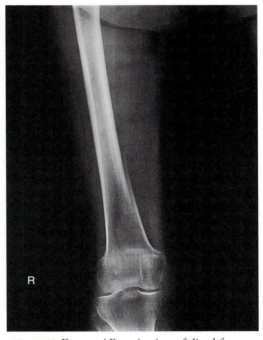

Fig. 14-68 Femur. AP projection of distal femur.

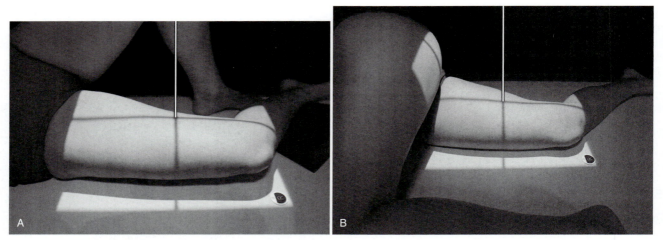

Fig. 14-69 Femur. Positions for lateral projection of distal femur. **A,** Unaffected leg posterior. **B,** Unaffected leg anterior and supported.

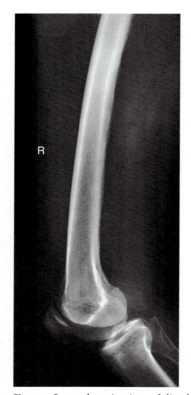

Fig. 14-70 Femur. Lateral projection of distal femur.

Proximal Femur

The routine examination of the proximal femur includes the AP and lateral projections.

IR: 14 × 17 inches (35 × 43 cm) lengthwise

Grid: Yes

SID: 40 inches minimum

Body position:

AP: Supine with affected femur aligned to center of table.

Lateral: Recumbent in oblique position on affected side with support under unaffected hip. Affected femur aligned to center of table. Knee and hip of unaffected limb are flexed and leg is supported posterior to body.

Part position:

AP: Leg is extended with sagittal plane perpendicular to IR. Rotate the limb internally 10 to 15 degrees to place the femoral neck in profile. Superior margin of IR is placed at level of ASIS (Fig. 14-71).

Lateral: Rotate pelvis posteriorly 10 to 15 degrees from lateral position to prevent superimposition. Sagittal plane of femur is parallel to IR as much as possible. Superior margin of IR is placed at level of ASIS (Fig. 14-73).

Central ray: Perpendicular to midpoint of IR.

Patient instruction: Do not move.

Structures seen: Hip joint and proximal three fourths of femur (Figs. 14-72 and 14-74).

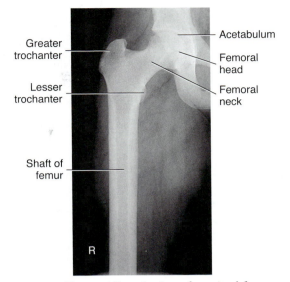

Greater trochanter — Acetabulum — Femoral head — Lesser trochanter — Femoral neck — Shaft of femur — R

Fig. 14-72 Femur. AP projection of proximal femur.

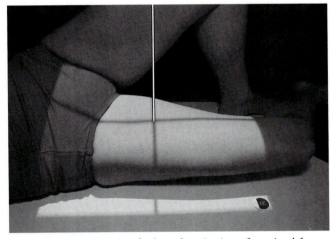

Fig. 14-73 Femur. Position for lateral projection of proximal femur.

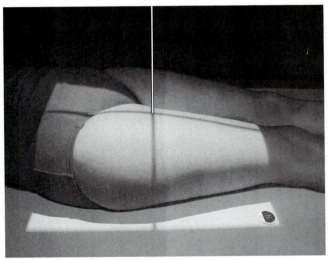

Fig. 14-71 Femur. Position for AP projection of proximal femur.

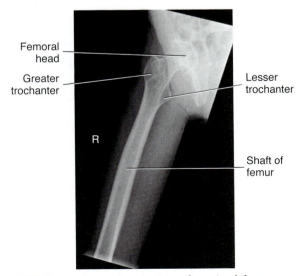

Femoral head — Greater trochanter — Lesser trochanter — Shaft of femur — R

Fig. 14-74 Femur. Lateral projection of proximal femur.

Pelvis

Routine Examination

The routine examination of the pelvis includes the AP projection.

IR: 14 × 17 inches (35 × 43 cm) crosswise

Grid: Yes

SID: 40 inches minimum

Body position: Supine on table. Coronal plane of body is parallel to IR (Fig. 14-75). If there is no suspicion of recent fracture, femurs are rotated medially 15 to 20 degrees to place femoral necks parallel to IR. The heels will be 8 to 10 inches apart (Fig. 14-76).

IR placement: Center IR midway between ASIS and pubic symphysis.

Central ray: Perpendicular to midpoint of IR.

Collimation: Adjust to 14 × 17 inches (35 × 43 cm) on the collimator.

Patient instruction: Stop breathing. Do not move.

Structures seen: Entire pelvis and proximal portion of femurs (Fig. 14-77).

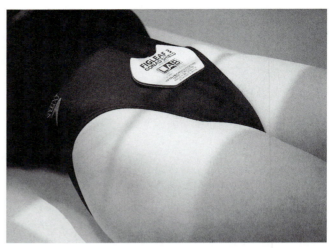

Fig. 14-75 Pelvis. Position for AP projection. (NOTE: A gonad shield is not used unless hips are of primary interest.)

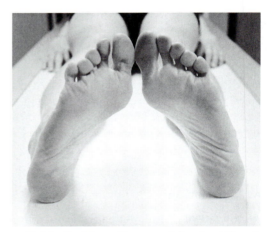

Fig. 14-76 Pelvis. Position of knees and feet for AP projection.

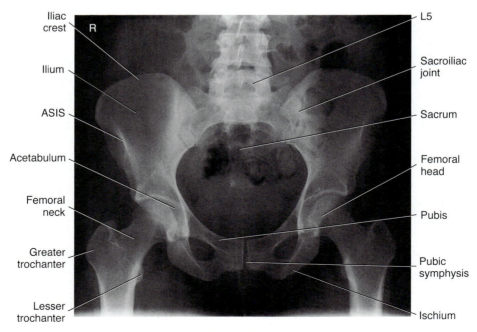

Fig. 14-77 Pelvis. AP projection.

Hip

When there has been recent trauma to the hip with a possibility of hip fracture, it is usual for the examination to begin with an AP projection of the entire pelvis. *Do not move the affected leg, regardless of its position,* until a physician has checked the pelvis image. If a lateral projection is needed in cases of recent hip fracture, an axiolateral projection is done without moving the affected leg.

Routine hip examinations are commonly performed as follow-up studies after treatment for hip fracture or for evaluation of chronic hip complaints.

Fig. 14-78 illustrates a method to locate the hip joint, the long axis of the femoral neck, and the centering point for hip radiographs. The midpoint of an imaginary line between the ASIS and the pubic symphysis marks the superior margin of the acetabulum. This area must be included in examinations of the proximal femur and in all hip studies. When a perpendicular line is drawn inferior to the center of this line, forming a T, this second line will indicate the long axis of the femoral neck. The center of the femoral neck is approximately 2.5 inches inferior to the junction and is the centering point for radiographic examinations of the hip.

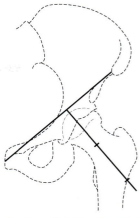

Fig. 14-78 Hip localization. Palpate the anterior superior iliac spine (ASIS) and the pubic symphysis. A line between these two points forms the crossbar of a T with the dome of the acetabulum at its center. The leg of the T is perpendicular to the crossbar and indicates the axis of the femoral neck. The midpoint of the femoral neck is the center point for hip radiographs. It is located along the leg of the T, approximately 2.5 inches inferior to its junction with the crossbar.

Routine Examination

The routine examination of the hip includes the AP and lateral projections.

IR: 10 × 12 inches (24 × 30 cm)

Grid: Yes

SID: 40 inches minimum

Body position: Supine on table.

Part position:

AP: Femur is medially rotated 15 degrees as for pelvis (Fig. 14-79).

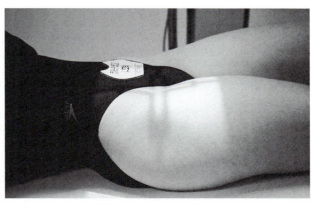

Fig. 14-79 Hip. Position for AP projection.

Lateral ("frog-leg" position): Hip is flexed as much as possible and femur abducted 45 degrees. If patient cannot abduct femur sufficiently from supine position, pelvis may be rotated toward affected side (Fig. 14-81).

Central ray: Perpendicular to midfemoral neck.

Collimation: Adjust to 10 × 12 inches (24 × 30 cm) on the collimator.

Patient instruction: Do not move.

Structures seen: Proximal fourth of femur, acetabulum, and portion of pelvis surrounding acetabulum (Figs. 14-80 and 14-82).

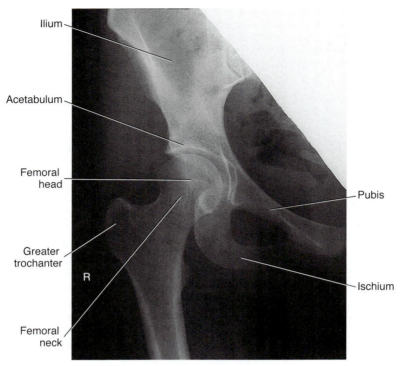

Ilium

Acetabulum

Femoral
head

Pubis

Greater
trochanter

R

Ischium

Femoral
neck

Fig. 14-80 Hip. AP projection.

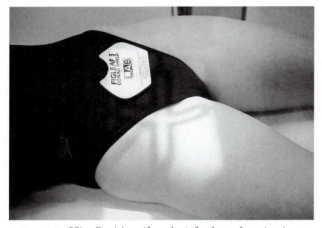

Fig. 14-81 Hip. Position (frog-leg) for lateral projection.

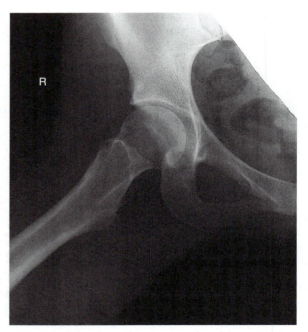

R

Fig. 14-82 Hip. Lateral projection (frog-leg position).

Alternative Lateral Projection

When a lateral projection is needed in cases of known or suspected recent hip fracture, the axiolateral projection (Danelius-Miller method), also called the *cross-table lateral* or *surgical lateral projection*, is substituted for the frog-leg lateral projection. This radiograph is taken without moving or rotating the affected leg.

IR: 10 × 12 inches (24 × 30 cm) crosswise

Grid: Yes

SID: 40 inches minimum

Body position: Supine on table.

Part position: The hip and knee of the unaffected limb are flexed 90 degrees and supported above the table. A 10 × 12 inch grid cassette is used or a stationary grid is attached to a 24 × 30 cm IR. The IR is oriented vertically and crosswise, angled parallel to the long axis of the femoral neck, and the medial margin of the IR is placed solidly into the soft tissue just proximal to the iliac crest (Fig. 14-83).

Central ray: Horizontal and perpendicular to the center of the IR, entering through the patient's groin.

Collimation: Adjust to 10 × 12 inches (24 × 30 cm) on the collimator.

Patient instruction: Do not move.

Structures seen: Proximal fourth of femur, acetabulum, and portion of pelvis surrounding acetabulum (Fig. 14-84).

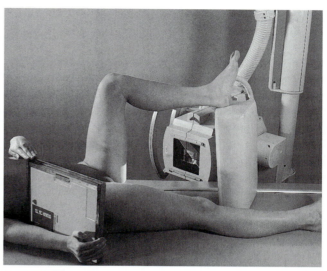

Fig. 14-83 Hip. Position for axiolateral projection (Danelius-Miller method). Also called a *cross-table lateral* or *surgical lateral projection*.

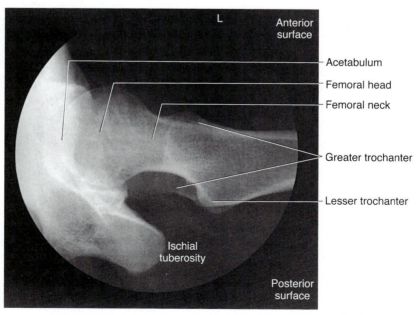

Fig. 14-84 Hip. Axiolateral projection (Danelius-Miller method).

PATHOLOGY

Probably the most significant pathology affecting the lower limb from the radiographer's viewpoint is trauma. Fractures and other conditions affecting this portion of the anatomy may vary greatly, and only those most commonly seen in radiography are discussed here.

Common Fractures

Stress fractures are most commonly seen in the feet, the result of stress to a bone from repeated injuries that would not cause fractures if they occurred only once. Stress fractures of long bones are usually simple, nondisplaced fractures (Fig. 14-85). They are common in the metatarsals and in the calcaneus as a result of running, jogging, or marching. They also occur in the tibia, fibula, femoral shaft, femoral neck, ischium, and pubis.

Sufficient force to cause a fracture of the tibia places a great strain on the fibula, often resulting in a fibular fracture as well. The associated fibular fracture may be in the same general region as the tibial fracture. One example is the bimalleolar fracture (Fig. 14-86). On the other hand, a distal tibia fracture may be associated with a fracture of the fibula at its weakest point, the proximal shaft, just distal to the head. When the shaft of the tibia is fractured with a twisting injury (common among skiers), the result is often a spiral fracture (Fig. 14-87).

Knee fractures in healthy individuals are relatively uncommon because the bones of the knee are very strong. When excessive force is applied to the knee joint, the result is more likely an injury to the meniscus cartilage and/or to one or more of the ligaments that connect the tibia to the femur. These soft tissue injuries are not visible on routine radiographs. Special imaging techniques, such as arthrography (joint studies involving injection of contrast media into the joint capsule) and magnetic resonance imaging studies, are used to evaluate soft tissue injuries to the knee.

The common fractures of the femur occur in the shaft, the neck, or the intertrochanteric region (between the trochanters). Fractures of the proximal femur (head, neck, and intertrochanteric region) are generally referred to as *hip fractures* (Fig. 14-88). Hip fractures associated

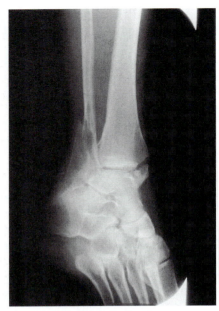

Fig. 14-86 Bimalleolar fracture.

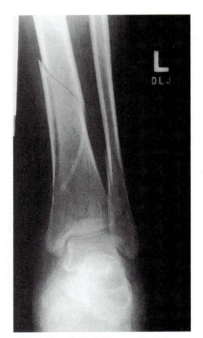

Fig. 14-87 Spiral fracture of tibia.

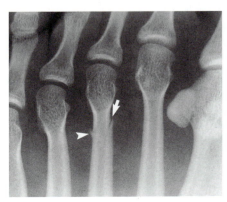

Fig. 14-85 Stress fracture of third metatarsal *(arrows)*.

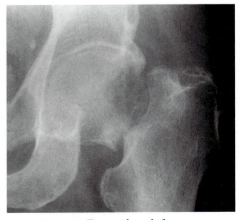

Fig. 14-88 Femoral neck fracture.

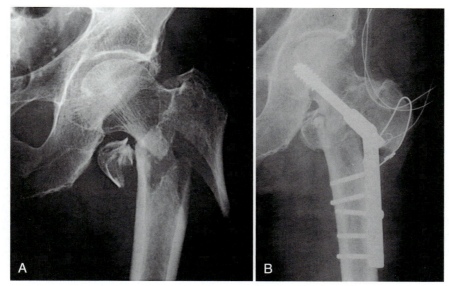

Fig. 14-89 A, Intertrochanteric hip fracture. **B,** Internal fixation of intertrochanteric fracture.

with weakened bone from osteoporosis are common among the elderly, particularly women. Most fractures of the femur are treated by means of internal fixation, surgical application of hardware to hold the bones in place. Fig. 14-89 shows internal fixation of an intertrochanteric hip fracture. When there is severe degeneration of the hip joint, the treatment may be a total hip replacement (Fig. 14-90). In Fig. 14-90, the **prostheses** (anatomic replacements) for both the femoral head and the acetabulum are made of metal. It is not uncommon, however, for the acetabulum prosthesis to be made of a plastic material. Because the plastic is not visible on a radiograph, a radiopaque wire is embedded in its rim.

Because the pelvis as a whole is a rigid ringlike structure, fractures of the pelvis often occur in pairs. The reason for this is apparent if you consider how unlikely it would be to break a Life Savers candy in only one place. The stress that causes one fracture creates an opposing stress, and two fractures result.

Nontraumatic Conditions

As previously mentioned, arthritis may affect any joint of the body, and there are a number of different types. Rheumatoid arthritis, discussed in Chapters 12 and 13, may also affect the joints of the feet. Gouty arthritis is a

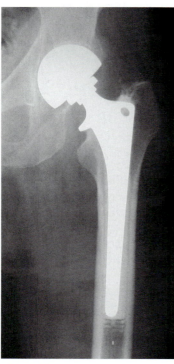

Fig. 14-90 Total hip replacement.

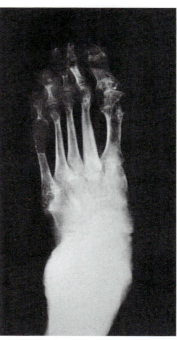

Fig. 14-91 Gout affecting the foot, particularly the great toe and first metatarsal.

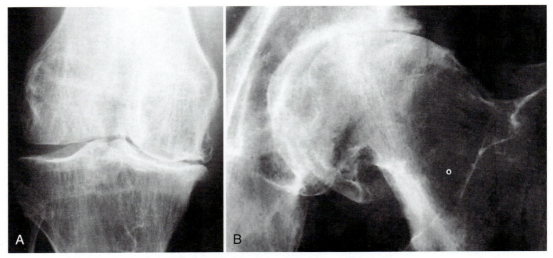

Fig. 14-92 Osteoarthritis. **A,** Knee. **B,** Hip.

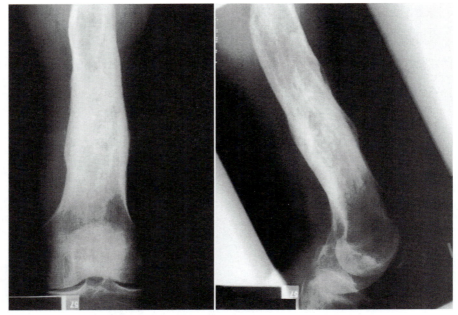

Fig. 14-93 Healed osteomyelitis of distal femur.

joint condition caused by gout, a systemic disorder that increases the uric acid content of the blood. Gouty arthritis commonly affects the feet, particularly the joints of the great toe (Fig. 14-91), although it may also involve the hands. Osteoarthritis may cause degeneration of any of the joints of the lower limb but is most common in the knee and the hip (Fig. 14-92). This condition is often associated with osteoporosis. Note the irregular contours of the articular surfaces and the bony hypertrophy at the margins of the joints.

Osteomyelitis, as introduced in Chapter 13, is an infection of the bone. In the acute phase of the disease, there is bony destruction. With healing, however, there is considerable new bone formation (Fig. 14-93).

Neoplastic and metastatic bone diseases may also affect the bones of the lower limb. Fig. 14-94 is an example of osteogenic sarcoma, one of several types of malignant bone tumors that occur in the lower limb. The typical lesions of osteogenic sarcoma occur in the distal ends of long bones and are both destructive and sclerotic (thickened and hardened). They are associated with a tumor mass within the soft tissues. The bony spicules (needle-like formations) that extend into the soft tissue mass create the classic sunburst pattern of this disease. Fig. 14-95 shows osteoblastic metastases of the pelvis and proximal femurs, secondary to carcinoma of the urinary bladder.

SUMMARY

The bones of the foot include the phalanges, metatarsals, and tarsals. The tibia and fibula form the lower leg,

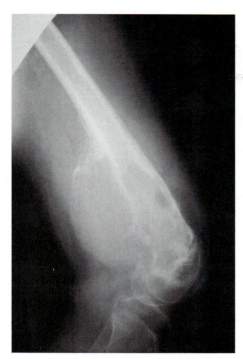

Fig. 14-94 Osteogenic sarcoma of the distal femur.

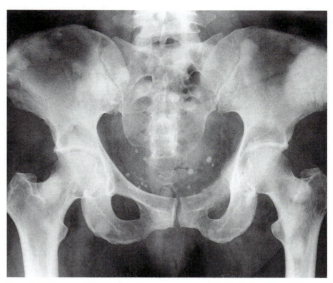

Fig. 14-95 Osteoblastic metastatic lesions of the pelvis and proximal femurs.

articulating at the ankle with the talus. The femur articulates with the tibia at the knee, and it forms the hip joint where it articulates with the innominate bone at the acetabulum. The two hip bones—each consisting of ilium, ischium, and pubis—form the pelvis. Important palpable bony prominences of the lower limb include the medial and lateral malleoli of the ankle, the condyles and greater trochanter of the femur, the iliac crest, the ASIS, and the pubic symphysis.

Radiography of the foot, heel, and ankle is done on the tabletop, without a grid. The patient is seated or recumbent on the radiographic table. Multiple projections are often done on a single IR. Examinations of the femur and pelvis, on the other hand, are done using grids or Buckys with the patient recumbent. Radiography of the knee may be done either with or without a grid.

The most common radiographic pathology occurring in this portion of the anatomy involves trauma, particularly fractures. Nontraumatic conditions, such as arthritis, osteomyelitis, and neoplastic disease, are also seen.

Chapter 15

Spine

Learning Objectives

At the conclusion of this chapter, you will be able to:

- Name the regions that make up the spine and identify each on an anatomic diagram and on a radiograph
- Identify on a diagram the parts of a typical vertebra
- Identify significant positioning landmarks for the spine by palpation
- Demonstrate correct body and part positioning for routine projections and common special projections of the spine
- Correctly evaluate radiographs of the spine for positioning accuracy
- Describe and recognize on radiographs abnormalities and pathology common to the spine

Key Terms

atlas
axis
cervical spine
coccyx
dens
facets
intervertebral disks
kyphosis
kyphotic curve
lamina (pl. laminae)
lordosis
lordotic curve
lumbar spine
pedicles
sacrum
scoliosis
stenosis
thoracic spine
vertebra (pl. vertebrae)

Most radiography of the spine may be accomplished successfully in either the upright or the recumbent position. In medical practices and hospitals, radiography of the spine is done in both the recumbent and upright positions. In chiropractic practices, spine radiography is almost always done in the upright position. This chapter provides instruction and illustration for both methods.

ANATOMY

The spine (Fig. 15-1) is the central portion of the skeletal system. It provides the supporting framework for the body. It also surrounds and protects the spinal cord. The spine is called the *vertebral column* because it is made up of many irregularly shaped bones known as **vertebrae.** The spine is divided into five regions: cervical spine, thoracic spine, lumbar spine, sacrum, and coccyx. The vertebrae are named according to spinal region and are numbered from the top down. For example, the third vertebra from the top of the thoracic region is simply called the *third thoracic vertebra*, abbreviated T3.

When viewed from the front, the normal spinal column is relatively straight. When seen from the side, however, the spine has four curves (Fig. 15-2). It arches anteriorly and posteriorly to provide a springlike flexibility that absorbs shock as we walk and run. A curvature that is convex (bowing outward) anteriorly is called a **lordotic curve,** or **lordosis.** One that is convex posteriorly is called a **kyphotic curve,** or **kyphosis.** An abnormal lateral curvature

is called **scoliosis** and results from rotation o and/or kyphotic curve (Fig. 15-3).

A typical vertebra is illustrated in Fig. 1 blocklike anterior portion is called the *body.* It co cancellous bone with a thin cortex. Posterior to th is a ring of bone called the *vertebral arch.* It is forn the **pedicles,** which attach to the body on either sid by the **laminae** posteriorly. The hole in the ring is called the *vertebral foramen.* It is the passage for the spinal cord.

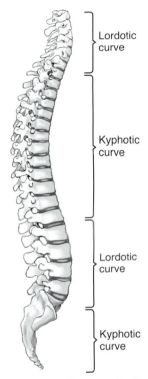

Fig. 15-2 Lateral aspect of spine.

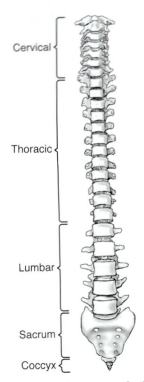

Fig. 15-1 Anterior aspect of spine.

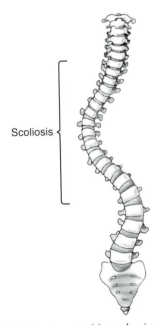

Fig. 15-3 Scoliosis: abnormal lateral spine curvature.

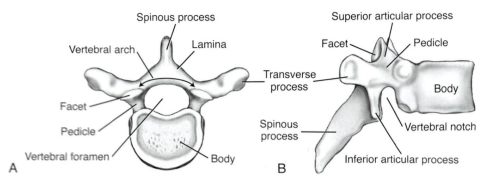

Fig. 15-4 Typical vertebra. **A,** Superior aspect. **B,** Lateral aspect.

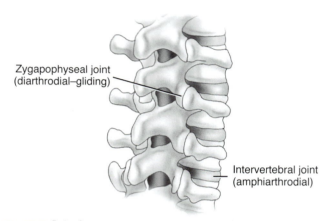

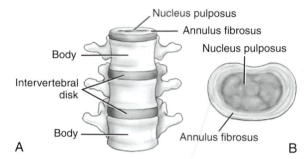

Fig. 15-6 Intervertebral disk. **A,** Anterior aspect. **B,** Superior aspect.

Fig. 15-5 Spinal joints. Intervertebral joints are between the bodies anteriorly, and zygapophyseal joints are between the articular processes posteriorly.

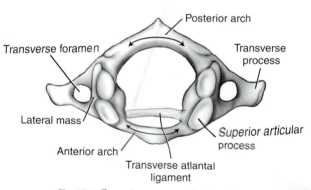

Fig. 15-7 Superior aspect of atlas (C1).

The concave superior and inferior surfaces of the pedicles are called *vertebral notches.* The spaces formed by joining with the vertebral notches above and below are the *intervertebral foramina,* which allow passage of spinal nerves and blood vessels. Two projections, extending laterally from the junction of the pedicles and lamina, are called the *transverse processes.* The spinous process projects posteriorly and inferiorly from the junction of the lamina. Four articular processes extend superiorly and inferiorly from the junction of the pedicles and lamina. The articular surfaces of these processes are called **facets.** They articulate with facets on the articular processes of the vertebrae above and below, forming the zygapophyseal joints. The zygapophyseal joints are diarthrodial joints of the gliding type. Fig. 15-5 illustrates typical joints of the spine.

The vertebrae are cushioned anteriorly, between the bodies, by pads of fibrocartilage called **intervertebral disks** (Fig. 15-6). These disks have a tough outer covering, the annulus fibrosus, and a soft, pulpy center called the *nucleus pulposus.*

Cervical Spine

The **cervical spine** is the most superior region of the vertebral column. It supports the head and the structures of the neck. The cervical spine consists of seven vertebrae and has a lordotic curve.

The first two cervical vertebrae differ in form from the others to accommodate the support and rotation of the skull. The first cervical vertebra (C1) is called the **atl** (Fig. 15-7). It is a ringlike structure with no verteb body and a very short spinous process called the *poste tubercle.* The atlas consists of two lateral masses nected by an anterior arch and a posterior arch. lateral mass has superior and inferior articular proc The superior articular processes articulate with th of the skull, and the inferior ones form joints with processes on the superior aspect of the second vertebra (C2). The transverse processes project and slightly downward from the lateral masse

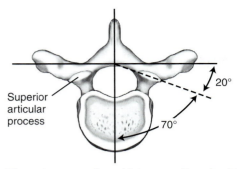

Fig. 15-13 Thoracic zygapophyseal joints are aligned at 70 degrees to the sagittal plane and are seen in oblique projections.

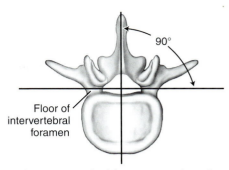

Fig. 15-16 Lumbar intervertebral foramina are aligned at 90 degrees to the sagittal plane and are seen in lateral projection.

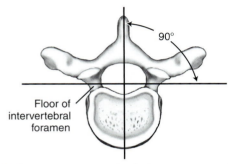

Fig. 15-14 Thoracic intervertebral foramina are aligned at 90 degrees to the sagittal plane and are seen in lateral projection.

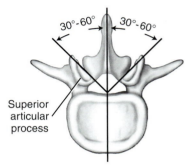

Fig. 15-17 Lumbar zygapophyseal joints are oriented 30 to 60 degrees to the sagittal plane and are seen in oblique projections.

Sacrum and Coccyx

At birth, the **sacrum** consists of five sacral vertebrae. In the adult, they are fused into a solid bony structure (Fig. 15-19). The sacrum articulates with the ilia of the pelvis on either side, forming the sacroiliac joints. Its broad, flat superior surface is called the *sacral base*. The lateral portions of the first sacral segment are winglike structures called the *alae*. The four pairs of sacral foramina are passages for nerves.

The **coccyx,** the most inferior portion of the spine, is approximately the size of the fifth finger. In lay terms, it is called the *tailbone*. The coccyx usually consists of four small vertebral segments, but it is not unusual for there to be three or five segments. The coccygeal segments tend to fuse in the adult. Two small bony projections extend superiorly from the posterior aspect on each side of the first coccygeal segment. These are called the *coccygeal cornua* (singular *cornu*, which means "horn"). They are joined to similar projections from the posterior inferior aspect of the sacrum, called the *sacral cornua*.

Together the sacrum and coccyx form a kyphotic curve. This curvature is more pronounced in females than in males. The sacral base slopes downward anteriorly, and the degree of slope is called the *sacral base angle*. This angle is greatest in females. It is greater when standing than when recumbent and is least when supine with the knees flexed. Average sacral base angles for males and females are listed in Table 15-1.

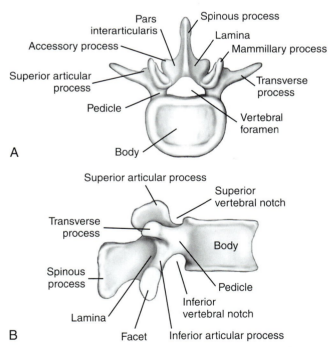

Fig. 15-15 Lumbar vertebra. **A,** Superior aspect. **B,** Lateral aspect.

When radiographed in the oblique projection, the lumbar vertebrae demonstrate a configuration that resembles a Scottie dog (Fig. 15-18). The superior articular processes form the ears of the dog, and the inferior articular process forms the front legs. The pars interarticularis corresponds to the dog's neck.

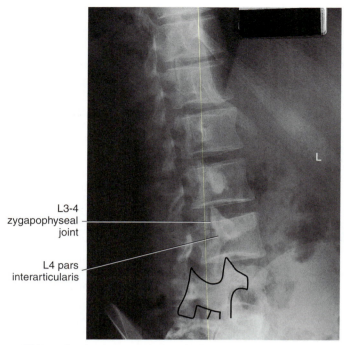

Fig. 15-18 Oblique lumbar spine radiograph showing Scottie dog configuration.

L3-4 zygapophyseal joint

L4 pars interarticularis

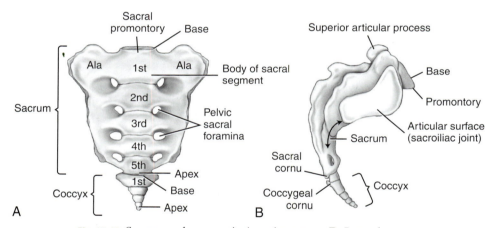

Fig. 15-19 Sacrum and coccyx. **A,** Anterior aspect. **B,** Lateral aspect.

Sacral promontory
Base
Ala   1st   Ala
Body of sacral segment
2nd
Sacrum
3rd
Pelvic sacral foramina
4th
5th
1st   Apex
Base
Coccyx
Apex
A

Superior articular process
Base
Promontory
Articular surface (sacroiliac joint)
Sacrum
Sacral cornu
Coccyx
Coccygeal cornu
B

Table 15-1

Average Sacral Base Angulation

Body Position	Sacral Base Angle in Males	Sacral Base Angle in Females
Standing	35 degrees	40 degrees
Supine with legs extended	30 degrees	35 degrees
Supine with knees fixed	25 degrees	30 degrees

POSITIONING AND RADIOGRAPHIC EXAMINATIONS

Many landmarks are used in positioning and alignment for various aspects of spine radiography. Fig. 15-20 illustrates the landmarks of the cranium and face that are helpful for radiography of the cervical spine. Fig. 15-21 shows the topographic anatomy that corresponds to specific vertebral levels of the spine. Memorizing these locations will enhance your ability to position patients accurately.

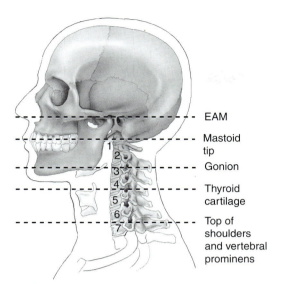

Fig. 15-20 Palpable landmarks for cervical spine positioning. *EAM,* External auditory meatus.

"Coned-down" radiographs, historically called *spot films,* may be requested for better visualization of specific areas of the spine. As discussed in Chapter 9, the use of a small radiation field, centered on the area of clinical interest, improves contrast while minimizing the negative effects of distortion and parallax. The most common areas for coned-down radiography are the upper cervical spine (C1 and C2) and the lumbosacral junction, but it may be helpful in any area of the spine. The limited operator must be able to correctly identify the location of any vertebra when a coned-down radiograph is necessary. When taking a closely collimated image of a vertebra that does not have a precise palpable landmark, it is helpful to have reference from routine radiographs. The limited operator can measure the distance from a palpable landmark to the vertebra of clinical interest on the radiograph and use this information to center properly.

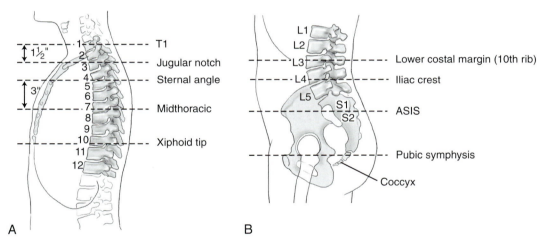

Fig. 15-21 Palpable landmarks for spine positioning. **A,** Thoracic region. **B,** Lumbar region. *ASIS,* Anterior superior iliac spine.

Cervical Spine

Two films are necessary to demonstrate the entire cervical spine in the AP projection. The AP axial projection of the lower cervical spine demonstrates C3 through C7, but the lower jaw and the teeth are superimposed over the atlas and axis. To demonstrate the upper cervical vertebrae, a second AP projection is taken through the open mouth. This projection is sometimes referred to as the *AP open-mouth* or the *odontoid* projection.

For the lateral projection, the inferior margin of the image receptor (IR) must be below the level of the upper surface of the shoulder to demonstrate all of C7. This results in a large object–image receptor distance (OID) between the neck and the IR. To minimize magnification and improve detail on this projection, a 72-inch source–image receptor distance (SID) is used. Detail is also enhanced by the use of the small focal spot.

Before undergoing cervical spine radiography, the patient must remove eyeglasses, earrings, hairpins, necklaces, and any clothing that has fasteners that might fall within the radiation field. Dentures and hearing aids should also be removed.

Routine Examination

The routine examination of the cervical spine includes the AP axial (lower cervical), AP (upper cervical), and lateral projections.

AP Axial Projection (Lower Cervical Spine)

IR: 8 × 10 inches (18 × 24 cm) lengthwise

Grid: Yes

SID: 40 inches minimum

Body position: Seated, standing, or supine.

Part position: Midsagittal plane of both body and head are aligned perpendicular to center of IR, with patient facing tube. Head position is adjusted so that a line between mental point and base of skull makes an angle of 15 degrees with horizontal plane (Fig. 15-22). When patient is recumbent, patient's head rests on table (Fig. 15-23). Head is placed firmly against IR holder when upright. If desired position cannot be attained in this way, a radiolucent wedge sponge is placed under/behind head for stability.

> **TIP:**   The upper margin of the collimator light field will fall across the patient's face at an angle of 15 degrees, which simplifies the adjustment of the head position.

Central ray: Centered with regard to IR at an angle of 15 degrees cephalad through thyroid cartilage.

Collimation: Adjust to 10 inches (25 cm) lengthwise and 1 inch (2.5 cm) beyond skin shadows on the sides.

Patient instruction: Stop breathing. Do not move.

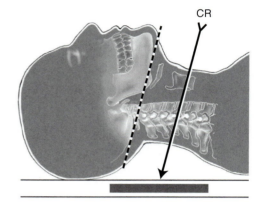

Fig. 15-22 Head position for AP axial projection of lower cervical spine. Chin is projected over base of skull. Angled x-ray beam is parallel to cervical disk spaces. *CR,* Central ray.

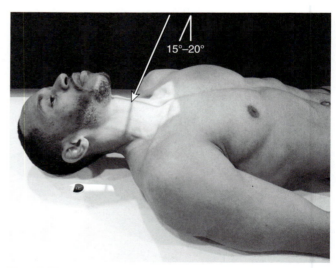

Fig. 15-23 Cervical spine (lower). Position for AP axial projection.

Structures seen: Vertebrae C3 through T2, including bodies, articular pillars, and intervertebral disk spaces (Fig. 15-24).

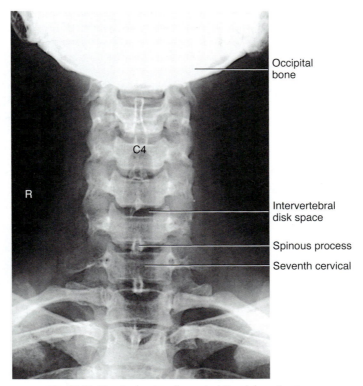

Occipital bone

C4

R

Intervertebral disk space

Spinous process

Seventh cervical

Fig. 15-24 Cervical spine (lower). AP axial projection.

AP Projection/Open Mouth Technique (Upper Cervical Spine)

IR: 8 × 10 inches (18 × 24 cm) lengthwise

Grid: Yes

SID: 40 inches minimum (30 inches may be used to increase the odontoid area field of view)

Body position: Seated, standing, or supine.

Part position: Patient faces tube with midsagittal plane of both body and head perpendicular to center of IR. Position of head is adjusted so that a line between lower surface of upper teeth (occlusal plane) and base of skull is parallel to horizontal plane (Figs. 15-25 and 15-26). When patient is upright, patient's head is placed firmly against IR holder or a radiolucent wedge sponge for stability.

Central ray: Perpendicular to center of IR, through midpoint of open mouth.

Collimation: Adjust to 5 × 5 inches (13 × 13 cm) on the collimator. Close collimation improves image quality and prevents unnecessary exposure to thyroid gland and eyes.

Patient instruction: Open mouth as wide as possible. Stop breathing. Do not move.

> **TIP:**   If the patient has closed the mouth following positioning and must reopen it before the exposure, it is wise to instruct the patient to "drop the lower jaw" as far as possible. When instructed to "open wide," patients may tend to extend the neck, which causes incorrect position of the head.

Structures seen: Lateral masses and transverse processes of atlas, dens, and upper half of body of axis, seen between upper and lower teeth (Fig. 15-27).

> **TIP:**   If the base of the skull is superimposed on the atlas and the dens, then the patient's neck was extended too far. If the upper teeth are superimposed on the atlas and the dens, then the patient's neck was flexed too much. If the lower teeth are superimposed on the upper half of the axis and the base of the skull is in the proper position, the patient's mouth was not open far enough.

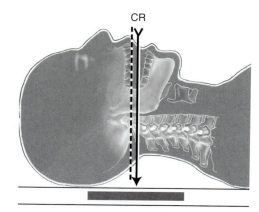

Fig. 15-25 Head position for AP projection of upper cervical spine. With mouth wide open, upper teeth are projected over base of skull, with atlas and axis projected between upper and lower teeth. *CR*, Central ray.

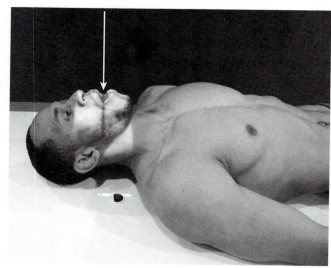

Fig. 15-26 Cervical spine (upper). Position for AP projection—open mouth technique.

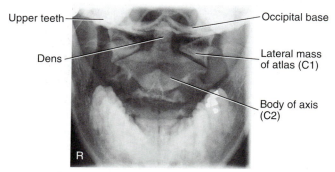

Fig. 15-27 Cervical spine (upper). AP projection—open mouth technique.

Lateral Projection (Grandy Method)

IR: 8 × 10 inches (18 × 24 cm) lengthwise

Grid: Yes

SID: 60 to 72 inches (152 to 183 cm) is recommended because of the increased OID

Body position: Seated or standing.

Part position: Midsagittal planes of body and head are parallel to IR with infraorbitomeatal line parallel to floor. Shoulders must be relaxed and depressed. IR is positioned so that upper margin is about 1 inch above the external auditory meatus (EAM) (Fig. 15-28).

> **TIP:** Patients with high, square shoulders may need to have sandbags of equal weight suspended from the wrists to place the shoulders below C7 (see Fig. 13-104). Alternatively, patient may stand on the center of a long strap, grasping the two ends to maintain downward tension on the shoulders.

Central ray: Perpendicular to center of IR through body of C4.

> **TIP:** Place your finger on the tip of the C7 spinous process and note the location of its shadow in the collimator light beam. It should be within the posterior margin of the IR and at least 2 inches above its inferior margin.

Collimation: Adjust to 8 × 10 inches (18 × 24 cm) on the collimator. Eyes should be excluded from field.

Patient instruction: Stop breathing. Do not move.

> **TIP:** Do *not* instruct patient to "take a deep breath" because doing so tends to elevate the shoulders.

Structures seen: All seven cervical vertebrae and soft tissues of anterior neck, including spinal alignment, bodies, disk spaces, spinous processes, and zygapophyseal joints (Fig. 15-29).

> **NOTE:** When a good effort has been made to lower the shoulders for the lateral cervical spine projection but the radiograph fails to demonstrate C7, it is necessary to supplement the examination with the lateral projection of the cervicothoracic region, described later in this chapter.

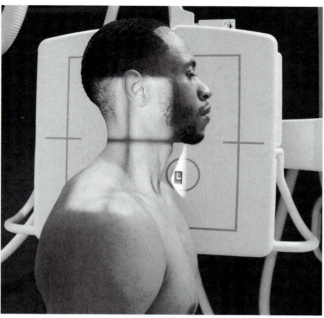

Fig. 15-28 Cervical spine. Position for lateral projection.

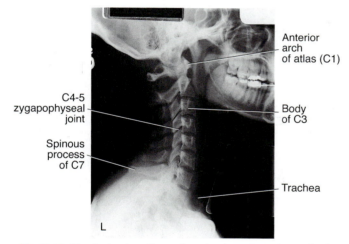

Fig. 15-29 Cervical spine. Lateral projection, Grandy method.

Supplemental Projections

Lateral Projection in Flexion and Extension

Lateral projections with the cervical spine in flexion and extension are performed to evaluate intersegmental stability.

> **NOTE:** When there has been recent trauma to the cervical spine, the lateral projection in the dorsal decubitus position should be evaluated by the physician before proceeding with flexion and extension lateral projections.

IR: 10 × 12 inches (24 × 30 cm) lengthwise

Grid: Yes

SID: 60 to 72 inches (152 to 183 cm) is recommended because of the increased OID

Position for flexion: Patient is positioned as for routine lateral projection. Patient is then instructed first to "tuck" chin close to neck and then to flex neck, attempting to look at a spot at midsternum (Fig. 15-30).

Position for extension: Patient is positioned as for routine lateral projection. Patient is then instructed to extend neck, looking at a spot on ceiling directly above head (Fig. 15-31).

> **NOTE:** *The radiographer must not force these positions. The desired degree of flexion or extension is the fullest extent that is tolerable for the patient.*

Central ray: Perpendicular to center of IR, through body of C4.

Collimation: Adjust to 10 × 12 inches (24 × 30 cm) on the collimator.

Patient instruction: Stop breathing. Do not move.

Structures seen: All seven cervical vertebrae and soft tissues of anterior neck, including spinal alignment, bodies, disk spaces, spinous processes, and zygapophyseal joints. Head tilted face down in flexion (Fig. 15-32) and tilted face up in extension (Fig. 15-33).

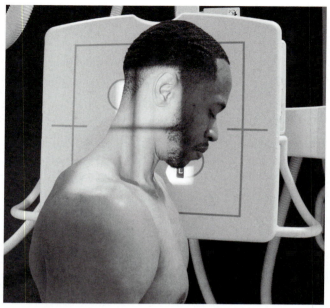

Fig. 15-30 Cervical spine. Position for lateral projection in flexion.

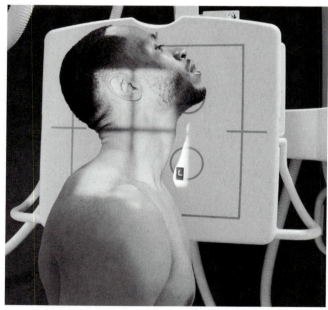

Fig. 15-31 Cervical spine. Position for lateral projection in extension.

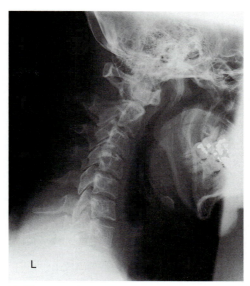

Fig. 15-32 Cervical spine. Lateral projection in flexion.

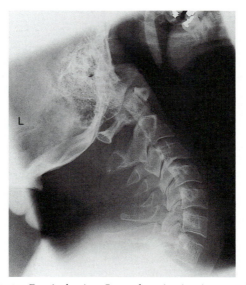

Fig. 15-33 Cervical spine. Lateral projection in extension.

Oblique Projections

Oblique projections are taken in left/right pairs. They may be done in a posteroanterior (PA) projection (right anterior oblique [RAO] and left anterior oblique [LAO] positions) or AP projection (right posterior oblique [RPO] and left posterior oblique [LPO] positions). They may be done recumbent, with a 40-inch SID, or upright, with either a 40-inch or a 72-inch SID. The available equipment and the preferences of the physician may dictate both the method and the positions used.

IR: 8 × 10 inches (18 × 24 cm) lengthwise

Grid: Yes

SID: 60 to 72 inches (152 to 183 cm) is recommended because of the increased OID

Body position: Seated, standing, or recumbent.

Part position: Coronal plane of body forms angle of 45 degrees with plane of IR. Sagittal plane of skull is perpendicular to coronal plane of body. Have patient elevate and, if necessary, protrude the chin so that mandible does not overlap spine.

Central ray:

AP obliques: Angled 15 degrees cephalad to center of IR through body of C4 (Figs. 15-34 and 15-35).

PA obliques: Angled 15 degrees caudad to center of IR through body of C4 (Figs. 15-37 and 15-38).

Collimation: Adjust to 8 × 10 inches (18 × 24 cm) on the collimator. Eyes should be excluded from field.

Patient instruction: Stop breathing. Do not move.

Structures seen: AP obliques demonstrate intervertebral foramina on side farthest from IR (Fig. 15-36). PA obliques demonstrate intervertebral foramina on side nearest IR (Fig. 15-39).

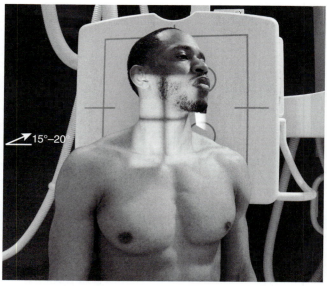

Fig. 15-34 Cervical spine. Position for AP axial oblique projection, patient upright.

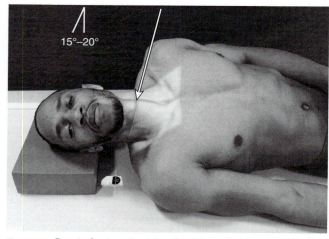

Fig. 15-35 Cervical spine. Position for AP axial oblique projection, patient recumbent.

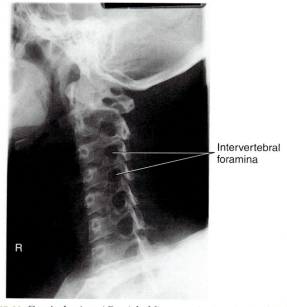

Intervertebral foramina

Fig. 15-36 Cervical spine. AP axial oblique projection (40-inch SID).

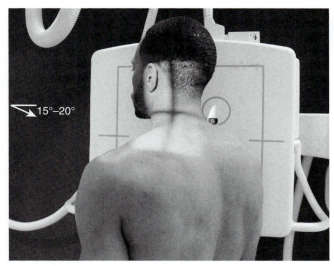

Fig. 15-37 Cervical spine. Position for PA axial oblique projection, patient upright.

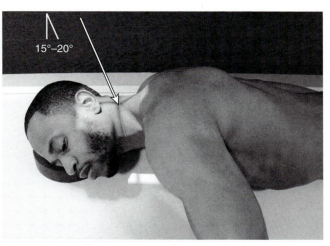

Fig. 15-38 Cervical spine. Position for PA axial oblique projection, patient recumbent.

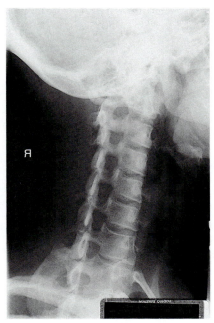

Fig. 15-39 Cervical spine. PA axial oblique projection (72-inch SID).

Lateral Projection of Cervicothoracic Region

The lateral projection of the cervicothoracic region is commonly called the *swimmer's technique*. It is used when routine lateral projections of either the cervical or the thoracic spine fail to demonstrate this area adequately. The shoulder positions create a small "window" between the shoulders, and the cervicothoracic spine is projected into this relatively open area.

IR: 10 × 12 inches (24 × 30 cm) lengthwise

Grid: Yes

SID: 40 inches minimum

Body position: Seated, standing, or recumbent.

Part position: Sagittal planes of body and head are parallel to IR. Arm nearest IR is raised above head and shoulder is rounded anteriorly. Opposite shoulder is depressed and slightly posterior (Figs. 15-40 and 15-41).

Central ray: Perpendicular to IR at C7-T1 interspace. Central ray enters at base of neck in midcoronal plane at level of C7 spinous process.

Collimation: Adjust to 10 × 12 inches (24 × 30 cm) on the collimator.

Patient instruction: Stop breathing. Do not move.

Structures seen: Vertebrae C6 through T3 (C5 through T5 with larger IR) in lateral projection without significant rotation. Bodies, disk spaces, spinous processes, and zygapophyseal joints are demonstrated between shoulders (Fig. 15-42).

> **TIP:** Take care when positioning the arms so that the midsagittal plane of the body remains parallel to the IR. The most common error associated with this position is rotation of the body so that the spine is oblique rather than lateral.

Compensating Filter: This projection will be improved with the use of a compensating filter because of the extreme difference between the thin lower neck and the very thick upper thoracic region. With the use of a specially designed filter, the C7-T1 area can be more clearly seen.

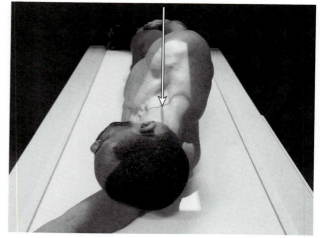

Fig. 15-40 Cervicothoracic region. Position for swimmer's lateral projection, patient recumbent.

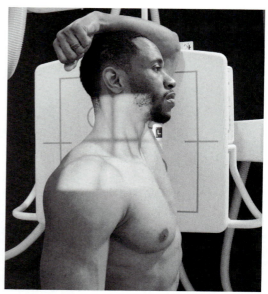

Fig. 15-41 Cervicothoracic region. Position for swimmer's lateral projection, patient upright.

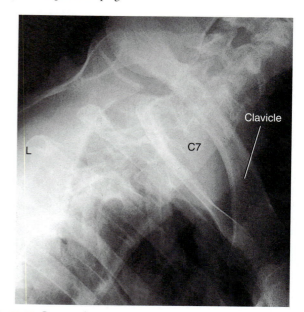

Fig. 15-42 Cervicothoracic region. Swimmer's lateral projection.

Thoracic Spine

There is significant tissue density variation between the extreme ends of the thoracic spine. Near the neck there is much less tissue to penetrate than at the level of T12 in the upper abdominal region. For this reason, it is desirable to use the anode heel effect (see Chapter 5). For recumbent studies, the patient should be instructed to lie on the table with the head toward the anode end of the x-ray tube. If use of the anode heel effect is insufficient to compensate for the extremes in tissue density, a wedge-type compensating filter may be placed in the x-ray beam so that its thick edge is over the upper thoracic spine.

In the lateral projection, the density variation is reversed. The proximal thoracic spine is more difficult to penetrate because of the bone and muscle mass of the shoulders, and there is little lung tissue in this area. The inferior portion is relatively easily penetrated because its mass is largely air-containing lung. For this reason, it may be desirable to reverse the position of the compensating filter for the lateral projection. In any case, the first three thoracic vertebrae are seldom visualized well on the lateral projection. When the area of clinical interest includes the upper thoracic vertebrae, it is usual for the examination to include a swimmer's lateral projection of the cervicothoracic region. This projection was explained and illustrated in the previous section. In some facilities, the swimmer's lateral projection is a routine part of the basic thoracic spine examination.

For this examination, the patient should undress down to the waist and don a gown that opens in the back. This will facilitate visualization and palpation of the spine. Any jewelry that would be in the radiation field should be removed. For standing examinations, the shoes should also be removed.

Routine Examination

The routine examination of the thoracic spine includes the AP and lateral projections.

AP Projection

IR: 14 × 17 inches (35 × 43 cm) lengthwise

Grid: Yes

SID: 40 inches minimum

Body position: Seated, standing, or recumbent.

Part position: Midsagittal plane of body is perpendicular to IR and centered on it, with patient facing tube. Superior border of IR is aligned 1.5 to 2 inches (3.8 to 5 cm) above the shoulders (Figs. 15-43 and 15-44). When patient is supine, it is helpful to place a bolster under knees. When patient is standing, feet should be shoulder-width apart with equal weight bearing, and patient's back should be firmly against IR holder.

Central ray: Perpendicular to center of IR at T7. This point is in midline at approximate midpoint of sternum.

Collimation: Adjust to 7 × 17 inches (18 × 43 cm) on the collimator. Close collimation improves visualization and reduces patient dose. When there is significant scoliosis, a wider field may be necessary.

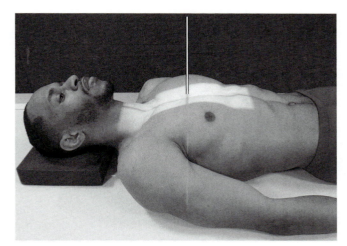

Fig. 15-43 Thoracic spine. Position for AP projection, patient recumbent.

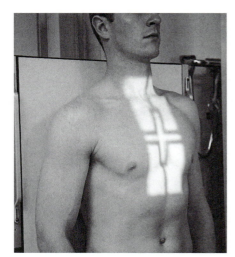

Fig. 15-44 Thoracic spine. Position for AP projection, patient upright.

Shielding: Lead half-apron.

Patient instruction: Do not move. Suspend breathing on expiration.

Structures seen: All 12 thoracic vertebrae, particularly the bodies, disk spaces, and transverse processes. C7 and at least a portion of L1 are usually also seen (Fig. 15-45).

Compensating Filter: The image quality of this projection can be improved significantly with use of a compensating filter. Various wedge filters are available to assist in providing a uniform density of the entire thoracic spine.

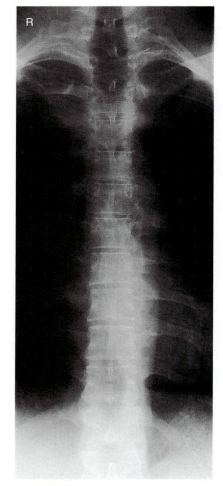

Fig. 15-45 Thoracic spine. AP projection.

Lateral Projection

IR: 14 × 17 inches (35 × 43 cm) lengthwise

Grid: Yes

SID: 40 inches minimum

Body position: Seated, standing, or recumbent.

Part position: Sagittal plane of body is parallel to IR. Center the posterior half of the thorax to the midline of the IR. Arms may be raised overhead (Fig. 15-46) or anterior to body with shoulders rounded anteriorly (Fig. 15-47). The superior border of the IR is adjusted to 1.5 to 2 inches (3.8 to 5 cm) above the shoulders. Take care that entire length of thoracic spine is parallel to IR. When patient is recumbent, this may require support of a radiolucent sponge under waist and/or hips.

Central ray: Perpendicular to center of IR at level of T7. Central ray enters at inferior angle of scapula through middle of posterior half of thorax.

Collimation: Adjust to 7 × 17 inches (18 × 43 cm) on the collimator. A wider field may be necessary if there is exaggerated thoracic kyphosis.

> **TIP:** Place a strip of lead or a lead rubber mask behind the patient so that its margin is aligned with the shadow of the patient's back in the collimator light. This absorbs backscatter and improves visualization of the spinous processes.

Patient instruction: Do not move. Perform shallow breathing during exposure.

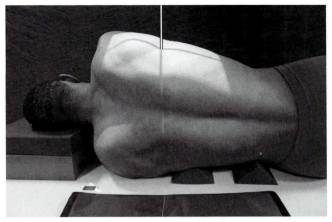

Fig. 15-46 Thoracic spine. Position for lateral projection, patient recumbent. Note the lead strip placed on table for absorption of scatter radiation.

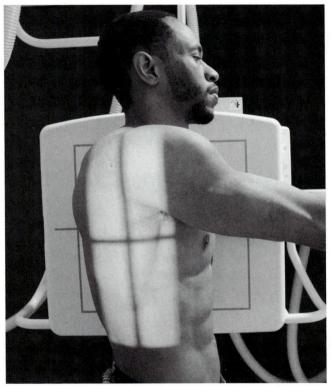

Fig. 15-47 Thoracic spine. Position for lateral projection, patient upright.

TIP: A low milliamperage (mA) setting that provides the desired milliampere-seconds (mAs) with an exposure time of 1 to 3 seconds is necessary for best results with breathing technique.

Structures seen: T3 through T12 with blurring of ribs and lung markings when breathing technique is used (Fig. 15-48).

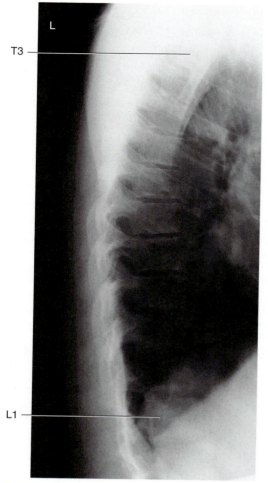

Fig. 15-48 Thoracic spine. Lateral projection. Note blurring of ribs and lung structures resulting from use of breathing technique.

Lumbar Spine

For lumbar spine radiography, patients should remove outer clothing from the torso and don a gown opening in the back. Female patients must remove bras. For upright studies, shoes are also removed.

Routine Examination

The routine examination of the lumbar spine includes the AP or PA and lateral projections.

AP or PA Projection

IR: 14 × 17 inches (35 × 43 cm) lengthwise

Grid: Yes

SID: 40 inches minimum

Body position: Standing or recumbent.

Part position:

AP: Patient faces tube with midsagittal plane perpendicular to IR and centered on it (Fig. 15-49). When patient is supine, knees are flexed and may be supported with a bolster. When patient is standing, feet are shoulder-width apart with equal weight bearing, and torso is stabilized against upright IR holder (Fig. 15-50).

PA: Patient stands facing IR or lies prone, with midsagittal plane perpendicular to IR and centered on it.

Central ray: Perpendicular to center of IR through L4, in midline at level of iliac crest.

Collimation: Adjust to 8 × 17 inches (20 × 43 cm) on the collimator or to 14 × 17 inches (35 × 43 cm) when a full abdomen image is requested. Ensure sacroiliac (SI) joints are included.

Shielding: Use gonad shielding for males. Shield females only if shield will not interfere with purpose of examination. Consider PA projection for reduced ovarian dose.

Patient instruction: Do not move. Suspend breathing on expiration.

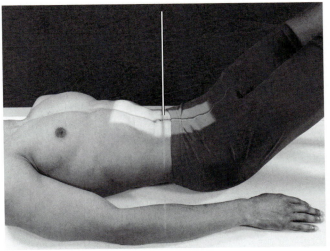

Fig. 15-49 Lumbar spine. Position for AP projection, patient recumbent. Note close collimation, which improves image quality and reduces patient exposure.

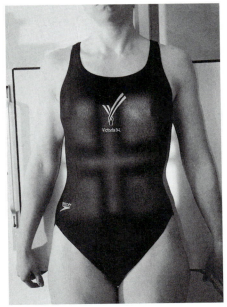

Fig. 15-50 Lumbar spine. Position for AP projection, patient upright. Note wide collimation to include entire abdomen.

Structures seen: All five lumbar vertebrae, intervertebral disk spaces, proximal portion of sacrum, and sacroiliac joints. This projection demonstrates the bodies, disk spaces, and transverse processes. The pedicles are seen on end. When a 35- × 43-cm IR is used, central pelvis and hip joints may be visualized if collimation is not too close (Figs. 15-51 and 15-52). Visualization of hip joints is particularly important to demonstrate pelvic tilt when an upright AP projection is taken.

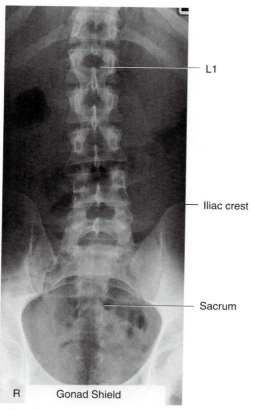

Fig. 15-51 Lumbar spine. AP projection, patient recumbent with knees flexed.

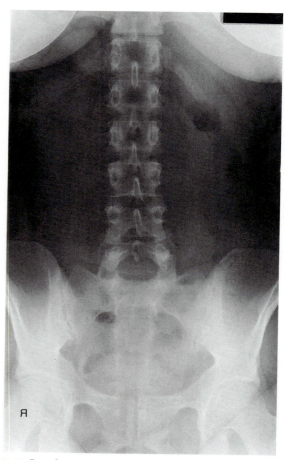

Fig. 15-52 Lumbar spine. PA projection, patient recumbent (same patient as Fig. 15-51). Note widening of intervertebral disk spaces and magnification of sacrum.

Lateral Projection

IR: 14 × 17 inches (35 × 43 cm) lengthwise

Grid: Yes

SID: 40 inches minimum

Body position: Standing or recumbent.

Part position: Sagittal plane is parallel to IR.

Recumbent: In lateral recumbent position, spine is aligned parallel to center of Bucky with arms anterior to body. Radiolucent sponges may be used to elevate waist and/or hip to keep spine level (Fig. 15-53). Knees are flexed. A pad between knees helps keep pelvis lateral and maintain lateral position of spine.

Upright: Feet are shoulder-width apart with equal weight bearing, and torso is stabilized against upright IR holder. Arms are crossed over chest with hands supported on shoulders. Alternatively, arms may be supported out of radiation field by having patient grasp a pole (Fig. 15-54).

Central ray: Perpendicular to center of IR through L4, in midaxillary line at level of iliac crest.

> **TIP:** Place a strip of lead or a lead rubber mask behind the patient so that its margin is aligned with the shadow of the patient's back in the collimator light. This absorbs scatter and improves visualization of the spinous processes.

Collimation: Adjust to 8 × 17 inches (20 × 43 cm) on the collimator.

Patient instruction: Do not move. Suspend breathing on expiration. (Respiratory phase is particularly important on the lateral projection. If exposed on inspiration, the posterior lung fields will superimpose the body of L1.)

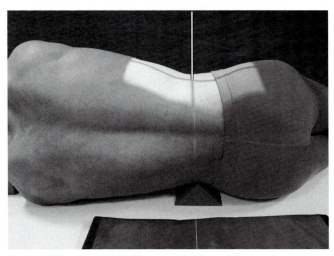

Fig. 15-53 Lumbar spine. Position for lateral projection, patient recumbent. Note the lead strip placed on the table for absorption of scatter radiation.

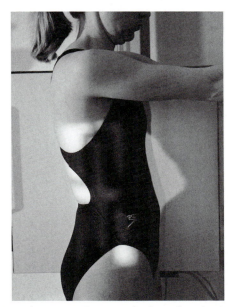

Fig. 15-54 Lumbar spine. Position for lateral projection, patient upright.

Structures seen: All five lumbar vertebrae and superior half of sacrum, including intervertebral foramina, spinous processes and profile of the bodies, and intervertebral disk spaces (Fig. 15-55).

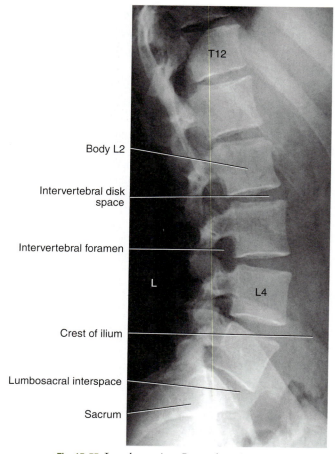

Fig. 15-55 Lumbar spine. Lateral projection.

Supplemental Projections

AP Oblique Projection

Bilateral oblique projections are taken. AP obliques (RPO and LPO positions), rather than PA obliques, are most commonly done because they demonstrate the zygapophyseal joints and pars interarticularis of the side nearest the IR, providing better detail.

IR: 14 × 17 inches (35 × 43 cm) lengthwise

Grid: Yes

SID: 40 inches minimum

Body position: Standing or recumbent.

Part position: Sagittal plane is aligned at angle of 45 degrees to IR.

Recumbent: From supine position, patient is rotated 45 degrees toward side being radiographed (Fig. 15-56). Position may be supported by a large 45-degree-angle radiolucent sponge. Take care that the entire spine is rotated the same amount so there is no torsion (twist) of spine.

Upright: From AP position, patient is rotated 45 degrees toward side being radiographed. Feet are shoulder-width apart with equal weight bearing, and torso is stabilized against upright IR holder (Fig. 15-57).

Central ray: Perpendicular to center of IR through L3. Central ray enters at point 2 inches medial to anterior superior iliac spine (ASIS) farthest from IR and 1.5 inches superior to iliac crest.

Collimation: Adjust to 9 × 14 inches (23 × 35 cm) on the collimator.

Shielding: Although gonad shielding is shown in Fig. 15-56, it is not recommended if the lower lumbar spine is of clinical interest.

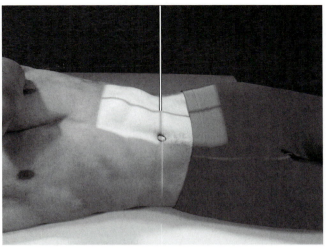

Fig. 15-56 Lumbar spine. Position for AP oblique projection, RPO position, patient recumbent.

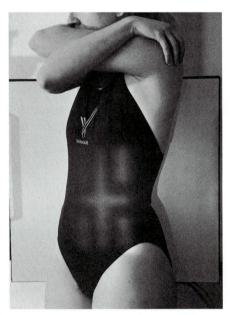

Fig. 15-57 Lumbar spine. Position for AP oblique projection, RPO position, patient upright.

Patient instruction: Do not move. Suspend breathing on expiration.

Structures seen: All five lumbar vertebrae and upper portion of sacrum, including zygapophyseal joints and pars interarticularis on the side nearest the IR (Fig. 15-58).

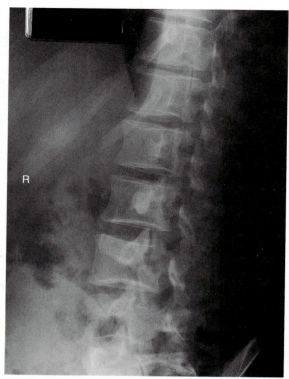

Fig. 15-58 Lumbar spine. AP oblique projection, RPO position.

Lateral Projection of L5-S1 Lumbosacral Junction

A coned-down radiograph of the lumbosacral junction in the lateral projection is helpful when there is poor visualization of this area on the routine lateral projection. This may occur as a result of insufficient penetration of this dense area. This projection is important because this junction is a common site of chronic low back pain. Although this projection may be taken with the patient upright, the result is usually superior when the patient is recumbent.

IR: 8 × 10 inches (18 × 24 cm) lengthwise

Grid: Yes

SID: 40 inches minimum

Body position: As for routine lateral lumbar projection, with care taken that spine is parallel to IR (Fig. 15-59).

Central ray: Directed perpendicular to center of IR through lumbosacral joint. This centering point is 2 inches posterior to ASIS and 1.5 inches inferior to iliac crest on coronal line midway between ASIS and posterior prominence of sacrum. When spine cannot be supported, angle 5 degrees caudad for males and 8 degrees caudad for females.

Collimation: Field size adjusted to 5 × 5 inches in the center of the IR.

Patient instruction: Do not move. Suspend breathing on expiration.

Structures seen: The lower one or two lumbar vertebrae, the upper sacrum, and an open lumbosacral junction (Fig. 15-60).

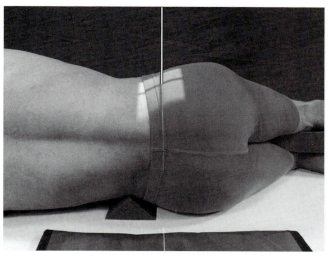

Fig. 15-59 L5-S1 Lumbosacral junction. Position for lateral projection.

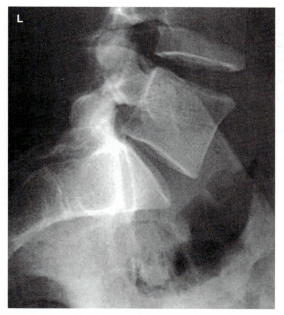

Fig. 15-60 L5-S1 Lumbosacral junction. Lateral projection.

Lumbar Spine and Sacroiliac Joints

AP Axial Projection of Lumbosacral Junction and Sacroiliac Joints

Because of the sacral base angle, the lumbosacral junction is not well seen on the routine AP projection of the lumbar spine. The AP axial projection directs the central ray parallel to the sacral base. See Table 15-1 for variations in sacral base angle. This projection is also useful for demonstration of the sacroiliac joints.

IR: 8 × 10 inches (18 × 24 cm) lengthwise

Grid: Yes

SID: 40 inches minimum

Body position: Supine, as for AP recumbent lumbar spine, with knees flexed and supported.

Central ray: Angled 30 degrees cephalad for males and 35 degrees cephalad for females. It is directed to center of IR through lumbosacral junction (Fig. 15-61). Central ray enters in midline, 1 inch inferior to the ASIS (Fig. 15-62).

Collimation: Adjust to 8 × 10 inches (18 × 24 cm) on the collimator.

Shielding: Gonad shielding for males. Ovarian shielding would interfere with purpose of examination.

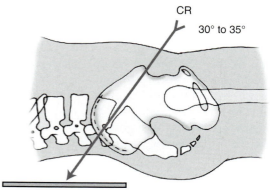

Fig. 15-61 Alignment of central ray (CR) for AP axial projection of lumbosacral junction and sacroiliac joints.

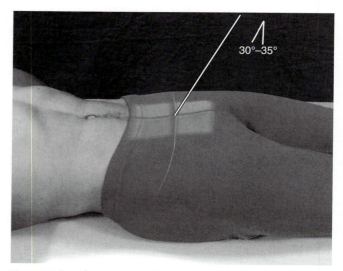

Fig. 15-62 Lumbosacral junction and sacroiliac joints. Position for AP axial projection.

Structures seen: Open lumbosacral junction, sacral alae, and sacroiliac joints (Fig. 15-63).

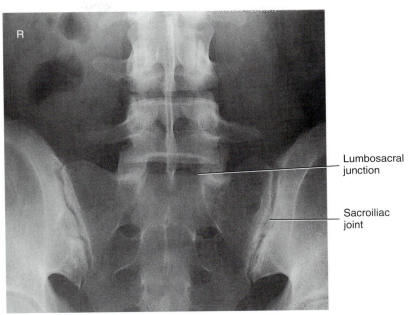

Lumbosacral junction

Sacroiliac joint

Fig. 15-63 L5-S1 Lumbosacral junction and sacroiliac joints. AP axial projection.

Sacroiliac Joints

Routine Examination

The routine examination of the sacroiliac joints includes the AP oblique projections. The AP axial projection of the lumbosacral junction and the sacroiliac joints may also be included.

AP Oblique Projection

Bilateral AP oblique projections are usually taken for comparison.

IR: 8 × 10 inches (18 × 24 cm) lengthwise

Grid: Yes

SID: 40 inches minimum

Body position: Recumbent.

Part position:

AP obliques (RPO, LPO positions): From supine position, body is rotated so that coronal plane is aligned at angle of 25 to 30 degrees to IR (Fig. 15-64). The side of interest is elevated, furthest from IR (Fig. 15-65). Position may be supported by radiolucent sponge under hip and lumbar area of elevated side. Take care the entire spine is rotated the same amount so that there is no torsion of spine.

PA obliques (RAO, LAO positions): From prone position, body is rotated so that coronal plane is aligned at angle of 25 to 30 degrees to IR. Side of interest is nearest the IR. This position may be supported by radiolucent sponge under hip and abdomen area on opposite side. Take care the entire spine is rotated the same amount so that there is no torsion of spine.

Central ray:

AP obliques: Perpendicular to center of IR through point 1 inch medial to ASIS farthest from IR.

PA obliques: Perpendicular to center of IR through point 1 inch medial to ASIS nearest the IR.

Collimation: Adjust to 8 × 10 inches (18 × 24 cm) on the collimator.

Shielding: Shield males with precision. Do not shield females.

Patient instruction: Do not move. Suspend breathing on expiration.

Structures seen:

AP obliques: Sacroiliac joint farthest from IR (Fig. 15-66).

PA obliques: Sacroiliac joint nearest IR.

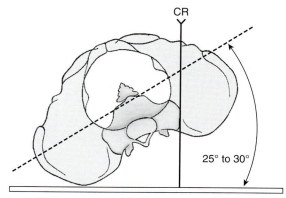

Fig. 15-64 When coronal plane is aligned to IR at a 25- to 30-degree angle, perpendicular central ray (CR) passes through sacroiliac joint on elevated side.

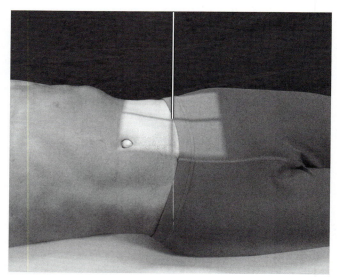

Fig. 15-65 Sacroiliac joint. Position for AP oblique projection, RPO position.

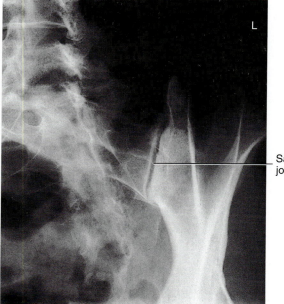

Sacroiliac joint

Fig. 15-66 Sacroiliac (SI) joint. AP oblique projection, RPO position, demonstrating left SI joint.

Sacrum

Routine Examination
The routine examination of the sacrum includes the AP axial and lateral projections.

AP Axial Projection

IR: 10 × 12 inches (24 × 30 cm) lengthwise

Grid: Yes

SID: 40 inches minimum

Body position: Recumbent or supine.

Part position: Midsagittal plane is perpendicular to IR and centered to it. Knees are flexed and supported with a bolster, if needed.

Central ray: Angled 15 degrees cephalad to enter body at midline, 1 inch inferior to the ASIS (Fig. 15-67).

Collimation: Adjust to 10 × 12 inches (24 × 30 cm) on the collimator.

Shielding: Shield males with precision. Do not shield females.

Patient instruction: Stop breathing. Do not move.

Structures seen: Entire sacrum and sacroiliac articulations (Fig. 15-68).

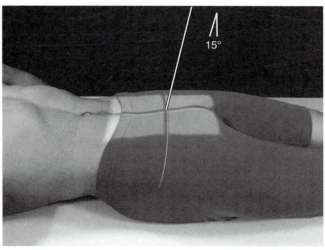

Fig. 15-67 Sacrum. Position for AP axial projection.

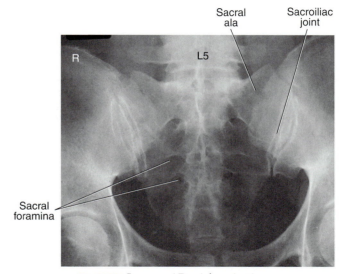

Fig. 15-68 Sacrum. AP axial projection.

Lateral Projection

IR: 10 × 12 inches (24 × 30 cm) lengthwise

Grid: Yes

SID: 40 inches minimum

Body position: Recumbent.

Part position: Sagittal plane is parallel to IR.

Recumbent: Spine is aligned parallel to center of Bucky with arms anterior to body. Radiolucent sponges may be used to elevate waist and/or hips to keep spine level (Fig. 15-69). Knees are flexed. A pad between knees helps maintain lateral position of pelvis and spine.

Central ray: Perpendicular to center of IR through center of sacrum. Central ray enters at point 3.5 inches posterior to ASIS (Fig. 15-70).

> **TIP:** Place a strip of lead or a lead rubber mask behind the patient so that its margin is aligned with the shadow of the patient's back in the collimator light. This absorbs backscatter and improves contrast resolution of the sacrum image.

Collimation: Adjust to 10 × 12 inches (24 × 30 cm) on the collimator.

Patient instruction: Do not move. Suspend breathing on expiration.

Structures seen: Entire sacrum and lumbosacral junction (Fig. 15-71). Coccyx is sometimes seen.

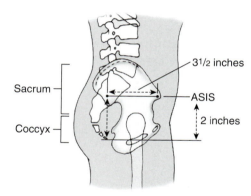

Fig. 15-69 Localization of sacrum and coccyx in relation to palpable landmarks. *ASIS,* Anterior superior iliac spine.

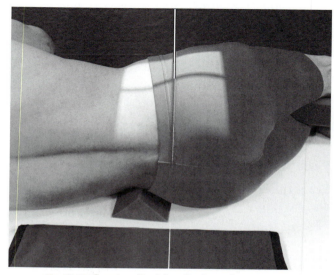

Fig. 15-70 Sacrum. Position for lateral projection.

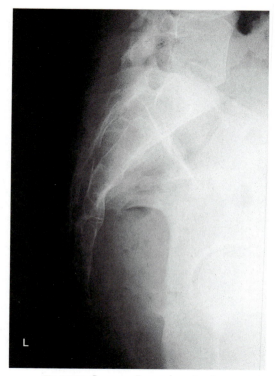

Fig. 15-71 Sacrum. Lateral projection.

Coccyx

Routine Examination

The routine examination of the coccyx includes the AP axial and lateral projections.

AP Axial Projection

IR: 8 × 10 inches (18 × 24 cm) lengthwise

Grid: Yes

SID: 40 inches minimum

Body position: Recumbent.

Part position: Coronal plane is parallel to IR with patient facing tube. Midsagittal plane is centered to midline of Bucky. When patient is supine, knees are flexed and supported with a bolster, if needed.

Central ray: Angled 10 degrees caudad to enter body in midline, 1 inch inferior to the ASIS (Fig. 15-72).

Collimation: Adjust to 6 × 8 inches (15 × 20 cm) on the collimator. Close collimation is required for adequate visualization.

Shielding: Precise gonad shielding for males. Do not shield females.

Patient instruction: Do not move.

Structures seen: Entire coccyx and distal portion of sacrum (Fig. 15-73).

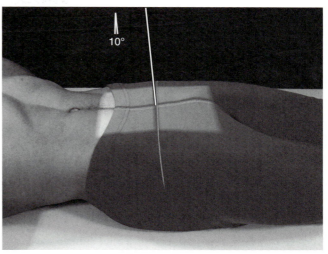

Fig. 15-72 Coccyx. Position for AP axial projection.

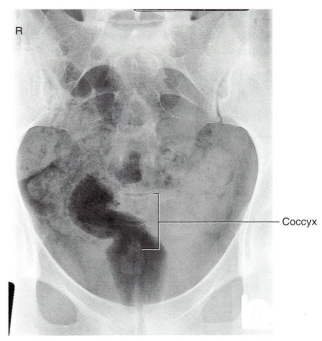

Fig. 15-73 Coccyx. AP axial projection.

Patient instruction: Stop breathing. Do not move.

Structures seen: Portion of mandible, entire spine, portion of pelvis (Figs. 15-77 and 15-78).

Compensating filter: The wide range of body part thicknesses and tissue densities in the thoracic and abdominal areas necessitates the use of specially designed compensating filters to create a more uniform radiographic brightness throughout the entire spine.

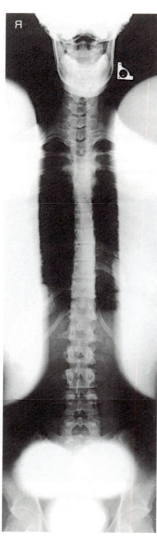

Fig. 15-77 Full spine. PA projection with breast and gonad shielding.

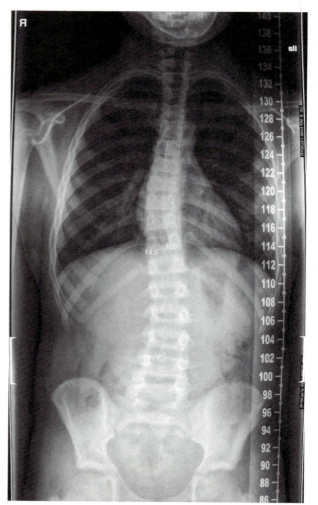

Fig. 15-78 Full spine. Image was made using two CR imaging plates and computer software to "stitch" the images together.

Lateral Projection

IR: 14 × 36 inches (35 × 90 cm), or 14 × 34 inches (35 × 86 cm) if using computed radiography, lengthwise

Grid: Yes

SID: 60 inches minimum

Position: Same as for upright lateral projection of thoracic spine. Shoulders are rounded anteriorly and arms are extended anterior to body and supported (Fig. 15-79).

Shielding: Lead aprons, upright shield stands, or shadow shield devices that attach to collimator.

Patient instruction: Stop breathing. Do not move.

Structures seen: Portion of mandible and skull, entire spine, portion of pelvis (Fig. 15-80).

Compensating Filter: The wide range of body part thicknesses and tissue densities in the thoracic and abdominal areas necessitates the use of specially designed compensating filters to create a more uniform radiographic density (brightness) throughout the entire spine.

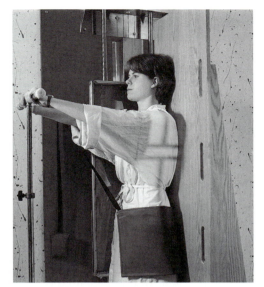

Fig. 15-79 Full spine. Position for lateral projection.

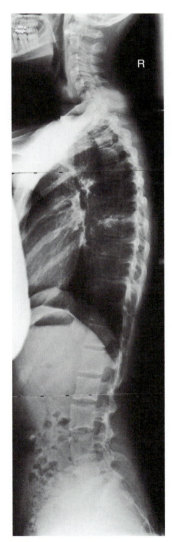

Fig. 15-80 Full spine. Lateral projection.

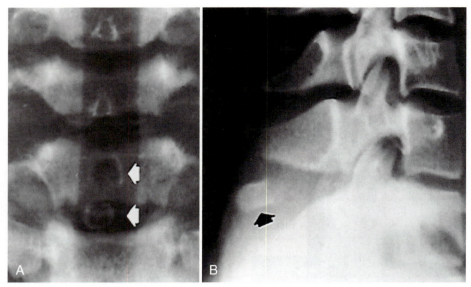

Fig. 15-88 Clay shoveler's fracture, an avulsion of the spinous process of C7. **A,** AP projection shows the classic "double spinous process" sign *(arrows)*. **B,** Avulsed fragment is clearly seen on the lateral projection *(arrow)*.

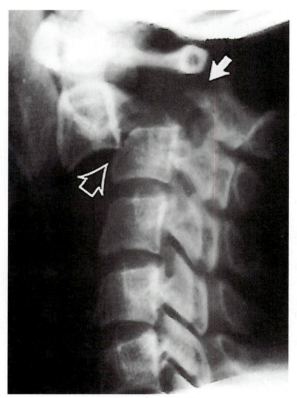

Fig. 15-89 Hangman's fracture is a fracture of the neural arch of C2 *(solid arrow)* with associated subluxation of C2-C3 *(open arrow)*.

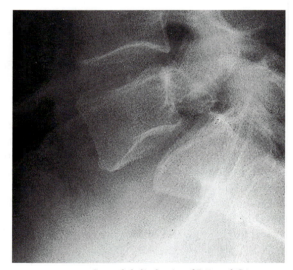

Fig. 15-90 Spondylolisthesis of L5 and S1.

a defect or a fracture of the pars interarticularis or of the pedicle.

Spondyloschisis is the term for a congenital fissure (split or cleft) in the neural arch. Spina bifida occulta, discussed and illustrated earlier in this chapter, is an example of spondyloschisis.

Disk Pathology

The pulpy center of intervertebral disks is normally gel-like, semiliquid, and very flexible. Its mass shifts to change the shape of the disk with the pressure of various spinal movements. With advancing age and repeated minor traumas to the spine, the disks tend to degenerate. The nucleus may dry out and become atrophied, which causes narrowing of the disk space. Without adequate cushioning, the joint becomes inflamed, and the surrounding bony structures show the characteristic signs of degeneration: sclerotic (hardened), irregular bone margins with hypertrophic lipping and spurring (Fig. 15-91). This condition is called *degenerative disk disease (DDD)* and is usually associated with osteoarthritis.

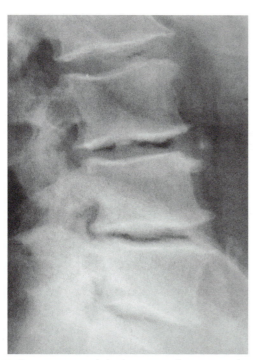

Fig. 15-91 Degenerative disk disease with associated arthritic changes. Note disk space narrowing and hypertrophic spurs on the anterior vertebral bodies. The dark linear shadows overlying two of the disks represent the "vacuum phenomenon" sometimes seen with severe disk degeneration.

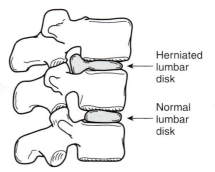

Fig. 15-92 When an intervertebral disk herniates, the annulus ruptures and the nucleus pulposus is forced out posteriorly and/or laterally. The herniated nucleus then occupies space in the spinal canal or intervertebral foramen, causing nerve pressure.

Disk herniation or herniated nucleus pulposus (HNP) is the condition often called, in lay terms, a *slipped disk*.

The annulus fibrosus ruptures, and the nucleus is forced into the area posterior to the disk space (Fig. 15-92). The displaced nucleus causes pressure on the spinal cord and/or the nerve roots in this area.

Disk herniation is caused by trauma to the disk. In the lumbar area, it may be caused by pressure from lifting a heavy object. Herniated cervical disks are often the result of motor vehicle accidents. Disk herniation may cause acute pain, chronic discomfort, or recurrent painful episodes involving the site of the herniation. There may also be pain, numbness, or altered sensation in areas remote from the spine.

Although the radiographic examination may show a decrease in the height of the disk space, special imaging techniques are necessary to demonstrate disk herniation definitively. Myelography, discography, computed tomography, and magnetic resonance imaging studies (Fig. 15-93) may be used to identify disk pathology.

Remote Symptoms of Spine Pathology

The nerves communicate messages of motion and sensation between the brain and all parts of the body by way of the spinal cord. The spinal cord is surrounded by the vertebral foramina, and nerves pass from the spinal cord to other parts of the body by way of the intervertebral

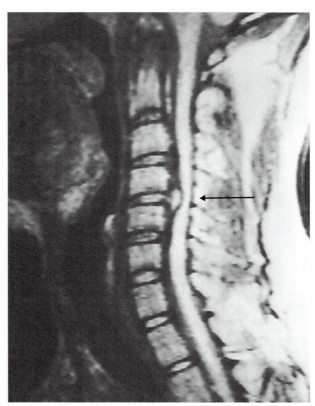

Fig. 15-93 Magnetic resonance image of the cervical spine in the sagittal plane shows herniation of the C4-C5 disk *(arrow)*. Note impression on the spinal cord.

foramina. This explains why changes in the vertebrae may cause symptoms in parts of the body remote from the spine. Such symptoms are indications of pressure on or irritation of the nerve roots.

Nerve root insult may cause pain, numbness, or altered sensation. Sciatica, for example, is pain along the path of the sciatic nerve in the buttock, posterior thigh, and leg. It is caused by nerve irritation in the lumbar region. Damage to nerve roots may cause weakness or paralysis. The function or control of organs may be affected as well. For example, nerves in the upper cervical region control vital functions such as breathing, and nerves in the lumbar region control bowel and urinary bladder function.

There are many possible causes of nerve root compression. Hypertrophic arthritic changes, such as bony spurs on the vertebrae, may cause **stenosis** (narrowing) of the intervertebral foramina. Misalignment of vertebrae, subluxation, or spondylolisthesis may cause crowding of the nerve pathways. Disk herniation is also a common cause of remote nerve symptoms.

SUMMARY

The vertebral column surrounds the spinal cord and is the supporting structure for the body. It consists of 33 vertebrae or spinal segments: 7 cervical, 12 thoracic, 5 lumbar, 5 sacral, and 4 coccygeal. Most vertebrae consist of an anterior body, a posterior vertebral arch, two lateral projections called *transverse processes*, and a posterior projection called the *spinous process.* The joints between the vertebral bodies are cushioned by intervertebral disks. Zygapophyseal joints between the posterior elements facilitate motion. Each region of the spine has either a kyphotic or lordotic curvature.

Limited operators must be familiar with the landmarks used to locate center points and individual vertebrae in each region of the spine. The zygapophyseal joints and the intervertebral foramina of each spinal region vary in their relationships to body planes. The limited operator must be familiar with these relationships to demonstrate these structures accurately.

Most spine radiography may be done with the patient either upright or recumbent. All of the basic examinations of the spine consist of at least AP or PA and lateral projections. Oblique and axial projections and coneddown radiographs are frequently taken to supplement routine examinations.

Congenital anomalies are common in the spine. Those most frequently seen include extra vertebrae, transitional vertebrae, and anomalous ribs. Many pathologic conditions of the spine are diagnosed radiographically. Trauma may require radiographs to identify fractures or significant displacements. Degenerative, inflammatory, and neoplastic diseases also affect the spine and are evaluated with radiography. Some spinal conditions cause nerve symptoms in areas of the body remote from the spine.

Chapter 16

Bony Thorax, Chest, and Abdomen

Learning Objectives

At the conclusion of this chapter, you will be able to:

- Name the bones that make up the bony thorax and identify each on an anatomic diagram and on a radiograph
- Name and identify on an anatomic diagram the principal organs located within the thoracic cavity
- Name and identify on an anatomic diagram the principal organs located within the abdominal cavity
- Identify significant positioning landmarks in the thoracic and abdominal areas by palpation
- Demonstrate correct body and part positioning for routine projections and common special projections of the bony thorax, chest, and abdomen
- Correctly evaluate radiographs of the bony thorax, chest, and abdomen for positioning accuracy
- Describe and recognize on radiographs pathology that is common to the bony thorax, chest, and abdomen

Key Terms

aorta	KUB
atelectasis	mediastinum
bronchus (pl. bronchi)	peritoneum
cardiophrenic angles	pleura
carina	pleural effusion
colon	pneumoconiosis
costophrenic angles	pneumonia
diaphragm	pneumothorax
duodenum	sphincter
emphysema	sternum
esophagus	thorax
ileum	trachea
jejunum	vena cava

Anatomy and positioning of the thoracic and abdominal cavities are covered in this chapter. Chest radiography is within the scope of practice for most limited x-ray machine operators (LXMOs), with the exception of those holding licenses that restrict practice to specific body parts. Radiography of the ribs and of the abdomen are less commonly within the LXMO scope of practice but are included in this chapter for educators and students in those states where imaging of these body parts is allowed.

Radiography of skeletal anatomy requires an approach that is quite different from that used for visualization of the soft tissues and organs. Examinations of the bony thorax and chest involve the same general part of the body, but they differ from each other considerably. This chapter details the positioning and techniques required for best demonstration of both types of thoracic tissue.

Although chest and abdominal radiography both involve soft tissue and organs, they are quite different. As explained in Chapter 7, subject contrast reflects tissue density differences within the body part. Differences in subject contrast require variations in technique to obtain optimal visualization on the radiograph. The subject contrast of the chest differs greatly from that of the abdomen. Subject contrast within the chest is provided by the radiolucency of the air in the lungs. The abdomen has tissues with very similar densities and therefore has relatively little subject contrast.

Chest radiographs provide diagnostic information about the heart, lungs, and other organs that lie in the area around the heart. Although chest radiography may seem to be the simplest and most familiar of all radiographic examinations, it is also the most likely to provide life-saving information for the patient's care. For this reason, the ability to take high-quality chest radiographs is an essential skill for limited operators.

Radiography of the abdomen, on the other hand, is less likely to be required of the limited operator. In some states, abdominal radiography is beyond the scope of limited practice. Even when there is no restriction on abdominal radiography, these examinations are not often performed in an outpatient setting. If you are using this book as a text in a formal course, the abdomen may not be included in the curriculum. Basic information on the anatomy, positioning, and pathology of the abdomen is included here so that the content will be comprehensive for those who need this information.

ANATOMY

Bony Thorax

The term **thorax** refers to the upper portion of the trunk, the chest. The thoracic cage (Fig. 16-1) is the bony structure that surrounds the organs of the chest and upper abdomen. It consists of the 12 thoracic vertebrae, 12 pairs of ribs, and the breastbone, which is called the **sternum.**

The sternum is a slender, flat bone located in the midline of the anterior thorax. It has three parts: the manubrium, the body or gladiolus, and the xiphoid process. The manubrium is the superior portion. Its upper margin is indented to form the jugular notch, also called the *manubrial notch* or *suprasternal notch*, which is a useful positioning landmark. The body is the long, middle portion of the sternum. The junction of the manubrium and the body forms a palpable bony ridge called the *sternal angle*. The xiphoid process is the distal tip and is also a useful positioning landmark. In childhood the xiphoid process is formed only of cartilage; it ossifies in adulthood.

The ribs are numbered 1 through 12, from the top down. They are attached posteriorly to the thoracic vertebrae, forming the costovertebral articulations. Ribs

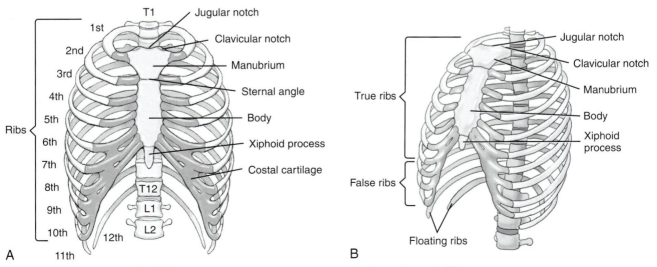

Fig. 16-1 Bony thorax. **A,** Anterior aspect. **B,** Anterolateral oblique aspect.

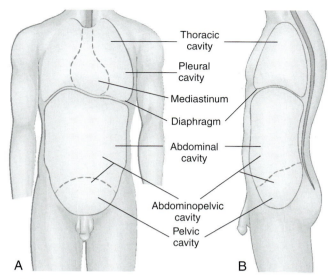

Fig. 16-2 Body cavities. **A,** Anterior aspect. **B,** Lateral aspect.

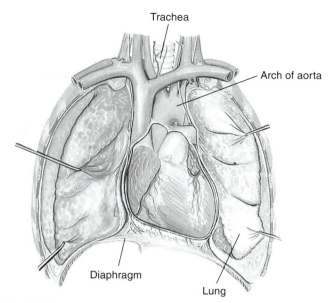

Fig. 16-3 Thoracic cavity is divided into three sections: right and left pleural cavities and mediastinum.

are long, flat, slender, curved bones, and most have costal cartilage at their anterior ends. The connection between the rib and its associated cartilage is called the *costochondral articulation.* The anterior end of each rib is approximately 3 to 4 inches inferior to its posterior end. When one is breathing, the rib articulations move gently, which allows expansion of the thorax with inspiration and contraction with expiration.

The first seven pairs of ribs are called *true ribs.* They attach anteriorly to the sternum, forming cartilaginous amphiarthrodial joints. The lower five pairs of ribs are called *false ribs* because they do not completely surround the thorax. Ribs 8, 9, and 10 attach to bands of costal cartilage that attach to the sternum. Ribs 11 and 12 are also called *floating ribs.* They have no cartilage and are not attached anteriorly.

Cavities of the Trunk

The interior of the trunk of the body is divided into two main cavities, the thoracic cavity and the abdominopelvic cavity (Fig. 16-2). The two cavities are separated beneath the lungs by the **diaphragm.** The diaphragm is a large sheath of muscle that expands and contracts with breathing. It forms an arching curve from front to back.

Chest

The thoracic cavity (Fig. 16-3) is divided into three parts: two pleural cavities that contain the lungs and the space between the lungs, which is called the **mediastinum.** The principal structures within the mediastinum are the heart, with its associated great vessels; the trachea or "windpipe"; and the **esophagus.** The **trachea** is a part of the respiratory system and connects the throat to the lungs. The esophagus is a part of the digestive system and connects the throat to the

stomach. Portions of the lymphatic system (the thymus gland and many lymph nodes) are also located within the mediastinum.

The heart (Fig. 16-4) is the principal organ of the circulatory system, introduced in Chapter 12. It occupies the inferior portion of the mediastinum in a sac of serous membrane called the *pericardium.* It is about the size of a fist and consists mainly of heart muscle tissue called *myocardium.* The heart is divided into four hollow chambers: the right and left atria, which are receiving chambers, and the right and left ventricles, which are discharging chambers. Blood enters the atria through veins and is pumped out into arteries via the ventricles. Valves between the chambers regulate blood flow.

The term *great vessels* refers to the veins and arteries that carry blood to and from the heart. The **vena cava** is the large vein that brings oxygen-depleted blood from the body to the right atrium. Venous blood contains carbon dioxide (CO_2), a gas that is a waste product of oxygen use. The blood then flows into the right ventricle and is pumped into the pulmonary arteries, which carry it to the lungs. In the capillaries of the lungs, CO_2 is exchanged for oxygen and the CO_2 is exhaled. Oxygenated blood returns from the lungs to the left atrium via the pulmonary veins. From the left atrium it flows into the left ventricle, which pumps it back out to the body via the **aorta.** The aorta is the largest artery of the body. It leaves the heart in a superior direction and makes a "U-turn" called the *aortic arch.* Arteries branching from the aortic arch supply blood to the head and upper body. The descending aorta passes in an inferior direction posterior to the heart, through the diaphragm, and through the abdomen. Its many branches supply oxygenated blood to the remainder of the body.

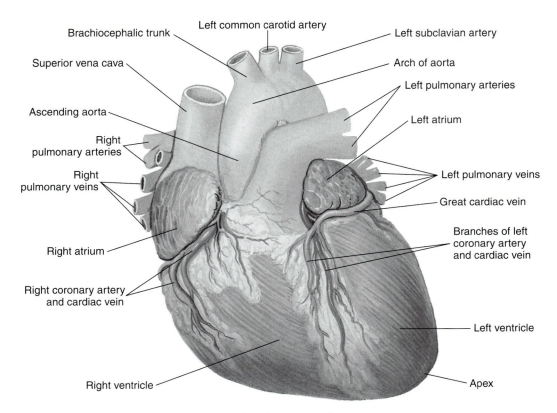

Fig. 16-4 Anterior aspect of heart.

Respiratory System

The respiratory system was introduced in Chapter 12. The principal organs of the respiratory system are the lungs (Fig. 16-5). The lungs are divided into sections called *lobes*. The right lung has three lobes: superior, middle, and inferior. The left lung has only two lobes: superior and inferior. Each lung is shaped somewhat like a tall pyramid. The broad lower surface is called the *base* and the angle at the top is called the *apex*. The inferior lateral corners are called the **costophrenic angles.** The

inferior medial corners are called the **cardiophrenic angles.** The left lung is slightly smaller and is narrower at the base than the right lung.

The other organs of the respiratory system include the mouth and nasal passages, the pharynx (throat), the larynx, the trachea, and the **bronchi** (singular, *bronchus*) (Fig. 16-6).

A small valve between the pharynx and the trachea, the epiglottis, closes off the trachea when one swallows so that food passes into the esophagus rather than the

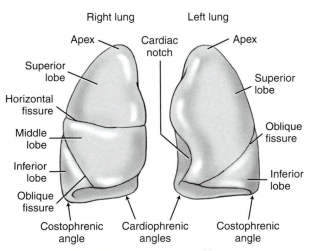

Fig. 16-5 Anterior aspect of lungs.

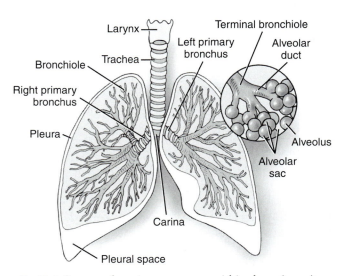

Fig. 16-6 Organs of respiratory system within thoracic cavity.

trachea. The trachea divides into right and left primary branches at the **carina** (tracheal bifurcation) at about the level of the sternal angle and the T4-T5 interspace. Each primary branch enters one lung and then divides into secondary branches, one for each lobe of the lung.

The membranes that line the pleural cavities and cover the lungs are called **pleura.** They secrete serous fluid that moistens and lubricates the surfaces so that the lungs can move smoothly against the walls of the pleural cavity with breathing motion. The space between the lungs and the cavity walls is called the *pleural space.*

Abdomen

The abdominopelvic cavity is divided into two sections: the abdominal cavity and the pelvic cavity. The abdominal cavity is the larger section, extending from the diaphragm into the upper portion of the bony pelvis. It contains the principal organs of the digestive tract: the stomach, small and large intestine, liver, gallbladder, and pancreas. The spleen, which is part of the lymphatic system, is also located within the abdominal cavity. Its location is immediately beneath the diaphragm on the far left and behind the stomach.

The abdominal organs are contained in a double-walled serous membrane sac called the **peritoneum.** Parietal peritoneum lines the walls of the cavity and visceral peritoneum is positioned over and around the organs in folds. The folds between the organs, the mesentery, hold them in position. The anterior fold of the visceral peritoneum is called the *omentum.*

The abdominopelvic cavity also contains the urinary system. The kidneys and ureters are located in the retroperitoneal space, posterior to the visceral peritoneum against the posterior wall of the abdominal cavity.

The pelvic cavity is inferior to the abdominal cavity and situated within the bones of the pelvis. It contains the urinary bladder, the distal portion of the large intestine, and the internal parts of the reproductive system.

There are two systems for dividing the abdominopelvic cavity into parts so that locations within it can be readily identified. The simplest system is that which divides the area into four quadrants (Fig. 16-7). More specific localization is provided by a system that divides the abdomen into nine regions (Fig. 16-8). The limited operator must learn the names of the quadrants and regions and the principal structures that lie within each. This knowledge will help you to communicate clearly the site of a patient's pain or wound or to locate the area of clinical interest on a radiograph.

Alimentary Canal

The digestive system was introduced in Chapter 12. The portions of the alimentary canal that are within the abdominopelvic cavity are the distal end of the esophagus, the stomach, the small intestine, and the large intestine, also called the **colon** (Fig. 16-9).

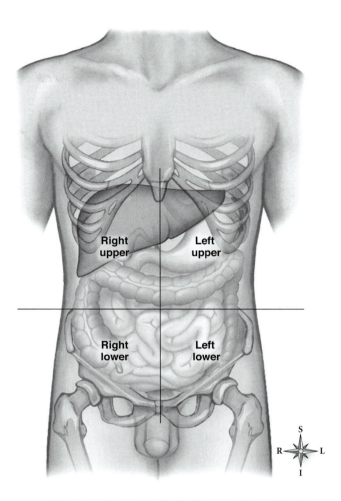

Fig. 16-7 Abdominopelvic cavity divided into quadrants. *I,* Inferior; *L,* left; *R,* right; *S,* superior.

From the mouth, food passes through the pharynx and into the esophagus at the epiglottis. The esophagus passes through the mediastinum and the diaphragm and into the abdominal cavity. Between the esophagus and the stomach is a round muscle called a **sphincter** that opens and closes the opening to the stomach.

The stomach is in the left upper quadrant of the abdomen. Its rounded upper portion is called the *fundus.* The large central curved portion is called the *body.* The lateral surface of the body is called the *greater curvature,* and the medial one is called the *lesser curvature.* The narrow distal portion of the stomach is called the *pylorus.* Another sphincter, the pyloric sphincter, joins the pylorus to the first portion of the small intestine.

Digestion and absorption of food occur in the small intestine. The adult small intestine is 20 to 22 feet in length. Its diameter ranges from 1.5 inches at the proximal end to about 1 inch at the distal end.

The small intestine has three parts. The proximal portion is the **duodenum.** It is about 8 to 10 inches long and forms the shape of the letter C. The rounded segment just distal to the pyloric sphincter is called the *duodenal*

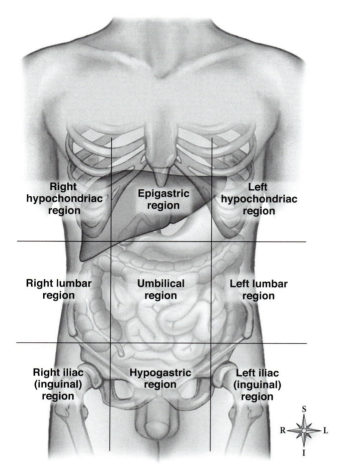

Fig. 16-8 Nine abdominal regions. *I*, Inferior; *L*, left; *R*, right; *S*, superior.

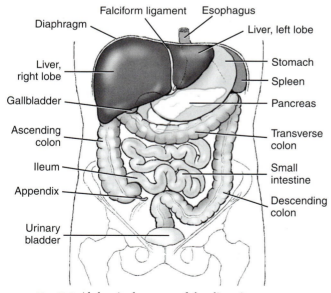

Fig. 16-9 Abdominal organs of the digestive system.

loop back and forth across the central and lower part of the abdominal cavity and are framed by the colon.

The principal functions of the large intestine or colon are to reclaim water from the intestinal contents and to eliminate solid food waste from the body. The first portion, the cecum, is located in the right lower quadrant. The terminal ileum attaches to the cecum at the ileocecal valve. The appendix is a small pouch attached to the cecum. From the cecum, the ascending colon extends superiorly to the right upper quadrant, where it makes a right-angle turn in the medial direction. This turn is called the *right colic flexure*. The transverse colon extends across the upper abdomen and turns inferiorly on the left side at the left colic flexure. From this flexure it extends inferiorly and is called the *descending colon*. In the left lower quadrant, the colon forms an S-shaped curve. This portion is called the *sigmoid colon* for the Greek letter sigma (Σ). The sigmoid colon extends toward the midline, where it turns inferiorly again and is called the *rectum*. The terminal portion of the rectum is called the *anal canal*. Food waste exits the body at the anal sphincter.

Other Digestive System Organs

The other organs of the digestive system that lie within the abdominal cavity are the liver, gallbladder, and pancreas (Fig. 16-10). The liver and gallbladder and their associated ducts are called the *biliary system*.

The liver is a large organ in the right upper quadrant. It fills the right hypochondriac region and part of the epigastric region. It is wedge-shaped, with its apex to the left of the midline. The liver has several important functions. It is a storehouse for energy, and it removes toxins from the blood. Its most important function from a radiographic standpoint is the production of bile. The

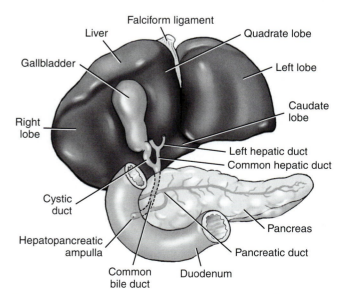

Fig. 16-10 Liver, gallbladder, and pancreas in relation to the duodenum.

bulb. There is no obvious division between the second and third portions of the small intestine. The first 8 feet or so past the duodenum are called the **jejunum,** and the remainder is called the **ileum.** The distal portion of the ileum is called the *terminal ileum.* The ileum and jejunum

liver manufactures and secretes bile, which the body uses to digest fats. The hepatic ducts of the liver collect the bile and come together to form the common hepatic duct.

The gallbladder is a storage sac for bile and is located on the undersurface of the liver. The cystic duct is the passage for bile between the gallbladder and the common hepatic duct. The common hepatic and cystic ducts come together to form the common bile duct. Following a meal that contains fats, the gallbladder contracts, releasing bile. The bile flows through the common bile duct and into the duodenum at the hepatopancreatic ampulla, also called the *ampulla of Vater*.

The pancreas is an elongated gland that lies transversely in the upper abdomen. It is attached to the posterior abdominal wall. The wide end, which is called the *head*, lies in the curve of the duodenum. The tail lies adjacent to the spleen. The midportion is called the *body*. The pancreas manufactures insulin and glucagon, enzymes that are essential to sugar metabolism. The pancreas also secretes pancreatic juices that aid digestion. The pancreatic juices flow through the pancreatic duct and empty into the duodenum at the hepatopancreatic ampulla.

BODY HABITUS

Accurate radiography of the chest and abdomen requires an awareness of body habitus, that is, the general shape of the patient's body. Organs vary greatly in size, shape, and location according to body types. The four basic types of body habitus are called *sthenic*, *hyposthenic*, *asthenic*, and *hypersthenic* and are illustrated in Fig. 16-11.

The sthenic body habitus is considered to be "average." About 50% of the population has this body type.

The size, shape, and location of organs correspond to classic textbook descriptions and illustrations.

The hyposthenic body type might be thought of as "slender normal." About 35% of the population has a hyposthenic build. The organs tend to be longer, narrower, and more vertical in position.

The asthenic body type is very slender. The organs are long and narrow, and the abdominal organs are located much lower in the body. About 10% of the population has this body type.

The hypersthenic body type is a massive, stocky build. About 5% of the population has this body type. The thorax is short, broad, and deep. The organs tend to be high and more horizontal in position.

POSITIONING AND RADIOGRAPHIC EXAMINATIONS

The radiographic examinations of the thorax and abdomen presented in this chapter are those that require no use of radiographic contrast media. They represent the positions and projections of those body structures most commonly employed in limited practice. They generally require use of large 14 × 17 inch (35 × 43 cm) image receptors (IRs). Variations in orientation and centering of the IR for thoracic and abdominal imaging are related to the location of the diaphragm, influenced by body habitus and respiratory phase. Although the thorax and abdomen may have a similar thickness, imaging requires application of different technical factors: high kilovoltage peak (kVp) for the large variations in tissue densities in the chest, moderate kVp to demonstrate the small differences in tissue densities in the abdomen, and low kVp for the thin bones of the thoracic cage.

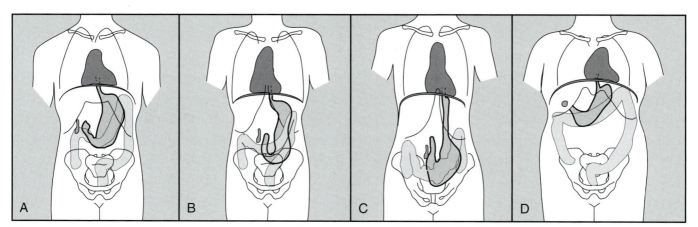

Fig. 16-11 Organ shape and location in relation to body habitus. **A,** Sthenic. **B,** Hyposthenic. **C,** Asthenic. **D,** Hypersthenic.

Chest

When physicians read chest radiographs, the diameter of the heart shadow is compared with the size of the thoracic cage. This is an important diagnostic measurement. Chest radiography is done at 72 inches (183 cm) source–image receptor distance (SID) to minimize magnification of the image of the heart. For the same reason, posteroanterior (PA) and left lateral projections are preferred to anteroposterior (AP) and right lateral projections. Keeping the heart as close to the IR as possible and using a 72-inch SID increases the accuracy of heart size measurements.

Exposures of the chest are most commonly made on inspiration to expand the lung fields. This expansion also results in separation of the pulmonary vasculature (the small vessels of the lungs), allowing a more complete evaluation of the lung. It is a good practice to have the patient take two deep inspirations, holding the breath in on the second inspiration. This practice often produces a deeper inspiration for the exposure. In addition, if deep inspiration causes a cough reflex, the radiographer will be less likely to expose the IR during a cough. The act of inspiration causes the diaphragm to move caudad (Fig. 16-12). The greater the inspiration, the greater the depression of the diaphragm. Evidence of a full inspiration is seen on a chest radiograph when 10 ribs can be counted superior to the diaphragm.

The upright position is important, both for maximum lung expansion (gravity aids in caudal movement of the diaphragm) and for the visualization of air-fluid levels or pleural effusions. The decubitus position is also used to evaluate the presence of excess fluid in the pleural cavity. Air-fluid levels and pleural effusion are discussed in the pathology section of this chapter.

The chest has a high degree of subject contrast because the lungs are air-filled and easily penetrated, whereas the mediastinum is a very dense structure. For this reason, chest radiography requires a high kVp

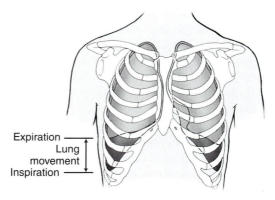

Fig. 16-12 Lung movement during respiration. Lungs expand during inspiration as the diaphragm moves caudad. Lungs contract on expiration as the diaphragm moves cephalad.

technique to create low radiographic contrast images and prevent the appearance of black lungs and white mediastinum with little detail visible in either area. In addition, this high kVp technique causes the ribs to appear less visible so the soft tissues are more easily evaluated. A grid is used to reduce fog from the high-energy scatter radiation that is produced with high kVp. Short exposure times are important because the heartbeat causes motion within the chest that blurs the image when the exposure is longer than 0.05 second.

A lead half-apron that wraps around the pelvis, front and back, is the ideal gonad shield for chest radiography. Collimation and the beam attenuation by posterior body structures provide gonad shielding from lower energy primary radiation and collimator scatter. The quantity of collimator scatter reaching the patient at 72 inches SID is minimal. However, for maximal protection, a lead shield should be used for all chest radiographs.

In preparation for chest examinations, the patient is instructed to remove all clothing and jewelry from the area between the neck and the waist and to don a gown that opens in the back.

Routine Examination

The routine examination of the chest includes the PA and left lateral projections. When a patient is unable to stand for the PA projection, the AP projection can be substituted.

IR: 14 × 17 inches (35 × 43 cm) lengthwise

Grid: Yes

SID: 72 inches (183 cm), if possible

Body position: Standing, facing IR holder.

Part position:

PA: Anterior surface of chest is against upright Bucky with coronal plane parallel to IR. Backs of hands are placed on hips, and shoulders are rotated anteriorly (Fig. 16-13*A*). The purpose of arm position is to rotate scapulae out of the way so that they will not be superimposed on lungs. As an alternative, patients who are unsteady may wrap their arms around the Bucky to prevent movement and decrease potential for a fall. IR is aligned so that upper margin is 1.5 to 2 inches (3.8 to 5 cm) above level of spinous process of C7.

> **NOTE:** Crosswise IR placement may be needed for patients with hypersthenic body habitus.

AP: Patient supine with arms at side (Fig. 16-13*B*). IR is aligned so that upper margin is 1.5 to 2 inches (3.6 to 5 cm) above level of shoulders.

Lateral: Both arms are raised overhead, with patient grasping opposite elbows. As an alternative, patients who are unsteady can grasp an overhead bar, if incorporated into the upright Bucky, or an IV pole to prevent movement and decrease potential for a fall. Left side of body is in contact with upright Bucky, and midcoronal plane of thorax is perpendicular to center of IR (Fig. 16-15). IR placement is unchanged from PA projection.

Central ray:

PA: Perpendicular to center of IR. Center point should be at the level of T7, which corresponds to the level of the inferior angle of the scapulae.

AP: Perpendicular to center of IR. Center point should be on the midsagital plane at a level 3 inches below the jugular notch.

Lateral: Perpendicular to center of IR. Center point should be on the midcoronal plane at the level of T7.

Collimation: Adjust to 14 × 17 inches (35 × 43 cm) on the collimator.

Patient instruction: Do not move. Stop breathing on second deep inspiration.

Structures seen: Heart, lungs, and mediastinum. No rotation of the sternoclavicular joints on the PA projection (Fig. 16-14). Superimposition of the posterior ribs, indicating no rotation, on the lateral projection (Fig. 16-16).

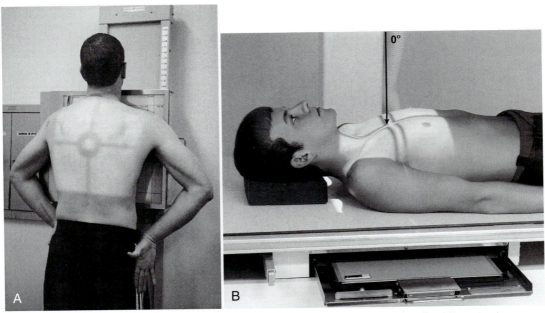

Fig. 16-13 Chest. **A,** Position for PA projection, patient upright. **B,** Position for AP projection, patient supine.

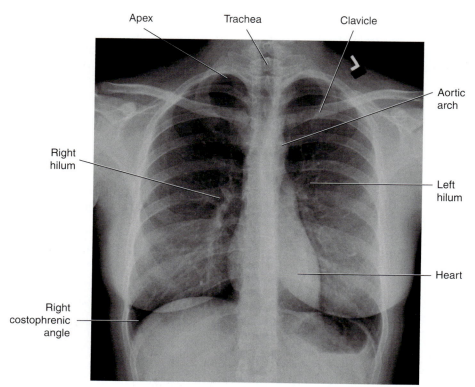

Apex   Trachea   Clavicle

Aortic
arch

Right
hilum

Left
hilum

Heart

Right
costophrenic
angle

Fig. 16-14 Chest. PA projection.

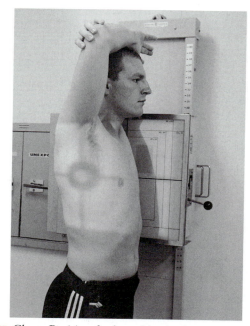

Fig. 16-15 Chest. Position for lateral projection, patient upright.

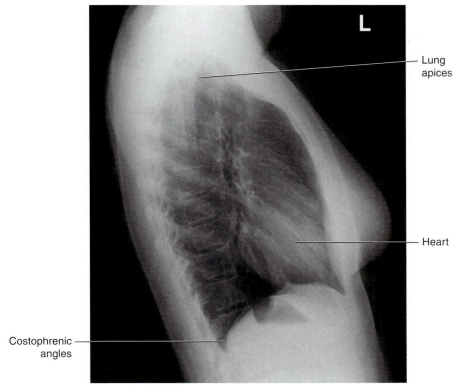

Lung
apices

Heart

Costophrenic
angles

Fig. 16-16 Chest. Lateral projection.

Supplemental Projections

AP or PA Projection (Lateral Decubitus Position)

IR: 14 × 17 inches (35 × 43 cm) lengthwise

Grid: Yes

SID: 72 inches (183 cm)

Body position: Recumbent, lying on side of interest.

Part position: Midsagittal plane of chest horizontal. Chest elevated 2 to 3 inches (5 to 8 cm) on radiolucent pad. Anterior or posterior surface of chest against a vertical grid device (Fig. 16-17).

Central ray: Horizontal and perpendicular to center of IR. Center point should be midsagittal and at the level of T7.

Collimation: Adjust to 14 × 17 inches (35 × 43 cm) on the collimator.

Patient instruction: Do not move. Stop breathing on second deep inspiration.

Structures seen: Heart, lungs, and mediastinum. Sternoclavicular joints equidistant from spine, which indicates no rotation (Fig. 16-18). Any free fluid present in the pleural space will be demonstrated along the dependent chest wall.

NOTE: Long axis of the IR is horizontal, placed lengthwise in relation to the long axis of the chest.

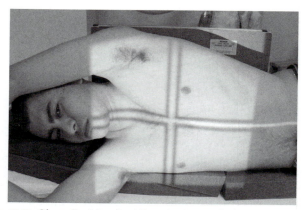

Fig. 16-17 Chest. Position for AP projection (right lateral decubitus position).

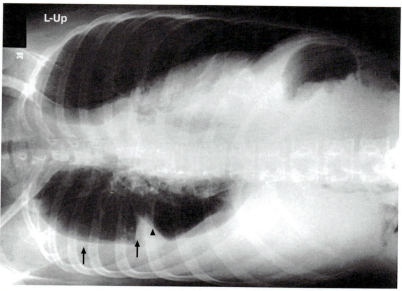

Fig. 16-18 Chest. AP projection, right lateral decubitus position. Fluid is visible in the right pleural cavity *(arrows)*. Note fluid in the fissure between lobes of the lung *(arrowhead)*. Note correct side marker placement, with the "up" side of the chest indicated.

Chest (Lung Apices)

AP Axial Projection (Lordotic Position)

IR: 14 × 17 inches (35 × 43 cm) lengthwise

Grid: Yes

SID: 72 inches (183 cm)

Body position: Standing.

Part position: Patient stands facing tube, 8 to 12 inches (20 to 30 cm) in front of upright Bucky. Patient then arches back and places shoulders against Bucky. Sagittal plane is perpendicular to IR. Backs of hands are placed on hips and shoulders rotated anteriorly (Fig. 16-19). The purpose of the arm position is to rotate scapulae out of the way anteriorly so that they will not be superimposed on lungs. IR is aligned so that upper margin is 3 inches above upper border of shoulder.

Central ray: Perpendicular to center of IR. Center point should be at the level of the midsternum.

> **NOTE:** If the patient is unable to assume the lordotic position, the central ray can be angled 15 degrees cephalad with the patient standing erect. A 30-degree angle may be needed for patients with a shallow chest (small AP diameter).

Collimation: Adjust to 14 × 17 inches (35 × 43 cm) on the collimator.

Patient instruction: Do not move. Stop breathing on second deep inspiration.

Structures seen: Apices of both lungs, free of superimposition by the clavicles (Fig. 16-20).

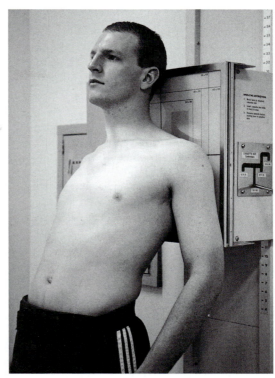

Fig. 16-19 Chest. Position for AP axial projection (lordotic position).

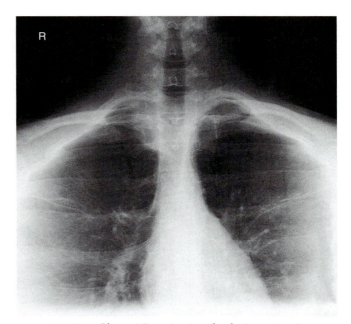

Fig. 16-20 Chest. AP projection (lordotic position).

Ribs

Rib studies may be done with the patient recumbent or upright. Upright positions are usually most comfortable for patients with painful rib injuries. Upright positions may also be safer, decreasing the possibility that pressure on rib fragments will cause puncture of the lung during positioning.

For purposes of radiography, ribs are named both by anatomic location and in relation to the diaphragm. Upper ribs are cephalad to the diaphragm, whereas lower ribs are below the diaphragm. The anterior aspects of the ribs are called the *anterior ribs*, whereas the posterior aspects are called the *posterior ribs*. The lateral aspects are referred to as the *axillary ribs* or *axillary portions*, because they are located within or near the axillary region.

A rib examination usually consists of AP or PA and oblique projections. Some physicians prefer to include chest radiographs because rib fractures may cause significant soft tissue injury that must be evaluated for proper patient care and treatment.

Both anterior and posterior ribs that are within the radiation field are seen on either AP or PA rib projections. However, the ribs nearest the IR are visualized with better detail. It is usual to take AP projections when the area of clinical interest is primarily posterior and to take PA projections for greater detail of the anterior ribs. Variations are acceptable when the preferred position would be too painful for the patient.

AP or PA projections demonstrate the anterior and posterior portions of the ribs, which are in the coronal plane. The axillary (lateral) portions of the ribs are oriented more or less in the sagittal plane and are seen "on end" on the AP or PA projection. For this reason, oblique projections are used to demonstrate the axillary portions of the ribs. Lateral projections are not useful because they result in the superimposition of right and left ribs.

For posterior ribs, the AP oblique projection is taken in the "same side" oblique position, with the side of clinical interest placed nearest the IR. That is, the right posterior oblique (RPO) position is used for right ribs and the left posterior oblique (LPO) position is used for left ribs. For anterior ribs, the correct PA oblique projection is that in which the side of interest is farthest from the IR. The right anterior oblique (RAO) position demonstrates the left ribs, and the left anterior oblique (LAO) position demonstrates the right ribs.

The ribs below the diaphragm require more exposure than the ribs above the diaphragm. This is because the air-containing lung tissues above the diaphragm are much more radiolucent than the dense abdominal tissues below the diaphragm. Separate exposure charts are used for the two areas. The lower ribs are radiographed on expiration to raise the diaphragm, ensuring a uniform tissue density.

Routine Examination

Upper Posterior Ribs: AP and AP Oblique Projections

IR: 14 × 17 inches (35 × 43 cm) lengthwise

Grid: Yes

SID: 40 inches minimum

Body position: Standing or recumbent.

Part position:

AP: Supine on table or upright with posterior surface of chest against upright Bucky or grid holder (Fig. 16-21). Coronal plane is parallel to IR. Upper margin of IR is 1.5 to 2 inches (3.8 to 5 cm) above level of spinous process of C7.

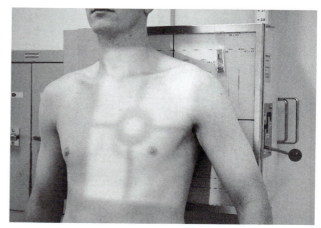

Fig. 16-21 Upper posterior ribs. Position for AP projection, patient upright.

AP oblique: RPO position for right ribs or LPO position for left ribs. Coronal plane forms an angle of 45 degrees with IR plane (Fig. 16-22). Upper margin of IR is 1.5 to 2 inches (3.8 to 5 cm) above level of spinous process of C7.

Central ray:

AP: Perpendicular to center of IR. Center point should be in midclavicular line at approximate level of axillary fold.

AP oblique: Perpendicular to center of IR. Central ray enters at a point on midline of anterior surface at approximate level of axillary fold.

Collimation: Adjust to 14 × 17 inches (35 × 43 cm) on the collimator.

Patient instruction: Do not move. Stop breathing on inspiration.

Structures seen: Ribs 1 through 10. Posterior portions are best seen on AP projection (Fig. 16-23); axillary portions are best seen on oblique projection (Fig. 16-24).

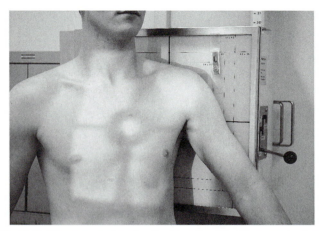

Fig. 16-22 Upper posterior ribs. Position for AP oblique projection, patient upright.

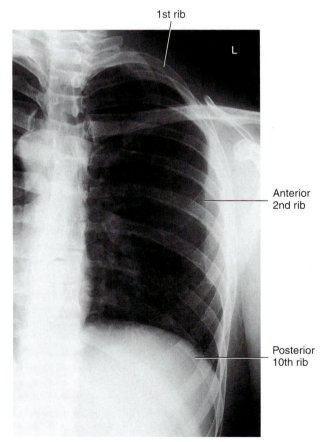

1st rib

L

Anterior 2nd rib

Posterior 10th rib

Fig. 16-23 Upper posterior ribs. AP projection.

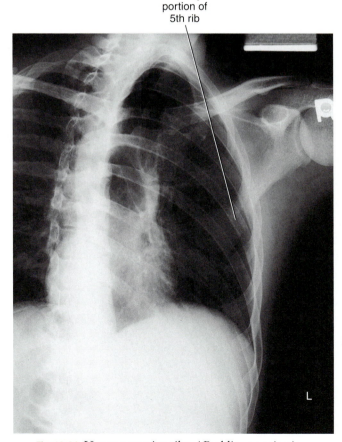

Axillary portion of 5th rib

P

L

Fig. 16-24 Upper posterior ribs. AP oblique projection.

Upper Anterior Ribs: PA and PA Oblique Projections

IR: 14 × 17 inches (35 × 43 cm) lengthwise

Grid: Yes

SID: 40 inches minimum

Body position: Standing or recumbent.

Part position:

PA: Prone on table or upright with anterior surface of chest against upright grid cabinet (Fig. 16-25). Coronal plane is parallel to IR. Upper margin of IR is 1.5 to 2 inches (3.8 to 5 cm) above level of spinous process of C7.

PA oblique: RAO position for left ribs or LAO position for right ribs. Coronal plane forms angle of 45 degrees with IR plane (Fig. 16-27). Upper margin of IR is 1.5 to 2 inches (3.8 to 5 cm) above level of spinous process of C7.

Central ray:

PA: Perpendicular to center of IR. Center point should be in midclavicular line at approximate level of axillary fold.

PA oblique: Perpendicular to center of IR. Central ray enters at point on posterior surface midway between spine and midaxillary line of affected side at approximate level of axillary fold.

Collimation: Adjust to 14 × 17 inches (35 × 43 cm) on the collimator.

Patient instruction: Do not move. Stop breathing on inspiration.

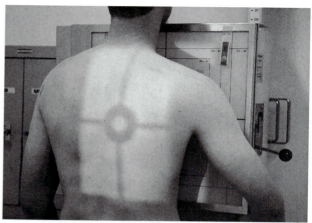

Fig. 16-25 Upper anterior ribs. Position for PA projection, patient upright.

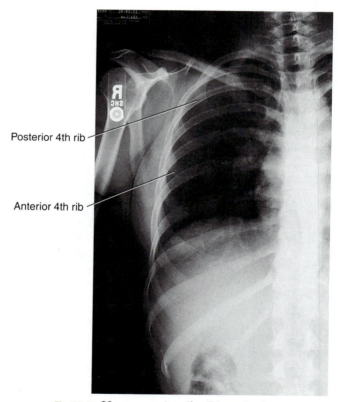

Posterior 4th rib

Anterior 4th rib

Fig. 16-26 Upper anterior ribs. PA projection.

Structures seen: Ribs 1 through 10. Anterior portions are best seen on PA projection (Fig. 16-26); axillary portions are best seen on oblique projection (Fig. 16-28).

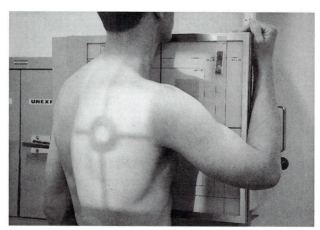

Fig. 16-27 Upper anterior ribs. Position for PA oblique projection, patient upright.

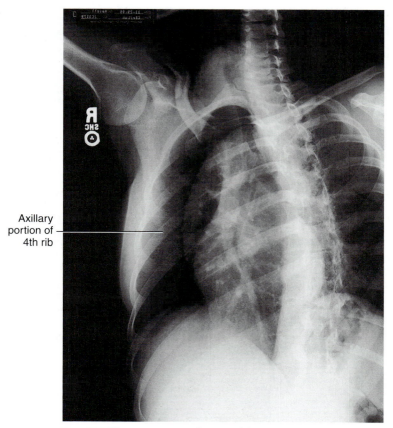

Axillary portion of 4th rib

Fig. 16-28 Upper anterior ribs. PA oblique projection.

Lower Posterior Ribs: AP and AP Oblique Projections

IR: 14 × 17 inches (35 × 43 cm) lengthwise

Grid: Yes

SID: 40 inches minimum

Body position: Standing or recumbent.

Part position:

AP: Supine on table (Fig. 16-29) or upright with posterior surface of chest against upright grid cabinet. Coronal plane is parallel to IR. Lower margin of IR is at level of iliac crest.

AP oblique: RPO position for right ribs or LPO position for left ribs. Coronal plane forms angle of 45 degrees with IR plane (Fig. 16-30). Lower margin of IR is at level of iliac crest.

Central ray:

AP: Perpendicular to center of IR. Center point should be in midclavicular line at approximate level of tip of xiphoid process.

AP oblique: Perpendicular to center of IR. Central ray enters at point on midline of anterior surface at approximate level of tip of xiphoid process.

Collimation: Adjust to 14 × 17 inches (35 × 43 cm) on the collimator. If smaller IR is used, collimate to the smaller size.

Patient instruction: Do not move. Stop breathing on expiration.

Structures seen: Ribs 8 through 12. Posterior portions of ribs are best seen on AP projection (Fig. 16-31); axillary portions are best seen on oblique projection (Fig. 16-32).

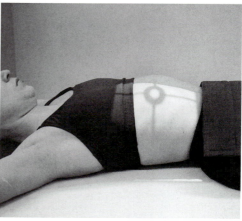

Fig. 16-29 Lower posterior ribs. Position for AP projection, patient recumbent.

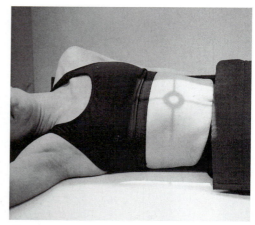

Fig. 16-30 Lower posterior ribs. Position for AP oblique projection, patient recumbent.

Diaphragm

8th rib

11th rib

R

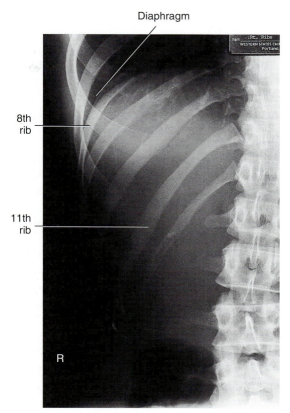

Fig. 16-31 Lower posterior ribs. AP projection.

Diaphragm

11th rib

R

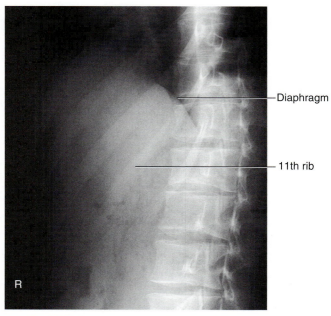

Fig. 16-32 Lower posterior ribs. AP oblique projection.

Abdomen

Radiographic examinations of the abdomen may consist of one or more projections, depending on the purpose of the examination. The basic projection, which is a part of any abdomen study, is the AP projection in the supine position, also called a **KUB.** Although *KUB* stands for "kidneys, ureters, and bladder," this projection is used in many cases in which the urinary tract is not of primary clinical interest.

A radiographic examination for patients with acute abdominal pain will likely include an AP projection in both the supine and upright positions. If the patient is unable to stand for the upright radiograph, the AP projection in the left lateral decubitus position is substituted. The purpose of including upright or decubitus positions is to demonstrate air-fluid levels in the intestines and to visualize free intraperitoneal air, if present. The significance of these findings is discussed in the pathology section of this chapter. For these findings to be most effectively demonstrated, the patient must maintain the upright or decubitus position for several minutes before the radiographer makes the exposure. An upright PA projection of the chest is often included in examinations for acute abdominal pain and can substitute for the upright abdomen position for demonstration of free intraperitoneal air.

In addition to the AP projection in the supine, upright, and decubitus positions, it may sometimes be desirable to take a lateral projection of the abdomen. The lateral projection is necessary to evaluate the abdominal aorta and to localize abdominal foreign bodies that are not within the gastrointestinal tract.

Gonad shielding is required for abdominal radiography of male patients. Properly placed, it does not affect visualization of the contents of the abdominopelvic cavity. Ovarian shields, on the other hand, obscure the pelvic cavity on females and should not be used for abdominal studies. Shielding may be used for females for upright radiographs when the suspected pathology is in the upper and middle portions of the abdomen, and the pelvic portion is well demonstrated on the KUB.

Routine Examination

The routine examination of the abdomen includes the AP projection in the supine position. Supplemental radiographs are produced in the upright and left lateral decubitus positions.

AP Projection (Supine Position)

IR: 14 × 17 inches (35 × 43 cm) lengthwise

Grid: Yes

SID: 40 inches minimum

Body position: Supine.

Part position: Sagittal plane is perpendicular to IR (Fig. 16-33) and knees may be flexed moderately and supported by a bolster. The IR is centered at the level of the iliac crests. Check that inferior margin of IR is at the level of the greater trochanter to ensure inclusion of pelvic floor.

Central ray: Perpendicular to center of IR through a point in midline at level of iliac crest.

Collimation: Adjust to 14 × 17 inches (35 × 43 cm) on the collimator.

Patient instruction: Do not move. Stop breathing on expiration.

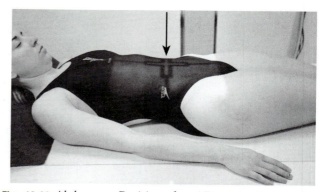

Fig. 16-33 Abdomen. Position for AP projection, patient recumbent.

Structures seen: Abdominal contents between diaphragm and pelvic floor (Fig. 16-34). When exposure is correct, psoas muscles, liver margin, and kidney shadows should be visible.

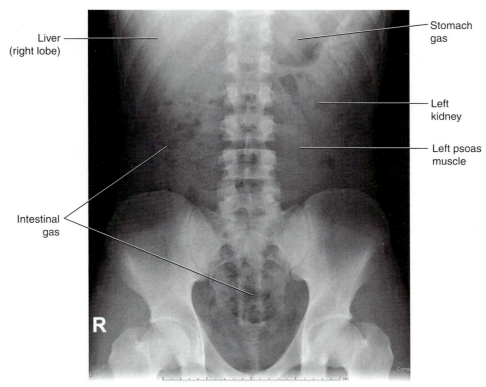

Liver (right lobe)

Stomach gas

Left kidney

Left psoas muscle

Intestinal gas

R

Fig. 16-34 Abdomen. AP projection, patient recumbent.

Supplemental Projections

AP Projection (Upright Position)

IR: 14 × 17 inches (35 × 43 cm) lengthwise

Grid: Yes

SID: 40 inches minimum

Body position: Standing, facing tube.

Part position: Midsagittal plane is centered to IR and perpendicular to it (Fig. 16-35).

Central ray: Perpendicular to center of IR through a point in midline approximately 2 inches superior to level of iliac crest.

Collimation: Adjust to 14 × 17 inches (35 × 43 cm) on the collimator.

Patient instruction: Do not move. Suspend breathing on inspiration.

Structures seen: Abdominal contents between diaphragm and pelvic floor, if included. Diaphragm must be seen at top of IR (Fig. 16-36). Air-fluid levels will be visible in intestines, if present. Free intraperitoneal air, if present, may be seen beneath diaphragm. See Pathology section for discussion of air-fluid levels and free intraperitoneal air.

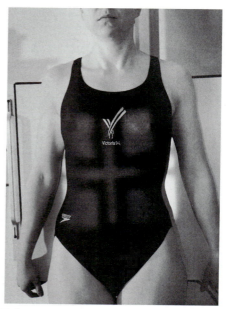

Fig. 16-35 Abdomen. Position for AP projection, patient upright.

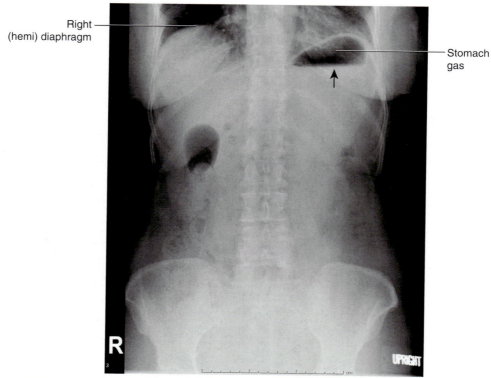

Fig. 16-36 Abdomen. AP projection, patient upright. Note fluid in stomach, visible as a horizontal light line just below the stomach gas *(arrow)*.

AP Projection (Left Lateral Decubitus Position)

IR: 14 × 17 inches (35 × 43 cm) lengthwise

Grid: Yes

SID: 40 inches minimum

Body position: Recumbent on left side on radiographic table or stretcher (Fig. 16-37). If stretcher is used, it is placed in front of upright Bucky. Patient is facing tube.

Part position: Midsagittal plane of abdomen is horizontal and is centered to vertically oriented IR and perpendicular to it.

Central ray: Horizontal and perpendicular to center of IR through a point in midline approximately 2 inches superior to level of iliac crest.

Collimation: Adjust to 14 × 17 inches (35 × 43 cm) on the collimator.

Patient instruction: Do not move. Suspend breathing on inspiration.

Structures seen: Abdominal contents between diaphragm and pelvic floor, if included. Diaphragm must be seen (Fig. 16-38). Levels of air-fluid, if present, will be visible in intestines. Free intraperitoneal air, if present, will be seen near top of IR, along right abdominal wall adjacent to liver. See Pathology section for discussion of air-fluid levels and free intraperitoneal air.

NOTE: Long axis of IR is horizontal, placed lengthwise in relation to the long axis of the abdomen.

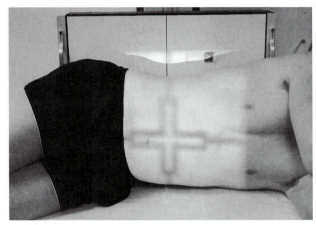

Fig. 16-37 Abdomen. Position for AP projection (left lateral decubitus position).

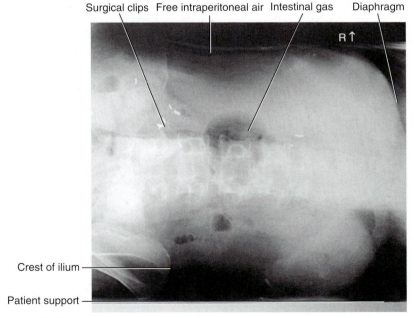

Surgical clips   Free intraperitoneal air   Intestinal gas   Diaphragm

Crest of ilium

Patient support

Fig. 16-38 Abdomen. AP projection (left lateral decubitus position).

PATHOLOGY

Bony Thorax

The most common reason for radiography of the bony thorax is trauma. The young boy in Fig. 16-39 was injured in a car accident. Trauma to the sternum is demonstrated in Fig. 16-40.

Nontraumatic pathology of the bony thorax includes malignant bone disease. Primary neoplastic lesions may occur in the bony thorax. Multiple myeloma is a fairly common example. Metastatic bone lesions also occur in the ribs, often secondary to lung tumors. Osteochondroma (exostosis), a benign bone tumor, is also seen in ribs.

Air-fluid Levels

When fluid is present in a space normally occupied by air, it is an important diagnostic sign of pathology. The interface between air and fluid is usually clearly visible radiographically. The possibility of abnormal air-fluid levels exists in the chest, the abdomen, and the paranasal sinuses (see Chapter 17).

Because fluid is heavier than air, the air will always be above the fluid, and the interface between the air and the fluid will be a horizontal line. *A horizontal x-ray beam is necessary to demonstrate air-fluid levels.* This is easily understood when you look at a glass that contains water. Seen from the top, it is not possible to tell how much water the glass holds. Seen from the side, however, the horizontal line of sight makes the air-fluid level clearly visible (Fig. 16-41). For this reason, upright and/or decubitus positions using a horizontal central ray are *necessary* for demonstration of air-fluid levels.

Chest

Many acute and chronic conditions may affect the organs of the chest, and most can be evaluated radiographically. The scope of this text permits only a very limited introduction to this subject, and examples of some of the common types are offered.

Trauma to the chest may result in lung collapse, called **atelectasis.** Air escaping from the collapsing lung may occupy space in the pleural cavity formerly occupied by the lung. The presence of air in the pleural cavity is called **pneumothorax.** This intrapleural air may also result from penetration of the chest wall. Atelectasis is always present when there is pneumothorax. The lung markings (bronchioles and blood vessels that create the threadlike lines of decreased radiographic density in the lungs) are compressed with atelectasis. The radiographic appearance is such that the lung appears lighter in the collapsed area because the lung markings are very close together. Pneumothorax appears as an absence of lung markings in an area where lung is normally present. Pneumothorax is seen in Fig. 16-42.

Atelectasis may affect a portion of a lung without pneumothorax (Fig. 16-43). The cause may be bronchial obstruction from foreign body or neoplasm. Abscess

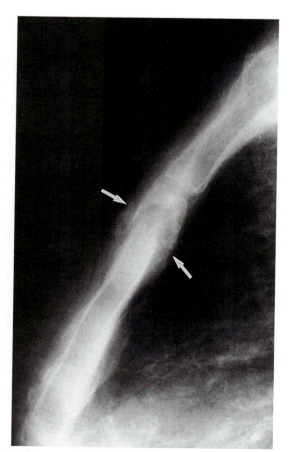

Fig. 16-40 Fracture of sternum (*arrows*) from striking steering wheel in car accident.

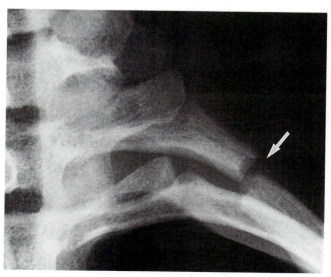

Fig. 16-39 Fracture of left first rib (*arrow*) posteriorly.

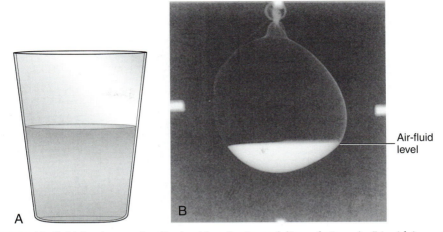

Fig. 16-41 Air-fluid levels are visualized with a horizontal line of view. **A,** Liquid in a glass. **B,** Radiograph of balloon showing air-fluid level.

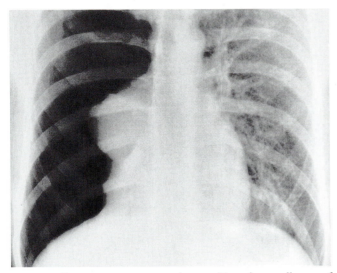

Fig. 16-42 Spontaneous pneumothorax. Complete collapse of right lung.

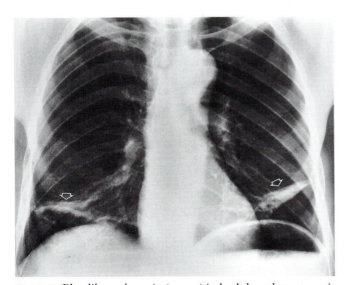

Fig. 16-43 Platelike atelectasis *(arrows)* in both lung bases associated with chronic bronchitis.

(localized infection), emphysema, and chronic bronchitis may also cause atelectasis.

Pneumonia is an inflammation of the lung that is usually caused by bacterial or viral infection. It may also be caused by the inhalation of chemical agents or the aspiration of vomitus. Acute pneumonia causes consolidation of the lung tissue, increased tissue density because of engorgement of the blood vessels, and fluid within spaces that are normally air-filled. Several types of pneumonia are illustrated in Fig. 16-44.

Emphysema, a chronic lung condition, is a type of chronic obstructive pulmonary disease. It is characterized by obstruction and destruction of the small airways and alveoli of the lungs, which results in overinflation of the lungs and the inability to exhale stale air effectively. Chronic overinflation of the lungs increases the AP diameter of the chest and causes depression and flattening of the diaphragm (Fig. 16-45). It is important for radiographers to recognize the outward physical signs of emphysema before performing radiography so that the exposures for chest radiographs may be adjusted appropriately. Patients with emphysema are often described as "barrel-chested." The difference between the PA and lateral chest measurements will be only 8 cm or less. There may be retraction of the costal muscles near the neck with prominence of the clavicles. Patients may practice positive pressure breathing, pursing their lips as they exhale. The large chest measurement does not require a large exposure because the chest volume consists predominantly of air. The milliampere-seconds (mAs) for chest radiographs must be reduced by 30% to 60% from the usual mAs for patients of similar measurement. The actual percentage of mAs reduction necessary depends on the severity of the disease.

Tuberculosis (TB) is an infectious lung disease (Fig. 16-46). Most persons exposed to the TB organism do not develop active disease. The body's immune system walls off the infection so that it becomes dormant. In this inactive stage, the individual has no symptoms and

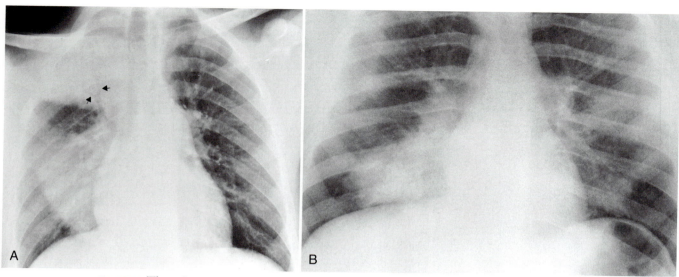

Fig. 16-44 There is great variation in the radiographic appearance of pneumonia. **A,** Bacterial pneumonia with consolidation of right upper lobe and medial and posterior segments of right lower lobe. The air bronchogram *(arrows)* is the air contrast of the upper lobe bronchus seen through the consolidated lung, a diagnostic sign. **B,** Bacterial bronchopneumonia producing ill-defined consolidation in right lung base.

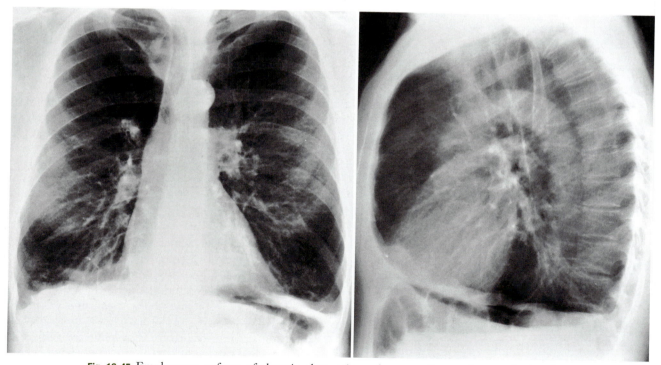

Fig. 16-45 Emphysema, a form of chronic obstructive pulmonary disease characterized radiographically by dark, overinflated lungs and flattened diaphragm.

cannot transmit the disease to others. TB may become active, however, when the immune system is depressed. Malnutrition, human immunodeficiency virus (HIV) infection, other disease processes, or advanced age may allow TB to become active. When dormant TB becomes reactivated, it is called *secondary tuberculosis.* It often affects the apices of the lungs. A chest radiograph in the

lordotic position may be ordered to better visualize this area of the lungs. The primary screening test for TB is the tuberculin skin test. Anyone who has ever contracted the disease will have developed antibodies to the TB organism and will have positive test results. When the skin test result is positive, chest radiographs are taken to rule out active disease. Sputum cultures for TB bacteria

Fig. 16-46 Tuberculosis has different radiographic appearances. **A,** Active, primary tuberculosis in right upper lobe. **B,** Secondary tuberculosis with fibrocalcific changes in both apices.

may be *necessary* to confirm the diagnosis of active disease. Precautions to prevent the spread of active TB are discussed in Chapter 21.

The term **pneumoconiosis** refers to a group of chronic occupational lung diseases caused by the inhalation of irritating dust. One type is silicosis (Fig. 16-47), which results from the inhalation of silicone dioxide. It affects workers in mines, foundries, and sandblasting operations. Other examples of pneumoconiosis include asbestosis and coal miner's disease (black lung).

Lung cancer may arise from the lung tissue, the pleura, or a bronchus. The radiographic appearance differs greatly, depending on the type of tissue involved and the stage of the disease. Fig. 16-48 provides examples of neoplastic lung disease.

Many different malignant diseases metastasize to the lungs. Metastatic lesions may be solitary or multiple and may display a wide variety of radiographic appearances. Fig. 16-49 provides examples of metastatic lung disease.

Congenital malformations, hypertension, and valvular disease may all cause inefficient heart function. The heart tends to become enlarged, and the aorta may become elongated and tortuous. Cardiac insufficiency causes pulmonary edema, the collection of fluid in the tiny spaces within the lung. Advanced cardiac insufficiency with pulmonary edema is called *congestive heart failure* (Fig. 16-50).

Pleural effusion is a collection of fluid in the pleural space (Fig. 16-51). This is a nonspecific radiographic finding with many possible causes. The most common causes are neoplastic disease, congestive heart failure, pulmonary embolism, infection, and pleurisy (inflammation of the pleura). When a patient is in the upright position, the fluid collects in the bottom of the pleural space and gives

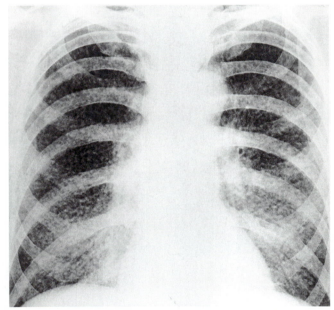

Fig. 16-47 Silicosis, characterized by miliary calcific nodules scattered throughout both lungs.

the appearance of blunting or rounding of the normally sharp costophrenic angles. This is an important reason why both costophrenic angles must always be included on PA chest radiographs.

Abdomen

Many abdominal structures, and particularly the internal contours of abdominal organs, cannot be seen radiographically without the use of contrast media. A contrast

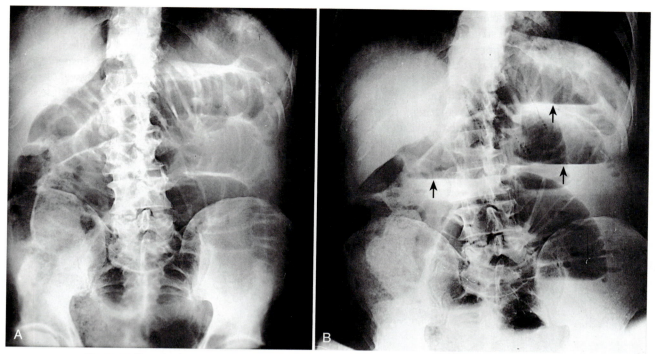

Fig. 16-53 Bowel obstruction. **A,** Supine position shows distended loops of small intestine. **B,** Upright position on the same patient shows air-fluid levels (*arrows*) within small intestine.

distended, gas-filled small intestine. On the upright abdomen radiograph, air-fluid levels are present (Fig. 16-53). The presence of large quantities of gas results in increased radiographic density if routine exposure factors are used. For this reason, it is desirable to decrease the mAs somewhat for abdominal radiography in cases of bowel obstruction.

The term *ruptured hollow viscus* refers to an opening between the gastrointestinal tract and the peritoneal cavity. A ruptured appendix and a perforated ulcer are examples. When this occurs, gas and intestinal contents leak into the peritoneal cavity, causing inflammation and a potentially life-threatening infection called *peritonitis.* Ruptured hollow viscus is diagnosed radiographically by the appearance of gas, or "free air," in the peritoneal cavity outside the gastrointestinal tract. Because gas rises, it is seen on upright position images just beneath the diaphragm (Fig. 16-54). In the left lateral decubitus position, free air rises to the right abdominal wall and is visible along the flank.

The accumulation of fluid in the peritoneal cavity is called *ascites.* When ascites is present, the abdomen tends to be distended and rigid. Ascites is a nonspecific finding that is indicative of serious disease. Examples of conditions that may be associated with ascites include cirrhosis of the liver, neoplastic disease of the intestine, and pelvic inflammatory disease, which is an infection involving the female reproductive organs. Ascites increases the tissue density of the abdomen, which requires an increase in mAs to obtain adequate radiographic density.

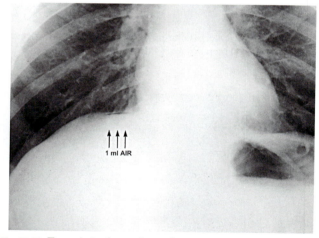

1 ml AIR

Fig. 16-54 Free air in the peritoneal cavity is seen as a thin, black horizontal line under the diaphragm on this upright radiograph.

SUMMARY

The bony thorax consists of the ribs, the sternum, and the thoracic spine. The ribs and sternum are radiographed using relatively low kVp techniques to avoid overpenetrating these small bones. Rib examinations consist of both AP or PA and oblique projections, and procedures vary depending on the region of clinical interest. Different exposures are required, depending on whether the ribs of interest are above or below the diaphragm. Lateral and RAO positions are used to demonstrate the sternum. Both rib and sternum examinations are often done upright for patient comfort and safety. These radiographs are usually taken to demonstrate fractures, but other abnormalities of these skeletal structures may be demonstrated as well.

Chest radiographs demonstrate the heart, lungs, and mediastinum and are commonly taken by limited operators. These radiographs may provide lifesaving information about the condition of vital organs. Routine chest radiography consists of PA and left lateral projections taken upright at 72 inches SID to minimize magnification of the heart. They are exposed on deep inspiration using a grid and high kVp exposure factors. Many inflammatory and neoplastic diseases are evaluated by means of chest radiography, as are conditions caused by trauma or heart problems.

Radiography of the abdomen is less common for limited operators to perform. The AP projection in the supine position, also called the *KUB*, demonstrates the outlines of some abdominal organs and may also reveal calcifications in the urinary or biliary system or abnormal gas patterns in the intestines. Upright or decubitus positions are used to demonstrate air-fluid levels that indicate intestinal obstruction or free intraperitoneal air that is diagnostic of ruptured hollow viscus.

Chapter 17

Skull, Facial Bones, and Paranasal Sinuses

Learning Objectives

At the conclusion of this chapter, you will be able to:

- Name the principal bones that make up the cranium and the face and identify each on an anatomic diagram and on a radiograph
- Name and identify the four sets of paranasal sinuses on an anatomic diagram and on radiographs
- Identify significant positioning landmarks of the skull and face by palpation
- Demonstrate correct body and part positioning for routine projections and common special projections of the skull, facial bones, and paranasal sinuses
- Correctly evaluate radiographs of skull, facial bones, and paranasal sinuses for positioning accuracy
- Describe and recognize on radiographs pathologic conditions that are common to skull, facial bones, and paranasal sinuses

Key Terms

acanthion
blowout fracture
cerebral concussion
contrecoup injury
cranium
external auditory (acoustic) meatus (EAM)
external occipital protuberance
foramen magnum
glabella
gonion
lacrimal bones

mandible
maxilla
mental protuberance (point)
multiple myeloma
nasal concha (pl. conchae)
nasion
orbits
palatine bones
sella turcica
sutures
vomer
zygomas

Skull radiography is much less common than it once was. Today, the first choice for diagnostic imaging in cases of head trauma is the computed tomography (CT) scan, which provides information about the condition of the brain that cannot be obtained with routine radiography. CT is now also the principal imaging modality for the paranasal sinuses and some types of facial injuries.

On the other hand, radiography of the bones of the head is still a useful diagnostic tool. When a CT scanner is not immediately available, radiography can provide much valuable information. In addition, some types of skull pathologic conditions and facial injuries are still best evaluated radiographically.

The anatomy of the bones of the skull and face is complex. A comprehensive understanding of these structures requires diligent study. You will find it helpful to use a model of the skull that allows you to see both the internal and external structures in three-dimensional perspective.

ANATOMY

The skull consists of 22 bones. It is divided into the cranium, which protects the brain, and the facial bones, which provide the facial structure. These bones also contribute to the oral and nasal cavities and form the orbits.

Cranium

The term **cranium** refers to the bones that surround the brain (Fig. 17-1). The portion of the cranium on which the base of the brain rests is the floor and the remainder that surrounds the brain is called the *calvaria*. The cranium consists of eight bones: frontal, occipital, right and left parietal, right and left temporal, sphenoid, and ethmoid.

The frontal bone is the bone of the forehead and also constitutes the anterior portion of the top of the skull. The bony prominence on the frontal bone between the eyebrows is a palpable positioning landmark called the **glabella.** On either side of the glabella, the frontal bone forms the superior portions of the **orbits** (eye sockets).

The occipital bone is at the lower part of the back of the skull and also forms the posterior portion of the cranial floor or base. In the approximate center on the outer surface of the occipital bone is a palpable bony prominence called the **external occipital protuberance.** The large round hole in the anterior portion of the occipital bone is called the **foramen magnum.** It is the passage for the spinal cord between the skull and the spine. Between the frontal and the occipital bones are the two parietal bones.

The ethmoid bone forms the anterior floor of the cranium. It articulates with the underside of the frontal bone, extending inferiorly and posteriorly behind the nose. The ethmoid bone also forms a portion of each orbit.

The sphenoid bone is a complex bone that makes up part of the floor of the cranium and also portions of its lateral outer shell. The sphenoid bone is posterior to the ethmoid bone and is shaped somewhat like a bat (Fig. 17-2).

The rounded fossa in the center of its anterior superior surface, called the **sella turcica,** is the location of the pituitary gland. The bilateral inferior projections are called the *pterygoid processes.*

The temporal bones (Fig. 17-3) also form portions of both the floor and the lateral outer surface of the cranium. They articulate with the sphenoid bone anteriorly and the occipital bone posteriorly. On the inferior lateral border is the **external auditory meatus,** also called the **external acoustic meatus.** Both terms are abbreviated **EAM.** The EAM is the opening to the ear canal and is an important positioning landmark. Extending medially from the EAM area is a dense pyramid of bone called the *petrous portion,* which contains the middle and inner ear structures. The mastoid portion of the temporal bone contains many small air cells, and the mastoid process is palpable just posterior to the earlobe. Just anterior to the EAM is the mandibular fossa, the socket that articulates with the condyle of the mandible. Just superior to the EAM is a long, slender, horizontal bony projection called the *zygomatic process,* which articulates anteriorly with the zygomatic (cheek) bone to form the zygomatic arch.

The joints that connect the bones of the cranium are synarthrodial (immovable) joints called **sutures,** which have individual names. The parietal bones are joined by the sagittal suture. Between the frontal bone and the parietal bones is the coronal suture. Between the parietal bones and the occipital bone is the lambdoidal suture. The joint that joins the parietal and temporal bones is the squamosal suture.

Facial Bones

The palpable bones of the face include the **maxilla, mandible** (jaw), **zygomas** (cheek bones), and nasal bones (Fig. 17-4).

The maxilla is actually two maxillary bones fused in the center beneath the nose. The maxilla is the largest immovable bone of the face and articulates with all of the other facial bones except the mandible. Its upper margins form the inferior medial orbital rims. Its inferior margin, called the *alveolar process,* contains the roots of the upper teeth. The junction of the two maxillary bones forms a superior prominence called the *anterior nasal spine.* This point, located at the junction of the nose and the upper lip, is a positioning landmark called the **acanthion.**

The nasal bones are situated between the orbits and articulate laterally with the maxillary bones and posteriorly with the ethmoid.

The zygoma or zygomatic bone can be palpated as the prominence of the cheek. Each zygoma articulates superiorly with the frontal bone, inferiorly with the

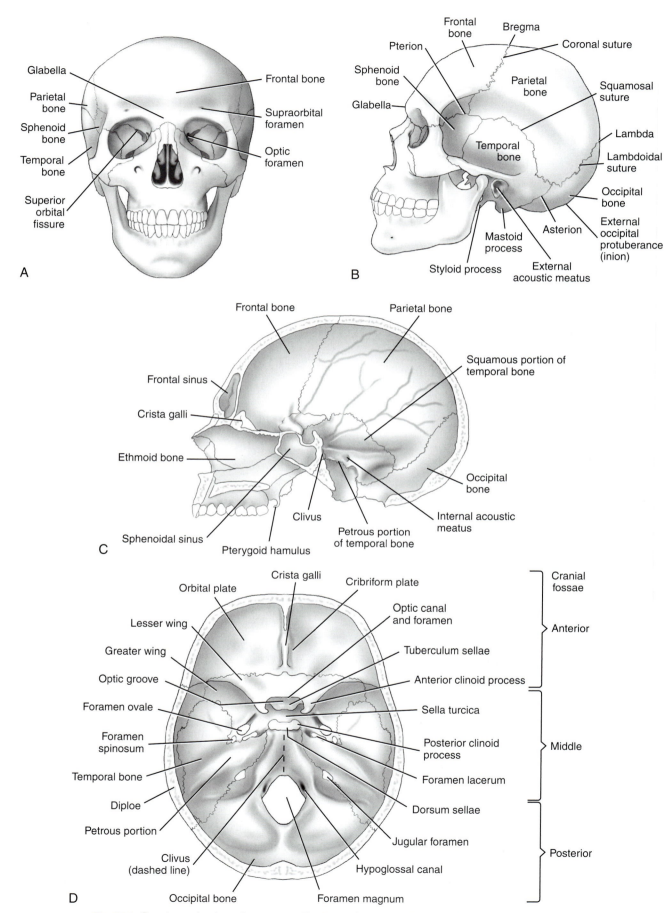

Fig. 17-1 Cranium. **A,** Anterior aspect. **B,** Lateral aspect. **C,** Lateral aspect of interior of cranium. **D,** Superior aspect of cranial base.

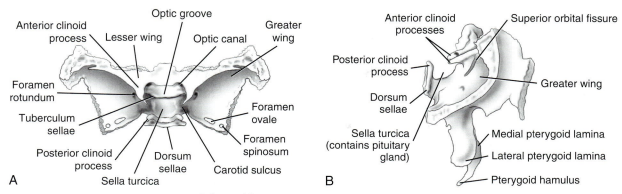

Fig. 17-2 Sphenoid bone. **A,** Superior aspect. **B,** Lateral aspect.

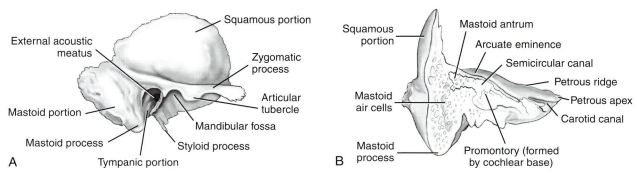

Fig. 17-3 Temporal bone. **A,** Lateral aspect. **B,** Coronal section through mastoid and petrous portions.

maxilla, and posteriorly with the zygomatic process of the temporal bone. The anterosuperior border forms the lateral rim of the orbit.

The mandible, or jaw, is the only movable bone of the face. The horizontal medial portion is called the *body*. Its superior margin is the alveolar process, which contains the roots of the lower teeth. The prominence in the center of its lower margin is called the **mental protuberance** or **mental point** and is a common positioning landmark. Extending superiorly from each end of the mandibular body is a large vertical projection called the mandibular *ramus* (plural, *rami*). The right angle formed by the contour of the inferior posterior ramus is called the *angle of the mandible*, or **gonion**, and is a common positioning landmark. The superior margin of the ramus forms a concave curve called the *mandibular notch*. On the anterior end of the notch is a pointed projection, the coronoid process. The rounded projection on the superior posterior ramus, the mandibular condyle, articulates with the mandibular fossa of the temporal bone to form the temporomandibular joint.

Seven additional small bones that are not externally palpable make up the remainder of the bony structure of the face: the **vomer,** two **palatine bones,** two inferior **nasal conchae,** and two **lacrimal bones.**

The vomer is posterior to the acanthion at the floor of the nasal cavity. It forms the inferior portion of the nasal septum, the wall that divides the nasal cavity. The two palatine bones, together with the maxilla, form the hard palate or roof of the mouth. Three pairs of nasal conchae—superior, middle, and inferior—are thin, curved bony projections that divide the nasal cavity, forming air passages lined with mucous membrane. The superior and middle conchae are projections of the ethmoid bone. The inferior conchae are separate bones that articulate with the maxilla on either side. The lacrimal bones are small, thin bones that form a portion of the medial wall of each orbit.

Paranasal Sinuses

The paranasal sinuses are air-filled cavities within the ethmoid, frontal, and sphenoid bones and within the maxilla (Fig. 17-5). They serve as resonating chambers for the voice and help to warm and moisten inhaled air. The sinuses develop during childhood and are not fully formed until age 16 to 18. At maturity, passages connect the sinuses to each other and to the nasal cavity.

The maxillary sinuses are also called the *maxillary antra* or the *antra of Highmore.* They are the largest paranasal sinuses and are located within the body of the maxilla on either side of the nasal cavity.

The frontal sinuses are the second largest paranasal sinuses and are located in the anterior frontal bone, superior

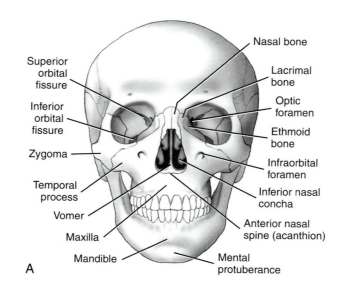

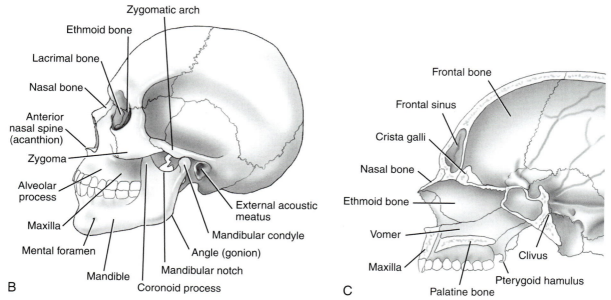

Fig. 17-4 Facial bones. **A,** Anterior aspect. **B,** Lateral aspect. **C,** Interior of facial bones, lateral aspect.

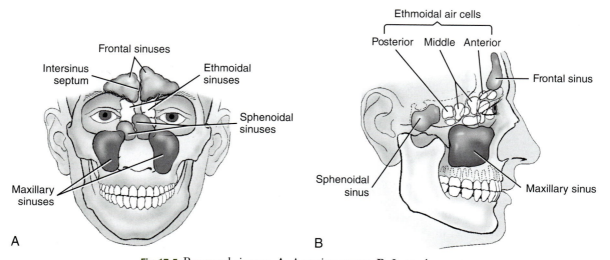

Fig. 17-5 Paranasal sinuses. **A,** Anterior aspect. **B,** Lateral aspect.

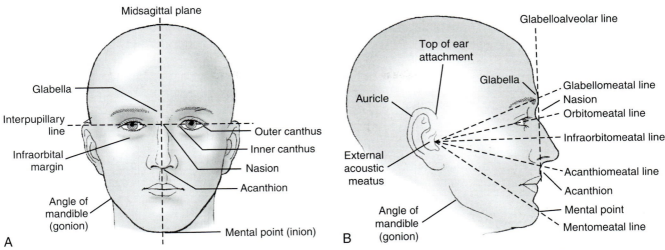

Fig. 17-6 Common landmarks for positioning of the cranium and facial bones. **A,** Anterior aspect. **B,** Lateral aspect.

to the nasal cavity. They are divided by a central septum into right and left compartments and are usually further subdivided. They are not symmetrical and may vary greatly in size and shape. Absence of frontal sinuses is a normal variant.

The sphenoidal sinuses occupy most of the body of the sphenoid bone and are located immediately inferior to the sella turcica. Although they normally occur as a pair of chambers, it is not unusual for only a single chamber to be present.

The two ethmoidal sinuses are located within the lateral masses of the ethmoid bone and consist of a varying number of small air cells. They are situated between and behind the orbits and anterior to the sphenoid sinuses.

POSITIONING AND RADIOGRAPHIC EXAMINATIONS

Fig. 17-6 illustrates the landmarks used for radiographic positioning of the cranium, facial bones, and paranasal sinuses. Note the locations of landmarks mentioned previously in this chapter: glabella, acanthion, gonion, and mental point. Another significant landmark is the **nasion,** the anterior depression in the midline of the skull between the orbits. Note also the positioning lines used to judge the degree of flexion or extension of the neck that is appropriate for skull positions. Those lines that are used in this text are the orbitomeatal line (OML), the infraorbitomeatal line (IOML), and the mentomeatal line (MML).

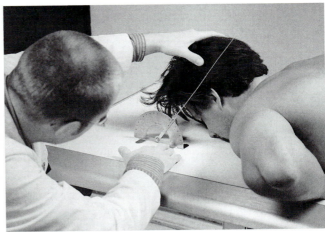

Fig. 17-7 Angligner assists in positioning skull with baselines correctly aligned with regard to IR.

Accurate positioning for radiographic examinations of the skull requires precise attention to all three body planes: coronal, sagittal, and transverse. The coronal and sagittal planes are adjusted by body position and rotation of the head. The transverse plane alignment depends on the flexion or extension of the neck. To determine the alignment between body planes or positioning lines and the image receptor (IR) plane, it is helpful to use a tool called an *Angligner* (Fig. 17-7). In the absence of such a tool, a simple protractor or triangles cut from cardboard provide a useful guide.

Cranium

The projections chosen for skull radiography depend on physician preferences and the ability of the patient to assume the required body positions. For example, either a posteroanterior (PA) or a PA axial projection (Caldwell method) will be included in the routine examination, but not both. The PA axial projection is most common.

Although the side nearest the IR is best demonstrated on the lateral projection, some physicians prefer a basic series that includes both right and left lateral projections. The anteroposterior (AP) or AP axial projection and PA axial projection (Haas method) can be substituted when the patient cannot assume the positions needed for the customary projections.

Routine Examination

The routine examination of the cranium includes the PA or PA axial (Caldwell method), AP axial (Towne method), and lateral projections.

PA and PA Axial Projection (Caldwell Method)

IR: 10 × 12 inches (24 × 30 cm) lengthwise

Grid: Yes

Source–image Receptor Distance (SID): 40 inches minimum

Body position: Prone or seated facing upright Bucky.

> **TIP:** When the prone patient crosses the arms under the chest, this elevation of the thorax allows greater flexion of the neck. This facilitates accurate positioning and relieves pressure on the nose.

Part position: Sagittal plane of skull is perpendicular to center of IR, with forehead and nose resting on table or against upright Bucky. Neck flexion adjusted to place OML perpendicular to IR (Fig. 17-8).

Central ray:

PA: Perpendicular to center of IR through nasion.

PA axial (Caldwell method): Angled 15 degrees caudad to center of IR through nasion (Fig. 17-10).

Collimation: Adjust to 10 × 12 inches (24 × 30 cm) on the collimator.

Patient instruction: Do not move. Stop breathing.

Structures seen: Frontal bone and outer contours of cranium from frontal perspective. When perpendicular central ray is used, petrous pyramids are projected within orbits (Fig. 17-9). When a 15-degree caudad angle with the Caldwell method is used, petrous pyramids are projected through the lower third of the orbit and the orbital margins are more clearly demonstrated (Fig. 17-11).

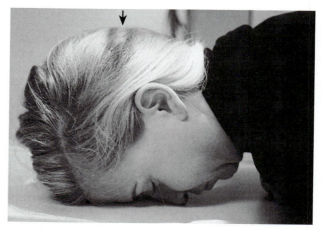

Fig. 17-8 Cranium. Position for PA projection.

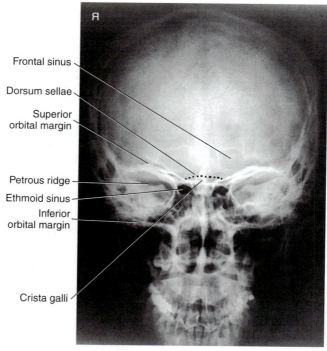

Frontal sinus
Dorsum sellae
Superior orbital margin
Petrous ridge
Ethmoid sinus
Inferior orbital margin
Crista galli

Fig. 17-9 Cranium. PA projection.

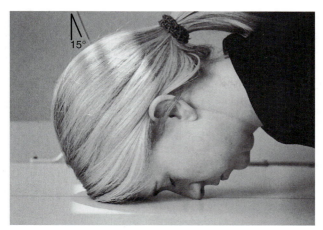

Fig. 17-10 Cranium. Position for PA axial projection (Caldwell method).

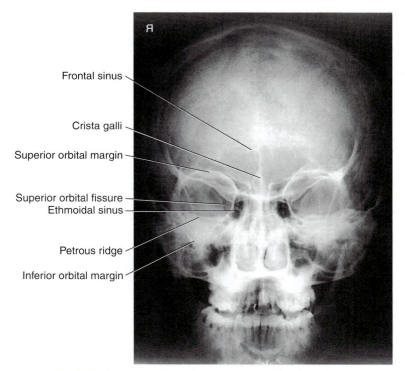

Frontal sinus

Crista galli

Superior orbital margin

Superior orbital fissure
Ethmoidal sinus

Petrous ridge

Inferior orbital margin

Fig. 17-11 Cranium. PA axial projection (Caldwell method).

AP Axial Projection (Towne Method)

IR: 10 × 12 inches (24 × 30 cm) lengthwise

Grid: Yes

SID: 40 inches minimum

Body position: Supine or seated.

Part position: Sagittal plane of skull is perpendicular to IR with back of head resting on table or against upright Bucky. Neck flexion adjusted to place OML perpendicular to IR (Fig. 17-12).

> **TIP:** If patient is unable to flex neck sufficiently to get OML perpendicular to IR, placement of a wedge sponge under the head may assist in attaining correct position.

Central ray: Angled 30 degrees caudad to center of IR through the foramen magnum at the level of the EAM. Central ray enters skull in midsagittal plane, approximately 2.5 inches superior to glabella.

> **TIP:** If the patient is unable to flex the neck sufficiently to get the OML perpendicular to the IR, the IOML can be placed perpendicular and the central ray angled 37 degrees caudad.

Collimation: Adjust to 10 × 12 inches (24 × 30 cm) on the collimator.

Patient instruction: Do not move. Stop breathing.

Structures seen: Occipital bone, posterior parietal bones, foramen magnum, and petrous portions of temporal bones (Fig. 17-13).

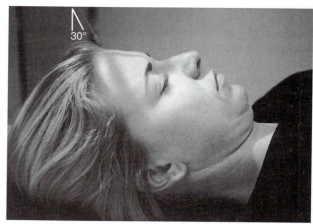

Fig. 17-12 Cranium. Position for AP axial projection (Towne method).

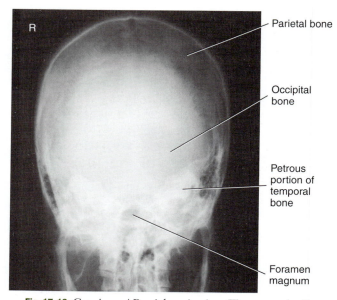

Fig. 17-13 Cranium. AP axial projection (Towne method).

Lateral Projection

IR: 10 × 12 inches (24 × 30 cm) crosswise

Grid: Yes

SID: 40 inches minimum

Body position: Recumbent or seated in an anterior oblique body position with side of interest nearest IR (Fig. 17-14).

Part position: Sagittal plane of head is parallel to IR and interpupillary line is perpendicular to it (Fig. 17-15). Support under mandible may assist in maintaining this position. Neck flexion is adjusted to place the IOML parallel to the long axis of the IR.

Central ray: Perpendicular to center of IR through a point approximately 2 inches superior to EAM.

Collimation: Adjust to 10 × 12 inches (24 × 30 cm) on the collimator.

Patient instruction: Do not move. Stop breathing.

Structures seen: Lateral image of entire cranium. Sella turcica is seen in profile. There should be no rotation or tilt of cranium, and paired structures should be superimposed (Fig. 17-16). Side nearest IR is most clearly seen.

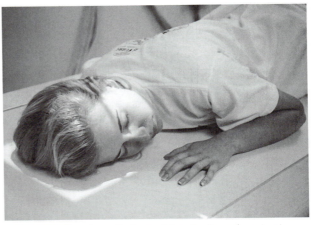

Fig. 17-14 Cranium. Body position for lateral projection.

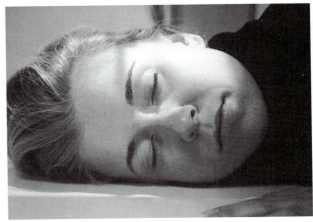

Fig. 17-15 Cranium. Position for lateral projection.

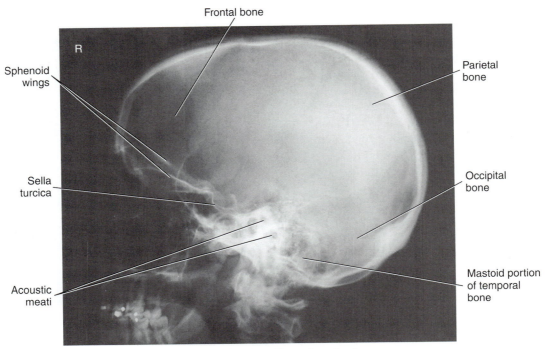

Fig. 17-16 Cranium. Lateral projection.

Alternative Projections

AP and AP Axial ("Reverse" Caldwell Method) Projections

When obesity or injury makes it difficult to position the patient prone, an AP projection may be substituted for the PA or PA axial (Caldwell method) projection. Radiation dose to the eyes and thyroid gland is increased compared with the PA projections.

IR: 10 × 12 inches (24 × 30 cm) lengthwise

Grid: Yes

SID: 40 inches minimum

Body position: Supine or seated.

Part position: Sagittal plane of skull is perpendicular to IR with back of head resting on table or against upright Bucky. Neck flexion adjusted to place OML perpendicular to IR (Fig. 17-17).

> **TIP:** If the patient is unable to flex the neck sufficiently to get the OML perpendicular to the IR, placement of a wedge sponge under the head may assist in maintaining the correct position.

Central ray:

AP: Perpendicular to center of IR through nasion.

AP axial ("reverse" Caldwell method): Angled 15 degrees cephalad through nasion.

Collimation: Adjust to 10 × 12 inches (24 × 30 cm) on the collimator.

Patient instruction: Do not move. Stop breathing.

Structures seen: Frontal bone and outer contours of cranium from frontal perspective. When a perpendicular central ray is used, petrous pyramids are projected within the orbits (Fig. 17-18). With the "reverse" Caldwell method, using a 15-degree cephalad angle, petrous pyramids are projected through the lower third of the orbit and the orbital margins are more clearly demonstrated. The orbits and other anterior structures are magnified in comparison to PA projections.

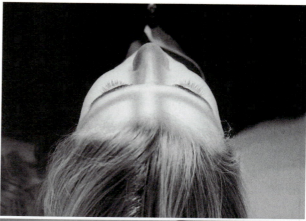

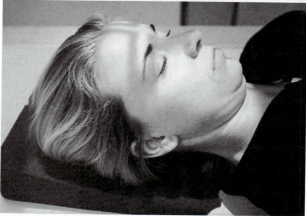

Fig. 17-17 Cranium. Position for AP projection.

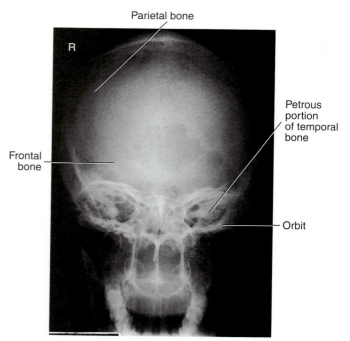

Fig. 17-18 Cranium. AP projection.

PA Axial Projection (Haas Method)

The PA axial projection (Haas method) may be used instead of the AP axial projection (Towne method). The Haas method is useful when obesity or exaggerated kyphosis of the thoracic spine makes it difficult for the patient to assume a supine position with the OML perpendicular to the IR or nearly so. Both the patient position and the tube angle are reversed. The resulting radiograph is similar to the AP axial projection (Towne method), but detail of the posterior structures is somewhat compromised because of the increased object–image receptor distance (OID).

IR: 10 × 12 inches (24 × 30 cm) lengthwise

Grid: Yes

SID: 40 inches minimum

Body position: Prone or seated facing IR.

Part position: Sagittal plane of skull is perpendicular to IR with forehead and nose resting on table or against upright Bucky. Neck flexion is adjusted to place OML perpendicular to IR (Fig. 17-19).

Central ray: Angled 25 degrees cephalad to center of IR through a point 1.5 inches below external occipital protuberance. Central ray exits skull in midsagittal plane at location approximately 1.5 inches superior to nasion.

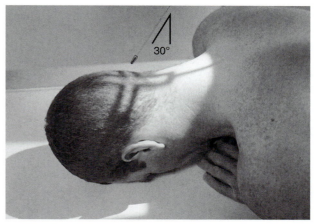

Fig. 17-19 Cranium. Position for PA axial projection (Haas method).

Collimation: Adjust to 10 × 12 inches (24 × 30 cm) on the collimator.

Patient instruction: Do not move. Stop breathing.

Structures seen: Occipital bone, posterior parietal bones, foramen magnum, and petrous portions of temporal bones (Fig. 17-20).

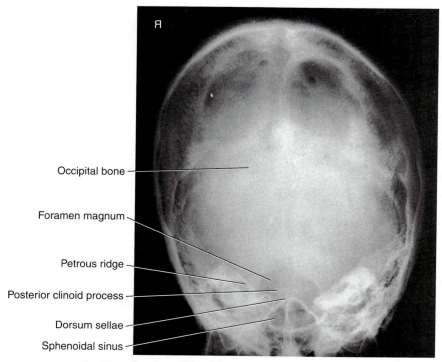

Occipital bone

Foramen magnum

Petrous ridge

Posterior clinoid process

Dorsum sellae

Sphenoidal sinus

Fig. 17-20 Cranium. PA axial projection (Haas method).

Supplemental Projection

Submentovertical Projection

The submentovertical projection is added to the routine examination when it is desired to demonstrate the structures of the cranial base more completely than they are seen with the Towne method. It is especially helpful for demonstration of the sphenoid bone and the cranial foramina.

IR: 10 × 12 inches (24 × 30 cm) lengthwise

Grid: Yes

SID: 40 inches minimum

Body position: Supine with shoulders and thorax elevated and supported to place top of head against table, or seated with back to IR and back arched to place top of head against upright Bucky.

Part position: Sagittal plane of head is perpendicular to IR. Neck is extended as much as possible with head resting on its vertex. Neck extension is adjusted to place IOML parallel to IR or as near parallel as possible (Fig. 17-21).

Central ray: Perpendicular to IOML through midline and passing through a point 0.75 inches anterior to the level of the EAM.

Collimation: Adjust to 10 × 12 inches (24 × 30 cm) on the collimator.

Patient instruction: Do not move. Stop breathing.

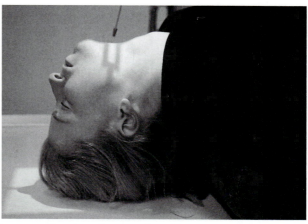

Fig. 17-21 Cranium. Position for submentovertical projection.

Structures seen: Cranial base, including occipital bone, foramen magnum, sphenoid and ethmoid bones, and petrous portions of temporal bone (Fig. 17-22). Foramina ovale and spinosum are also demonstrated on this projection.

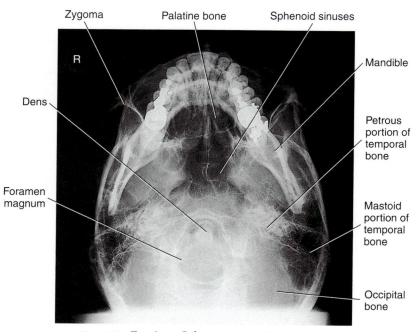

Fig. 17-22 Cranium. Submentovertical projection.

Facial Bones

Routine Examination

The routine examination of the facial bones includes the PA axial (Caldwell method), parietoacanthial (Waters method), and lateral projections.

PA Axial Projection (Caldwell Method)

The PA axial projection (Caldwell method) is performed the same as the PA axial projection of the cranium (Caldwell method) described earlier.

Structures seen: Orbits, zygomatic bones, maxilla, nasal septum, and a portion of the mandible (Fig. 17-23). The petrous ridges are projected into the lower third of the orbits.

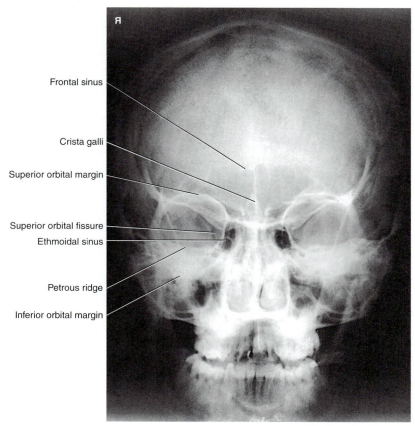

Frontal sinus

Crista galli

Superior orbital margin

Superior orbital fissure
Ethmoidal sinus

Petrous ridge

Inferior orbital margin

Fig. 17-23 Facial bones. PA axial projection (Caldwell method).

Parietoacanthial Projection (Waters Method)

IR: 8 × 10 inches (18 × 24 cm) lengthwise

Grid: Yes

SID: 40 inches minimum

Body position: Standing, seated, or recumbent, facing IR.

Part position: Neck is extended with chin resting on table or upright Bucky. Neck flexion is adjusted so that MML is perpendicular to IR and OML forms a 37-degree angle to IR (Fig. 17-24). Sagittal plane is perpendicular to IR.

> **TIP:** When patient is correctly positioned, the distance between the table or upright Bucky and the tip of the nose should be about 0.75 inches or the width of the index finger.

Central ray: Perpendicular to IR to exit at the acanthion.

> **NOTE:** Should be done upright, with a horizontal beam, to show air-fluid levels.

Collimation: Adjust to 8 × 10 inches (18 × 24 cm) on the collimator.

Patient instruction: Do not move. Stop breathing.

Structures seen: Maxilla, orbits, zygomatic arches, and nasal septum (Fig. 17-25).

> **TIP:** The petrous portion of the temporal bone should be projected beneath the maxillary sinus. If it is superimposed over the floor of the sinus, a greater degree of neck extension is necessary.

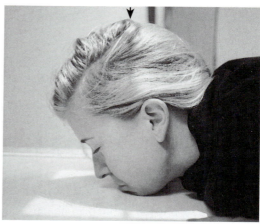

Fig. 17-24 Facial bones. Position for parietoacanthial projection (Waters method).

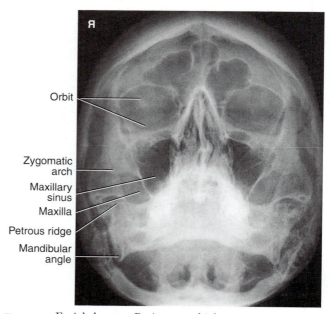

Orbit

Zygomatic arch

Maxillary sinus

Maxilla

Petrous ridge

Mandibular angle

Fig. 17-25 Facial bones. Parietoacanthial projection (Waters method).

Lateral Projection

The lateral projection is performed the same as for the lateral projection of the cranium described earlier, with the following exceptions.

IR: 8 × 10 inches (18 × 24 cm) lengthwise

Central ray: Perpendicular to center of IR through a point approximately halfway between outer canthus and EAM (Fig. 17-26).

Collimation: Adjust to 8 × 10 inches (18 × 24 cm) on the collimator.

Structures seen: Lateral image of all facial bones, with superimposition of paired bones (Fig. 17-27).

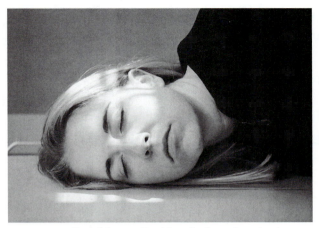

Fig. 17-26 Facial bones. Position for lateral projection.

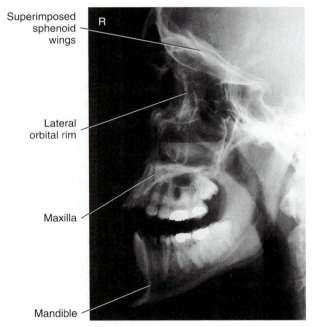

Fig. 17-27 Facial bones. Lateral projection.

Supplemental Projections

Verticosubmental Projection of Zygomatic Arches

The zygomatic arches are seen on the submentovertical projection of the skull. Alternatively, the position may be reversed to provide a verticosubmental projection.

IR: 8 × 10 inches (18 × 24 cm) crosswise

Body position: Prone or seated facing IR.

Part position: Neck is extended with chin resting on table or upright Bucky. Neck flexion is adjusted to place IOML nearly parallel to IR (Fig. 17-28). Sagittal plane is perpendicular to IR.

Central ray: Angled caudad, perpendicular to the IOML and passing through the midsagittal plane 1.5 inches posterior to the level of the outer canthus.

Collimation: Adjust to 8 × 10 inches (18 × 24 cm) on the collimator.

Patient instruction: Do not move. Stop breathing.

Structures seen: Zygomatic arches free of superimposition (Fig. 17-29).

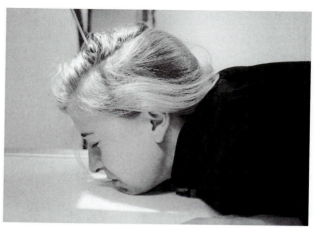

Fig. 17-28 Zygomatic arches. Position for verticosubmental projection.

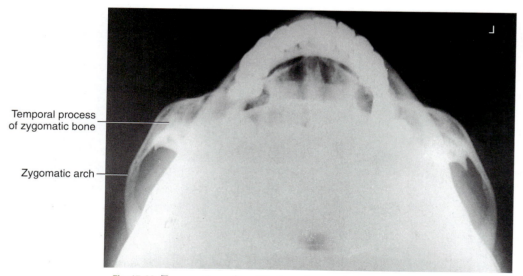

Temporal process of zygomatic bone

Zygomatic arch

Fig. 17-29 Zygomatic arches. Verticosubmental projection.

Lateral Projection of Nasal Bones

The nasal bones are very thin, so exposure factors similar to those used for a finger are used. Both lateral projections may be performed on a single IR, because these are paired bones.

IR: 8 × 10 inches (18 × 24 cm) crosswise for two exposures on one IR

Grid: No

SID: 40 inches minimum

Body position: Same as for cranium and facial bones.

Part position: Same as for cranium and facial bones (Fig. 17-30).

Central ray: Perpendicular to IR to midpoint of nasal bone.

Collimation: Adjust to 3 × 3 inches (8 × 8 cm) on the collimator, with the field extending from the glabella to the acanthion and 0.5 inches (1.3 cm) beyond the tip of the nose.

Patient instruction: Do not move. Stop breathing.

Structures seen: Lateral image of the nasal bone closest to the IR, the anterior nasal spine, and associated soft tissue (Fig. 17-31). Both lateral projections are usually taken.

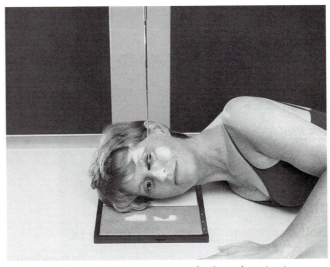

Fig. 17-30 Nasal bones. Position for lateral projection.

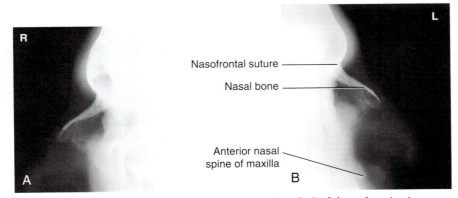

Nasofrontal suture

Nasal bone

Anterior nasal spine of maxilla

Fig. 17-31 Nasal bones. **A,** Right lateral projection. **B,** Left lateral projection.

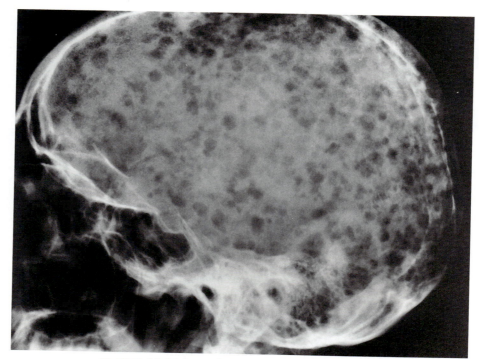

Fig. 17-56 Multiple myeloma as manifested in the skull.

illustrates multiple lytic lesions of **multiple myeloma,** a malignant bone disease that may involve many bones of the body.

SUMMARY

Radiography of the skull, facial bones, and paranasal sinuses is less common than it once was, having been replaced in many cases by CT studies and sometimes MRI. Radiography of the head is most common today for evaluation of bone disease in the skull, for screening for facial fractures, and for evaluation of the paranasal sinuses when CT is not readily available.

The bones that make up the cranium and facial structures are complex and require careful study. All are immovable, with the exception of the mandible, and are joined by synarthrodial joints called *sutures.* Proper positioning

requires attention to all three body planes and the use of bony landmarks and positioning lines. The most common positioning line for alignment of the transverse plane is the OML between the midpoint of the lateral orbital margin and the EAM.

The basic projections for radiography of the skull, face, and sinuses are AP, PA, lateral, submentovertical, and parietoacanthial (Waters method). Variations in tube angle are used to project structures of interest with the least distortion and free of superimposition by structures that could compromise visualization. The submentovertical and verticosubmental projections are used to demonstrate the cranial base, the zygomatic arches, and the sphenoid sinuses.

There are four sets of paranasal sinuses, named for the bones in which they are located: maxillary, frontal, ethmoid, and sphenoid. The sinuses are radiographed with the patient in the upright position to visualize air-fluid levels.

Chapter 18

Radiography of Pediatric and Geriatric Patients

Learning Objectives

At the conclusion of this chapter, you will be able to:

- Demonstrate appropriate levels of communication with children of any age
- Immobilize an infant or toddler for a radiographic examination
- Compare the characteristics of the developing skeleton with those of the mature skeleton
- Formulate exposures for pediatric radiographic techniques
- Identify pediatric radiographic examinations that vary in method from adult examinations
- List signs that suggest the possibility of nonaccidental trauma in children
- List considerations that improve communication and compliance when dealing with older patients
- Describe changes that occur to the skeleton and the soft tissues as a result of aging
- Adjust radiographic exposures appropriately for patients with osteoporosis and/or advanced age
- List and describe three pathologic conditions common to pediatric patients
- List and describe three pathologic conditions common to geriatric patients

Key Terms

Alzheimer disease
aspiration
battered child syndrome
decubitus ulcers
demineralization
diverticulitis
geriatrics

nonaccidental trauma (NAT)
organic brain syndrome
osteopenia
osteoporosis
Parkinson disease
pediatrics
valid choice

The term **pediatrics** refers to the care of children. **Geriatrics** is the term for the care of elder adults. This chapter is divided into two parts, one devoted to the special needs of infants and children and the other to the requirements of older adults. Pediatric and geriatric patients have the same needs as other patients: confidence and reassurance, safety and security, and comfort and competent care. It is in the ways these needs are met that their requirements differ.

This chapter offers strategies for effective communication with both pediatric and geriatric patients in the clinical setting. It also covers variations in the skeletons and soft tissues of these patients and the exposure adjustments required for successful radiography. Instructions are provided for immobilizing infants and small children. Pediatric procedures that vary from the methods used for adults are addressed as well. Pathologic conditions unique or especially common to the very young and the very old are also presented.

PEDIATRICS

Communication

Relating to a child can be difficult for those who have little experience with children. Even successful parents sometimes have problems relating to other people's children. This is a skill that improves with practice. If relating to children does not come easily for you, experience with children without the stress of the workplace may help. Consider spending an afternoon at the park with children of a relative or friend. Make it a point to get acquainted with a neighbor's child. When introduced to a child, make a special effort to relate in a comfortable way.

Children tend to be more intuitive than adults. They can usually sense when you really care about them. If your real concern is whether you will get off duty on time or whether your employer will be satisfied with the images, the child will not be fooled by your pretended interest. To gain a child's trust, your interest and concern must be genuine.

Effective communication is age appropriate and shows both respect and concern. We communicate both verbally and nonverbally. Research indicates that about 70% of communication received by adults is nonverbal. That is, we learn far more from posture, body language, facial expression, and tone of voice than from what is actually said. Positive touch is both firm and gentle and is also an important aspect of nonverbal communication. There are no available figures for the percentage of communication received by children that is nonverbal, but it is presumed to be even higher than for adults.

Children are more likely to have a positive attitude about radiography if they perceive your facility to be a child-friendly place. Some small furniture and an assortment of books and games (Fig. 18-1) will help them feel welcome and will keep them occupied if they must wait. At the very least, it is helpful to have a few toys or interesting objects that can capture the attention of children of different ages (Fig. 18-2). One inexpensive item that appeals to a wide age range is stickers. They may be used as a get-acquainted gift and/or a reward for good behavior.

Neonate and Infant (Birth to 1 Year)

The neonatal period includes the first month of life (Fig. 18-3). During this stage, infant behavior is mostly reflexive and is influenced by your face, voice, and touch.

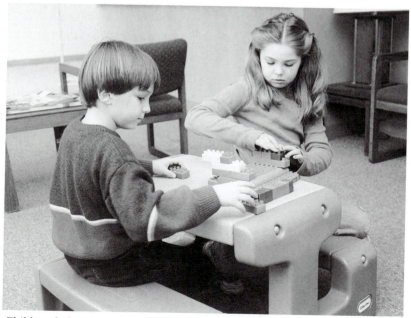

Fig. 18-1 Children feel welcome when the clinic waiting room has an area in which they can play.

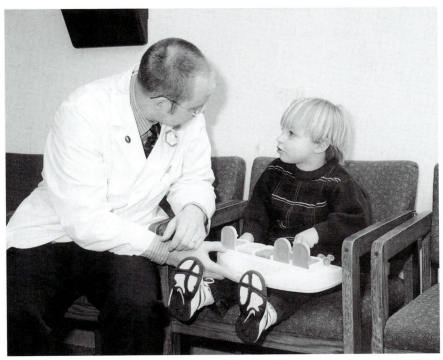

Fig. 18-2 Toys or other interesting objects may serve to distract a frightened child.

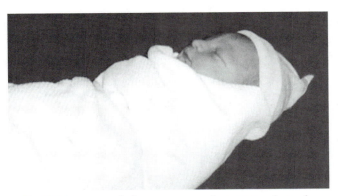

Fig. 18-3 Neonates feel most secure when wrapped snugly.

Some important things to remember when dealing with infants in the first month of life include the following:
1. They like to be bundled up. They feel more secure when they are warm and snugly wrapped.
2. They like to be held firmly and gently. It may help settle them if you rock them or walk around with them.
3. They relate to faces. They like eye contact, but they cannot focus very far away, so closeness is good.
4. They respond to the sound of voices long before they can understand words. Talk to them softly as you work.

The period from 1 month to 1 year of age is characterized by rapid physical growth and development. There is a progression from reflexive to more purposeful behavior. Two- and three-month-old infants smile because it elicits a response from others. Sucking, chewing, and vocalizing

are important oral activities. By 8 months of age, infants begin to differentiate themselves from others. They recognize familiar persons, such as their parents, and they fear strangers and unfamiliar situations. At 9 months, infants experience separation anxiety. Keep infants and parents together as much as possible, limit the number of staff, and provide familiar objects, such as a blanket, toy, or pacifier. Employing familiar objects and incorporating play will serve to distract the infant during the exam.

Always provide a safe environment. Never leave an infant on a flat surface unattended, keep the crib rails up at all times, and immobilize the infant during the exam whenever it is necessary.

Toddler (1 to 2 Years)

Toddlers start walking between 10 and 14 months of age and start to communicate using two- and three-word sentences. They like to explore and manipulate their environment.

Strange adults are often intimidating to children because of their stature, so try to speak to children at their own eye level (Fig. 18-4). You will find that this is especially helpful when you approach the child to "make friends" before the radiographic procedure. If you are calm, cheerful, and unhurried, the toddler is much less likely to respond negatively to the strange surroundings and machines. Allowing the toddler to take a favorite blanket or toy to the radiology department can help promote a feeling of security. Talk to toddlers and play with them to distract them during the exam and reduce their stress. Even if they do not understand all you say, a cheerful voice is reassuring. Prepare the toddler shortly before

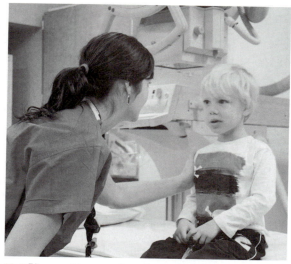

Fig. 18-4 Use positive touch and eye contact at the child's eye level.

the procedure and use demonstration in addition to spoken instructions. When directions are given, keep them short and simple, giving one direction at a time, because toddlers have a short attention span. They need lots of reminders and lots of patience.

Toddlers are quite attached to their parents, but are also beginning to assert their independence because they are mobile and have the ability to do more for themselves. Resistance to control by parents or health care workers can result in negative behaviors, such as temper tantrums. Respond to these behaviors using a friendly but firm approach, and set limits by stating, "You must lie still." Allow the toddler choices when possible and, when necessary, explain to parents that immobilization techniques will need to be used to obtain the child's radiographic images.

Preschooler (3 to 5 Years)

Children at this age (Fig. 18-5) require somewhat different approaches to care and communication. They are demonstrating increasing independence, they are conversational and able to share information with you, and they can cooperate more fully, but they also fear a loss of self-control and need to make valid choices even more than adults do. A **valid choice** is one in which either alternative is acceptable to you. For example, you might ask, "Would you like to wear a blue gown or a red one?" or "Would you like to get up on the table by yourself or would you like me to help you?" Asking, "Would you like to lie down here?" is *not* a valid choice. If the child must lie down for the procedure, there is no choice involved, and if the child answers "No," you have placed yourself in an awkward position. Although children have no choice about submitting to the examination, they should be encouraged to cooperate as much as possible. Apprehensive children do not feel reassured by such statements as, "This won't hurt a bit." All too frequently, the only word they assimilate is "hurt," and they become even more frightened. Asking, "Have you ever had your picture taken by x-ray?" allows you to add whatever simple explanation is necessary. The statement "We're going to take a picture of your leg with this special big camera so

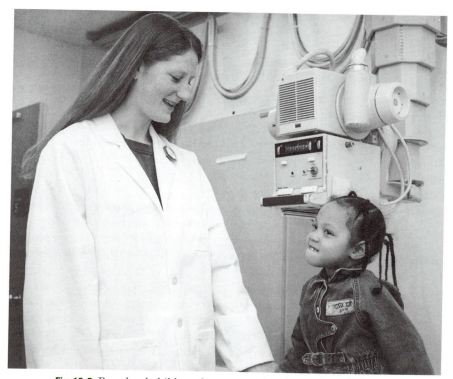

Fig. 18-5 Preschool children demonstrate increasing independence.

your doctor can see why it hurts" is understandable to most children in this age group.

Preschoolers will want to understand what you are doing. They are curious and will probably ask questions. Keep your explanations simple, direct, and honest. Too much detail may be frightening or boring, especially if they do not understand all you say. Avoid stating how many pictures you plan to take. These children will count, and if additional images are necessary, you may lose credibility. Honest praise is a good motivator.

School Age (6 to 12 Years)

Children in this age group can think logically about anything that can be touched and seen. Give specific information about the examination (Fig. 18-6); be explicit about the body areas or parts that will be involved. Be honest and let them know whether or not they will experience any pain or discomfort. Although they have an increased attention span and reasoning skills, continue to use demonstrations or models to explain the examination. They want to be brave and are usually willing to help (Fig. 18-7). Most respond readily to humor. If pain or fear causes them to revert to the behavior of a younger child, the techniques for dealing with younger children may be applied. Valid choices, positive expectations, and honest praise will usually ensure success.

Adolescent (13 to 18 Years)

Special sensitivity is required to deal with the emotional needs of younger adolescents. Although they may act quite adult under normal circumstances, they can become frightened and confused and may revert to childlike behavior when ill or in stressful situations. Show empathy if the adolescent loses control of his or her emotions. Adolescents fear threats to their physical appearance and loss of control and independence. Avoid using an authoritarian approach and involve them in as much decision making as possible.

You can establish rapport and reduce adolescents' anxiety about the procedure by talking with them about their hobbies, favorite sports, school, or friends before beginning the exam. Prepare the adolescent for the procedure away from parents and peers, if possible. If parents are present, involve them, but do not talk to parents "about" the adolescent, and include the patient in all discussions. This age group has moved past the physical or concrete properties of a situation and is capable of understanding abstract principles. Provide thorough explanations and the rationale for procedures using proper medical terminology.

Young teens usually behave much like adults, but the hormonal changes of puberty can make them subject to mood swings. When hurt or frightened, they may behave somewhat like toddlers; they may act self-centered and their attention span may be short. When this happens, appropriate praise and/or disapproval are effective strategies. One important characteristic of most young teens is an exaggerated sense of modesty. They are in the process of coming to terms with the physiologic changes of puberty and can be easily embarrassed by any attention to their bodies. Girls may feel "naked" if asked to remove their bras. The x-ray may be perceived as an "all-seeing eye," ready to reveal their innermost secrets. Special sensitivity is needed. If undressing is required, provide one

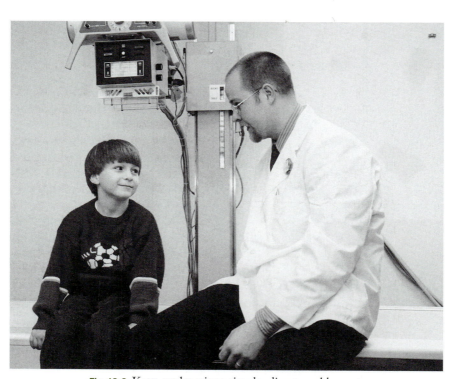

Fig. 18-6 Keep explanations simple, direct, and honest.

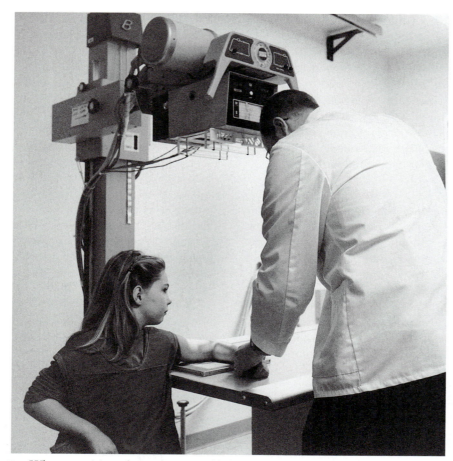

Fig. 18-7 When a positive relationship is established, children are more likely to cooperate.

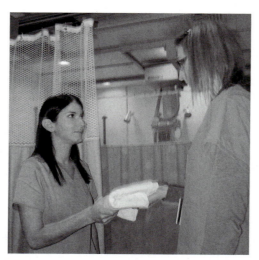

Fig. 18-8 Sensitivity to privacy improves relationships with young teens.

or more gowns (Fig. 18-8) so that the patient is modestly covered during the examination. If you must inquire about sensitive subjects, such as bowel habits or menstrual periods, discuss these topics in a matter-of-fact way and do it privately.

A professional approach, coupled with warm reassurance, promotes a more positive attitude in both children and adolescents. Many of the poor attitudes toward health care displayed by adults can be traced to a lack of sensitivity in the care given by health professionals during their formative years.

Parents in the X-ray Room

One question that limited operators must answer when small children are radiographed is whether or not to allow parents in the x-ray room. Experts disagree on this subject, and there are good arguments on both sides of the issue.

The principal argument in favor of a parent's presence is that separating parent from child creates anxiety in both the child and the parent. Having the parent close may be reassuring to the child. In addition, parents often have skills for calming their children and gaining their cooperation. If help is needed to hold a child in position during an exposure, a parent is the logical person to assist.

The opposing argument holds that a parent's presence may create anxiety for both parent and child. The child may appeal to the parent for "rescue" from the procedure, creating a dilemma for the parent: rescue and comfort the child or support the continuation of the procedure. This argument tends to support the idea that if the parent is not visible, the child is more likely to accept the procedure. If the child is distressed and must be immobilized, the parent will be less upset if waiting out of sight and out of earshot. The parent can comfort the child as soon as the procedure is completed.

Each approach has merit under certain circumstances. The duty of the limited operator is to evaluate the circumstances and make a judgment call. Consider the age of the child. Babies may be calmed by hearing the mother's voice nearby. Toddlers that usually get their way with their parents may behave better if taken into the x-ray room alone. Consider the state of mind of both the parent and the child. Even the best parents sometimes behave irrationally when their children are sick or injured. The parent may feel helpless and have a strong need to control everything. The presence of a parent who is not calm is likely to upset the child. When both parents are present, it is usually best for only one to accompany the child into the x-ray room. If you choose to have a parent present, try to select the one with the most matter-of-fact attitude.

At this point, there are two important things to remember, and both should be reassuring to you. You can change your mind, and you can ask for help. Whatever you decide, if you make the wrong decision, it is reversible. If a parent is a problem in the room, you can say, "I think little Sara and I can work this out by ourselves. Please wait in the waiting room, and I'll bring her out just as soon as we're finished." And if you begin without the parent and change your mind, you can say, "I think Jason needs his mommy. Would you mind giving me a hand?" Finally, if the situation seems unmanageable, do not hesitate to ask for help. A more experienced staff member can sometimes save the day. As a last resort, consult the physician, who may decide to postpone the procedure or to sedate the patient.

Immobilization

Infants and small children can be immobilized for most examinations without the need for someone to hold them. Whenever possible, mechanical immobilization of some type is the best answer. This section introduces some of the commercial devices available for this purpose. If pediatric patients are frequently seen in your facility, it is wise to invest in commercial immobilization devices to meet your needs. Noncommercial devices and the use of items commonly found in the x-ray room or the clinic are also illustrated in this section.

When circumstances require that someone hold a child during an exposure, remember that this *must not* be done by a limited x-ray machine operator. Occupationally exposed persons such as radiographers are prohibited from holding either patients or image receptors (IRs) during exposures. A non–occupationally exposed person must be recruited for this duty, and the best candidate is usually the child's parent, provided that person is not pregnant. Provide a lead apron. Lead gloves should be

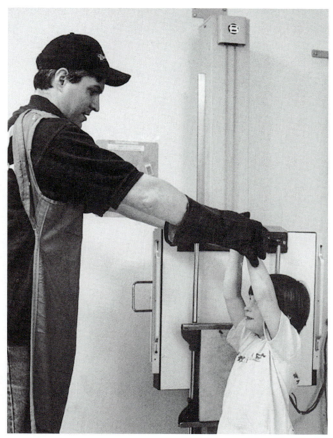

Fig. 18-9 Take appropriate precautions for radiation safety when holding is required.

worn if the hands will be in the radiation field. Demonstrate precisely how the child should be held and how to sit or stand to minimize exposure to primary radiation. Using extended arms so that the holder's body is at arm's length from the child will reduce exposure from scatter radiation (Fig. 18-9). To avoid the need for repeat exposures, take care to ensure that the holder has a comfortable and *firm* grip on the child in the correct position.

Commercial Immobilization Devices

Table restraints are common accessories for radiographic tables. These wide bands attach to the sides of the table and may be adjusted for placement at various locations along its length. Wide strips of Velcro secure the bands around the patient. Similar devices called *compression bands* consist of a single band of cloth that is secured to rails on both sides of the table. The band is tightened using a ratchet roller. Although originally designed to provide abdominal compression for specific procedures, compression bands are also useful to provide immobilization and security from falls.

Many radiographic devices designed for pediatric immobilization are modifications of the original designs for circumcision boards. They are frames to which the child is attached by Velcro straps at strategic locations. Figs. 18-10, 18-11, and 18-12 illustrate a variety of these

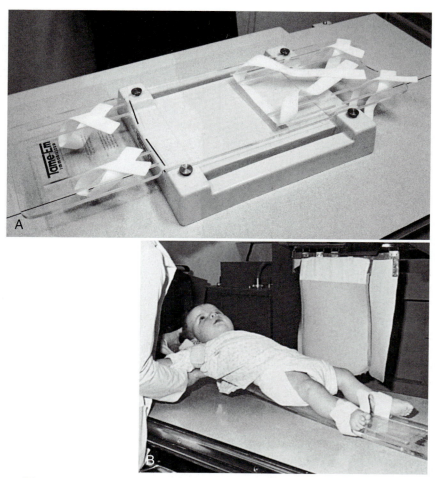

Fig. 18-10 Tame-Em adjustable infant restraining device. **A,** Device is made of Lucite with Velcro straps. **B,** Device in use.

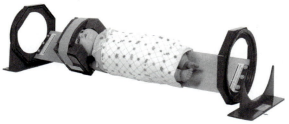

Fig. 18-11 Octastop restraint board. Device features octagonal end plates and Velcro restraining straps to hold child securely in oblique position, shown here, plus seven other positions.

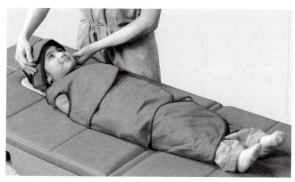

Fig. 18-12 Olympic Papoose Boards come in several sizes to provide selective immobilization for infants, children, and adults. Wide fabric straps with Velcro secure the patient's torso and legs.

products. Some come in several different sizes; others are adjustable in size. Each has some advantages and disadvantages. For example, the Octastop restrainer has octagonal end pieces that allow the child to be placed in eight different positions. Once the child is secured in the device, anteroposterior (AP), posteroanterior (PA), right and left lateral, and four oblique positions of the torso are obtainable without readjustment of the attachments. The disadvantage of this device is that object–image receptor distance (the distance between the patient and the imaging plane) is greater than usual.

Radiography of the skull, face, and neck requires precise immobilization of the head. The devices described earlier have head straps that aid in this process, but specific devices for head immobilization can be very helpful if they are available. Fig. 18-13 illustrates head clamps for this purpose.

The Pigg-O-Stat (Fig. 18-14) is a unique device for upright chest radiography of infants and small children. Its saddle-like seat is mounted in a disk that rotates for various projections. An adjustable clear plastic sheath

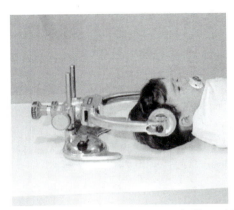

Fig. 18-13 Adjustable head clamp secures skull positions with cushioned contacts.

surrounds the child's upper body and is fastened securely with leather straps behind the waist and the head. This plastic portion supports the body upright and holds the arms overhead. The unit incorporates gonad shielding and a holder for the IR. The Pigg-O-Stat is not inexpensive, but it is a worthwhile investment where there is a high volume of pediatric chest radiography.

Noncommercial Devices and Methods for Immobilization

The principal objective of most immobilization is to prevent motion from flailing arms and kicking legs. When the extremities are under control, it is nearly impossible for a child to turn over or move about. In the absence of a commercial immobilization device, the extremities can be controlled by using a "mummy wrap." A sheet is used to secure the arms at the sides of the body and to hold the legs together. This technique is illustrated in Fig. 18-15. Infants wrapped in this way, with a lead apron placed over the pelvis, are both immobilized and shielded. Older children may still be able to "buck," flexing their knees and necks to bounce the torso up and down. Fig. 18-16 shows the use of the mummy wrap in conjunction with the table restraint strap across the knees, which is very effective.

The use of tape to maintain position is illustrated in Fig. 18-17. Note that the adhesive surface of the tape is not in contact with the patient's skin. The tape can be twisted so that the nonadhesive side is against the skin, or a gauze pad may be placed between the tape and the skin. Tape is not effective if applied to the tabletop or the flat surface of the IR. It must be wrapped around the edge of the IR or table so that lifting pressure does not loosen it.

Stockinet is a tubular knitted fabric placed on extremities before the application of a cast. It is also useful for securing arms or legs together (Fig. 18-18). Velcro straps may also be used to hold the legs together and in position. Sandbags, too, can be used to hold extremities in place. Another convenient way to hold extremities in place is to use a flexible sheet of Plexiglas (Fig. 18-19). This plastic material is available at reasonable cost from plastics dealers.

When the head must be precisely positioned and head clamps are not available, tape is not the only answer. Two or three large books may be placed on each side of the head. Radiolucent sponges are placed between the books and the head, and the books are moved close enough to hold the head firmly (Fig. 18-20). Another option is to use large, heavy "bookends" made from angle iron in

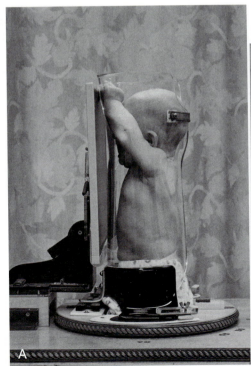
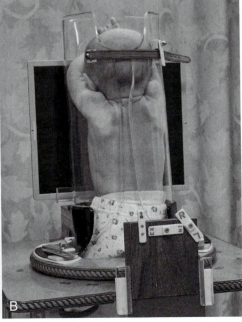

Fig. 18-14 Pigg-O-Stat positioning chair for upright pediatric chest radiography.

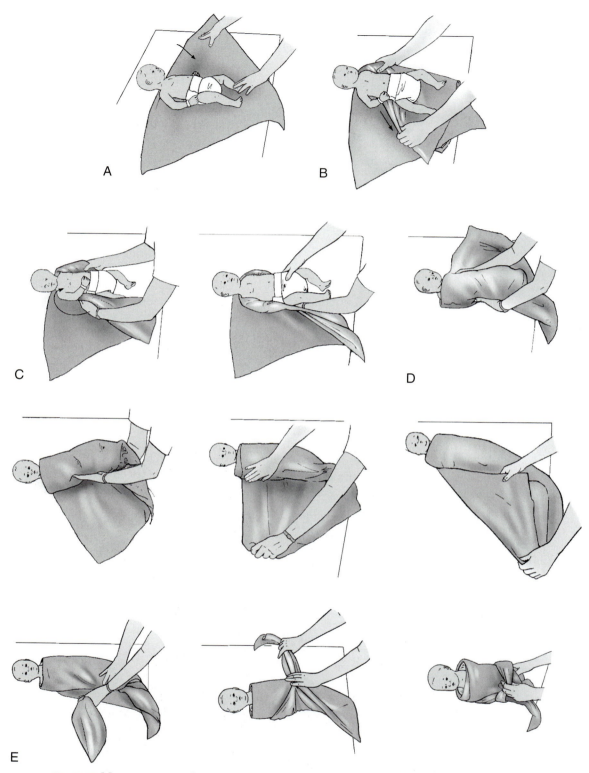

Fig. 18-15 Mummy wrap technique. **A,** Fold the sheet on the diagonal to make a triangle. Place the child on the sheet with wide edge under neck. **B,** Wrap one corner up over an arm, tuck it under the body, and pull it through. **C,** Wrap the first corner over the second arm and tuck it under the body. **D,** Wrap the second corner over the chest and secure it under the body. **E,** Complete mummy wrap by securing the second corner around the child.

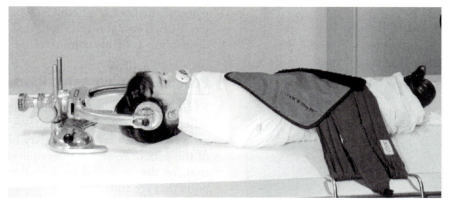

Fig. 18-16 Mummy wrap used in combination with other immobilization methods.

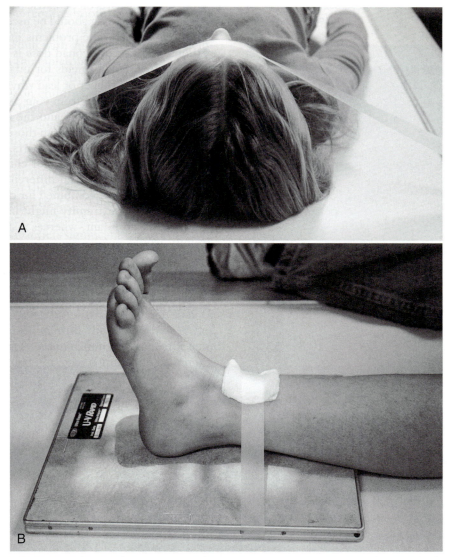

Fig. 18-17 Tape is often used to maintain pediatric positions. **A,** Tape is twisted to avoid adhesive contact with skin. **B,** Gauze is used to prevent adhesive contact with skin.

Much of the information in this chapter is not new. Facts from many chapters are brought together here and considered with respect to the evaluation of image quality.

Critical image review is an important contribution to your patients care and to the physician who will interpret (read) the images. It is also essential to your continuing education as a limited operator. Image evaluation is the process by which you determine whether each projection is correctly identified and marked and whether it has sufficient diagnostic quality to meet the minimum requirements of the order or if it must be repeated. When a projection must be repeated, your review provides information to ensure that the new radiograph is satisfactory.

Up to this point, the text has dealt primarily with the science of radiography and the basic procedures involved in the application of that science. Radiography is also an art, and your ability to take consistently high-quality radiographs will only develop with time and practice. Every radiograph you take is an opportunity to learn; each image you review can teach you something that will improve your ability. Your skills will develop most rapidly if you pay close attention to the results of your work, always striving for excellence.

VIEWING RADIOGRAPHS

Viewing Conditions

Unless you are working in a practice that still uses screen-film imaging, you will be viewing images on a computer monitor. It is likely that your viewing monitor will have less resolution than the one used by the physician when interpreting the images you produce. If an image is of questionable quality on your monitor, it may still be acceptable on the physician's monitor. It is essential that you solicit feedback from the physician when he or she finds images to be unacceptable. That is an important component of improving your knowledge of appropriate image quality.

It is not necessary to view images in a fully darkened room, but a low light level in the viewing area is necessary. Too much light causes the pupils of the eyes to contract, admitting less light to the eye, and therefore causing radiographs to appear dark. A black frame, called a mask, usually surrounds each image, enhancing your ability to perceive its detail accurately. Inappropriately placed lights may cause an unacceptable glare on the monitor screen. If the area where you view images is brightly lit, that must be taken into account when judging image brightness. An image may appear dark to you, but may be perfectly acceptable when viewed by the physician under an appropriately lower light level.

Image Orientation

Radiographs are generally viewed "right side up," with the most superior aspect of the anatomy at the top. Regardless of the patient's position when the image receptor (IR) is exposed, it is customary to view both anteroposterior (AP) and posteroanterior (PA) projections as if the patient were facing the viewer in the **anatomic position.** This is the position in which the patient is standing erect, with the face directed forward, arms extended by the sides with the palms facing forward, and the toes pointing anteriorly (Fig. 19-1). The patient's right side is toward the viewer's left. You will notice that radiographic markers will appear backward on PA projections because the image must be flipped, from left to right, for it to be oriented in anatomic position for viewing. Oblique projections are viewed using the same general rules. Lateral projections are usually viewed in the same position as they are taken; for example, a left lateral projection is oriented with the patient facing toward the viewer's right.

Exceptions to these general rules are made for examinations of the distal upper limb and the foot and for decubitus projections. Radiographs of the fingers, hand, wrist, forearm, and foot are usually viewed with the distal aspect pointing to the ceiling. Decubitus projections are often viewed horizontally, in the same position as they are taken.

The radiographs in this text are presented using these rules for viewing.

Some chiropractors and surgeons prefer to view AP and oblique spine projections from the same perspective used to examine the patient, as if they were facing the patient's back. In this case, the radiograph is oriented so that the patient's left side is on the viewer's left.

SYSTEMATIC IMAGE REVIEW

With practice, you will learn to evaluate an image quite rapidly. However, it is important not to rush this process or significant details may be overlooked. An accurate assessment of image quality requires a systematic approach. You may find it helpful to use the acronym *I AM ExpERT*. These letters stand for *identification, anatomy, marking, exposure, esthetic considerations, radiation safety*, and *troubleshooting*.

- **Identification.** First, check the image identification. Is it clear and complete? Does it match the identification on the requisition?
- **Anatomy.** Is the pertinent anatomy included on the projection and clearly visible? Was the patient properly positioned? Look for missing anatomy, evidence of rotation, or superimposed structures that indicate improper position.
- **Marking.** Is the correct right or left side marker clearly visible and in the proper location? If your facility's protocol requires additional markers for images,

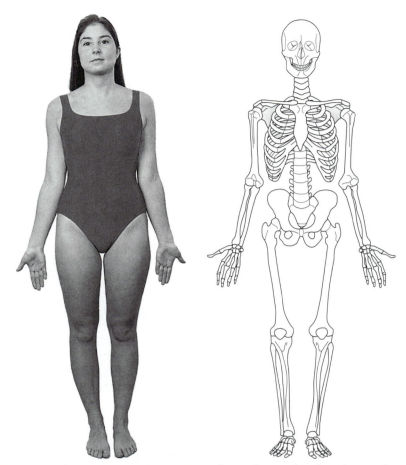

Fig. 19-1 Patient in the anatomic position. Most radiographs are placed on the view box with the body part matching this position.

such as flexion, weight bearing, or upright, check for placement and clear visibility of these additional markers as well.

- **Exposure.** Were the exposure factors appropriate? Are the essential features of the anatomy sharp and distinct? For a digital imaging system, is the exposure indicator number within the appropriate range? For a film-screen system, is the image too dark? Too light? Does it have sufficient contrast? Too much contrast?
- **Esthetic considerations.** Does the image have artistic merit? Do artifacts, misalignments, or other features of the image detract from its general appearance?
- **Radiation safety.** Is there evidence of collimation on at least three margins of the image? Where appropriate, is shielding apparent and correctly placed?
- **Troubleshooting.** Identify the cause of any problems noted on the image. Are they so significant as to require the image to be repeated? If so, what changes are necessary for the repeat to be successful? Regardless of whether a repeat is required, what steps are necessary to improve image quality in the future?

Each of these aspects of image evaluation is discussed in greater detail later in this chapter.

IMAGE IDENTIFICATION AND MARKERS

The first thing to check when reviewing a radiograph is the patient identification. This information must be complete and legible. Certainly, it is a good practice to be aware of the need for accurate radiographic identification and to cultivate a habit of identifying images properly. However, errors sometimes occur. Your facility should have a policy regarding images that are not properly labeled and a method of rectifying the mistake.

Check to be certain that the correct right- or left-side marker (and any other required marker) is clearly visible and properly located. Correct marker placement is discussed in Chapter 12. All radiographic markers should be placed so they are recorded on the image during the exposure. Although digital radiography systems allow the addition of "electronic markers" during image review and postprocessing, this practice is not recommended. Although electronic marking may not be illegal, the practice is not considered the standard of care and can call into question the quality of the imaging process.

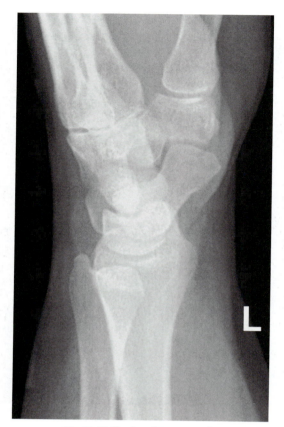

Fig. 19-22 Review image no. 3.

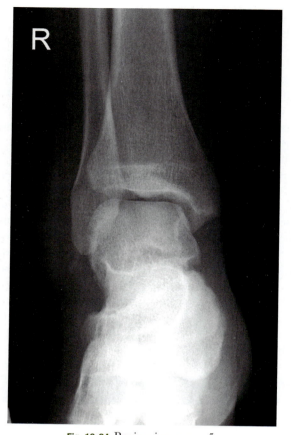

Fig. 19-24 Review image no. 5.

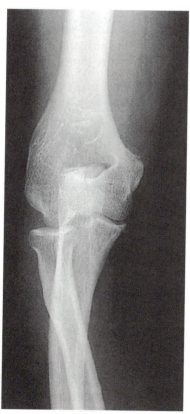

Fig. 19-23 Review image no. 4.

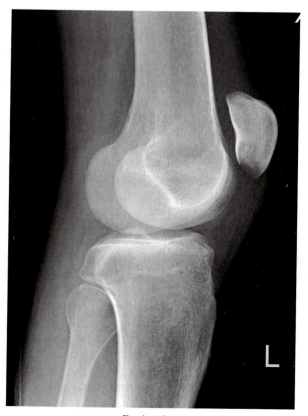

Fig. 19-25 Review image no. 6.

PART IV

Professionalism and Patient Care

Chapter 20

Ethics, Legal Considerations, and Professionalism

At the conclusion of this chapter, you will be able to:

- Discuss reasons why a study of professional behavior is important to the limited x-ray machine operator
- Apply ethical concepts to typical situations that arise in the health care setting
- Explain the rationale for confidentiality of professional communications and list precautions for maintaining confidentiality
- Demonstrate respect for patient rights that the limited operator is responsible for protecting
- List specific acts of misconduct and malpractice that could occur in the practice of radiography and describe the most frequent circumstances that cause patients to initiate litigation
- List aspects of self-care that demonstrate responsible behavior by the limited operator
- Demonstrate effective communication skills, including listening skills, nonverbal skills, and validation of communication; discriminate between assumed and validated statements
- Suggest positive strategies for both verbal and nonverbal communication with patients who have hearing and/or visual impairments and with patients from other cultures
- Demonstrate communication strategies that promote teamwork in the workplace
- Demonstrate professional skills in handling messages sent and received on paper and by telephone, voice mail, and fax
- Demonstrate the use of patient charts for both obtaining and recording information; state the essential characteristics of good medical records
- Explain requirements for maintaining radiographic images and procedures for lending them

Key Terms

aggressive	intentional misconduct
assault	invasion of privacy
assertive	libel
battery	malpractice
chart	morals
charting	negligence
defamation of character	reasonably prudent person
empathy	*respondeat superior*
ethics	rule of personal responsibility
ethnic	slander
false imprisonment	values
informed consent	

How does a profession differ from a job? Many different definitions have been advanced for *profession*. Generally speaking, a profession is more than a field of study; it is the application of specialized knowledge in a way that benefits others and carries a high degree of responsibility to the community it serves. A profession is organized to govern itself: to effectively set standards of professional behavior, education, and qualification to practice and to enforce those standards within its ranks. Having a peer-reviewed journal or publication is also expected of a profession. This allows the profession to advance and to continually review and challenge the basis of knowledge on which it functions.

Limited operators are taking the first steps toward making limited radiography a profession, and they have not yet attained true professional status. On the other hand, their work is closely associated with that of physicians, nurses, and other health care professionals. The public does not usually distinguish between limited x-ray machine operators (LXMOs) and professional radiologic technologists. Any person who cares for the sick or injured, and who uses equipment that produces ionizing radiation, has a duty to perform competently and professionally. For these reasons, a high level of professionalism in both attitude and behavior is expected of the limited operator. Strict adherence to professional standards by limited operators will hasten the day when professional status is achieved. As a limited operator, your work must be focused on the patients in your care, and your efforts must be devoted to providing quality service. It is a primary goal of this text to assist you in this effort.

ETHICS, MORALS, AND VALUES

Correct behavior or "right action" may be dictated by moral, legal, or ethical considerations. **Morals** are right actions based on religious teachings. Most religions have similar guidelines for the proper conduct of life and relationships. Such concepts as honesty, fairness, and compassion are cultural standards based on moral principles. When principles are in conflict—for instance, in a situation in which it may not seem compassionate to be honest—**values** will determine which concept prevails. Values refer to the priority that is placed on the significance of various moral concepts. Values differ among individuals; morals, although they are matters of individual choice, are largely dictated by the culture.

Laws, on the other hand, are legal requirements for behavior. In this way, the government can control the behavior of groups and individuals. Laws govern health care delivery, the practice of radiography, and certain interpersonal interactions. Legal matters that are important to limited operators are discussed in the section on legal considerations that follows.

Ethics are rules that apply values and moral standards to our actions. Professional ethics define what is meant by correct behavior within a profession. A code of ethics is a document that sets forth these professional standards. A code of ethics is a hallmark of a profession because it signifies high principles of professional behavior and willingness by the profession to control its own conduct. Limited operators have yet to develop a code of ethics that applies specifically to this group. This does not mean, however, that there are no applicable standards. State laws and licensing boards may limit the scope of practice and prohibit "unprofessional conduct."

Standards of Ethics for Radiography

As the employee of a physician or health care organization, the limited operator must strive to support and uphold the ethics that apply to all health care personnel. In general, the ethics of health care require that *all* patients receive respectful, competent, and compassionate care. The dignity and confidentiality of each patient must be respected by those who provide health care.

The *Standards of Ethics* for the profession of radiologic technology is a two-part document that consists of a Code of Ethics and Rules of Ethics. Both are developed and adopted by the American Registry of Radiologic Technologists (ARRT) (see Chapter 1). They are published by the ARRT and are available on the ARRT web site at www.ARRT.org. The Code of Ethics is an aspirational document that establishes a high standard of professional conduct and assists the members of the profession in practicing ethical principles. It is reproduced in Box 20-1. The Rules of Ethics are mandatory standards of minimally acceptable professional conduct for all registered radiologic technologists and applicants for certification by the ARRT.

Although both the Code and the Rules apply directly to those who are certified by the ARRT, they are very important to limited operators as well. Until such time as limited operators have established themselves professionally and have their own code of ethics, *this is the standard by which all who practice radiography will be judged.*

American Registry of Radiologic Technologists Code of Ethics

The 10 principles of the ARRT Code of Ethics are self-explanatory. Some of these concepts are expanded in other sections of this chapter. Principles 3, 5, 7, and 9, however, deserve additional attention.

Principle 3 requires radiographers to put aside all personal prejudice and emotional bias when rendering professional services. This is more difficult than it may at first appear. Most of us can easily identify prejudice in others, but our own biases or judgments may be beyond our awareness or may seem to be fully justified or "only common sense." All of us have some natural preferences that may result in discriminatory treatment if we are not fully aware of them. With what patients do you feel most

Box 20-1

American Registry of Radiologic Technologists Code of Ethics

The Code of Ethics forms the first part of the *Standards of Ethics*. The Code of Ethics shall serve as a guide by which Certificate Holders and Candidates may evaluate their professional conduct as it relates to patients, healthcare consumers, employers, colleagues, and other members of the healthcare team. The Code of Ethics is intended to assist Certificate Holders and Candidates in maintaining a high level of ethical conduct and in providing for the protection, safety, and comfort of patients. The Code of Ethics is aspirational.

1. The radiologic technologist acts in a professional manner, responds to patient needs, and supports colleagues and associates in providing quality patient care.
2. The radiologic technologist acts to advance the principal objective of the profession to provide services to humanity with full respect for the dignity of mankind.
3. The radiologic technologist delivers patient care and service unrestricted by the concerns of personal attributes or the nature of the disease or illness, and without discrimination on the basis of sex, race, creed, religion, or socio-economic status.
4. The radiologic technologist practices technology founded upon theoretical knowledge and concepts, uses equipment and accessories consistent with the purposes for which they were designed, and employs procedures and techniques appropriately.
5. The radiologic technologist assesses situations; exercises care, discretion, and judgment; assumes responsibility for professional decisions; and acts in the best interest of the patient.
6. The radiologic technologist acts as an agent through observation and communication to obtain pertinent information for the physician to aid in the diagnosis and treatment of the patient and recognizes that interpretation and diagnosis are outside the scope of practice for the profession.
7. The radiologic technologist uses equipment and accessories, employs techniques and procedures, performs services in accordance with an accepted standard of practice, and demonstrates expertise in minimizing radiation exposure to the patient, self, and other members of the healthcare team.
8. The radiologic technologist practices ethical conduct appropriate to the profession and protects the patient's right to quality radiologic technology care.
9. The radiologic technologist respects confidences entrusted in the course of professional practice, respects the patient's right to privacy, and reveals confidential information only as required by law or to protect the welfare of the individual or the community.
10. The radiologic technologist continually strives to improve knowledge and skills by participating in continuing education and professional activities, sharing knowledge with colleagues, and investigating new aspects of professional practice.

comfortable? Men? Women? Those of your own race? Those over 16? Under 65? Middle class? Do you feel greater compassion for a patient with a heart problem than for one with a sexually transmitted disease? Once we identify those areas in human relationships where we are most at ease, it becomes apparent that we are less comfortable in some situations or would prefer to avoid these situations altogether. It is instructive to pay attention to how we deal with patients who are outside our "comfort zone." Sometimes we tend to act more friendly or solicitous to cover up feelings. At other times we may remain aloof, appearing to be preoccupied because we are in a hurry. Lack of interest and concern is unacceptable, and feigned concern or pretended interest is never the same as the real thing. Faithfulness to the spirit of principle 3 requires a high degree of self-awareness and presents a serious professional challenge.

Principle 5 deals with the question of professional responsibility. It implies that radiographers are sufficiently educated and experienced to be capable of independent discretion and judgment. Within the scope of their professional activity, they are expected to be both capable of making decisions and accountable for the decisions they make. A very important aspect of assuming this responsibility is awareness and acceptance of your limitations.

Although responsibilities may vary with the working environment, regular duties should be specified in job descriptions and must be consistent with the permitted scope of practice. It is in no one's best interest to perform tasks without adequate knowledge or to undertake a responsibility without proper qualification. This principle also holds individuals accountable for errors committed under the orders of another person, if the responsible person knew, or *should have known*, that the order was in error.

Principle 7 requires that radiographers adhere to accepted practices and make every effort to protect themselves and all patients and staff from exposure to unnecessary radiation. The ethical implications of this issue are very important. When this principle is violated, there is no telltale evidence. The negative consequences of other breaches of ethics might be immediate, but the latent effects of unnecessary radiation exposure may not be apparent for 10 to 20 years, and genetic effects may not manifest themselves for several generations. Making every effort to minimize radiation exposure—even when the patient is difficult to handle, even when you are really in a hurry, and even when no one is watching—requires both good habits and a strong ethical commitment to radiation protection.

Principle 9 relates to the confidentiality of information in a health care setting, which is one of the cardinal concepts in all codes of ethics relating to health care. The confidentiality of conversations between patients and their physicians is considered so important that, along with communications to lawyers and the clergy, it is protected by "legal privilege." This means that the professional cannot be required to divulge such information, even when doing so might be of material value in a court of law. Limited operators and radiographers often hear conversations between patients and their physicians, and they have access to information contained in patient records. Patients may confide in them, and they may be present in circumstances in which patients are unable to preserve their dignity and may behave in ways that would cause them shame or embarrassment if known to friends or family. All of this information is considered confidential. Many patients do not want it known that they are ill. Some may wish to keep the diagnosis confidential. Information that seems of no consequence to you may constitute a very sensitive issue for the patient. Any breach of confidence, even if no names are mentioned, may rightly be interpreted by others as an indication that the limited operator does not respect professional confidence. Betrayals of confidence cause individuals to lose faith in health care providers and may prevent them from revealing facts essential to their care.

The patient's right to confidentiality is not violated by appropriate communications among health care workers when the information is pertinent to the patient's care. It is justifiably assumed in such a case that the transfer of information is for the patient's benefit and that all personnel involved are bound by the ethics regarding confidentiality. Appropriate communications are those directed privately to those who have a need for the information. Conversations about patients must never be held in public areas such as waiting rooms, elevators, or cafeterias.

The ethics of patient-staff communication also require the exercise of sound judgment and restraint to avoid exposing patients to the health care worker's personal concerns or the problems of the staff. Using the patient as a sounding board for complaints or gossip is inexcusable.

Ethical Judgments and Conflicts

The process of ethical analysis is a method of evaluating situations in which the correct action is in question. Although some situations may be obviously unethical and unacceptable to almost everyone, circumstances often occur that present conflicts between values, and the best solution is not immediately apparent. In the face of an ethical dilemma, you must be prepared to assess the problem objectively and come to a conclusion that you can implement and defend. Ethical analysis is a process involving the following four basic steps:

1. Identify the problem
2. Develop alternate solutions
3. Select the best solution
4. Defend your selection

You may realize that there is a problem before you have fully identified it. Identifying the problem means that you can state the conflict clearly. It may be helpful to write it down. It is important to consider every aspect of the problem, to be certain that you have all the pertinent information, and to be confident that your information is accurate. Do not rush this process. A competent identification of the dilemma is essential to its successful resolution.

Once the problem is well-defined, the next step is to proceed with the development of alternative solutions. In this part of the process, think of as many potential solutions as possible. This is a brainstorming exercise in which no judgments are made. View the problem from the perspective of everyone involved. Include not only the interests of individuals, but also those of your institution, your profession, and society as a whole.

Only after you have an exhaustive list of possible resolutions does the next step in the process begin: the selection of the *best* alternative. This is the most stimulating and challenging part of the analysis, in which you weigh the alternatives and render a judgment as to which is best. In this process, you will need to eliminate choices that have positive attributes and possibly one or two that you particularly like.

When the best alternative has been selected, you should be prepared to explain your choice based on the standards that affected your decision. By what standard, then, should the alternatives be judged and defended?

Both moral principles and ethical theories provide guidelines for determining whether actions are right or wrong. No one system serves adequately for all occasions. Although religious literature and educational systems may have instilled moral rules, there is no comprehensive list of moral principles that is universally accepted and available as a resource. Ethical theorists have tried to codify moral rules into sets of generally accepted principles, but they are not all in agreement.

Principle-based ethics, also called *principlism*, is a widely accepted standard for selecting and defending solutions to ethical dilemmas in health care communities. Six moral principles, sometimes called *ethical principles*, are accepted as guides to right action that should be respected unless there is a compelling moral reason not to do so. The six principles are the following:

1. *Beneficence:* Goodness. Actions that bring about good are considered right.
2. *Nonmaleficence:* No evil. An obligation not to inflict harm.
3. *Veracity:* Truth. An obligation to tell the truth.

4. *Fidelity:* Faithfulness. An obligation to be loyal or faithful.
5. *Justice:* Fairness. An obligation to act with equity.
6. *Autonomy:* Self-determination. Respecting the independence of others and acting with self-reliance.

Now let us consider the dilemma of Jackie Webber and evaluate her problem using ethical analysis.

For over a year Jackie Webber has worked for Dr. Savage in his clinic. Recently Jackie has noticed that Dr. Savage has been returning to the office later and later after the lunch hour. Several times she was certain that he smelled of alcohol, and he often seemed distracted and unfocused after lunch. This afternoon, as Dr. Savage was performing a minor sterile procedure, he dropped an instrument on the floor and bent over to pick it up. Jackie stepped forward, picked up the instrument, and brought another sterile instrument from the supply cabinet, but she sensed that if she had not intervened, Dr. Savage would have picked up the instrument and continued with the procedure.

1. **Identify the problem:** Jackie suspects that her employer may be treating patients and performing invasive procedures while under the influence of alcohol.
2. **Develop alternate solutions:** Jackie considers the dilemma and lists the following possible actions:
   • Do nothing at all.
   • Ask around the clinic and see if any of her co-workers have noticed that Dr. Savage seemed drunk.
   • Tell Dr. Savage that she suspects he is treating patients under the influence of alcohol and see what he says.
   • Warn Dr. Savage that if he does not stop drinking at lunch she will have to report him.
   • Discuss the issue with the office manager, who is Dr. Savage's wife.
   • Discuss the issue with Dr. Savage's partner, Dr. Melcher.
   • Send an anonymous letter to the Board of Medical Examiners.
   • Send a signed letter to the Board of Medical Examiners.
   • Resign her position and look for another job without mentioning the issue of Dr. Savage's drinking.
3. **Select the best solution:** Is there a solution that will protect Dr. Savage's reputation if Jackie's suspicion is unfounded? How might the rights or the care of Dr. Savage's patients be affected by Jackie's actions? Does Jackie have a duty to judge Dr. Savage's actions? Is there any way to confirm or refute her suspicions without spreading rumors or slandering Dr. Savage?
4. **Defend your selection:** The basic principle of nonmaleficence is often expressed as, "First, do no harm." Because the potential for harm to Dr. Savage's patients may be great, Jackie must act. Principle 5 of the ARRT Code of Ethics states, "The radiologic technologist assesses situations; exercises care, discretion

and judgment; assumes responsibility for professional decisions; and acts in the best interest of the patient." This is clearly a case in which Jackie's discretion, judgment, and responsibility are called for. Which course of action best fits this description? Defend your answer.

Ethical analysis is being used increasingly to solve institutional problems. When several individuals have analyzed the situation, the next step may be to seek resolution through discussion that leads to consensus. Once the question is resolved, action can be taken. The one responsible for implementing the ethical decision is called the *moral agent.*

Ethical conflicts may trouble us when the ethics of the group are not compatible with our personal beliefs. For example, there are health professionals who find that caring for some patients with acquired immunodeficiency syndrome (AIDS) offends their personal sense of morality because they disapprove of the homosexual lifestyle. For others, the conflict between their religious beliefs and the legal right of a patient to receive an abortion may present a problem. Professionals must not permit issues of personal morality to supersede the group moral duty to provide quality patient care. Although ethical standards might pose personal moral challenges, these standards assure us that professional ethical judgments will hold true for everyone in similar circumstances. They test whether a specific behavior will support the values and duties of the profession. If you experience frequent ethical conflicts that cannot be resolved, you may need to find a new position or career that conforms more closely to your own moral standards.

Patient Rights

Considerable emphasis is placed on consumer advocacy in our society, and this value is especially significant in the field of health care. As a result, many organizations and health care institutions have written statements listing patient rights. The American Hospital Association publishes a patient information pamphlet about patient rights entitled *The Patient Care Partnership: Understanding Expectations, Rights and Responsibilities.*[h] Although some of these concepts apply specifically to physicians or hospitals, several of them are especially pertinent to the work of radiographers and limited operators.

Considerate and Respectful Care

Foremost among patients' rights is the right to high-quality care. This statement is self-explanatory and applies to every patient, regardless of current status. This is essentially the same professional behavior prescribed by principles 2 and 3 of the ARRT Code of Ethics.

---

[h]www.aha.org/advocacy-issues/communicatingpts/pt-care-partnership.shtml.

The right to considerate and respectful care implies the expectation that the patient's modesty will be respected and that every effort will be made to assist the patient in maintaining a sense of personal dignity. The limited operator must remember that many health care procedures may threaten the patient's modesty and dignity. Patients are likely to be much more sensitive in these situations than the health care workers, for whom the procedures are an everyday occurrence.

Somewhat related to this right is the generally accepted practice of ensuring that a patient and a physician or other health care worker of the opposite sex are not left alone together in a setting that requires undraping of the patient or examination of the genitals or female breasts. A chaperone, preferably of the same sex as the patient, should be present when possible. The objective of this practice is not to prevent the health professional from violating ethical principles, although this may be a consideration. The main purpose is to ease the patient's mind if he or she fears such an encounter and to provide a witness in case the patient later claims to have been assaulted or touched in an unprofessional manner. Many health care organizations have policies that apply in these situations, and many physicians prefer to be chaperoned, even when no such policy exists. The limited operator should be aware of any such policies and be sensitive to others' needs in this regard. Similar considerations may affect decisions about whether to allow parents to observe the care provided to their minor children.

Note that students and others not required for a procedure must have the patient's permission to be present. The taking of photographs, other than for the sole purpose of the patient's care, also requires consent.

A Clean and Safe Environment

Health care facilities have a duty to provide an environment that is both clean and safe, and patients have a right to expect that this duty will be carried out. Your responsibilities with respect to cleanliness and safety are discussed in detail in Chapter 21.

Information

The patient also has a right to information, but this does not place an obligation on you to provide any and all information that may be requested. Limited operators must be prepared to offer explanations of radiographic procedures and to identify themselves and the physicians with whom they work. Patients have a right to know whether those involved in their care are students or trainees. They also have a right to be involved in their care and to receive answers to questions about their diagnosis, treatment, and other aspects of care; responding to these questions is the duty of the physician. Your duty in this regard is simply to refer the patient to his or her doctor.

Confidentiality

The right of confidentiality was discussed earlier in this chapter. The Health Insurance Portability and Accountability Act (HIPAA) was enacted in 1996 and has two main provisions. Title I provides for continuing health care coverage for workers and their families when there is a loss or change of employment. Title II, which concerns us here, requires the U.S. Department of Health and Human Services (HHS) to protect the privacy rights of patients and increase health care system efficiency by drafting rules and creating standards for the use and dissemination of health care information. These rules are intended to provide for the protection of patient privacy as health care information is maintained electronically and transmitted from one agency to another. Since April 2003, hospitals have been required to provide protection for patients concerning the release of individual financial and medical information without the written consent of the patient. No information may be released to employers, financial institutions, or other medical facilities without specific permission by the patient. In brief, this law requires the following:

1. The patient must receive a clear written explanation of how the health provider may use the disclosed information.
2. The patient will be able to see and copy records and request amendments.
3. A history of routine disclosures must be available to the patient.
4. Health care providers must obtain consent before sharing routine information about treatment, payment, and health care operations. Separate authorization is needed for nonroutine disclosures and nonhealth purposes.
5. Patients have the right to request restrictions on uses and disclosures of their information.
6. Patients may file complaints with a covered provider or with the HHS about violations of these rules.

Your health care facility will have specific written procedures to ensure compliance with HIPAA standards. It is your duty to be familiar with these procedures and to apply them conscientiously. The following practices are examples of specific applications of HIPAA standards as used in some institutions:

- No schedules or other documents that include patients' names may be posted in public areas.
- Use only patients' first names when summoning them from public areas. Avoiding the use of last names is preferred to preserve a degree of anonymity.
- All health record information used for statistical or research purposes must be de-identified by eliminating any names, numbers, codes, or biometric identifiers that are associated with a specific person.
- When the release of medical information is authorized, only the specific information designated in the authorization may be included in the release. A copy of the authorization must be kept on file.

- Only specific individuals trained in HIPAA compliance are allowed access to protected health care information.
- All computer files that contain or may contain patient information must be encrypted. Secure access is required for this data.

Refusal of Treatment or Examination

All patients have the right to refuse treatment, which also implies the right to refuse examination. If a patient chooses to exercise this right, you must not proceed with the study. Signing an informed consent document does not invalidate the patient's right to refuse treatment once the procedure has begun. Consent may be revoked at any time during the procedure. If this occurs, take time to explore the reason why the patient is unwilling to continue. This may be a response to a temporary discomfort and not an objection to the procedure itself. Experience with these situations will allow you to respond with tact and concern, calming the patient so that the examination can be resumed. If the patient still refuses to complete the procedure, comply gracefully and notify the physician. When patients wish to leave a clinic or outpatient facility, they must not be prevented from doing so.

Informed Consent

Although patient consent to routine procedures is implied by the continued acceptance of care, **informed consent** is necessary for any procedure that is considered experimental or that involves substantial risk. Certain imaging procedures require that the patient receive an explanation of both the procedure and the potential risk and sign a consent form. This is particularly true for procedures involving the use of contrast media. When informed consent is required for complex procedures or surgery, the physician will provide the information and obtain the consent. For patients undergoing more routine procedures, a staff member may provide the necessary form and explanation (Fig. 20-1).

Most procedures commonly performed by limited operators do not require informed consent. When it is your duty to obtain informed consent, be sure that you are prepared with a full understanding of the procedure and its risks so that you can give an adequate explanation to the patient and answer any questions. If the patient asks a question for which you are not prepared, seek the correct answer before continuing. An improper response can invalidate the consent. The legal implications of informed consent cannot be overemphasized. Successful lawsuits against health care providers have been based on lack of compliance with the following guidelines:

- Patients must receive a full explanation of the procedure and its risks and sign the consent form before being sedated or anesthetized.
- A patient must be legally competent to sign an informed consent.

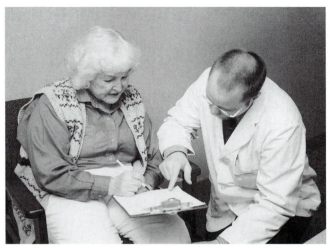

Fig. 20-1 Limited operator obtaining informed consent.

- Only parents or legal guardians may sign for a minor.
- Only a legal guardian may sign for a mentally incompetent patient.
- Consent forms must be completed before being signed. Patients should never be asked to sign a blank form or a form with blank spaces "to be filled in later."
- Only the physician named on the consent form may perform the procedure. Consent is not transferable from one physician to another, even an associate.
- Any condition stated on the form must be met. For example, if the form states that a family member will be present during the procedure, the consent is not valid if the family member is not in attendance.
- Informed consent may be revoked by the patient at any time after signing.

It is your responsibility to be aware of which procedures require written consent and to be certain that these forms are in order before proceeding with the examination.

LEGAL CONSIDERATIONS

Violations of Local and Institutional Standards

It is essential to maintain all required credentials. In states that require a current license or permit to practice radiography, practicing outside the legal requirements may result in fines, loss of credentials, or even imprisonment. Failure to maintain the qualifications required by your employer may result in termination of your employment. Infractions of laws or professional rules may make it impossible for you to obtain professional standing and/or employment as a limited operator in the future.

Intentional Misconduct

Personal injury lawsuits are becoming more and more common in the field of health care, and all fall into one of two categories: **intentional misconduct** or **negligence.** The types of intentional misconduct that may occur in a health care setting include assault, battery, false imprisonment, invasion of privacy, and libel or slander (defamation of character).

Assault may be defined as the *threat* of touching in an injurious way. The person need not be touched in any way for assault to occur. If the patient feels threatened and has cause to believe that he or she will be touched in a harmful manner, justification may exist for a charge of assault. To avoid this, the limited operator must explain what is to occur and reassure the patient in any situation in which the threat of harm may be an issue. *Never use threats to gain a patient's cooperation.* This statement applies both to pediatric patients and to adults.

Battery consists of an unlawful touching of a person without consent. This should not prevent the radiographer from placing a reassuring hand on the patient's shoulder when there is no intent to harm or to invade the patient's privacy. Nevertheless, if the patient refuses to be touched, that wish must be respected. Even the most well-intentioned touch may constitute battery if the patient has expressly forbidden it. A radiograph taken against the patient's will or on the wrong patient could also be construed as battery. This emphasizes the need for consistently double-checking patient identification and for being certain that proper informed consent has been obtained for procedures that require it. The accepted standard for checking identification is to ask the patient to state his or her full name and birth date and to check these identifiers against the order and any written documents that pertain to the procedure.

False imprisonment is the unjustifiable detention of a person against his or her will. This becomes an issue when the patient wishes to leave and is not allowed to do so. Inappropriate use of physical restraints may also constitute false imprisonment. Reasonable judgment must be used to decide whether restraints are necessary for safety. *Physical restraints that tie down an adult patient's hands or legs are applied only on the order of a physician.* It is rare for restraints to be used in outpatient facilities.

Invasion of privacy charges may result when confidentiality of information has not been maintained or when the patient's body has been improperly exposed or touched. Respect for the patient's modesty is vitally important. The significance of confidentiality is re-emphasized here. Health care facilities, physicians, and their employees may be liable if they disclose confidential information obtained from a patient or contained in the medical record. If the information disclosed reflects negatively on the patient's reputation, there may also be justification for a claim of **defamation of character.** Liability for invasion of privacy can result if photographs are published without a patient's permission.

Libel and **slander** refer to the malicious spreading of information that results in defamation of character or loss of reputation. *Libel* usually refers to written information, and *slander* is more often applied to information spread verbally. It should be clear that any breach of confidentiality is not only unethical but could also cause the limited operator to be sued for slander and/or invasion of privacy.

Intentional misconduct as discussed in this section often causes emotional distress in addition to any harm caused directly by the misconduct. For this reason, charges of intentionally inflicting emotional distress may be added to any of these other charges. Occasionally, such a charge may be made on its own merit without being accompanied by other charges of misconduct.

Negligence and Malpractice

Negligence refers to the neglect or omission of reasonable care or caution. The standard of reasonable care is based on the doctrine of the **reasonably prudent person.** This standard requires that a person perform as any reasonable person would perform under similar circumstances. In the relationship between a professional person and a patient or client, the professional has a duty to provide reasonable care. An act of negligence in the context of such a relationship is defined as professional negligence or **malpractice.** The LXMO is held to the standard of care and skill of the "reasonably prudent limited operator."

There has long been a tendency to place legal responsibility on the highest authority possible. For instance, according to the legal doctrine of *respondeat superior* ("let the master respond"), the employer is liable for employees' negligent acts that occur in the course of their work. In recent years, however, the **rule of personal responsibility** has been increasingly applied. This means that each person is liable for his or her own negligent conduct. Under this rule, the law does not allow the wrongdoer to escape responsibility, even though someone else may be legally liable as well.

Malpractice lawsuits against physicians, hospitals, and health care workers are becoming increasingly common. As a result, rates for malpractice insurance coverage have soared, and this topic is a serious concern to all health care professionals.

There has been much discussion about whether radiographers and limited operators should carry malpractice insurance. Health care facilities carry liability insurance, which covers them in the case of negligence by employees acting in the course of their employment. This coverage may also apply to employees individually. Limited operators should learn the extent and provisions of malpractice coverage provided by their employers.

Malpractice lawsuits have resulted in unfavorable judgments against radiographers as individuals. In rare cases, insurers who have paid malpractice claims have successfully recovered damages from negligent employees by filing separate suits against them. Some believe these are sufficient reasons to be protected by their own liability insurance policies. Others argue that the potential for a large insurance settlement is an incentive to sue, and that if the limited operator has no means of paying a large claim, no suit will be filed. The possibility of losing personal assets, such as one's home, may provide motivation for considering the purchase of malpractice insurance.

Lawsuits can result in conflict, expense, professional embarrassment, and loss of public confidence, even when the patient is denied any award. For these reasons, it is very important to use caution, both in the interest of quality patient care and in the avoidance of possible malpractice claims. Research indicates that lawsuits are most likely to occur when patients feel alienated from the people providing their care. When a trusting professional relationship is established, suits are less likely. The Seven *C*'s of malpractice prevention (Box 20-2) is a list of considerations to reduce the likelihood of lawsuits and legal liability for negligence in the health care setting.

Proper patient identification, accuracy in medication administration (see Chapter 23), and compliance with patient safety requirements (see Chapter 21) are positive steps the limited operator can take to prevent malpractice suits. Harm may result when medications or contrast media are administered without proper precautions or when drug reactions are not immediately identified and appropriately treated. Poor image quality creates a potential for misdiagnosis that may have serious consequences for both patient and limited operator. The potential for harmful error is often greatest in stressful situations. Appropriate responses in an emergency ensure the least possible risk. You must understand and accept that an appropriate response depends on your level of experience and education. Do not hesitate to ask questions and receive help when needed.

The limited operator can also protect patients and the employer by reporting illegal or unethical professional activities to the proper authority. In such a situation you must take care to be neither too zealous nor too hesitant. A simple, written statement that includes the facts (dates, times, names, and places) but avoids judgments or conclusions should be prepared as soon as possible after the occurrence. This statement should be submitted to the appropriate person, probably your immediate supervisor unless he or she was involved in the incident. The supervisor receiving such a report is responsible for seeing that it is given to the proper authority, who must then follow up by investigating. A single report may not produce change, but it may add strength to other reports or lead to increased supervision where necessary.

PROJECTING A PROFESSIONAL ATTITUDE

Think for a moment of a physician, nurse, or other health care worker that you have encountered when you were a patient. If this person had a neat, appropriate appearance, spoke in a way that was friendly and concerned but not too familiar, and projected an air of confidence and competence, you probably perceived that this person demonstrated a professional attitude. Patients expect professionalism in health care workers and will be most likely to respond with cooperation and confidence when these expectations are met. A professional attitude also promotes positive relationships with co-workers and employers.

Self-care

A limited operator who is not healthy is not a good health role model and cannot function effectively for both physical and psychologic reasons. Health is a state of physical, mental, and social well-being. To help others, we must first meet our own physical and mental needs. Certain needs are common to everyone and can be listed and ranked in importance (Fig. 20-2). Any unmet need causes stress and prevents us from experiencing a state of well-being.

Needs on the most basic level are foremost until these needs are adequately satisfied. As satisfaction occurs on one level, the needs of the next higher level occupy our attention. Self-actualization is the state in which we can express ourselves with a high degree of creativity. Constructively meeting your own needs for well-being, knowledge, and self-esteem enables you to function more fully, free from personal concerns when the patient requires full attention.

Box 20-2

The Seven C's of Malpractice Prevention

Competence. Knowing and adhering to professional standards and maintaining professional competence reduce liability exposure.

Compliance. The compliance by health professionals with policies and procedures in the medical office and hospital avoids patient injuries and litigation.

Charting. Charting completely, consistently, and objectively can be the best defense against a malpractice claim.

Communication. Patient injuries and resulting malpractice cases can be avoided by improving communications with patients and among health care professionals.

Confidentiality. Protecting the confidentiality of medical information is a legal and ethical responsibility of health professionals.

Courtesy. A courteous attitude and demeanor can improve patient rapport and lessen the likelihood of lawsuits.

Carefulness. Personal injuries can occur unexpectedly on the premises and may lead to lawsuits.

Reprinted with the permission of David Karp, loss prevention manager for the Medical Insurance Exchange of California.

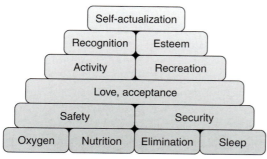

Fig. 20-2 Hierarchy of needs.

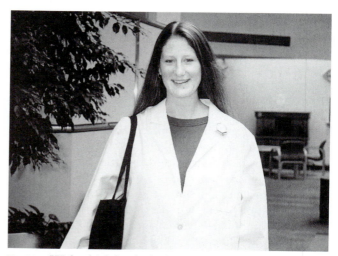

Fig. 20-3 With a high level of job satisfaction, a limited operator begins the day with a positive outlook.

Because many patients have a lowered resistance that makes them especially vulnerable to infection, you should not work when you are ill. However, because you are counted on to be present when scheduled, it is even better to prevent the onset of illness. Everyone experiences grief and acute anxiety occasionally, and such stresses can make you susceptible to illness. Whenever possible, you should stay at home to deal with such problems until a resolution is reached. Severe anxiety and stress can prevent you from properly fulfilling your responsibilities.

Do not overlook the importance of good nutrition and exercise habits. These practices pay off in an increased sense of well-being and in less time lost from work. Knowledge and practice of the principles of body mechanics (Chapter 21) will help prevent the types of injuries that can result from lifting and moving patients or equipment.

Preventive health measures are equally important. For example, health care facilities are required to offer hepatitis B vaccine without charge to employees who are at risk of exposure to this disease. If your work places you at risk of infection from needle sticks or other exposure to potentially contaminated blood, you are responsible for taking advantage of this important protection. The infection control precautions discussed in Chapter 21 have been developed to help prevent transmission of diseases from patient to patient and from patient to you. Your health and that of your patients depend on your commitment to understanding and applying these principles. Minimizing the spread of disease in a health care setting is a primary responsibility of all health care personnel.

Radiation exposure over the course of a career can have serious health consequences if proper precautions are not observed. Chapter 11 provides instruction in radiation protection. Adhering to radiation safety practices is another important aspect of self-care for limited operators.

Job Satisfaction

Most health care workers enter the field with a desire to help and to provide excellent patient care. Sometimes, however, the demands of clinical practice may tend to overshadow your best intentions. Patient needs may be overlooked in the stress of coping with technical demands

unless you make a conscious effort to learn, from the beginning, to handle both at once.

Your work will be the most satisfying when your contributions and the personal contacts they involve are genuine and sincere. When you do things because you *want* to do them and you enjoy doing them, you will do them well, and your work will be much less stressful (Fig. 20-3).

Appearance

Appearance can communicate how we feel about ourselves and our work. Everyone we meet forms an instant impression of who we are. What does your appearance tell patients about you? Similar to many health care workers, limited operators wear uniforms to present a simple, neat appearance. The uniforms are washable and plain to make them easy to keep clean. They should fit comfortably and be worn with simple, appropriate accessories. Avoid jewelry on hands or arms that could injure patients. Although fads and fashions change over time, a professional image will continue to be conservative.

Personal cleanliness and grooming are essential. Keep your fingernails reasonably short and smooth. Wear shoes that are comfortable and quiet to walk in and keep them clean. Use fragrances sparingly. Some patients have an allergic response to perfumes; others find heavy fragrances offensive. Strong fragrances can cause nausea in patients who are ill.

The appearances of the x-ray room and the public areas of your work environment are also important. An untidy, cluttered room does not show respect for patients. It suggests that personnel may be too pressured, too disorganized, or too uncaring to perform competently.

Teamwork

Teamwork is defined as the cooperative effort by the members of a group to achieve a common goal. The pressures of work may sometimes make this concept hard to apply. Your goal should be to provide the best possible patient care, and it is easier to do this when you work cooperatively with others.

Teamwork is a two-way street. If you appreciate help when schedules are tight, you need to be sensitive to the needs of your co-workers as well. The essence of teamwork is found in good communication among co-workers. Communication that promotes teamwork is discussed later in this chapter.

Empathetic Care

As stated earlier in this chapter, patients are entitled to considerate and respectful care. This statement applies to every patient, regardless of current status. Dealing effectively with clinical situations involves several abilities. One is the ability to show **empathy,** a sensitivity to the needs of others that allows you to meet those needs constructively, rather than merely sympathizing or reacting to their distress. Understanding and compassion are accompanied by an objective detachment that enables you to provide an appropriate response. For example, you could express sympathy for the victim of a tragic accident by crying or by smothering him with expressions of pity. A more productive expression of empathy would be to show concern and care while quickly and accurately providing the images that could aid in rapid diagnosis and treatment.

Beginners in the care of patients often express concerns such as, "What shall I do if the patient vomits? I just know I'll get sick, too!" or "I faint at the sight of blood." As you gain experience and confidence, you will learn to cope by focusing on the patient rather than on yourself. Thoughts of how you can meet the patient's needs will enable you to project a calm, reassuring attitude.

A focus on patient needs will also help you to respond calmly and assertively when the actions of a patient are inappropriate. It may seem strange or frightening that some individuals respond to stress and anxiety by becoming hostile or even threatening. These are often people who cope with stress by controlling the situation. Preserving a calm, objective attitude is most effective in dealing with these patients.

Overt expressions of sexuality by patients are encountered very infrequently. These events are usually a reflection of anxiety by patients who no longer feel functional as sexual human beings because of their current physical state. With this in mind, you can be less judgmental while setting limits on patient behaviors. In other words, you can refuse to accept the behavior while continuing to reassure and care for the patient.

Care of Supplies and Equipment

Health care facilities must stock large quantities of supplies to function effectively. In such an environment, it is easy to assume that free access implies free use. In truth, however, someone must pay the bill. The value of each inventory item includes an overhead factor that may be two or three times the item's basic cost. For example, when a sterile item is accidentally contaminated, the loss includes not only the cost of the item but also the costs involved in ordering, accounting, shipping, and storage. Medical supplies and equipment are expensive, and proper care is required to ensure that their value is preserved so that they are available for use when needed. The misuse of equipment or supplies, or their diversion for personal use, wastes funds and increases health care costs. The limited operator who avoids such waste is demonstrating a high standard of professional behavior.

Continuing Education

In radiography, as in any rapidly changing technical field, continuing education is necessary to learn about current trends and to maintain competencies. For this reason, limited operators must place a priority on acquiring new skills and expanding their knowledge. Textbooks often contain information that is valid when the manuscript is completed but outdated by the time the book is published. Standard practice changes rapidly, and today's knowledge will soon be out of date. Some states require continuing education as a condition of license or permit renewal, but continuing education is an important professional responsibility whether it is required or not.

Many opportunities for continuing education are available to the limited operator. Hospitals, colleges, and professional organizations provide educational opportunities that meet the need to stay abreast of current developments and expand skills. Education may take the form of courses, classes, workshops, seminars, and other group experiences, but there is also a variety of materials available for individual learning and self-study, including web-based instruction and correspondence courses.

When you are required to provide evidence of continuing education, be sure to determine in advance whether the education you plan to receive is approved and accredited for this purpose. Keep an accurate record of your continuing education activities and any documentation of participation that you receive. These documents are valuable even if they are not immediately required. Evidence of continuing education may assist your professional advancement by helping you to qualify for a promotion or a new position.

Failure to maintain competence and required certifications places both the employer and the employee at risk and may result in loss of employment and professional reputation. Knowing the credentials required in a given situation and maintaining current credentials are important professional responsibilities.

PROFESSIONAL COMMUNICATION

Communication is an interchange of ideas and information with others. How we communicate involves our attitudes and our manners. Attitude is a state of mind or an opinion that can be revealed by body position, tone of voice, facial expression, and other nonverbal signals. Manners are customs that express respect; they are sometimes referred to as the oil that makes daily contacts run smoothly.

Accurate communication is essential to quality patient care. The ability to give instructions depends on the speaker's being clear and precise. The listener, on the other hand, is equally responsible for attentive and receptive behavior. The need to establish rapport with both patients and co-workers by listening attentively and responding in a meaningful way can easily be overlooked under the pressures of a busy schedule. Stress in the workplace increases when interpersonal communication breaks down and good manners are neglected.

Nonverbal Communication

Although we perceive verbal language as our primary means of communication, nonverbal behaviors reveal a great deal about how we feel. Cultural background largely determines how nonverbal communication is interpreted. Most of us learn to respond to common cues in childhood. We perceive frowns or pursed lips as disapproval. Refusal to look directly into an individual's face while speaking conveys avoidance, submission, or rejection, whereas clenched teeth or fists suggest angry feelings under rigid control. Patients in pain may present a tight and rigid protective posture. Leaning forward while listening to another gives the appearance of intense interest in the subject being discussed.

As a rule, a positive and caring attitude naturally results in nonverbal behaviors that are also positive. The reverse is also true. A negative attitude will be unconsciously revealed, no matter what is said. What common nonverbal language do you recognize (Fig. 20-4)?

Eye Contact

In the United States, eye contact is considered a positive behavior. When you make direct eye contact with an individual while speaking, it is usually perceived as an expression of interest, concern, or honesty. As you will learn in a later section on culture and communication, it is important to remember that direct eye contact is not welcome in all cultures.

Touching

Touch is a means of communication, too. An abrupt or tentative touch may be perceived as distaste or reluctance to care for the individual. A positive touch is firm but gentle and reassures the patient that you are both capable and caring. People touch one another for a variety of reasons, including:

* To provide reassurance, support, encouragement
* To imply domination, anger, frustration
* To form a positive connection, as in a handshake or shoulder pat
* To perform professional services, such as those provided by a doctor, hairdresser, or masseuse

Remember that the brief hug around the shoulder that is so reassuring to many Americans may be an upsetting invasion of personal space and privacy to those whose culture does not include a casual embrace. In some cultures and religions, touch by a stranger or a member of the opposite sex is unacceptable or strongly frowned on.

When you must touch a patient, you are much less likely to unintentionally offend if you tell the patient in advance what you are about to do and then use a firm, appropriate touch. It is important that your touch has a professional purpose that is clear to the patient.

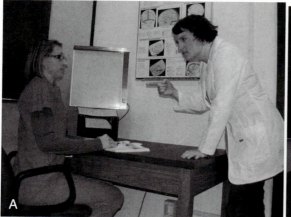 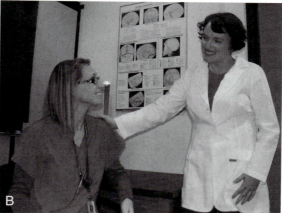

Fig. 20-4 More than 70% of communication received by adults is nonverbal. **A,** What message is this supervisor sending? **B,** Warmth is not conveyed with words.

Verbal Communication

Clear, distinct speech habits help to ensure accurate communication. Try to tailor the content of your speech to the comprehension level of the listener. Chapter 18 provides specific suggestions for communication with children and older adults. Use good eye contact and speak face to face. This approach assures others that they have your full attention and concern.

It is an asset to cultivate an ability to be **assertive**. This does not imply that you need to be **aggressive**. Expressions of aggression involve anger or hostility, whereas assertion is the calm, firm expression of feelings or opinions. You have the right to be assertive when you require assistance in a patient care situation that is beyond your ability. Employers may be assertive in requiring employees to maintain the level of competence required by their job descriptions. In dealing with patients who are reluctant to cooperate, pleasant assertiveness is the attitude that is most productive in obtaining compliance.

Listening Skills

How do you feel when you are interrupted or when the listener looks out the window while you attempt to make your point? Are you irritated when others "put words in your mouth" or change the subject without responding to what you have just said? Good communication is a two-way street. A good listener does more than wait his or her turn to speak. Listening skills involve the ability to focus on the speaker and to project an attentive attitude. When you give the speaker full attention, you can respond to what has been said rather than make a quick switch to the next item on your own agenda. In discussion, patients often give us clues about a physical problem that can be easily overlooked if we rush to get on to the next question.

Validation of Communication

Good communication requires validation of understanding. An informal response, such as a smile, nod, or brief "okay," may be perfectly satisfactory in a social situation, but when essential information is being presented, the response must reflect clear understanding. This is particularly true with all instructions that involve your professional activities. As a listener, you can be sure that you have understood the message by reflecting or repeating the essential elements of the speaker's statement in your response. When you are imparting information and do not receive a validating response, continue the conversation by asking your listener to restate the information. The conversation that follows is an example of a valid communication between a physician and a limited operator:

Physician: I think Mrs. Kirkland may have a right scaphoid fracture. Please take the routine exam and a Stecher view and let me see them right away.

Limited operator: That's a routine right wrist plus a Stecher view on Mrs. Kirkland, and I'll bring them to you as soon as they're ready.

Physician: Right. Thank you.

The lesson for both speakers and listeners is that messages must be both clear and complete and that comprehension of the message must be confirmed. Without such validation, neither party can be certain that all elements of the message have been understood.

Communication Under Stress

Any situation that disturbs our everyday activities imposes stress. Most health care involves some anxiety and often proves stressful to patients, families, and health care workers alike. This is especially true in a crisis when speed is a factor or when a complex situation causes disagreement about priorities.

Stress interferes with our ability to process information accurately or appropriately. A classic example is the victim of a house fire who flees with the nearest object, such as a rubber plant, rather than essential papers or treasured family possessions. In a stressful situation, accurate communication can be difficult. The principles of communication already discussed are always important, but these additional suggestions can improve your effectiveness under stress:

- Lower your voice and speak slowly and clearly.
- Be nonjudgmental in both verbal and nonverbal communication.
- Do not allow the inappropriate actions or speech of an upset individual to goad you into a similar response.
- When you are uncertain whether the listener has understood you, request an answer. For example, "Did you read the consent form? What did it ask you about allergies?"

Communication With Patients

The first contact with a patient is usually an introduction. In many social situations today, given names are used as soon as introductions are made. Although this may seem to project an air of friendliness and informality, it also poses certain problems. "Good morning, Mr. Robles. I'm Lisa McCall, the x-ray machine operator," is more than an example of good manners. It shows respect and concern and allows the patient to choose how he wishes to be addressed. In an effort to show friendliness, some staff may address adults as "honey" or "sweetie" instead of calling them by name. Others, who are focused on the work routine, may refer to "the diabetic in room 2" or "that sprained ankle in the hall." Talking down to adults or treating them impersonally diminishes their self-esteem and raises feelings of resentment. Such feelings can diminish the ability of the patient to understand and follow directions. These feelings may also prevent retention of information and could actually hinder recovery.

Resentment is destructive of the trusting relationship that is essential to quality care.

A helpful way to show respect and elevate patients' self-esteem is to involve them in their own care by giving them opportunities to make choices. Offering a valid choice, as discussed in Chapter 18, requires some thought, but the rewards in terms of patient satisfaction are well worth the effort. The choice does not need to be an earth-shaking decision. Questions such as, "Would you like a blanket over your knees?" or "Would you like to stop in the restroom before we begin?" can reassure patients who would like to feel capable of making decisions and who need to have a share in their own care. Treating patients as individuals, allowing them to make valid choices, and using good nonverbal skills are tools that alleviate fear and promote cooperation.

In determining why patients fail to follow instructions, one factor frequently encountered is the assumption that the patient understands the procedure. Such an assumption is really just a guess. For example, we could assume that because you are reading this text, you are a student in a radiography or medical assisting program. That could be true, or perhaps you are a nurse who is expanding your professional skills. You might also be an instructor or the proofreader for this book. Making assumptions about patients implies that you might also guess about physical status or mental ability, or even about willingness to cooperate. Can you assume that Mr. White, who may have broken his ankle, can be positioned flat on the radiographic table? No. Although his ankle injury might not prevent such positioning, he may have emphysema, which could interfere with his ability to breathe while lying supine.

Conversing with patients allows you to use your powers of observation. Is the patient alert or confused? How well does the patient hear? Is English comprehension a problem? From observation, you can often make a tentative assessment of the patient's ability to get on and off the examination table, walk unassisted to the bathroom, and so forth. Patient assessment is discussed in depth in Chapter 22, but assessment begins with communication. You should learn from this chapter that good communication with patients can help you establish a spirit of trust and cooperation that will assist in both patient assessment and patient care.

Special Circumstances in Communications

Deafness

The deaf patient presents a set of problems unlike those of patients with a hearing loss discussed in Chapter 18. Many totally deaf individuals live in a cultural setting that has its own social structure, language, and even "inside" jokes. Certain cues help in differentiating between the patient with a hearing loss and the deaf patient, especially in an emergency. You may become aware that a seemingly alert patient is totally deaf when he or she does one of the following things:

- Does not respond to noises or words spoken out of the range of vision
- Uses lip movements without making a sound or speaks in a flat monotone
- Points to the ears and mouth while shaking the head in a negative motion
- Uses gestures or writing motions to express the need for paper and pencil

Some deaf people are adept at lip reading and are able to speak, at least to a limited degree. More often the deaf are educated in American Sign Language (ASL), which is the most common sign language and is distinctly different from English. It has unique grammar, syntax, and rules. Learning a few basic signs may aid in establishing rapport with deaf patients. A card showing the alphabet and some common signs in ASL should be available through your local hospital's nursing service department or from community service agencies that assist the deaf. An interpreter is essential in any situation that requires complex instruction or an exchange of important information. Deaf patients have the right to choose the most preferred method of communication, which might be pencil and paper. Be sure that writing materials are available and that the patient's writing arm is free.

The health care setting can seem overwhelming, especially when the patient is a deaf child. If possible, allow the child and parents to tour the area before the examination begins. Take time to fully explain the procedure so the parents can help the child understand what to expect. If the child is distressed, you might consider allowing a parent to stay in sight or near the child while following appropriate radiation safety precautions.

Blindness

Most of us depend on our eyes to become familiar with our surroundings and to ensure our safety as we move about. Vision enables us to recognize individuals and locate items of daily living. The ability of a person who is blind to accomplish these same tasks without vision can seem astounding. People who are blind rely on hearing and touch to a much greater extent than sighted persons. With the aid of a cane or guide dog, many people who are blind lead very independent lives. Having learned to work outside the home, use public transportation, and maintain their own households, these patients may be insulted by attitudes that are too solicitous. They may be quite capable of proceeding confidently after a quick description of a room and the obstacles in it. You might say, "This is a square room, Mrs. Lord. The x-ray table is about 5 feet in front of you, and a chair is at 7 o'clock. After you're on the table, I'll be in a booth to your left." On the other hand, patients who are blind may welcome some special help in a strange environment. Some will prefer to follow you by listening to your footsteps and using a cane, whereas others may wish to place a hand on your shoulder or elbow. Those who are infirm may prefer your arm around their waist while you reassure and direct them verbally. Take care that obstacles such as step stools do not present a safety hazard as blind people move about. None of these approaches applies to all people who are blind. Good communication is the key to determining which form of help is acceptable and appropriate.

Remember that loss of the ability to see, hear, or speak is a communication impairment and not a reflection of the individual's intelligence or ability to think. Patients with sensory deprivation challenge us to be more flexible and innovative in the ways we offer explanations and reassurance.

Impaired Mental Function

Special sensitivity is needed when dealing with adult patients who are mentally or emotionally handicapped. Such patients may include those with congenital defects such as Down syndrome, those with illnesses or injuries affecting the brain, and those with severe emotional disorders that affect comprehension. As with children, you must assess the patient's ability to understand and follow instructions, because this ability may vary from a near infantile response to a functional capability close to normal. In general, the same clear, simple, and direct instructions offered to children are appropriate. You may need to repeat instructions if the attention span is short. Use the adult form of address, and treat these patients with the respect and dignity due anyone their age.

Communication With Patients' Families

When we are sick or injured, the presence of those who care about us is very reassuring and may be essential to our ability to cope. It is natural that family members rush to the emergency room after an accident, visit patients during hospital admissions, and accompany patients to their appointments. You may have to deal with family members who want to hold the patient's hand during a radiographic examination or who eagerly await the results of a diagnostic procedure. When you are busy and the patient is your primary concern, family members may appear as obstacles to your work. Dealing sensitively with families is often necessary and helps your patient in ways that may not be apparent.

Your communication with families often involves the transfer of practical information. Those waiting for a patient want to know how long the procedure will take, and they appreciate an update from you when a delay occurs. When the wait is prolonged, your attention to the waiting family's comfort might include directions to services, such as the restrooms, cafeteria, or telephone.

If the patient is a minor, is incompetent, or is sedated, you may need to provide instructions to a family member regarding preparations or follow-up care. Be sure you are speaking to the person who will actually assist the patient, because information can be lost when it is passed from person to person.

Questions often arise regarding the immediate presence of family members during a procedure. The family must usually stay outside the room, preferably in a waiting area or lobby that is out of hearing range. This is done not only because of radiation safety precautions but also because it allows the staff to proceed without interruptions from concerned family members who may not understand what is happening and may require explanations and reassurance. Procedures that involve patient discomfort or some blood loss may be very unsettling to loved ones. If families are waiting nearby, you should be aware of this and avoid making statements within hearing range that might alarm them or betray a professional confidence.

Occasionally a family member may need to stay with the patient in the procedure room, for example, as with a deaf child as mentioned earlier. In these situations, only one family member should be selected, and this person should receive a clear explanation before the procedure. You should answer questions at this point and clarify the role of family members. Provide radiation protection as necessary.

Sometimes dealing with families can be especially difficult. In an emotionally charged situation, we all use different means to cope with our anxiety. Some of us become dependent and wait for others to make decisions and give us instructions. Others maintain self-control by withdrawing or denying the importance of the situation. Anxiety causes some individuals to be quite aggressive or controlling when communicating about patients who are dear to them. Fear frequently engenders anger. If you can understand aggressive demands for service and attention as being an expression of fear, you can concentrate on reassuring rather than responding with anger yourself. Although you should refer inquiries about diagnosis or prognosis directly to the physician, an expression of concern can demonstrate empathy. "I know how worried you must be about Cynthia, Mr. Roth. I've let the doctor know you're waiting for the results."

Communication With Co-workers

The ability to relay information to other health professionals is essential. The kinds of problems we encounter when dealing with patients may also arise when communicating with co-workers. The pressures of time and workload may compound the personality conflicts that occur in any group. Good interpersonal relationships are built on the ability to make others feel good about themselves (Fig. 20-5). The nonverbal behaviors that we use with patients, such as touch and appearance, are equally effective with co-workers. Be a good listener. Use praise and appreciation as positive reinforcements when work is well done or when others go out of their way to provide assistance. Demonstrate respect for your

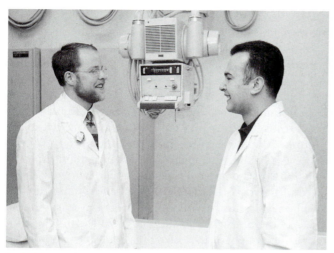

Fig. 20-5 Good interpersonal relationships are built on the ability to make others feel good about themselves.

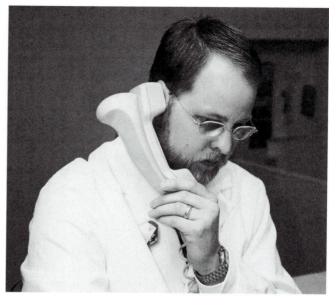

Fig. 20-6 A professional approach to telephone communication improves patient care.

co-workers as individuals by avoiding cliques and gossip. Especially avoid revealing personal information about your employer and your co-workers to patients or others.

One other concern regarding your interpersonal relationships with co-workers has ethical and legal implications. The pressure of work may make it difficult to find time to exchange general information. For this reason, break or lunchtime is often used to catch up on recent developments and share information. *Never discuss patients in a public setting.* It is acceptable to talk about changes in schedules, the holiday party, or the new computer system, but discussions of interesting cases, celebrity patients, or possible treatment errors can be overheard and used in damaging litigation. Such conversations are invasions of the personal rights and privacy of patients.

In a modern health care facility, a great amount of information is exchanged. Although much of the technical communication is conveyed using charts and forms, it can be equally important to relay informal messages accurately. Attention to details, such as adding your name and the date to telephone message forms and notes for the bulletin board, can help keep information retrieval pertinent.

Most businesses and health care facilities have voice mail systems to facilitate messaging when personnel are away from their telephones. When you receive a voice mail message, it is courteous to call back and confirm that you have received the message. Playing "telephone tag" can be very frustrating to the caller, and the problem is worsened when there is no way to know if the message has been received. When leaving a voice mail message (Fig. 20-6), be sure to identify yourself and your position or facility. State the date and time and your telephone number clearly. If you want your call returned so that you can talk to the person, suggest a convenient time to return the call. Here are some

additional guidelines for avoiding problems with telephone communications:

- Be familiar with your telephone system, including forwarding and hold functions.
- Identify yourself and your facility or department when calling or answering a call.
- Keep paper handy and make notes during the call to avoid losing details.
- Use a pleasant, receptive tone of voice.
- Validate the message before concluding the call.
- When receiving a call for someone else, avoid disclosing personal information. Simply state that the person is unavailable or out of the office and offer to take a message. Be sure the message is relayed to the proper person or department promptly.

Written communication is valuable only if it is received in good time. Whether this is a telephone message, a personal note, or a change in schedule, try to see that such messages are given directly to the intended individual or posted in plain sight in a predetermined spot. Be sure to identify yourself, your department (if appropriate), and the time the message was sent or received. If a response is needed, remember to include the return address and/or telephone number.

Facsimile transmissions, or faxes, are often used to send information between health care facilities. Physicians may use the convenience of fax transmission to prevent the errors that can occur with verbal telephone orders. If you are responsible for faxing information to another institution, remember to fill out the cover sheet first. Confusion about where the information is needed or who is to receive it can cause needless delays in patient care. When confidential information regarding a patient is to be sent by fax, it should be preceded by a phone call to alert the recipient. Confidentiality is difficult to preserve at best, and such information should be treated in a responsible manner. Most fax machines print out a record of the fax transmission. If it is your duty to transmit information by fax, know the procedure for maintaining this record. It may be attached to the original copy of the document or you may need to note the document's content on the fax record and file it separately.

ISSUES OF CULTURAL DIVERSITY

Non–English-speaking Patients

Language barriers are not handled very effectively in the United States. Federal legislation addresses the patient's right to understand and communicate effectively in health care situations, regardless of language barriers. Most large hospitals now have a service that will arrange for an interpreter when necessary. In a clinic setting, translation is most often handled by family members. If patients who do not speak English are commonly seen in your facility, you should become familiar with the policies in place for ensuring that communication meets the needs of these patients.

The difference between a certified interpreter and a friend or family member who assumes this role may be significant. The interpreter is trained to translate only what has been said, both by the patient and to the patient, and not to explain what is implied. Family and friends may tend to add inappropriate information or to edit the conversation in an effort to be cooperative or to save time. For example, a complete explanation of positioning and instructions for breathing may be abbreviated in translation to, "It's okay, mama. Just hold still." Family members may hesitate to reveal information about the patient that they believe is private or embarrassing. The patient may hesitate to reveal personal information through family or friends. Family members whose command of English is limited may have good intentions but be unable to provide adequate translation of complex information. The services of a trained interpreter provide a professional bridge in difficult communication situations. As with deaf clients, official interpreters must be used when complex and important information is being exchanged, so that interpersonal relationships will not interfere and the parties to the conversation can be certain that the translations are accurate.

When using an interpreter, look directly at the patient and speak as though the patient were able to understand you. The interpreter will translate as you speak or as soon as you have finished a sentence. Speaking to the interpreter directly tends to make the patient feel left out or talked about rather than involved in the process.

If a translator is unavailable, use demonstrations or pencil sketches to validate whether the individual understands and make extensive use of nonverbal encouragement. A friendly smile and a warm touch may be worth many words.

Scope of Diversity

American society today, both urban and rural, is far more culturally diverse than in our great grandparents' day. Data from the U.S. Census Bureau indicate that today the ratio of nonwhites to whites is 1:4 and that by 2070 half of all Americans will be African American, Hispanic, Native American, or Asian/Pacific Islander. Although this diversity poses certain social problems, it also creates a vast richness and creative potential.

Cultural diversity is a global health care issue. Research suggests that there are differences in outcomes of health care treatments that are related to race and ethnicity. Lawmakers have passed legislation to address cultural inequities in health care.[i] Your health care facility must plan for transcultural care and will expect staff to develop the attitudes and the knowledge required to help implement these plans.

The subject of ethnic and cultural diversity is complex and fills numerous textbooks. It is impossible within the scope of this book to anticipate the many diverse ethnic and cultural situations you will encounter in your work. We hope that the limited examples in the discussion that follows will help to raise your awareness of those situations in which sensitivity is needed.

The racial and **ethnic** (national) characteristics of individuals originally were identified with specific areas of the globe. Africans came from Africa, Chinese from China, and so forth. In many cases, racial characteristics such as skin color, hair texture, and the shapes of facial features were identified with specific cultures as well as with ethnic origins. As opportunities for emigration and travel increased, it became more difficult to identify the national origin of a specific individual. For example, not all patients with Asian features speak an Asian language.

Culture is determined by language and by the customs commonly observed. It can be misleading to generalize about the cultural attitudes and practices of any ethnic group because individual variations within a group depend on so many factors. In addition, the physical appearance of an individual may have no relationship to how extensively he or she has integrated culturally into the mainstream of American life. A person who has recently arrived from Eastern Europe wearing the latest athletic shoes, a baseball cap, and blue jeans may speak little or no English, whereas a patient wearing a turban and a dashiki may have been born in Chicago of ancestors who have lived there for generations.

When cultural diversity is mentioned, customs relating to nationality may be the first things that come to

---

[i]The Healthcare Equality and Accountability Act—Family Care Act of 2005 (S 1580/HR 3561) and the Faircare Act of 2005 (S 1929).

mind. Our society consists of many different groups in addition to ethnic groups, and each has unique characteristics that can affect the values and perceptions of individuals within the group. Historically, certain groups have been subjected to discriminatory treatment, which causes some individuals to have a high level of sensitivity about their group identity. Examples of such cultural groups include the following:

- Gender groups: male/female
- Racial groups: distinguished by skin color and other physical characteristics
- Generational groups: generation Y (millennials), generation X, Baby Boomers, and the elderly
- Geographic groups: North/South; East Coast/West Coast; native cultures in Hawaii, Alaska, and on and around reservations, plus areas where ethnic culture endures because large numbers of immigrants from a certain country have settled there (Mexican influences along the southern borders of Texas and California, and Scandinavian heritage in Minnesota, for example)
- Sexual preference groups: heterosexual, gay, lesbian, bisexual, and transgender
- Religious groups
- Groups based on nonracial physical characteristics: the blind, the deaf, the disabled, the obese
- Socioeconomic groups: low income (unemployed, welfare recipients, uninsured, underinsured), middle income, affluent
- Groups with various types of family structure: singles, unmarried couples with and without children, traditional nuclear families, single mother/single father heads of households, parents with children and grandchildren, and large, close-knit extended families

Culturally Significant Attitudes That May Impact Communication

The relationship between culture and communication is an integral part of our everyday lives. Our reactions and habits are learned from our parents, are passed down to our children, and largely govern the way we conduct our daily activities. Each society develops unwritten rules regarding such ordinary things as how close we stand when talking to another, where we touch another person in public, and other reflections of courtesy to those around us.

For example, it is important in many Asian societies to avoid placing another person in an embarrassing position. Harmony is to be promoted, and loud or aggressive behavior is considered a sign of poor manners. Such patients may respond more positively to a soft, quiet tone of voice than to the brisk, assertive commands so easily adopted by many Americans when in a hurry. When apprehensive or nervous, Asian patients may become reticent and unsociable, which can hinder effective communication.

The cultural differences in nonverbal behaviors are also highly significant. For example, a Vietnamese patient may smile to cover up disturbed feelings. Repeated head nods may indicate respect for the individual speaking, rather than agreement with the subject being discussed. Gestures, eye contact, and touch may have unintended meanings when perceived by someone from a culture that assigns different meanings to the same signals. For example, many Native Americans avoid direct eye contact, considering it a mark of disrespect. Many Asian societies use no eye contact during verbal communication and may resent direct eye contact, perceiving it as being impolite and an invasion of personal space. In countries with a high-density population, eye contact and touch are less acceptable among adults than in the United States. Pointing directly at an individual can be considered insulting in many cultural groups, including our own, but it can be especially offensive to Native Americans and certain Asian groups. Beckoning with the index finger is insulting to Filipinos and to Koreans.

In Hispanic culture, embracing, touching, and close proximity are easily accepted from familiar people. This may seem to contrast with a strong sense of modesty that can be demonstrated during physical examinations, so it is important to provide both men and women with ample gowns and covering during examinations in the imaging department. To Native Americans, personal space is very important, and although patients may embrace or touch others with whom they feel close, touching should be confined to that needed to provide health care.

An old superstition of Mediterranean origin is occasionally seen among Hispanic clients. The "evil eye" or *mal ojo* is thought to bring bad luck or illness if children are praised or admired without also being touched. Eye contact with adults is perfectly acceptable, but when praising a child, it is wise to give a touch or pat while expressing admiration. Although the parents may no longer express belief in the "evil eye," the ability of individuals to cause illness in a child by looking admiringly without touching is a very strong superstition.

The best way to understand people of another culture is to learn to know them personally. We hope that this discussion will heighten your awareness, not only of differences in ethnic backgrounds, but also of diversity within your own cultural group. The more sensitive you become to the reactions of all your patients, the more comfortable your interpersonal contacts will be.

How Cultural Issues May Affect Care

Although this discussion is limited in scope, it should help to increase your awareness of the diversity of needs, expectations, and fears that may influence your patients in the health care setting. Box 20-3 provides some examples of how various ethnic cultural groups approach both communication and health care and how their cultural status may affect the outcome of their contacts with

Box 20-3

Suggestions for Improving Communication and Care With Specific Ethnic Groups

Note that these are broad generalizations that may not apply to all members of a culture.

Anglo-American

- Patients expect to know and understand details of their conditions and treatments.
- Direct eye contact is expected; avoid excessive direct eye contact with members of the opposite sex to avoid any hint of sexual connotation.
- Emotional control is expected. Privacy is important and must be respected. Caregivers are usually welcome and expected to provide psychosocial care in addition to physical care.
- Decisions are made by individuals for themselves and may be made by either parent for a child.
- Independence is valued, and self-care concepts are generally accepted.
- Patients tend to be stoic when in pain but may also feel comfortable requesting pain medication when needed.
- Patients may prefer to be left alone when they do not feel well.
- An aggressive biomedical treatment of illness is generally preferred, but complementary and alternative medicine may also be used. Germs are thought to be the cause of illness and antibiotic treatment may be expected.

African American

- Because of a history of slavery and discrimination, African American patients may not trust "white institutions" such as hospitals and may be very easily upset by what they perceive to be discrimination. Be especially sensitive to this issue.
- Do not refer to a man as a "boy" or a woman as a "gal." These terms are often perceived as insulting. Address individuals using their titles and last names.
- Family structure may be nuclear, extended, or matriarchal. Close friends may be a significant part of the support system. The father or eldest male may be the spokesperson and/or primary decision maker, although this authority may lie with the eldest female in a matriarchal family.
- Patients may believe that disease is caused by improper diet, exposure to cold or wind, punishment by God for sin, or voodoo spells. Cultural lore prescribes appropriate treatments for these causes. There is a rich African American tradition of herbal and home remedies.
- Many have a present time orientation that can impede the implementation of preventive medicine and follow-up care.
- Blood or organ donation may not be acceptable except to meet the needs of family members.

Asian

- Agreement may be indicated with no intention to follow through, so it is important to explain reasons for compliance with instructions and to ask open-ended questions instead of those that can be satisfied with a yes or no answer.
- Avoid direct eye contact and hand gestures.

- Because there are no pronouns in most Asian languages, references to "he" or "she" may be confused.
- Wives may defer to husbands in decision making.
- Tremendous respect is accorded to the elderly.
- There is reluctance to admit pain.
- Traditional healing methods include coining and cupping, the use of herbs, and changes in temperature.
- Stigma is associated with mental illness, and emotional problems are not discussed with strangers. Mental or emotional problems may manifest as physical illness.

East Indian

This group includes Hindus and Muslims from India, Pakistan, Bangladesh, Sri Lanka, and Nepal.

- Direct eye contact may be perceived as rude or disrespectful, especially among the elderly.
- Silence may indicate acceptance or approval.
- Head movements may confuse those from Western cultures. A side-to-side head motion may indicate agreement or uncertainty, whereas an up-and-down nod may indicate that the listener acknowledges what the speaker is saying but does not agree.
- Husbands may answer questions addressed to their wives.
- A man should avoid shaking hands with an East Indian woman unless the woman extends her hand first.
- The father or eldest son usually has decision-making power after other family members have been consulted. Patients may not wish to participate in health care decisions, considering health care professionals to be the authorities in these matters. This may affect their willingness to sign consent forms.
- Same-sex caregivers may be preferred for reasons of modesty.
- Patients may be either stoic or expressive when in pain. Muslim patients may not want pain medication except under extreme circumstances.

Hispanic

- Because of the emphasis on personal relationships, it is helpful to ask about a patient's family and interests before focusing on health issues.
- Family members are likely to want to stay with the patient and to assist the patient with activities of daily living rather than allow these tasks to be done by professional caregivers.
- Modesty is very important, especially to older women.
- Traditional wives will defer to their husbands for decisions that involve care for themselves or their children.
- Many have a present time orientation that can impede the implementation of preventive medicine and follow-up care.
- Patients may respond to pain with loud outcries, depending on the audience. Males may be more expressive around family members than with health professionals.
- Patients may refuse certain foods or medications that they believe will upset the body's hot/cold balance. Avoid ice water unless requested. A high fat content in food may be perceived as healthy.

Continued

Box 20-3

Suggestions for Improving Communication and Care With Specific Ethnic Groups—cont'd

Middle Eastern

- Islam is a dominant force in the lives of most Middle Easterners. Devout Muslims pray several times a day facing Mecca (east) and appreciate privacy for this practice. They may have a fatalistic attitude about life, death, and health, believing that these matters are in the hands of Allah and that health-related practices are of little consequence.
- There is a tendency to be loud and expressive, especially during childbirth, when someone has died, and when in pain.
- Family members may feel responsible for ensuring the best care possible and so may make emphatic demands of health care personnel.
- Sexual segregation is extremely important, so whenever possible, same-sex caregivers should be assigned. Every effort must be made to maintain a woman's modesty at all times. Women do not wish to remove their head scarves (hijabs), especially in the presence of men.
- Women tend to defer to their husbands for decision making involving their own and their children's health care. Husbands may answer questions addressed to their wives. When important information is sought or provided, it is considered appropriate to speak first with the family spokesperson.
- Organ donation or autopsy may not be permitted for religious reasons.
- Damp, cold drafts and strong emotions are sometimes thought to cause illness. The "evil eye of envy" may also be thought to cause illness or misfortune, and amulets may be worn to prevent this; the amulet should not be removed.
- Muslims do not eat pork.

Native American

- Stories and metaphors may be used to communicate ideas. For example, a story about a neighbor who is ill may be a patient's way of describing his or her own symptoms.
- Long pauses in a conversation usually indicate that careful consideration is being given to a question. Do not rush the patient.
- Direct eye contact should be avoided, both as a show of respect and because some may feel that this threatens the loss or theft of the soul.
- Loud or aggressive behavior is considered very offensive and should be avoided.
- Historical mistreatment of Native American groups by white people, and especially the misuse of signed documents in this regard, may cause Native Americans to be leery of documents or unwilling to sign informed consents or advance directives.
- Illness of one member is a concern to all members of the family, and the extended family is very important. Patients usually make decisions for themselves, but this may vary with tribal and kinship structures. Hopi, Navajo, and Zuni tribes are matrilineal; in these groups descent is reckoned through the female line, and women or their brothers make the important decisions.
- Orientation to time is based on activities rather than the clock.
- Stoicism is valued, and patients may not express their pain other than to say they do not feel well. When a patient complains of discomfort and is not given relief, the complaint may never be repeated.
- Before cutting or shaving hair, check to see whether the patient or the family wants to keep it. In some tribes, cutting hair is associated with mourning.
- A medicine bag may be worn. Do not treat this casually or remove it without the patient's permission. If it must be removed, allow a family member to do so, keep it close to the patient, and return it as soon as possible.
- Native foods tend to be high in fat content. Foods that have been blessed (in either the traditional religion or Christianity) are believed to be free from harm.
- Use of traditional healers may be combined with the use of Western medicine. Allow traditional healers to perform rituals when possible and do not touch or casually admire their ritual objects.

Russian

The cultures of countries near Russia, particularly those of the Ukraine and Eastern Europe that were once part of the Soviet Union, are often quite similar to that of Russia today.

- Family members will be anxious about patients and will expect frequent updates about progress, treatments, and tests.
- A warm, caring attitude on the part of caregivers is especially welcome.
- Loud, abrasive demands for attention may be a reflection of the fact that this attitude was necessary to meet one's needs in the Russian health care system.
- Most patients are comfortable with direct eye contact and a firm, respectful attitude. Address patients using titles and last names. Hand gestures and facial expressions may be used by patients, especially when not proficient in English. Gestures and facial expressions may also supplement understanding when used by caregivers.
- The gender of the caregiver is not usually an issue, but it may be desirable to have a family member of the same gender present when performing personal care.
- There is a tendency to have a high tolerance for pain and to be stoic in this regard.
- Many, especially the elderly, believe that illness results from cold. Therefore keep the patient covered, close windows, keep the room warm, and avoid iced drinks.

From Ehrlich RA, Coakes D: *Patient care in radiography*, ed 9, St Louis, 2016, Mosby.

health care organizations. This listing is not comprehensive for all health care, but offers insight into the cultural issues that may affect patient care in imaging departments. For example, family structure may determine who makes decisions, who expects to receive information, and who usually signs documents. Although specific practices are described here in association with specific cultural groups, it is important that you understand these descriptions as broad generalizations and not use them in any way that would stereotype individuals.

Some ethnic cultures have a high level of sensitivity surrounding modesty and physical contact in health care. This may apply to any situation but is most often an issue when the patient and the health care provider are not of the same gender, especially if the patient is female and the health care professional is male. These attitudes are particularly prevalent in both Hispanic and Islamic cultures, but are certainly not limited to these groups.

Religion can be a significant factor in health care as well. Religion is almost synonymous with culture in some countries. For instance, the Muslim religion predominates in the Middle East, Roman Catholicism is prevalent in Latin America, and Hinduism influences the culture of India, but all of these regions have some religious diversity as well, so it may be misleading to make assumptions about religion based on national origin. Some religious groups dictate or prohibit specific health care practices. For example, some religions do not condone blood transfusions, some prohibit any practice that punctures the skin, and others oppose the practice of vaccination. Prayer and other religious healing practices may need to be accommodated in combination with medical treatments. Religious practices may influence the acceptability of certain diets or treatments and may dictate specific actions with respect to matters of life and death. Religious dietary requirements, such as kosher meals for orthodox Jews, may affect a patient's choice of medical facilities and may affect compliance with recommended health practices.

Professional Responsibility and Ethics in Relation to Diversity

You will recall from an earlier section of this chapter that issues of cultural diversity have significant ethical dimensions. The ARRT Code of Ethics requires radiographers to put aside all personal prejudice and emotional bias, rendering services to humanity with *full respect for the dignity of mankind*. Specifically, they are to conduct themselves in a professional manner, support their colleagues and associates, respond to patient needs, and deliver patient care and service unrestricted by concerns of personal attributes or the nature of the disease or illness and without discrimination on the basis of sex, race, creed, religion, or socioeconomic status.

Those who study the sociology of ethics tell us that the development of high moral and ethical standards does not come naturally to most people and is unlikely to be attained by simply reading a code of ethics or a chapter in a textbook. It is a process that begins with a commitment and continues with each encounter that presents an opportunity to listen, reflect, and learn. We must open our minds to the possibility that our own perceptions are not universal and that the differing perceptions and values of others have validity and importance.

Although understanding people of another culture is best accomplished by getting to know them personally, this may not always be practical. Many books are available on transcultural health care that can help you to bridge cultural gaps. If your geographic area has a significant number of individuals from another culture, you can enrich your life and provide better care by learning as much as possible about ethnic groups with which you come in frequent contact.

Nonverbal behaviors such as eye contact and touching are not interpreted in the same way by all those within our own society, and the differences are even greater between one culture and another. We hope that this discussion of transcultural issues has heightened your awareness, not only of different ethnic backgrounds, but of differences within American culture as well. The more sensitive you are to the reactions of all your patients, the more comfortable your interpersonal contacts will become.

MEDICAL INFORMATION AND RECORDS

Efficient record keeping, accomplished through effective documentation of information about patients and their care, is a vital aspect of meeting patients' needs (Fig. 20-7).

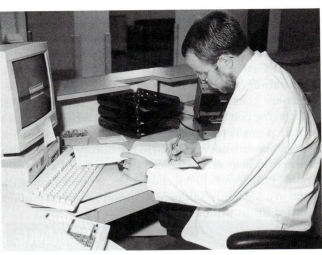

Fig. 20-7 All medical records you initiate must be pertinent, accurate, and legible.

radiologic technologists is prescribed by the *ARRT Standards of Ethics*. Many states have laws and regulations that define the scope of practice and provide guidelines for the professional conduct of limited operators. Ethical practice is essential to good patient care. Such conduct safeguards patient rights and reduces the likelihood of medicolegal difficulties.

Our success in any endeavor depends largely on our ability to communicate with one another. In a health care setting, many factors can cause anxiety in both patients and staff. When we approach patients with compassion and empathy, we find greater personal satisfaction in our work and improve the quality of care. The same principles of communication that increase the effectiveness of our relationships with patients and their families will enhance our relationships with co-workers.

Federal legislation addresses the patient's right to understand and communicate effectively in health care situations, regardless of language barriers. Both legal and ethical standards require attention to the needs of patients with their cultural backgrounds taken into account. Therefore health care workers must have a general knowledge of the customs of their patients and be sensitive to any needs they may have that differ from those of the culture of the majority.

Limited operators must respect the importance of medical records and strive to keep records that are pertinent, accurate, and legible. An understanding of patient charts provides a valuable resource to validate information. The ability to chart competently is essential if the job description requires making entries in these records. Diagnostic images are a part of the legal medical record and belong to the facility in which they are taken.

Safety and Infection Control

Whether your job description involves only radiography or includes other back office clinic functions, patient care skills will be essential to your work. In this chapter, you will learn some basic principles of patient care and ways to ensure the safety of your patients while also preventing injury to yourself and others.

Gathering places for the sick are often focal points for the transmission of disease. Anyone with a health problem is more susceptible to infection, and therefore infection control is of critical importance in patient care. It is your professional duty to follow established infection control procedures. This will promote the safety of your patients, yourself, and your co-workers.

Health care facilities that are affiliated with hospitals or government agencies are required to have policy and procedure manuals that provide protocols for many procedures discussed in this chapter. Small, private facilities may have less formal policies but should also have written protocols. It is your duty to be familiar with these protocols and to know where to find answers to questions about procedures.

As stated in Chapter 1, this text assumes that most limited operators will not be employed in hospitals and will not perform procedures involving contrast media. If your work involves hospital care or contrast procedures, a comprehensive text on patient care is recommended.

HAZARD CONTROL

Fire Prevention

The first consideration in fire safety is fire prevention, because it is obviously preferable to practice prevention than to cope with a fire. An awareness of potential hazards is the first step toward prevention.

Three components must be present for a fire to burn: a flammable substance (fuel), oxygen, and heat (Fig. 21-1). Fire can be prevented by ensuring that these three elements never occur in the same place at the same time. Conversely, a fire can be stopped if one of the elements can be removed from the situation. We use this principle when

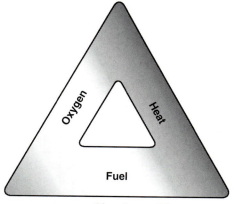

Fig. 21-1 Chemistry of fire.

we fight a fire by adding water (lowering the temperature) or by smothering (removing oxygen, as when we wrap a blanket around a person whose clothing has ignited). Most accidental fires are traceable to one of four causes: (1) spontaneous combustion, (2) open flames, (3) smoking, and (4) electricity.

Spontaneous combustion occurs when a chemical reaction in or near a flammable material causes sufficient heat to generate a fire. This is a relatively infrequent cause of fire in health care facilities, because local safety regulations control the types of chemicals and cleaning products in general use. Spontaneous combustion can occur when paint products, solvents, or oily cleaning rags are stored in a closed environment or too near a heat source. Oily or paint-soaked waste should be placed in tightly covered containers outside the building. Storage areas for dangerous products must meet the safety standards of the local health department.

Open flames that burn out of control are a common source of fires in homes but are less likely to cause problems in health care facilities. Take appropriate precautions in kitchens and laboratories where open burners are used. Precautions include keeping flammable substances a safe distance from the burner, using strict standards of cleanliness in kitchen areas, and never leaving open burners untended when they are in use. Do not burn candles.

Health care providers promote positive health habits by prohibiting smoking, so most hospitals, clinics, and physicians' offices are designated as nonsmoking facilities. Although this prohibition has reduced the incidence of smoking-based fires, some smokers may be tempted to smoke covertly. Smoking is especially dangerous in facilities that are not equipped to accommodate smoking. Be alert for the smell of smoke. Direct smokers to the designated smoking area, which will usually be outside the building.

Limited operators use a wide variety of complex electric equipment. Do not let familiarity with electric items lull you into a false sense of security. Electric fires are potential sources of fire hazard and are of special concern in radiology departments where there is much electric equipment. Box 21-1 lists precautions for avoiding electric hazards. Adherence to these rules greatly reduces the risk of both electric fire and electric shock. These principles apply in any area where electric equipment is used. When the building is not occupied, x-ray machines and all equipment that does not require constant power should be turned off or unplugged.

Short circuits in older x-ray control panels can generate enough heat to cause a fire. This is usually preceded by smoldering wire insulation, which causes smoke and an unpleasant odor and is readily detectable before an actual fire. If a short circuit occurs, turn off the electricity at the main power source, call for qualified assistance, and stand by with the proper fire extinguisher.

Oxygen by itself does not burn, but it does support combustion. Because the presence of oxygen greatly increases the fire hazard, it is important to exercise extreme

Box 21-1

Electric Safety Rules

- All electric equipment and appliances must be approved for their intended use and used as intended.
- Follow equipment manufacturers' instructions.
- Equipment used on or near patients or near water must have grounded plugs.
- Inspect equipment regularly, paying attention to cords and plugs. Arrange for repairs as necessary.
- Do not overload circuits by connecting too many devices to a single outlet or outlet group.
- Unplug or turn off electric equipment before exposing internal parts.
- Do not attempt to repair equipment unless you are trained to do so.
- Do not use extension cords. If necessary, use an approved power strip that is equipped with a circuit breaker.
- In case of electric fire, use a class C or carbon dioxide fire extinguisher.

care when oxygen is being used. There should be no smoking, no open flames, and no ungrounded appliances near areas where oxygen is in use.

Preparedness

Limited operators must be familiar with the fire plan for the facility. Be sure you know the evacuation route from your area and at least one alternate route. In addition, have a general knowledge of your facility's floor plan. It is your duty to know the locations of fire extinguishers and fire alarms. Knowledge of the procedure for reporting a fire is also essential.

In the event of a fire, large facilities use a coded communication to notify the staff without alarming the patients. This is usually a code number or code name announced over the paging system: "Attention all staff, there is a code 100 in the west wing." The same code is commonly used to signal fire drills. Take advantage of fire drills and in-service classes on fire safety to gain confidence in evacuation procedures and the use of fire extinguishers. If you are ever involved in an actual fire, your preparation and self-confidence will allow you to function effectively and will reassure those around you.

In small offices or clinics there may not be a formal fire plan or fire drills. Although the potential for fire within the facility may be small, there can be risk of fire from adjacent offices or buildings. Some sort of plan is essential. Local fire departments provide safety inspections and instruction in fire safety.

According to professional fire marshals, the most frequent infractions of fire safety rules include the following:
- Blocked fire exits
- Doors blocked open
- Equipment stored in corridors

- Improper storage of flammable items
- Improper use of extension cords

Doors should never be blocked open. Closed doors help prevent the rapid spread of fire. Wheelchairs, carts, and other equipment must be placed to avoid obstructing passages and doorways. Pay particular attention to passages and doors that are not often used. They may be the only safe exits in case of fire. Corridors should not be used to store equipment. If some items must be placed there temporarily, keep them all on the same side with room to pass easily. Ask yourself the question, "If we had to evacuate this area, would this equipment be a problem in this location?"

In Case of Fire

If you discover a fire, your primary responsibility is to evacuate everyone from the immediate area to a safe location. Second, report the fire and location, using the prescribed procedure. A small wastebasket blaze may be extinguished with a nearby pitcher of water or smothered with a pillow, but do not waste precious minutes in futile attempts. Your responsibility is the safety of patients and yourself.

An aid to help you recall the correct response in the event of a fire is the acronym RACE, which stands for rescue, alarm, contain, and evacuate/extinguish. Box 21-2

Box 21-2

In Case of Fire

Remain calm and remember the acronym RACE.

R—Rescue
- Remove patients from danger by moving them to a safe area. In large buildings, move patients past at least two fire doors within the facility.
- For larger fires, follow the instructions of coordinating personnel.

A—Alarm
- Activate the alarm system directly or use the established code for fire.
- Make sure that all personnel in the area are aware of the fire, being careful not to alarm patients.

C—Contain
- Close any open doors to limit the oxygen supply to the fire and to prevent the spread of smoke and heat.
- Check to make sure oxygen valves and electric circuit breakers are turned off.
- In inpatient facilities, close the doors to patient rooms. If a patient is still in a room, place the room's trash can in front of the door.

E—Extinguish/evacuate
- For small fires, use the available fire extinguisher to put out the fire or smother the fire with a blanket.
- For larger fires, evacuate the area of all personnel and wait for fire personnel.

lists the steps to follow in case of fire using the RACE concept.

During *any* emergency, it is important to remain calm and use a low voice. During a fire evacuation, try to avoid using the word *fire*. Instead, you might say, "Mrs. Jensen, there is a little smoke in one of the rooms, and we are going to move you outside until we can see how serious it is."

Fire Extinguishers

Fire extinguishers are marked to indicate the class or classes of fire for which they are appropriately used.

- Class A fires involve combustibles, such as paper or wood.
- Class B fires involve flammable liquids or gases.
- Class C fires involve electric equipment or wiring.

A multipurpose dry chemical extinguisher is suitable for all three classes of fires and is the type most often found in public buildings.

Fig. 21-2 shows a close-up view of a typical fire extinguisher mechanism. To use the fire extinguisher correctly, remember the acronym **PASS**:

Pull the pin.

Aim the nozzle.

Squeeze the handle.

Sweep. Use a sweeping motion from side to side.

Do not aim the fire extinguisher steadily at the flame; a sweeping motion is more effective and covers a wider area. This decreases the likelihood that the fire will spread. Fire extinguishers have considerable force and are effective at a safe distance from the fire. Stand back so as not to endanger yourself (Fig. 21-3).

Fire extinguishers must be inspected regularly and recharged periodically. A tag attached to the unit should indicate the date of the last inspection and the last recharge. The last inspection should have been no longer than 1 year earlier. When an extinguisher has been used, it must be recharged. It should be replaced immediately with a fresh unit.

Electric Shock

Electric shock may pose a serious hazard to both patients and personnel if safety precautions are not observed. This is especially true with x-ray equipment, which carries an electric potential in excess of 100,000 V. The hazard of lesser circuits should not be underestimated, however, because shocks from standard 120-V outlets can prove fatal under certain circumstances. Basic rules of electric safety are listed in Box 21-1. Caution is especially important when using electricity around water. *Never stand on a wet floor or use wet hands to perform tasks involving the use of electricity.*

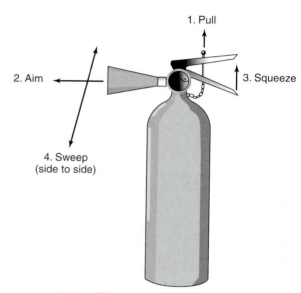

Fig. 21-2 Fire extinguisher mechanism.

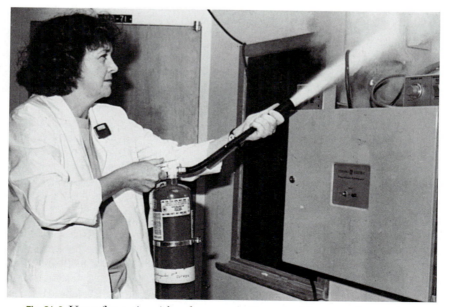

Fig. 21-3 Use a fire extinguisher from a safe distance with a sweeping motion.

Falls and Collision Accidents

Reducing the risk of falls and collisions is an important safety concern. Caution is needed for the safety of both patients and personnel. Be especially conscious of hazards when moving wheelchairs and other mobile equipment, and do not store or park equipment where it might cause a problem. Too narrow a passageway is unsafe for patients who must use walkers or crutches. Equipment too close to a corner may be an unseen obstruction to someone hurrying from an intersecting hallway or carrying a bulky object.

Storage areas are common sources of accidents when items are not placed there properly, including being secured when necessary. Heavy items should be placed near the floor. Do not be tempted to stack things precariously. Any object that could cause harm should be situated so that its position will not shift unexpectedly. To access items that are above your reach, use a secure stool or stepladder. *Never* stand on tables or chairs with wheels.

Electric cords should not be strung across doorways or other traffic patterns. Try to position equipment as close as possible to a suitable outlet. If a cord must cross a traffic path temporarily, secure it to the floor with tape to minimize the possibility of someone tripping over it. If hazardous, makeshift electric connections are a common problem, discuss this with your supervisor or employer and suggest a safe, permanent remedy.

Spills

Spills deserve special attention. Depending on the nature of the substance, spills may pose a chemical hazard in addition to a risk of injury from falls. Familiar substances such as household bleach or concentrated darkroom chemicals can cause eye damage or skin injury.

Hazardous liquids should be converted into solid waste and placed in plastic bags for removal. An absorbent material in the form of clay pellets (cat litter) or an absorbent mat is used to soak up the liquid before it is placed in a suitable plastic container. Your work area should have a spill kit that includes absorbent material and heavy plastic bags. If pellets are used, a broom and dustpan should be included. You can assemble your own spill kit or choose a suitable kit from the many that are commercially available. You will also need personal protective equipment. Nitrile gloves are special gloves that are impervious to most chemicals and are recommended for contact with many types of hazardous chemicals, including concentrated processing chemicals. Protective aprons and eye protection in the form of splash-proof goggles or face shields should be available.

The Occupational Safety and Health Administration (OSHA), a federal agency governing safety in the workplace, requires that all chemicals be properly labeled and that material safety data sheets (MSDSs) for all hazardous materials be on file and easily accessible to personnel. The MSDS for any chemical will spell out the required equipment and procedure for safe handling in the event of a spill. The developer and fixer solutions used to process radiographs are classified by OSHA as hazardous materials. OSHA requires that personnel wear protective aprons, splash-proof goggles, and nitrile gloves when pouring or cleaning up film processing solutions.

Appropriate cleaning measures are needed to avoid potentially serious problems whenever a spill involves a hazardous material.

The following steps help to ensure safety when a spill occurs:

- Limit access to the area.
- Evaluate the risks involved.
- Obtain both the information and the equipment to clean up the spill safely.
- Clean up the spill.
- If you lack the necessary skill or equipment, call your supervisor.

WORKPLACE SAFETY

Ergonomics

Ergonomics is the study of the human body in relation to the working environment. Ergonomic awareness and education in the workplace have reduced job injuries in recent years, but there is still cause for concern. The U.S. Bureau of Labor Statistics reports that workplace injury rates for health care workers are similar to those for industrial workers. The most common injuries reported by health care workers are musculoskeletal disorders (MSDs). Subcategories of MSDs as classified by OSHA include repetitive motion injuries, repetitive strain injuries, and cumulative trauma disorders (CTDs). Repetitive motion injuries and repetitive strain injuries, as their names suggest, are the result of performing repeated motions or applying pressure extensively. Stress caused by performing repetitive motion, overreaching, or maintaining the same positions for long periods causes microtrauma to muscle tissue. This microtrauma is the basis of CTDs that may produce chronic discomfort and lead to more significant musculoskeletal injury. The symptoms of CTDs include pain, numbness, tingling sensations, clumsiness, swelling (especially in the hand and wrist), weakness, loss of function, and overdevelopment of muscle groups.

Each year thousands of health care workers suffer occupational illness or injury that causes them to miss work. All health care workers are at risk for MSDs caused by back strain from lifting and moving patients and equipment. In addition, radiographers often experience neck and shoulder strains and rotator cuff tears from reaching overhead to move the x-ray tube. Workers who use computers extensively are more likely to experience spinal stress from sitting at a console for long periods and repetitive strain injury from intensive keyboard work. Keyboard stress can affect the hands and wrists with CTDs such as tendinitis, ganglion cyst, and carpal tunnel syndrome. Those whose work involves extended periods of viewing cathode ray tube monitors are also subject to vision problems.

Work injury is minimized when proper equipment is available and is used correctly, and when workers help one another. Frequent break periods and changes in position help to minimize both positional and repetitive stress. Studies indicate that ongoing education programs and appropriate responses by employers to the ergonomic concerns of their workers are effective strategies.

Body Mechanics

The principles of proper body alignment, movement, and balance are referred to as *body mechanics*. The application of these principles minimizes the energy required to sit, stand, and walk. Your effective strength is increased when you use these principles to perform tasks that require stooping, lifting, pushing, pulling, and carrying.

Applied body mechanics also prevent muscle and back strain. Such strains are a common problem among health care workers, causing much discomfort and reduced efficiency. When you injure yourself on the job, you place a greater burden on your co-workers. If you injure yourself while assisting a patient, you may injure the patient as well.

Three concepts are essential to understanding the principles of body mechanics (Fig. 21-4):
1. Base of support—This is the portion of the body in contact with the floor or other horizontal surface. A broad base of support provides stability for body position and movement.
2. Center of gravity, or center of body weight—This is the point around which body weight is balanced. It is usually located in the midportion of the pelvis or lower abdomen, but the location may vary somewhat depending on body build. The body is most stable when the center of gravity is nearest the center of the base of support.
3. Line of gravity—This is an imaginary vertical line passing through the center of gravity. The body is most stable when the line of gravity bisects the base of support.

Using these concepts, the principles of body mechanics can be stated in the five simple rules listed in Box 21-3. Memorize them and practice them, both at work and at home.

Bending and twisting the back while lifting is the most common cause of back strain (Fig. 21-5). A broad and stable base of support is ensured by standing with feet apart and one foot slightly advanced. Remember that your thigh muscles are among the strongest in your body. When you use good body mechanics, the combined strength of your legs, arms, and abdomen protects the shorter, more vulnerable back muscles. Think ahead and

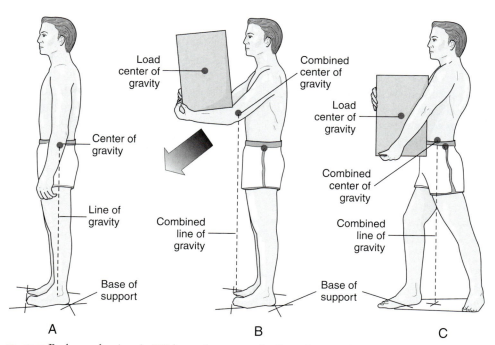

Fig. 21-4 Body mechanics. **A,** With good posture, the line of gravity bisects the base of support. **B,** When the load is held away from the body, the line of gravity does not bisect the base of support. **C,** A wide stance with the load held close to the body allows the combined line of gravity to bisect the base of support.

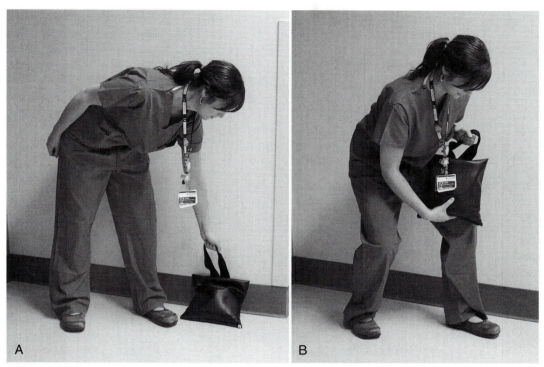

Fig. 21-5 Good body mechanics helps avoid fatigue and prevent back strain. **A,** Wrong. Back is bent and twisted. **B,** Right. Knees are flexed and back is straight.

Box 21-3

Rules of Body Mechanics

1. Provide a broad base of support.
2. Work at a comfortable height.
3. When lifting, bend your knees and keep your back straight.
4. Keep your load well balanced and close to your body.
5. Roll or push a heavy object. Avoid pulling or lifting.

use the tools available to you when anticipating a task that may cause muscle strain. Adjust the height of your work surface, use a cart to move a heavy load, and obtain help to lift heavy objects.

ASSISTING PATIENTS WITH POSITIONS AND MOVEMENTS

Body Positions

Common body positions have names, and it is easier to communicate and to follow physicians' orders if you understand these terms. You are already familiar with the terms for body positions used in radiographic positioning, such as *recumbent*, *supine*, and *prone* (see Chapter 12). In addition, there are specific positions most commonly associated with patient care situations (Fig. 21-6). The

Fowler position is a modification of the supine position in which the patient's upper body is elevated. This position provides more comfort and safety than the supine position for patients who are short of breath or experiencing nausea. The Sims position is a recumbent oblique position. In the Trendelenburg position, the patient's head is lower than the feet; usually the table is tilted approximately 15 degrees. This position is used during some fluoroscopic procedures and is helpful in the treatment of patients suffering from shock. The knee-chest position and the lithotomy position are not commonly used in radiography but are standard positions used for diagnostic examinations and therapeutic procedures.

Support and Padding

When lying on a hard surface, such as a radiographic table, patients are more comfortable with radiolucent sponges or cushions placed for support. If a pillow under the head will not be a hindrance to the examination, it can enable the patient to see what is occurring and thus help relieve apprehension. Elevation of the patient's head also relieves neck strain, allows easier breathing, and helps avoid the uncomfortable sensation that the head is lower than the feet.

A bolster under the knees of a supine patient relieves lumbosacral stress by straightening the lordotic lumbar curve. This is especially comforting to arthritic and kyphotic patients and to most elderly persons. It is essential for patients with spine injuries and those who have

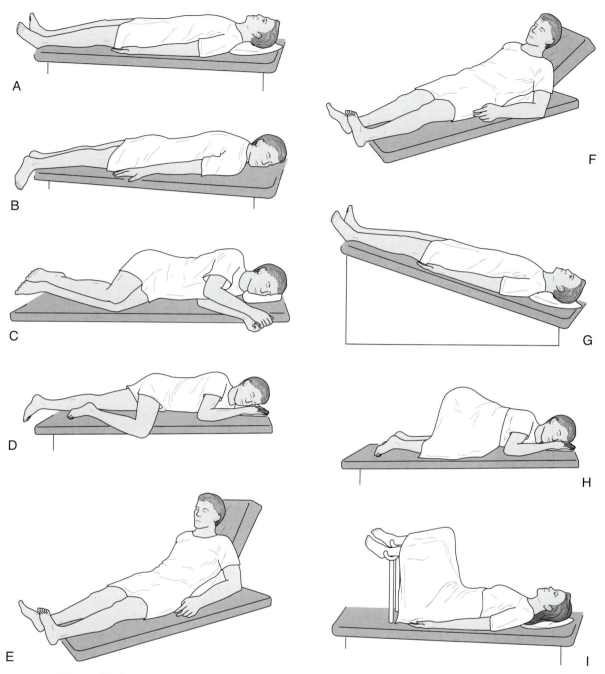

Fig. 21-6 Body positions. **A,** Supine. **B,** Prone. **C,** Lateral recumbent. **D,** Sims. **E,** Fowler. **F,** Semi-Fowler. **G,** Trendelenburg. **H,** Knee-chest. **I,** Lithotomy.

recently undergone spinal or abdominal surgery. Patients with abdominal pain must have the head elevated and a bolster under the knees to relieve strain on the abdomen.

Placement of padding under bony prominences, such as the sacrum, heels, and mid-thoracic curvature, can be important for many patients. One reason is that when patients are reasonably comfortable they are better able to maintain the positions needed for an effective examination, even on a hard surface. The measures used to promote comfort are frequently the same interventions that prevent complications. For example, as explained in Chapter 18, older or debilitated patients may develop

decubitus ulcers over prominent bony structures when pressure is exerted for even a short period of time.

Another safety consideration in positioning is the patient's ability to breathe. When the body is supine, the weight of the abdominal contents pushes the diaphragm up into the thoracic cavity, which makes it more difficult to take a deep breath. This is no problem for most people, but patients with **dyspnea** (difficulty breathing) or **orthopnea** (inability to breathe lying down) may be unable to lie supine. A patient who becomes short of breath when supine must be assisted to sit up immediately.

Patients who are nauseated also need to have their heads elevated. This position helps control nausea and vomiting and decreases the possibility that the patient will aspirate **emesis** (vomit). Patients who become nauseated and cannot be assisted to the Fowler position should be placed in a lateral recumbent position.

Positioning is one area in which your learning will be enhanced by acting out the patient's role. Practice positioning with your classmates until comfort and positioning are part of the same action.

Assisting Patients to Change Position

You will probably assist patients in sitting, standing, lying down, and moving about many times each day. Use of the correct technique is least likely to cause discomfort or injury to either the patient or yourself.

To help a seated patient stand up, stand facing the patient. Reach around the patient's upper body and place your hands firmly over the scapulae. The patient's hands may rest on your shoulders. If the patient has weakness on one side of the body, position yourself to brace the patient's weak leg with your knee as the patient stands. This will help to keep the patient's leg from bending and giving way with weight bearing. On your signal, lift upward while the patient rises to a standing position (Fig. 21-7). Remember to use a broad base of support and keep your back straight. This method may be reversed when assisting a standing patient to sit down. Be certain that the seat is secure and will not move as the patient sits.

Patients seated on the edge of the radiographic table often find it easier to lie down with some help. Place one arm under the knees and the other around the patient's shoulders. Lift the legs as you pivot the patient and rest the legs on the table (Fig. 21-8). At the same time, ease the shoulders down so that the patient is supine. This method is reversed when assisting a supine patient to sit up. It is much easier to sit up when the legs have been lowered somewhat than when they are extended on the table.

Patients suffering from recent back injuries and those recovering from spinal surgery will find it difficult to lie down and sit up. Moving from a supine position to a sitting position, or from sitting to supine, places considerable stress on the spine. It is preferable for these patients to sit from the lateral recumbent position. When lying down, the patient should lie first on one side and then turn to the supine position with the knees flexed. Provide support and assistance to the patient while extending the legs, and place a bolster or pillow under the knees for support when supine.

Some patients experience **orthostatic hypotension** when rising from a recumbent position. This condition is a temporary state of low blood pressure that causes patients to feel lightheaded or faint when they first sit up. A pause before assisting them to stand will give them an opportunity to regain their sense of balance.

Assisting Patients to Move About

Some patients who are weak or cannot bear their full weight easily on both legs may use a cane or a walker for support to move about. A walker is a lightweight metal frame with four legs and bars at the front and sides on which the patient may lean for support (Fig. 21-9). The patient moves the walker ahead before taking each step. Patients with ample strength who cannot bear weight on one leg will usually walk with crutches (Fig. 21-10). Patients who are accustomed to using crutches or a walker do not need other assistance to walk. Your responsibility is to show them the way and to make sure there are no obstacles in the path.

A gait belt, also called a *transfer belt*, should be used when assisting patients who are weak or unsteady. These belts are heavy fabric straps with a strong buckle. When placed snugly around the patient's waist, the belt provides a secure handhold for you to use in helping the patient to stand and walk.

Patients who cannot walk alone and who do not use a walker or crutches will need physical support to walk. Some patients have weakness of one side of the body. This is typical of stroke victims and those who have had injury or surgery to a lower extremity. Determine which is the patient's weak side and position yourself next to it.

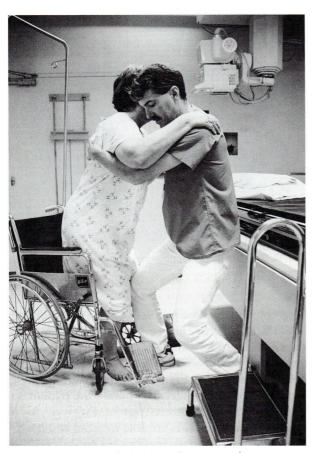

Fig. 21-7 Assisting patient to stand.

Significant diseases caused by bacteria include tuberculosis and streptococcal pharyngitis (strep throat), as well as infectious diarrhea and kidney disease caused by a particular strain of *Escherichia coli* (*E. coli* 0157:H7).

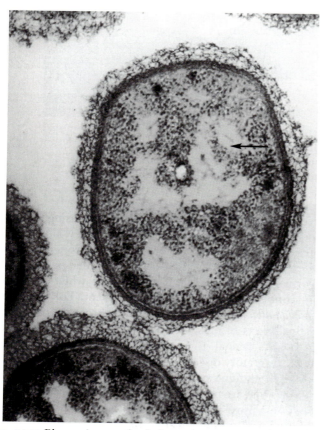

Fig. 21-18 Photomicrograph of a bacterium. Note the absence of a nuclear membrane.

Viruses

Viruses are subcellular organisms. They are among the smallest known disease-causing organisms. To be studied, they must be viewed with an electron microscope. Examples of viruses include influenza virus, human immunodeficiency virus (HIV), herpes virus, hepatitis virus, and rhinovirus. Rhinoviruses cause the common cold. Other common viruses are Epstein-Barr virus, which causes infectious mononucleosis, and varicella-zoster virus, which causes chickenpox.

Viruses cannot multiply independently. A virus invades a host cell, stimulating it to participate in the formation of additional virus particles. Each type of virus is specific to a particular type of cell. For example, the hepatitis virus attaches to liver cells. Because viruses reside in the host cell and use it to replicate, it has been difficult to develop antiviral drugs that are not also harmful to the host cell. Only a few antiviral agents exist, and these are useful against only a limited number of viruses.

Protozoa

Protozoa are complex, single-cell animals that generally exist as free-living organisms (Fig. 21-20). A few, however, are parasitic and live within the human body. Most parasitic protozoa produce some type of resistant form, such as a cyst, to survive in the environment outside the host. Other protozoa have complicated life cycles involving alternate existence in the human body and in insects. This is true of the protozoan that causes malaria. Protozoa can infect the gastrointestinal, genitourinary, respiratory, and circulatory systems.

Fungi

Fungi (singular, *fungus*) occur as single-celled yeasts or as filament-like structures called *molds* that are composed of

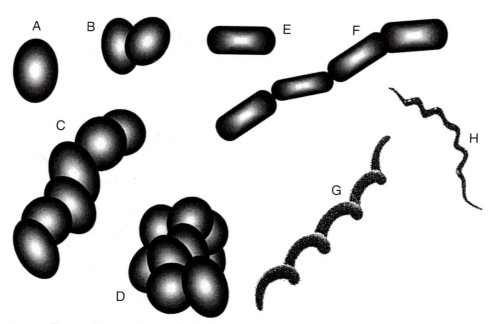

Fig. 21-19 Bacterial forms. Cocci: **A**, Single coccus. **B**, Diplococcus. **C**, Chain formation (*Streptococcus*). **D**, Cluster (*Staphylococcus*). Bacilli: **E**, Single bacillus. **F**, Chain. Spiral bacteria: **G**, Spirillum. **H**, Spirochete.

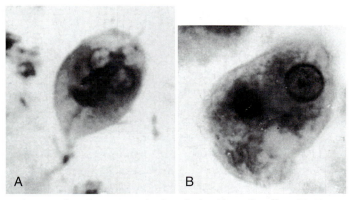

Fig. 21-20 Photomicrographs of protozoa. **A,** *Giardia lamblia*, a flagellate. **B,** *Entamoeba histolytica*, an ameba.

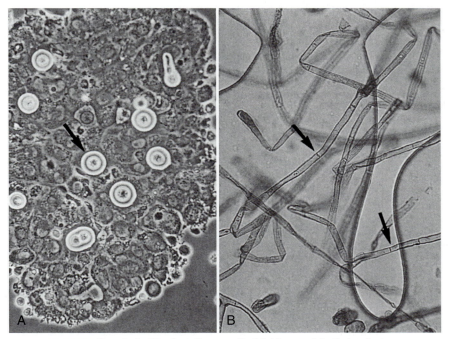

Fig. 21-21 Fungi. **A,** Single-cell yeast. **B,** Mold, a multicellular fungus.

many cells (Fig. 21-21). There are more than 100,000 diverse species of fungi, and many have useful purposes. They assist in the production of alcoholic beverages, are responsible for the flavor of cheese, give bread its lightness, and produce the antibiotic penicillin. In humans, fungi cause skin infections, such as athlete's foot and ringworm; respiratory infections, such as histoplasmosis; and infections in individuals with compromised immune systems.

Prions

The smallest and least understood of all infectious agents is the prion, which was discovered in 1983. Scientists believe that prions are infectious protein particles. Their method of replication is not understood. They were first identified as the cause of scrapie, a degenerative disease affecting the nervous systems of sheep. Prions also cause mad cow disease and a human variant called Creutzfeldt-Jakob disease, a disorder that causes brain damage with

a rapid decrease of mental function and movement. Perhaps other conditions that are characterized by slow deterioration of the nervous system are attributable to prions as well. There is early speculation that further research into the nature of prions may help us to better understand the cause of Alzheimer disease.

Reservoir of Infection

The reservoir, or source, of infection may be any place where pathogens can thrive in sufficient numbers to pose a threat. Such an environment must provide moisture, nutrients, and a suitable temperature, all of which are found in the human body. A source of infection might be the patient with hepatitis, a health care worker with an upper respiratory tract infection, or a visitor with staphylococcal boils.

Because some pathogens live in the bodies of healthy individuals without causing apparent disease, a person may be the reservoir for an infectious organism without realizing it. These persons are called **carriers.** Many people have throat culture results that are positive for *Staphylococcus aureus* (staph) but do not have a sore throat. A susceptible patient with an open wound could contract a life-threatening infection if sufficiently contaminated with this organism. A common example of a carrier of infection is the individual infected with HIV who has no symptoms and who spreads the disease through sexual intercourse or by sharing contaminated needles with intravenous drug users.

Although the human body is the most common reservoir of infection, any environment that will support the growth of microorganisms has the potential to be a secondary source. Such sources include contaminated food or water or any damp, warm place that is not cleaned regularly.

Susceptible Host

Healthy individuals have a high level of natural resistance to infection. Fatigue, stress, malnutrition, illness, and injury tend to tax and weaken the immune response, reducing natural resistance. In a health care setting, susceptible hosts are frequently patients whose natural resistance to infection is diminished. In addition to the primary problems that caused them to seek care, they may develop **iatrogenic** (health care–related) infections.

Infections also pose a threat to health care workers because their work results in exposure to many pathogens. In a single day, you may care for patients with pneumonia, hepatitis, and wound infections. Hepatitis B and C are the biggest concerns. Both are spread by blood and blood products and are most often transmitted to health care workers by accidental needle sticks. Those who must work when resistance is low because of fatigue, stress, or a low-grade infection have increased susceptibility to infection. Maintain your resistance to infectious illness by keeping your body healthy and well-rested.

Disease Transmission

The most direct way to intervene in the cycle of infection is to prevent transmission of the infectious organism from the reservoir to the susceptible host. To accomplish this successfully, you must understand the six main routes of transmission.

Direct Contact

The first route is by means of direct contact. In this transmission mode the host is touched by an infected person in such a manner that the organisms are placed in direct contact with susceptible tissue. For example, syphilis and HIV infections may be contracted when infectious organisms from the mucous membranes of one individual are placed in direct contact with the mucous membranes of a susceptible host. Also, skin infections often occur among health care workers because of frequent contact with patients who have bacterial diseases. The five other principal routes of transmission are indirect and involve transport of organisms by means of fomites, vectors, vehicles, airborne particles, and droplet contamination.

Fomites

An object that has been in contact with pathogenic organisms is called a **fomite.** Examples of fomites in the radiology department are the x-ray table, upright Bucky, image receptors, calipers, and positioning sponges that have been contaminated with infectious body fluids.

Vectors

A **vector** is an arthropod (insect, spider, or similar form) in whose body an infectious organism develops or multiplies before becoming infective to a new host. Some examples of vectors are mosquitoes that transmit malaria and dengue fever, fleas that carry bubonic plague, and ticks that spread Lyme disease and Rocky Mountain spotted fever. In these examples, the bites of infected insects transmit diseases to humans.

Vehicles

A **vehicle** is any medium that transports microorganisms. Examples include contaminated food, water, drugs, and blood.

Airborne Contamination

Airborne contamination is spread by dust containing either endospores or droplet nuclei (tiny infectious particles from evaporated droplets that contain microorganisms). Contaminated dust may remain suspended in the air for long periods. These particles may be dispersed by air currents and may be inhaled by a susceptible host. Special ventilation and airflow control are required to prevent airborne transmission of these infective particles. Tuberculosis, rubeola (measles), and varicella (chickenpox) are examples of infections spread by airborne particles.

Droplet Contamination

Droplet contamination often occurs when an infectious individual coughs, sneezes, speaks, or sings in the vicinity of a susceptible host. Droplet transmission involves contact of the mucous membranes of the eyes, nose, or mouth of a susceptible person with droplets containing microorganisms. These particles are relatively large and do not remain suspended in the air. They travel only short distances, usually 3 feet or less. Influenza, meningitis, diphtheria, pertussis (whooping cough), and streptococcal pneumonia are examples of illnesses spread by droplet contamination.

Although most microorganisms are fragile, requiring continuous warmth, moisture, and nutrients to exist, some are resistant to destruction and can remain viable for long periods of time. Bacteria that are capable of forming endospores may live in this form for many years. They are often carried in invisible dust particles in the atmosphere. Research has shown that some viruses can resist drying, remaining infectious for weeks. This is true of the viruses that cause herpes, both oral and genital. These examples indicate that some microorganisms can float through the air and lurk in dusty corners, waiting for the opportunity to invade a susceptible host. This should emphasize to you the need for cleanliness as a defense against infection.

INFECTIOUS DISEASES

Disease Information

There are many new diseases in the world, and some old ones are returning in epidemic proportions after years of low-level incidence. The wide and inappropriate use of broad-spectrum antibiotics has led to the development of drug-resistant infections in hospitals and in the community. Some of these infections are untreatable because the causative organisms are resistant to the available drugs. Development of a new drug takes time, is costly, and does not seem to be a lasting solution to this complex problem. As a worker in the health care field, you may be on the front line of exposure to infectious diseases. The Centers for Disease Control and Prevention (CDC) monitors and studies the types of infections occurring in the nation, compiles statistical data about these infections, and publishes this information in both a weekly report and an annual surveillance summary report. The CDC also provides information about prevention and treatment of specific infections. When questions arise regarding current information on disease prevention and infection control, the best source for answers is the CDC.[j]

Human Immunodeficiency Virus Infection and Acquired Immunodeficiency Syndrome

According to the CDC,[k] more than 1 million people in the United States are living with HIV infection, and approximately 25% of these infections are undiagnosed and/or untreated. The global annual mortality rate is 3 million, and the worldwide cumulative death toll could reach 100 million by 2020.

Although the incidence of acquired immunodeficiency syndrome (AIDS) has dropped significantly since 1990, the total number of HIV patients continues to rise. This is not only because of new cases but also because of the increasing number of HIV-infected individuals who have avoided converting to AIDS by the use of new, more effective drugs.

In the early 1980s, HIV was identified as the cause of AIDS. Two major types of HIV have been found to infect humans: HIV type 1 (HIV-1), the predominant type throughout the world, and HIV type 2 (HIV-2), found primarily in heterosexual populations in West Africa.

An HIV-infected individual can transmit the virus to others a few days after infection, even though antibodies to the virus may not be detected in the blood for 3 to 6 months. Without therapy, this individual will pass through several phases of infection over a span of months to years before exhibiting the immunosuppression of full-blown AIDS.

In the early stages of the infection, there is usually a brief period of flulike symptoms, often followed by years without symptoms. During the asymptomatic phase, the virus is silently replicating in the body and decreasing the number of CD4 lymphocytes. At the end of the asymptomatic period, before the full development of AIDS, the individual will experience night sweats, oral infections, weight loss, persistently enlarged lymph nodes, and low-grade fever. The appearance of AIDS is characterized by the occurrence of multiple **opportunistic infections** and malignant diseases. Opportunistic infections are caused by pathogens that do not cause disease in individuals with healthy immune systems. Some of the opportunistic infections observed are *Jiroveci* pneumonia (formerly termed *Pneumocystis carinii*), mucocutaneous *Candida*, disseminated herpes, and cytomegalovirus infection. There is also increased risk of contracting tuberculosis and developing active disease. Kaposi sarcoma, a malignancy of pigmented skin cells, is the most common form of cancer affecting AIDS patients.

Although drugs have been developed that prolong the time required for HIV infection to progress to AIDS, at this time no known cure exists. The primary problem in producing a successful vaccine has been the high mutation rate of this virus, but there is continued hope that a vaccine will be developed.

Fortunately, the AIDS virus is not acquired by casual contact. Touching or shaking hands, eating food prepared by an infected person, and contact with drinking fountains, telephones, toilets, or other surfaces do not result in transmission of HIV. The routes of transmission are sexual contact, contaminated blood or needles, fluids containing blood, or from mother to fetus via the placenta. Infection can also be transmitted to infants through breast milk. Men who have sex with other men still account for the largest number of cases of AIDS in this country, followed by intravenous drug users and persons engaging in high-risk heterosexual contact (unprotected contact with a person known to have or be at high risk for HIV). AIDS is increasing at a faster rate in the same groups in which HIV infection is increasing: non-Hispanic blacks, Hispanics, and women. The higher rate of AIDS in these groups has

---

[j]www.CDC.gov/.
[k]http://www.cdc.gov/hiv/library/reports/surveillance/2013/surveillance_Report_vol_25.html.

been attributed to poor access to health care, which has improved in the last few years, and/or failure to follow prescribed drug regimens. This means that a continued decline in AIDS diagnoses and deaths in the future will depend on better access to health care, simpler drug regimens, and the development of more effective antiretroviral drugs.

As a health care worker in today's world, you must expect to encounter unidentified or undiagnosed cases of AIDS and other blood-borne diseases. Controversy currently surrounds the patient's right to confidentiality regarding the AIDS diagnosis within the clinical setting, preventing you from being informed about diagnosed cases. Diagnosed patients are only the tip of the iceberg, however, because many undiagnosed cases exist for every known case. Anxiety about HIV infection is typical and understandable among health care workers, but the occupational risk is not great. The vast majority of health care workers infected with HIV were exposed as a result of activities unrelated to their work. The most common occupational exposure is the needle stick, but according to the CDC, the probability of infection following a needle stick injury exposing the injured person to blood containing HIV is only 3 out of 1000 exposures, or 0.3%. Thousands of needle sticks have been reported over the years, but as of December 2001, only 57 health care workers with no other identified risk factors had been diagnosed as HIV positive. Of these 57 cases, 26 had developed AIDS. Recent statistics for health care workers are not available, but it is projected that the percentages would be similar. The implications here are obvious. Although prevention at work is essential, self-care in terms of safe sexual practice and avoiding intravenous drug use is equally crucial.

Hepatitis

The five common types of hepatitis are classified A through E. Hepatitis A and E are transmitted through food and water contaminated with feces. Hepatitis B, C, and D are blood-borne. Hepatitis E is uncommon in the United States, and hepatitis D appears only as a co-infection with hepatitis B. Hepatitis B virus can be spread through contact with blood or blood products; contact with body fluids such as saliva, semen, and vaginal secretions; and maternal-fetal contact. Hepatitis C is primarily spread by contact with blood or blood products. The risk for contracting this virus is greatest for persons with large or repeated percutaneous exposures to blood, such as intravenous drug users, whose risk is 60%. The risk is lowest for those who are subject to sporadic percutaneous exposures such as health care workers, whose risk following a needle stick is 1% to 2%. The risk is 15% to 20% for sexual transmission and 5% to 6% for maternal-fetal transmission.

The manifestations of all forms of hepatitis are similar: jaundice, fatigue, abdominal pain, loss of appetite, nausea, vomiting, and diarrhea. Hepatitis C is a more silent infection and may not cause symptoms or awareness of the infection until there is liver damage. Both hepatitis B and hepatitis C have the potential to develop into chronic infections and cirrhosis, although the risk is greater with hepatitis C. After infection with hepatitis C virus, about 85% of individuals develop chronic infection, approximately 70% develop liver disease, 10% to 20% develop cirrhosis, and 1% to 5% develop liver cancer. These sequelae take place over a 10- to 20-year period.

The number of new cases of hepatitis B and C has decreased because of immunizations for hepatitis B, decreased needle sharing among intravenous drug users, and blood donor screening for both B and C viruses. However, the incidence of hepatitis A has shown periodic increases. Large nationwide outbreaks of type A usually occur once each decade, with the last major outbreak occurring in Pittsburgh in 2003. Small outbreaks were reported in Colorado and New York in 2010. The nationwide incidence has decreased dramatically since the turn of the twenty-first century.

Health care workers can protect themselves against hepatitis B by taking a vaccine, which usually provides immunity for 7 to 10 years. There is also a vaccine for hepatitis A, but it is indicated only in certain situations, namely for individuals with medical, behavioral, occupational, or other indications, such as travelers to Third World countries. Protection from hepatitis A and C can be achieved by following the established infection control practices in your institution. Hepatitis A remains the most common form of the disease and is best controlled by practicing good personal hygiene, especially hand hygiene.

Managing Occupational Exposures to Blood-borne Pathogens

If an accidental needle stick occurs or the skin is broken by a contaminated object, allow the wound to bleed under cold water and wash with soap. If the mucous membranes of your eyes, nose, or mouth are splashed with body fluids, rinse the affected area immediately with water. An incident report must be filed, even though the injury or incident might seem insignificant. In addition to completion of an incident report, most hospitals now ask that a baseline blood sample be drawn to help rule out infection acquired before the occupational exposure. You will also be advised by the medical provider about postexposure prophylactic (PEP) therapy following a puncture with a contaminated needle. If treatment is recommended, it should be administered within 2 hours of the blood exposure. Currently, for most HIV exposures that warrant PEP, a 4-week, two-drug regimen is recommended, and several drug options are available. At the same time you are tested for HIV, you will also be tested for hepatitis B and C. If you have not had the hepatitis B vaccine series, it will be initiated along with hepatitis B immune globulin for immediate immunity. There is no effective prophylactic therapy for hepatitis C at this time, so if testing reveals you were exposed to a hepatitis C virus–positive source, follow-up hepatitis C virus testing will be necessary to see if infection develops. Because HIV infection may not be apparent in the blood for approximately 3 months, another sample is tested for HIV at 6 months.

Tuberculosis

Tuberculosis (TB) is a disease of the lungs caused by the acid-fast bacillus *Mycobacterium tuberculosis*, also referred to as *tubercle bacillus*. Historically, this disease was called *consumption* because of the victim's tendency to "waste away." In the past, the incidence of TB in the United States was spread across all economic levels of society, but today the highest rate of active cases is seen among the homeless, recent immigrants, and immunosuppressed individuals. Although the incidence of cases in this country is much lower now than it was in the years before 1950, recent outbreaks of TB have raised grave concern because of the appearance of drug-resistant strains of the bacteria.

Pulmonary TB is spread through airborne droplet nuclei that are generated when an infected person coughs or speaks. These particles are easily transmitted because they are extremely tiny (1 to 5 μm in size) and air currents keep them airborne. The probability that a susceptible person will be infected depends on the concentration of the infectious droplet nuclei in the air.

Most people who become infected with tubercle bacilli do not develop a clinical disease or become infectious to others. In the vast majority of cases, the body's immune system walls off the infection within 2 to 10 weeks, preventing its multiplication and spread. The walled-off disease is inactive or dormant, but the infection can be reactivated at any time. Reactivation may occur with lowered resistance because of immunodeficiency, malnutrition, other illness, or old age.

In a weakened or immunosuppressed state, such as with HIV infection, patients progress rapidly to active disease. Symptoms of active disease include productive or prolonged cough, fever, chills, loss of appetite, weight loss, fatigue, and night sweats. As the bacilli multiply, they cause tissue necrosis that results in cavities in the lung. These spaces are major reservoirs of the infectious organisms, which can then be spread by coughing. Severe cases can be fatal. Examples of radiographs showing various stages of TB are presented in Chapter 16, Fig. 16-46. Extrapulmonary TB, infecting bone or organs other than the lung, accounts for a small percentage of TB infections. Patients with extrapulmonary infection and no active pulmonary disease do not transmit the disease through airborne contamination.

The simplest and most common method of testing for TB infection is the tuberculin skin test, also called a *Mantoux test* or *PPD test* (*PPD* stands for purified protein derivative, obtained from killed tubercle bacilli). This test involves an intradermal injection on the anterior forearm. The injection produces a raised area on the skin, similar to an insect bite, called a *wheal*. The wheal is inspected 48 to 72 hours after injection to determine whether the individual has been infected with TB. A negative test result indicates that the person has never been infected. A positive result indicates that a person has at one time been infected and has developed **antibodies** (resisting proteins) to the organism. Because few people who become infected ever develop clinical symptoms or become infectious to others, many people have a positive skin test result without having active disease. This test is administered when a person is known to have been exposed to TB and has not already tested positive for it.

If the skin test result is positive, or if symptoms are present, a chest radiograph is ordered to rule out active disease. When there are symptoms and/or positive radiographic findings, sputum smears and cultures are tested for acid-fast bacilli. Positive results are definitive proof of active disease and are an indication to begin treatment.

TB screening is often required for those who work in contact with vulnerable or high-risk populations. For example, schoolteachers, corrections officers, and health care workers are often required to have preemployment tuberculin skin tests.

The CDC reports that the current number of reported TB cases is the lowest since national reporting began in 1953.[1] Although TB rates have declined in both American-born and immigrant populations, this decline has been substantially less among immigrant and foreign-born populations. The continued decline in the number of reported cases since 1992 reflects improvements in TB prevention and control programs by state and local health departments but falls short of the national goal the CDC has set to eventually eliminate this disease from our population.

Early identification, isolation, and treatment are required to minimize transmission of TB. Health care workers are at risk of contracting this disease only when a patient is exhibiting symptoms of active TB. According to OSHA's standard on TB, infection control experts within the health care facility are to assess the actual risk for transmission of TB in inpatient and outpatient settings. If the findings reveal risk, they are to develop TB infection control interventions. These include free TB skin tests, the provision of personal respirator equipment, the operation of one or more isolation rooms with negative air pressure and special ventilation or circulation, annual employee training about the disease, and implementation of effective work practices. OSHA estimates that the average lifetime occupational risk of TB infection may be as high as 386 infections per 1000 workers exposed to TB on the job.

---

[1]www.cdc.gov/tb/statistics/default.htm.

Health Care–associated Infections

Approximately 2 million patients each year acquire infections within the health care setting. These are called **health care–associated infections (HAI).** Those that are contracted in the hospital setting are also known as **nosocomial infections.** Although many of these infections are not life threatening, the CDC estimates that 90,000 patients die each year of HAIs and that most of these are preventable. Although the clinic or office setting provides substantially less risk, the same problems exist wherever health care is provided, and you should be aware of these types of infections and of the ways in which they are transmitted.

Medical settings provide an ideal environment for the development and transmission of HAIs. Typical sources of these infections include the contaminated hands of health care providers and contaminated instruments and urinary catheters, which can allow microbes to gain easy entrance into the body. Invasive procedures permit pathogens to enter the bloodstream and overcome the defense mechanisms of **immunocompromised patients** (those with deficient immune systems, such as those with HIV infection and those taking antirejection drugs following organ transplants).

There are several HAIs that greatly concern health care providers and their patients because they are multi-drug-resistant. This means that they are resistant to more than one antibiotic. Methicillin-resistant *S. aureus* (MRSA) and vancomycin-resistant enterococci (VRE) both contribute to surgical wound, urinary tract, and bloodstream infections. MRSA can also cause respiratory infections. Penicillin-resistant *Streptococcus* and *Pseudomonas aeruginosa* cause respiratory infections. The overuse of antimicrobial agents and poor infection control practices have been implicated in the emergence and spread of these multidrug-resistant organisms. These pathogens are very difficult to treat, and intensive infection control is required to limit their spread.

MRSA has been recognized as a problem in the health care setting for the last 20 years. More recently, MRSA has also become a problem in the community and is referred to as *community-associated* or *CA-MRSA.* According to the CDC, infection with this variant has been associated with recent antibiotic use, sharing of contaminated personal items, living in crowded settings, and poor hygiene. This form of MRSA is associated with skin and soft tissue infections that are treatable with alternate antibiotics. The following groups have been affected: injection drug users, men who have sex with men, inmates, military recruits, children in childcare facilities, and athletes. Even as we write, other organisms are adapting to the drugs used to treat them and will soon emerge to present new infection control threats in health care facilities and possibly communities, so this problem will be with us for some time.

Another type of HAI that is very common in the hospital environment is *Clostridium difficile* colitis, a gastrointestinal infection that causes diarrhea. *C. difficile* is especially difficult to control because it is a spore-forming bacterium that is not eliminated by the usual routine methods of asepsis. Patients receiving antibiotic therapy are particularly susceptible to developing this infection because antibiotics tend to upset the normal balance of intestinal flora. About 20% of hospital patients receiving antibiotics develop *C. difficile* infections. Treatment is usually quite successful, but about 20% of treated patients relapse, sometimes developing a chronically recurring disease.

PREVENTING DISEASE TRANSMISSION

Until about 30 years ago, infection transmission was minimized by keeping infected persons separated from others. In acknowledgment that many patients with blood-borne infections are not recognized, the CDC introduced a system in 1985 known as *Universal Precautions (UP).* In this system, all patients are treated as potential reservoirs of infection. It is based on the use of barriers for all contacts with blood and certain body fluids known to carry blood-borne pathogens. The need to use barriers, such as gloves and masks, depends on the nature of the interaction with the patient rather than on the specific diagnosis.

Because UP placed emphasis on blood-borne infections and did not include precautions for contamination by feces, nasal secretions, sputum, urine, and vomitus (unless contaminated with visible blood), a new system was introduced in 1987 called *Body Substance Precautions (BSP),* also called *Body Substance Isolation (BSI).* This system focused on the use of barriers to prevent contact with all moist and potentially infectious body substances from all patients. The system was developed to protect health care workers from acquiring and transmitting infections from all pathogens. As of 1996, however, the CDC has recommended a new system that synthesizes the features of UP and BSP. This most recent system is called **Standard Precautions** and incorporates guidelines for isolation in hospitals. As applied in an outpatient setting, Standard Precautions are essentially the same as BSP.

Standard Precautions

Standard Precautions involve the use of barriers whenever contact is anticipated with any of the following:
- Blood
- Any body fluid or wound drainage
- Secretions and excretions (except sweat), regardless of whether they contain visible blood
- Nonintact skin
- Mucous membranes

Standard Precautions, as applied in an outpatient setting, are summarized in Box 21-4. They are designed to reduce the risk of transmission from unrecognized sources of pathogens in health care facilities, whether

Box 21-4

Standard Precautions for All Patient Care

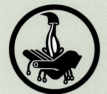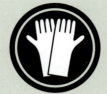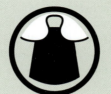

- Wash hands often and well and use alcohol-based hand rubs between washings.
- Wear protective gloves when likely to touch body substances, mucous membranes, or nonintact skin.
- Wear a plastic apron or a protective gown when clothing is likely to be soiled.
- Wear mask and eye protection when likely to be splashed.
- Place intact needle-syringe units and sharps in designated disposal containers. Do not break, bend, or recap needles.

blood-borne or not. If unanticipated contact with any body substance occurs, thoroughly wash the contact area as soon as possible. Use gloves to wipe up after all blood spills and disinfect using 1 part bleach to 10 parts water or the disinfectant specifically recommended for potential blood-borne pathogen contamination in your facility.

Standard Precautions require that each individual use judgment in determining when barriers are necessary. Each individual must establish his or her own standards for consistent use of barriers. These personal standards should be based on the individual's skills and the anticipated interactions involving the patient's body substances, nonintact skin, and mucous membranes. You will be making frequent decisions about when to take the extra time to protect both yourself and your patients. In the beginning, your level of precautions should be very high. Although you may observe more experienced workers taking fewer precautions, do not think you must follow their example. At this stage it is far better to take too many precautions than to take too few.

Be aware of the specific infection control policies in place at your facility. The key to effective protection is a consistent approach to *all contact* with *all body substances* of *all patients* at *all times*.

Medical Asepsis

Medical **asepsis** is the process of reducing the *probability* of infectious organisms being transmitted to a susceptible individual. The healthy human body has the ability to overcome a limited number of infectious organisms. This resistance can be overwhelmed by a massive exposure. On the other hand, a reduced resistance caused by disease, cancer chemotherapy, immunosuppressants, or extremes in age may result in infection after only minimal exposure. The fewer the organisms to which an individual is exposed, the more likely that he or she will resist infection. The process of reducing the total number of

organisms is called **microbial dilution** and can be accomplished at several levels.

Simple cleanliness measures prevent the transmission of organisms when proper cleaning, linen handling, and hand-washing techniques are used. The second level is **disinfection** and involves the destruction of pathogens by chemical agents. The third stage is surgical asepsis, or **sterilization.** This involves treating items with heat, gas, or chemicals to make them germ free. They are then stored in a manner that prevents contamination.

You can easily find examples of poor aseptic technique in most clinical settings. Unfortunately, the results of carelessness are seldom traced to the culprit. It is the patient acquiring an infection who suffers. Armed with the knowledge of disease transmission, how can you fight the spread of infection?

- Stay home when you are ill, if possible. Definitely avoid contact with immunocompromised patients.
- Cover your mouth with a tissue when you sneeze or cough or cover your face with your arm so that you cough into your elbow rather than your hand.
- Wear a clean uniform daily and remove it immediately when you go home.
- Follow hand hygiene recommendations.
- Use established precautions when handling patients, linens, or items contaminated with body substances.
- Practice good housekeeping techniques in your work area.
- When in doubt about the cleanliness of any object, do not use it.
- Immediately dispose of linens, instruments, or other items that touch the floor because the floor is always considered contaminated.
- When patients are coughing or sneezing, provide tissues and ask them to cover their mouth and nose.

Hand Hygiene

The first three principles listed earlier are simple and self-explanatory. Hand hygiene also may seem obvious, but this is the rule most consistently ignored in many health care settings. Hand hygiene refers to decontamination of the hands using soap and water, an antiseptic hand wash, or an alcohol-based hand rub. *Frequent hand hygiene is the single best protection against disease.* It should be followed explicitly before and after work, before meals, and often during the day.

The use of alcohol-based hand rubs takes less time and is often more convenient than hand-washing. Some individuals find hand rubs less irritating to the skin. The CDC believes that the use of hand rubs has greatly improved hand hygiene compliance in the health care setting and recommends that this method of hand hygiene be used

before and after patient contact, before donning gloves, after removing gloves, and after contact with equipment or objects that may have been in contact with a patient. Alcohol rubs are very effective against most microorganisms, including multidrug-resistant organisms. Alcohol-based rubs will not destroy endospores, however. Hand-washing with soap and water is still recommended to physically remove spores from the surfaces of contaminated hands. Use of alcohol-based hand rubs should not replace hand-washing with soap and water when hands are visibly soiled or contaminated with blood or body secretions or excretions. Aseptic hand-washing technique is both simple and effective. The technique is illustrated in Fig. 21-22.

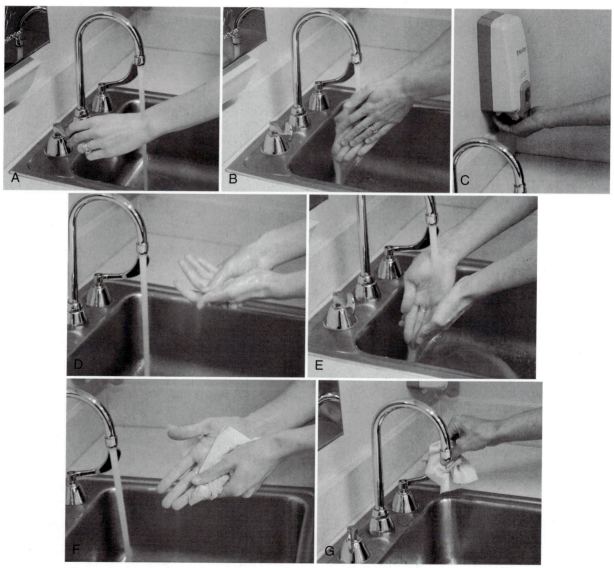

Fig. 21-22 Handwashing. **A,** Turn on water and adjust temperature. **B,** Wet hands thoroughly. Keep hands lower than elbows so water will drain from clean area (forearms) to most contaminated area (fingers). **C,** Apply antimicrobial soap. **D,** Lather well. Rub hands and fingers together with firm rotary motion for 20 seconds. *Friction is more effective than soap in removing microorganisms from skin.* Rub palms, backs of hands, and areas between fingers. **E,** Rinse, allowing water to run down over hands. Repeat steps to cleanse wrists and forearms. **F,** Use paper towel to dry thoroughly from fingertips to wrist. **G,** Turn off water with paper towel to avoid contaminating hands.

Gloves should always be worn to prevent contact with the patient's blood or other body fluids. Always perform hand hygiene following the removal of gloves.

Studies reveal that health care workers who wear artificial nails are more likely to harbor bacteria at the fingertips below the nails, both before and after handwashing, than those who have natural nails. For this reason, many health care facilities do not permit health care workers to wear artificial nails. According to the CDC, artificial fingernails or extenders should not be worn by health care workers who have direct contact with patients at high risk. The tips of natural nails should be kept smooth and short, less than 0.25 inch in length.

Housekeeping

Good housekeeping in the workplace reduces the incidence of airborne infections and the transfer of pathogens by fomites. A clean, dry environment discourages the growth of all microorganisms. A custodian or cleaning service may do much of the cleaning in the office or clinic at night, but you are responsible for inspecting the work area regularly and maintaining high standards of medical asepsis.

Several general principles apply whenever cleaning is required:
- Always clean from the least contaminated area toward the more contaminated area and from the top down.
- Avoid raising dust.
- Do not contaminate yourself or clean areas.
- Clean all equipment that comes in contact with patients after each use using a cloth moistened with disinfectant.

For a cleaning agent for decontaminating environmental surfaces, the CDC recommends either a diluted solution of sodium hypochlorite bleach (e.g., Clorox) or a disinfectant registered by the Environmental Protection Agency (EPA) as effective against HIV, hepatitis B virus, and the TB bacterium. Dilute the bleach by mixing 1 part bleach with 10 parts water. Mix fresh bleach daily because its effectiveness declines rapidly when diluted. EPA-registered disinfectants are available as liquids, spray foams, and disposable wipes. Your facility may have written procedures with detailed instructions concerning preferred cleansing agents and the extent of responsibility for disinfecting rooms. Consult the policy and procedure manual.

Handling Linens

Objects or linens soiled with body secretions or excretions are considered contaminated and may serve as fomites even though stains may not be apparent. For this reason, many clinics use disposable gowns and linens. Any linens used by patients should be handled as little as possible. To prevent airborne contamination, fold the edges to the middle without shaking or flapping and immediately place loosely balled linens in a hamper or a lined trash container. *Never use any linen for more than one patient.*

Handling and Disposal of Contaminated Items and Waste

A modern health care facility uses many disposable items, from simple objects (e.g., paper cups and tissues) to more complex items (e.g., trays for minor surgical procedures). Disposable items are designed to be used only once and then discarded. The only exception to this rule involves the immediate reuse of an unsterile item, such as an emesis basin, by the same patient.

Your facility will have a protocol for the discard of disposable items. Some place glass, plastic, and paper into separate covered containers. Others place everything together. Regulations demand that objects contaminated with blood or body fluids be discarded in a suitable container and marked with the **biohazard symbol** (Fig. 21-23). Used bandages and dressings are assumed to be contaminated. They are handled with gloves and placed directly into waterproof bags, which are then sealed and discarded. Do not remove anything from a hazardous waste container once it has been placed inside, and do not place any object in a plastic biohazard bag that could puncture the bag. Specific regulations vary by state with respect to what constitutes biohazardous waste and how these wastes must be handled.

Needles, syringes, and contaminated items capable of puncturing the skin are disposed of in a **sharps container.** Sharps containers are made of tough material that cannot be punctured by needles or glass and are designed to receive syringes and attached needles without recapping. They are discussed further and illustrated in Chapter 24. *Never recap a used needle.* This is how most finger punctures occur.

Before specimens are sent to the laboratory, they should be placed in clean containers with secure caps and

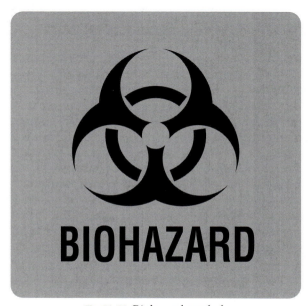

Fig. 21-23 Biohazard symbol.

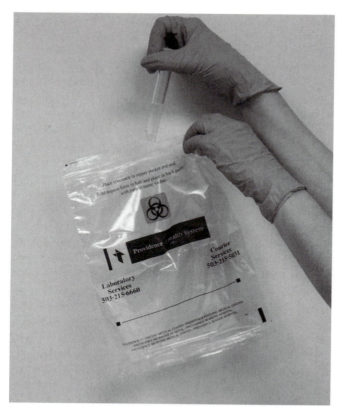

Fig. 21-24 Laboratory specimens are placed in a plastic bag labelled with a biohazard symbol.

slipped inside a plastic bag labeled with a biohazard symbol (Fig. 21-24).

Always wear gloves when assisting patients with bedpans or urinals. Collect any specimen needed and empty the bedpan or urinal immediately. Rinse it well over the toilet; discard it if disposable, or put it in the proper place to be sterilized.

SURGICAL ASEPSIS

Earlier in this chapter, we defined *medical asepsis* as a method of reducing the number of pathogenic microorganisms in the environment and intervening in the process by which they are spread. *Surgical asepsis*, on the other hand, is the complete removal of all organisms and their spores from equipment used to perform specific procedures. The linens, gloves, and instruments used in surgery may be the first examples brought to mind, but many other procedures, such as injections and the drawing of blood samples, also require sterile equipment, and some procedures demand an assortment of sterile equipment and supplies arrayed in a sterile field. In addition, some procedures require special skin preparation to prevent pathogens from entering the body.

Sterile items used in clinics and physicians' offices, such as syringes and needles, are usually disposable items. They are sterile when purchased and are protected by a paper or plastic wrap. Reusable items such as instruments and glass syringes are wrapped, sterilized, and stored in a clean, dry location.

Sterilization

Although you are unlikely to be directly involved in the process of sterilization, it is helpful to understand the methods that may be used. Chemical, gas, and steam sterilization are most common.

Chemical sterilization involves the immersion and soaking of clean objects in a bath of germicidal solution. Sterilization depends on solution strength and temperature and the immersion time, all of which are difficult to control accurately. Contamination of the solution or the object being sterilized may occur and is not easily detectable. For these reasons, chemical sterilization is not the most satisfactory method for providing surgical asepsis and is not recommended. If chemical sterilization must be used, be certain to follow the chemical manufacturer's instructions completely.

Items that would be damaged by moist heat are sterilized by means of conventional gas sterilization or by gas plasma technology. The conventional method uses a mixture of gases (Freon and ethylene oxide) heated to 135° F (57° C). Gas sterilization is too expensive and time consuming for general use and is used primarily for electric, plastic, and rubber items and for optical ware. Telephones, stethoscopes, blood pressure cuffs, and other equipment may be sterilized in this manner. This treatment sterilizes very effectively but has one drawback: because the gases used are poisonous, they must be dissipated by means of aeration in a controlled environment. Aeration is a slow process, so it is important to send items for conventional gas sterilization well in advance of the time they will be needed.

A safer method of sterilizing items that are sensitive to heat or moisture is the use of gas plasma technology. Items are cleaned, wrapped, and placed in a compact mobile unit where low-temperature hydrogen peroxide gas plasma diffuses through the wrappings and effectively kills both microorganisms and spores. Because the gas plasma system uses very low heat and moisture, it can effectively sterilize endoscopes, fiber optic devices, microsurgical instruments, and powered instruments.

Another advantage is greater safety for supply department workers because there are no toxic fumes, byproducts, or residues and no handling of hazardous chemicals. Gas plasma technology has significantly reduced the use of ethylene oxide, but it cannot completely replace this method because it is not effective for instruments that have long, narrow lumens and cannot be used for powders, liquids, or any cellulose materials, such as paper, cotton, linen, or muslin.

Hospitals usually have equipment for both gas and gas plasma sterilization, but these methods are not usually

PART V

Ancillary Clinical Skills

available in outpatient facilities. Items of value that have become contaminated may have to be sent out for gas sterilization.

An **autoclave** is an electric steam chamber that seals tightly to achieve high temperatures under pressure. Autoclaving, or steam sterilization, is the quickest and most convenient means of sterilization for items that can withstand heat. Higher temperatures can be achieved under pressure, which makes this an extremely effective method. Clinics that need to sterilize reusable equipment will have a small autoclave for this purpose.

An advantage of both steam and gas sterilization is that indicators can be used to identify that a pack has been sterilized. Indicators are placed inside the pack and outside to show that the gas or steam has penetrated to all surfaces. Indicators change color when the required conditions have been met. You are responsible for correctly recognizing the sterilization indicators used in your clinical facility.

Suppliers of commercial packs use ionizing radiation to destroy microorganisms and spores. Commercial packs also contain expiration dates and indicators to confirm their sterility.

Sterile Fields

If your job description includes assisting the physician with sterile procedures, you will need to know how to prepare a sterile field. A sterile field is a germ-free area prepared for the use of sterile supplies and equipment. The principles of surgical asepsis used in establishing and working with a sterile field are stated in Box 21-5. The first step in preparing a sterile field is to confirm the

sterility of packaged supplies and equipment. Packages are considered sterile if they meet the following criteria:

- They are clean, dry, and unopened.
- Their expiration date has not been exceeded.
- Their sterility indicators have changed to a predetermined color, confirming sterilization.

Proper preparation is essential to any procedure that requires sterile technique. You may be responsible for assembling the necessary equipment. Most procedures today use disposable equipment that is wrapped in paper or plastic. Directions on the packages are usually clear and precise. Taking time to read them well in advance increases self-confidence when assisting the physician. Nondisposable equipment that has been sterilized is double-wrapped in cloth or heavy paper and sealed with indicator tape. All packs are wrapped in a standardized manner and are always opened using the following method (Fig. 21-25):

- Check the pack to be certain it is the correct item and that all sterility indicators are positive as listed in the previous paragraph.
- Place the pack on a clean surface within reach of the physician.
- Just before the procedure begins, break the seal and open the pack.
- Unfold the first corner away from you, and then unfold the two sides.
- Pull the front fold down toward you and drop it. Do not touch the inner surface.
- The inner wrap, if there is one, is opened in the same manner.
- You have now established a sterile field.

Nondisposable sterile items wrapped separately may now be added to the sterile field. Standing back from the table, grasp the object through the wrapper with one hand. With the other hand, unseal the wrapper, allowing it to fall down over your wrist. Hold the edges of the wrapper with your free hand, and drop the object onto the sterile field without releasing the wrapper (Fig. 21-26).

Disposable sponges, gloves, and other small items are supplied in "peel-down" paper wraps and may be added to the sterile field. Following the instructions, separate the paper layers, invert the package, and allow the object to fall onto the sterile field without contaminating the object or the sterile field (Fig. 21-27).

It may be necessary to add a liquid medium, such as povidone-iodine (Betadine; a skin disinfectant), to a sterile tray. After double-checking the label, position the label toward your hand, open the spout, and squirt the first few drops into the wastebasket or sink. Then pour the required amount into the sterile receptacle on the tray, show the physician the label, and close the spout. By discarding the first small amount poured, you rinse the container's lip with the liquid and avoid the possibility of contaminating the tray (Fig. 21-28).

When a limited operator must manipulate items in a sterile field without wearing sterile gloves, a sterile

Box 21-5

Standard Principles of Surgical Asepsis

- Any sterile object or field touched by an unsterile object or person becomes contaminated.
- Never reach across a sterile field. Organisms may fall from your arm into the field. Also, reaching increases the chance of brushing the area with your uniform.
- If you suspect that an item is contaminated, discard it. This includes items that are damp (moisture permits the transfer of bacteria from the outside to the inside of a wrapped set) and items that have had the seal broken or on which the indicator tape has not assumed the correct color.
- Do not pass between the physician and the sterile field.
- Never leave a sterile area unattended. If the field is accidentally contaminated, for example, by a fly or a patient reaching for her glasses, no one would know.
- A 1-inch border at the perimeter of the sterile field is considered to be a "buffer zone" and is treated as if it were contaminated.

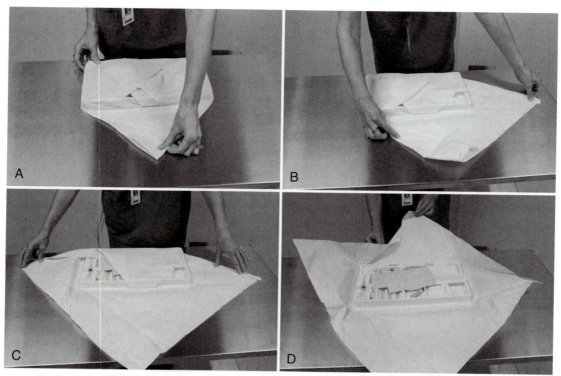

Fig. 21-25 Sterile field. **A,** After checking the sterilization indicator and expiration date on the pack, open the first corner away from you. **B,** Open one side by grasping its corner tip. **C,** Open second side in the same manner. **D,** Pull remaining corner toward you. If there is an inner wrap, open it in the same manner. A sterile field is now established.

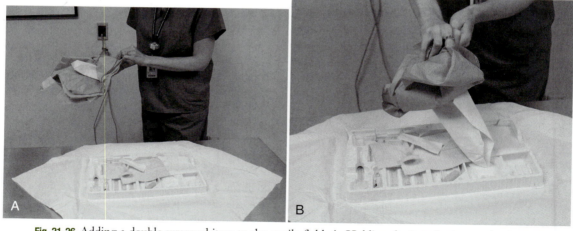

Fig. 21-26 Adding a double-wrapped item to the sterile field. **A,** Holding the item in the nondominant hand, open the outer wrap, opening the first fold away from your body. **B,** Avoid contamination of the field by holding the corners of the outer wrap while dropping the item onto the tray.

transfer forceps is used. Unwrap the forceps, grasping the handles firmly without touching the remainder of the instrument. Keep the forceps above your waist and in your sight at all times. After use, place the tips in a sterile field with the handles protruding so you can use them again. Do not reach across the sterile field.

If a procedure must be postponed, do not open the tray. If it is already open, cover it immediately with a sterile drape or discard it, because airborne contamination is just as serious as a break in sterile technique.

When the sterile procedure is completed, don protective gloves and thoroughly clean all reusable items to be sterilized. Items must be free of all residue so that the sterilizing agent can penetrate to all surfaces. Thorough cleaning is very important and is most easily accomplished when done promptly. Discard disposable items; place needles in the sharps container and put bloody sponges and other biohazardous waste in a biohazard bag. Remove your gloves and perform hand hygiene.

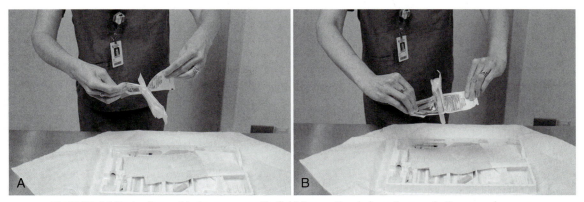

Fig. 21-27 Adding a disposable item to a sterile field from a "peel-down" wrap. **A,** Separate the wrap according to package instructions. **B,** Invert the package, allowing the item to drop onto the field.

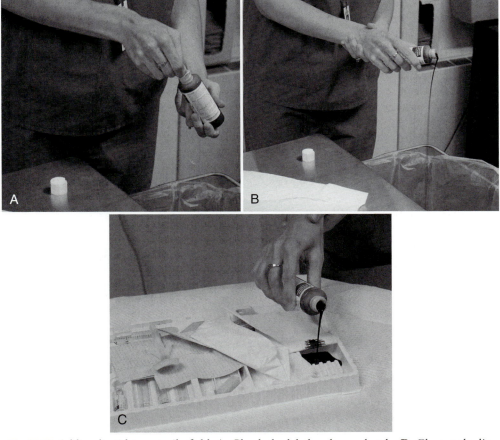

Fig. 21-28 Adding liquid to a sterile field. **A,** Check the label and open bottle. **B,** Cleanse the lip of the container by squirting a small amount into a waste container. **C,** Pour the required amount into a receptacle on the tray, taking care not to contaminate the field.

Anyone whose work involves sterile fields must have a "sterile conscience." This refers to an awareness of sterile technique and the responsibility for telling the person in charge whenever you contaminate a field or observe its contamination by someone else. You may feel reluctant to speak out about apparent breaks in technique because of the inconvenience of reestablishing a sterile field. Physicians and co-workers may not seem to appreciate your challenge at the moment, but your professionalism and concern for the patient's welfare will be reflected in the confidence they place in your aseptic technique.

Gloving

It is unlikely that you will be required to don sterile gloves. This skill may be important, however, if you are needed to assist with certain sterile procedures or to apply a sterile dressing. The technique is illustrated in Fig. 21-29.

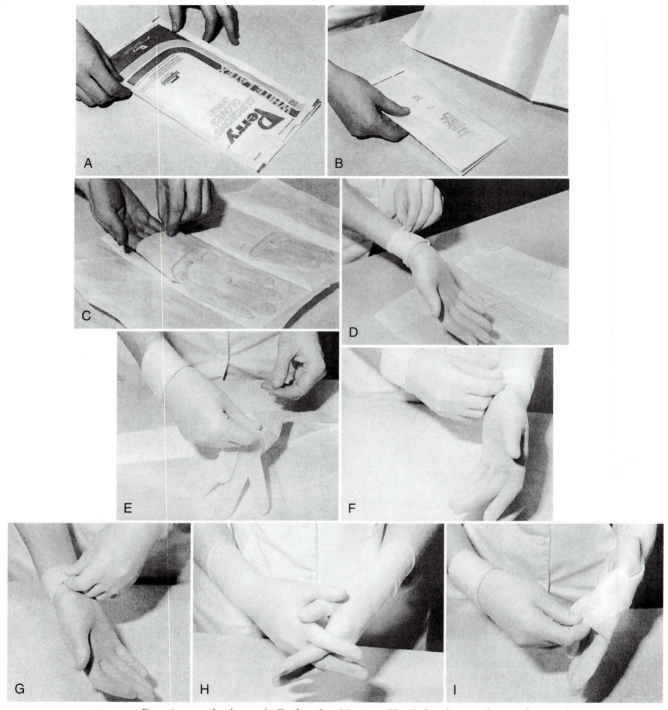

Fig. 21-29 Donning sterile gloves. **A,** *Perform hand hygiene.* Check the glove package to be certain that the size is correct and open the package. **B,** Open the outer wrap to expose the folded inner wrap. **C,** Open the inner wrap, touching only the outer surface. Expose the gloves with the open ends facing you. **D,** Put on the first glove, touching only the inner surface of the folded cuff. **E,** Using the gloved hand, grasp the second glove *under* the cuff. **F,** Put on the second glove and unfold the cuff. **G,** Insert the fingers under the cuff on the first glove and unfold the cuff. **H,** Gloving is complete. Keep your hands in front of your body at a safe distance from your uniform to prevent contamination. **I,** Remove the gloves by inverting them as you pull them off. Perform hand hygiene.

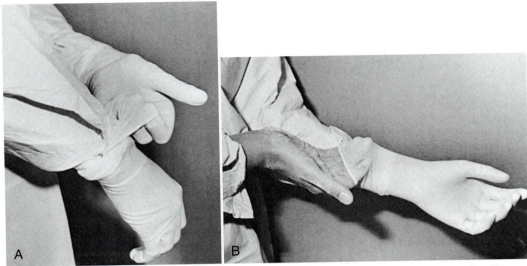

Fig. 21-30 Removing contaminated gloves. **A,** Grasp the first glove from the outside and pull it off. **B,** Insert your clean fingers inside the cuff of the second glove and remove it. Perform hand hygiene.

The technique for removing contaminated gloves is shown in Fig. 21-30. This method avoids contamination of your arms or sleeves and also of your ungloved hand.

Always perform hand hygiene before gloving and after removing gloves.

Removing and Applying Dressings

In many health care facilities today, limited operators and medical assistants are called upon to perform tasks that were once performed solely by nurses. For example, you may be directed by a physician to remove a patient's dressing. It may also be your duty to apply a fresh dressing when the examination has been completed.

When a dressing is to be removed, perform hand hygiene, don protective gloves, and inform the patient of what you are about to do. Use care in removing the dressing to prevent cross-contaminating the wound and yourself. Remove the dressing gently to avoid hurting the patient. Place the soiled dressing in a plastic bag and seal it before adding it to the biohazard container. Remove your gloves and repeat hand hygiene.

The application of a new dressing requires sterile technique. Begin by preparing your supplies: sterile gloves, sterile drape, sterile gauze, and tape. You may also need some normal saline solution to clean the area around the wound. When everything you will need has been assembled, proceed as follows:

- Tell the patient what you plan to do.
- Perform hand hygiene.
- Tear several strips of tape to a convenient length.

- Open the sterile drape pack, placing the drape near the patient.
- Partially open the drape by pulling from the corners. This creates a small sterile field for your other sterile items.
- Open the dressing package and add the sterile dressing to the sterile field.
- If you will need to cleanse around the wound, drop sterile gauze sponges into your field for this purpose.
- To moisten the gauze sponges, open a small vial of sterile normal saline solution. Recheck the label and pour a small amount of the saline over the sponges. Do not allow liquid to soak through to the sterile towel. Check the label for the third time before discarding the vial.
- Don sterile gloves using the method described for sterile gloving.
- Use the moist sponges to clean gently around the wound.
- Allow the area to dry completely.
- Apply the dressing over the wound and secure it in place with tape.
- Cover the patient.
- Dispose of any waste.
- Remove your gloves and repeat hand hygiene.

SUMMARY

The principle underlying everything discussed in the first part of this chapter is safety. You must be alert to potential hazards from fire, falls, spills, and electric shock and be prepared to respond appropriately when these hazards pose a threat. Safety is ensured when you use correct techniques for positioning patients and for assisting their movements. The objective is to protect patients when they are unable to protect themselves and to do so without personal injury.

Despite the "miracle drugs" developed over the past 60 years, infectious diseases are still a significant public health problem, and some are growing alarmingly worse. There are still no medications to treat most viral infections. Other organisms are changing rapidly and becoming immune to medications that were once highly effective.

Asymptomatic carriers of HIV and hepatitis B virus pose a significant threat to members of the community, including health care workers, who may be exposed to infectious blood or body fluids without being aware that the infection is present.

For all of these reasons, the safety of patients and health care workers requires conscientious infection control practices. Standard Precautions protect health care workers from infectious body fluids, both known and unsuspected. Aseptic techniques begin with a commitment to proper practices and are implemented through the conscientious application of knowledge and skill.

Chapter 22

Assessing Patients and Managing Acute Situations

At the conclusion of this chapter, you will be able to:

- List four personal comfort needs common to most patients and describe appropriate responses to meet these needs
- Assist patients who need to use bedpans or urinals
- Obtain and record a patient history
- Accurately observe patients' physical status and report status using appropriate terminology
- Take and record temperature (oral, rectal, and axillary), pulse rate (at four common sites), respiration rate, and blood pressure; state normal values for each
- Administer oxygen or suction appropriately in an emergency
- Recognize acute life-threatening conditions, such as shock, heart attack, respiratory arrest, and cardiac arrest, and respond appropriately
- List the four levels of consciousness and discuss possible causes for changes in level of consciousness
- Demonstrate correct handling of patients with extremity fractures and recently applied casts
- Assist patients who experience asthma attack, hyperventilation, nausea and vomiting, epistaxis, hypoglycemia, vertigo, seizures, or syncope

Key Terms

anaphylaxis
angina
anoxia
apex
asthma
cerebrovascular accident (CVA)
cyanotic
diabetic coma
diaphoretic
diastolic
dyspnea
epistaxis
erythema
fibrillation
hemorrhage

hypertension
hyperventilation
hypoglycemia
hypotension
incontinence
shock
sphygmomanometer
syncope
systolic
tachycardia
thready pulse
transient ischemic attack (TIA)
urticaria
vertigo

This chapter addresses basic principles involved in meeting patient needs, but before these needs can be met, they must be clearly identified. Observation, evaluation, and assessment are the skills needed to determine patient needs. When these skills are consciously practiced in the clinical area, they increase your value as a limited operator. They help you become more sensitive to the safety of the environment and the conditions of your patients.

The dictionary defines an *emergency* as a serious event that happens unexpectedly and demands immediate attention. Sudden deterioration in the status of any patient under your care is an acute situation requiring an appropriate response. Whether such a situation leads to a more serious problem may depend on whether you are prepared to act quickly and efficiently. Seen from this perspective, no patient problem can be considered trivial. Acute situations are bound to occur when you are dealing with patients who are ill or injured, and you must be prepared to cope in a way that will minimize the possibility of further injury or complication.

ASSESSING THE PERSONAL CONCERNS OF PATIENTS

Uncertainty about the coming procedure, fear of a possible diagnosis, or concern about the effect of illness on family members can cause varying reactions in patients. Sometimes these concerns are expressed as anger and demonstrated by inappropriate speech or rude behavior toward personnel. Other expressions of anxiety may be a need to talk constantly or, conversely, a tendency to become quiet and withdrawn. You may observe fidgeting or other nervous mannerisms.

Anxiety can also be caused by a concern over modesty, especially when patients must undress for examinations or treatments. Reassure patients by displaying a matter-of-fact attitude while providing ample cover and an explanation of the procedure.

Your presence is comforting to the anxious patient. Touch patients reassuringly and tell them what to expect. Let them know when you leave the area and when you expect to return. Escort ambulatory patients to the bathroom or back to the waiting area. It can be very distressing to patients if they must wander about in an examination gown wondering where to go. Once you start a procedure, try to remain near the patient. If patients must wait in an x-ray room or dressing room, let them know that you are within hearing distance and that they may call on you for help. If a call button is available, show patients how to use it and assure them that someone will assist them promptly if they call. If no call signal is available, check with patients frequently while they wait.

Physical discomfort adds to tension as well. Remember that most patients will find it hard to remain still during a long procedure on a hard surface. This is especially difficult for a thin patient or an elderly person with kyphosis. Note whether an obese patient has difficulty

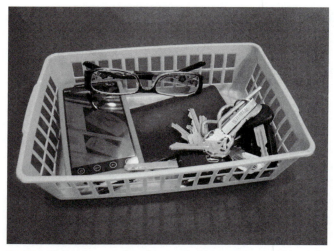

Fig. 22-1 Valuables are placed in a suitable container within sight of the patient.

breathing when lying flat on the table. Note skin temperature when you touch the patient and inquire whether the patient is warm enough. If the patient feels chilled, provide a blanket and tuck it around the patient to provide both warmth and a sense of security. As you move briskly around the room the temperature may seem warm enough to you, but elderly or frail patients may not be active enough to keep warm. If the patient is coughing or sniffling, offer paper handkerchiefs and position a waste container within reach for the soiled tissues.

If dentures must be removed, provide a suitable disposable container and place it in a safe and visible location. Dentures slide in much more easily when wet, so add water to the container or direct the patient to a sink when dentures are replaced. Eyeglasses and hearing aids are also items essential to activities of daily living and are difficult and expensive to replace or repair. A bright-colored plastic box or basket is a useful container for these items and other small valuables (Fig. 22-1). Choose a safe location in view of the patient. Use the same place consistently and point out the location to the patient.

PHYSIOLOGIC NEEDS

Water

A dry mouth can be caused by thirst but can also result from anxiety or medication. A drink of water, offered with a straw if the patient is lying down, may be very comforting. Because some tests require that the patient have nothing by mouth, even water, it is wise to check that water is permitted.

Elimination

An urgent need to void can be very distressing to a patient. A full bladder may cause discomfort, irritability, and difficulty remaining still during the procedure. If this need is ignored in an older or debilitated patient, **incontinence** (loss of bladder control) may result, causing embarrassment for the patient and cleanup problems for you. Be especially sensitive to the need for bathroom facilities when procedures are prolonged.

Before a patient uses the bathroom, check to see if a specimen of urine or feces should be collected. If so, provide instructions and the correct container. Urine collection procedure is explained in Chapter 24. When a patient needs to defecate or urinate and is unable to walk or be taken to the bathroom in a wheelchair, a bedpan or urinal is used. This is not a common requirement in most outpatient facilities, but assisting patients with bedpans or urinals is a basic clinical skill.

When a bedpan is necessary, follow the procedure outlined in Box 22-1. Be sure that the patient is adequately covered for privacy. When a female patient is placed on the bedpan, the upper torso needs to be slightly elevated to prevent urine from running up her back. When a patient is restricted in mobility, two people may be needed to assist the patient onto the bedpan. If the patient is on the x-ray table, one person should stand on each side of the table to prevent the patient from falling.

When the patient is finished, you may have to assist with wiping. Wear gloves and have toilet tissue, a wet washcloth, and a dry towel conveniently placed. Assist the patient to lift the hips or roll away from you onto one side while you steady and remove the pan. Place it safely aside and, if necessary, help the patient by wiping from front to back with paper first, and then with a wet cloth before drying. Offer the patient a disposable moist towelette or a clean wet cloth and towel to cleanse the hands.

Male patients may need to use a urinal. Usually this is simply a matter of providing the urinal and removing it again when the patient is finished. If the patient is unable to use it himself, don protective gloves and spread the patient's legs; lift the sheet with one hand and slide the penis into the urinal with the other. It may be advisable to hold the urinal in position until the patient is finished.

Patients may find it difficult to use a bedpan or urinal if they feel that they are under observation. If possible, you should remain out of the patient's line of sight while staying close enough to ensure patient safety.

Empty the bedpan or urinal carefully into the toilet to avoid splashing. Remember to perform hand hygiene after removing your gloves.

Placing a patient on the bedpan or offering the urinal is not a complex task. Once you are familiar with this procedure, the chief obstacle to overcome is embarrassment. A cheerful, matter-of-fact attitude will make the process easier for you and for the patient.

Sanitary Supplies

Occasionally a patient requires a sanitary napkin. Know where these are kept. If a soiled napkin is to be removed, direct the patient to a bathroom or place a paper bag within reach. Dispose of the bag with the soiled napkin in the appropriate container.

TAKING A HISTORY

It is important for you and the physician who interprets the images to know why an examination is being done. If the images are sent out to a radiologist, this information must accompany them. If the requisition does not provide complete and accurate information about the patient's history and condition, you will need to obtain this information from the patient. The answers you receive may influence how the examination is conducted. The history also aids the radiologist in focusing the interpretation to meet the referring physician's needs. This does not need to be a detailed medical history, but rather a thoughtful consideration of the patient's current status and why this particular radiographic study is being done.

The process of taking a history presents an opportunity for you to give the patient individual attention and build rapport. In addition, your ability to gain the patient's confidence will influence the amount of relevant information you obtain. Remember to introduce yourself, call the patient by name, and deal with immediate patient concerns as soon as possible.

Begin the history by asking a general question about the nature of the problem, such as, "Do you know why

Box 22-1

Assisting Patients With the Bedpan

1. Assemble your equipment. You will need a bedpan and bedpan cover (a towel or pillowcase may be used), toilet tissue, washcloth and towel, and sheet or blanket.
2. Perform hand hygiene and don disposable gloves.
3. Close the door to provide privacy.
4. If the patient is on the x-ray table, elevate the upper torso with pillows or angle sponges. Cover the patient.
5. Ask the patient to bend the knees and raise the hips.
6. Assist the patient by lifting with one hand under the small of the back while you slide the bedpan under the buttocks with the other.
7. Ask the patient to call when finished. If the patient is on the x-ray table, remain nearby but out of the patient's line of sight.
8. When the patient is finished, provide toilet tissue, then a wet washcloth and towel or a moist towelette for the patient's hands.
9. Ask the patient to raise the hips and remove the bedpan.
10. Cover the bedpan and place it aside until the patient is settled and secure.
11. Dispose of the contents in the toilet; remove the gloves and perform hand hygiene.

Dr. Chen wants you to have an x-ray of your chest?" Be realistic in the scope of your questions. Focus on expanding the information provided on the x-ray requisition. This is especially important when the request or order does not indicate the rationale for ordering the procedure. Most requisition forms have a place for this information, but in practice the history is often absent or is so limited that it does not seem relevant without further explanation. The information you obtain is most useful when recorded on the appropriate form. You may also need to enter it into the computer record.

History requirements vary with the nature of the examination. Table 22-1 provides history questions and observations pertinent to many patient complaints. You can use it to become familiar with the types of information that will be most useful in specific situations. The history examples in this table use common abbreviations that are also used in charting and other medical recording.

Patients may have been asked to complete a history questionnaire on their initial visit, but this information may be out of date. In facilities that perform procedures using contrast media, a special history questionnaire that includes questions about allergies and kidney function may need to be filled out and signed before each procedure that involves injection of an iodinated contrast medium.

Table 22-1

Guidelines for Taking a History of a Patient's Chief Complaint

Type of Examination	Questions	Observations	Example of History*
Orthopedic, acute injury	How did the injury occur? When? Can you show me exactly where it hurts?	Swelling, deformity, discoloration, laceration, abrasion	Twisting injury, L ankle, while skiing today; swelling & pain over lateral malleolus.
Orthopedic, not involving acute injury	Where does it hurt? How long has it been bothering you? Were you ever injured there? How was the injury treated (cast, surgery)? Has there been any recent change?	Deformity, scars, range of motion, weight bearing	Chronic pain, R knee 2 yr, worse since building fence Sat. Prev Rx c̄ cortisone inj. No known injury.
Neck	Did you injure your neck? How? When? Where does it hurt? Do you have any pain, numbness, or tingling of the shoulder or arm? Which side?	Range of motion	MVC 10/12/15; lower neck pain & L shldr pain c̄ numbness & tingling, L hand.
Spine	Did you injure your back? How? When? Do you have pain, numbness, tingling, or weakness of the hip or leg? Which side? Any bowel or bladder problems?	Gait, range of motion	Lifting injury 2 wk ago. LBP radiating to R hip.
Head	Were you injured? When? How? Do you have pain? Where? Did you lose consciousness? For how long?	Speech: clarity, confusion; gait	Severe HA, blurred vision, dizziness, & gen'l weakness, 24 hr. No known injury. Speech slurred.
Chest	Do you know why your doctor ordered this examination? Are you short of breath? Do you have a cough? Do you cough up anything? Do you cough up blood? Have you had a fever? Do you have any heart problems?	Respirations, cough	SOB, wheezing, & R chest pain since resp flu 4 wk ago. Moderate, nonproductive cough.
Abdomen, gastrointestinal examinations	Do you know why your doctor ordered this examination? Do you have pain? Where? Do you have nausea? Diarrhea? Have you had any other tests for this problem (lab tests, ultrasound)? Do you know the results? Have you ever had abdominal surgery? When? Why?		LLQ pain, incr over past mo. ? mass seen on US done here 10/21/11.
Urology	Do you know why your doctor ordered this examination? Do you have any pain? Where? For how long? Do you have trouble passing urine? Pain? Urgency? Frequency? Have you ever had this problem before? Do you have high blood pressure?		2 prior episodes of UTI; current malaise, fever, & mid back pain.

*&, and; ?, question of; *inj*, injection; *shldr*, shoulder; *gen'l*, general; *resp*, respiratory; *US*, ultrasound. To identify other common abbreviations used in charting (e.g., *MVC*, motor vehicle crash), see Appendix L.

Examinations for patients with chronic conditions or those receiving posttreatment follow-up may require a comparison with prior imaging studies. If these are not part of the current file, your history should contain information on previous relevant examinations, including when and where they were done.

Some medical assistants take preliminary histories before the physician sees the patient. Although the physician is responsible for taking the official medical history, a preliminary history can save time, allowing the physician to focus quickly on details of the patient's problem. If taking patients' preliminary histories is one of your accepted responsibilities, the standard format that follows can serve as a guide. Using this outline will allow you to elicit the greatest amount of information about the patient's chief complaint in the least amount of time and will help you avoid missing relevant facts.

Onset: How did it start? What happened? When did it first trouble you? Was it sudden or a complaint that gradually got worse?

Duration: Have you ever had it before? If so, when? Has it been continuous? Does it bother you all the time? How long has this attack been bothering you?

Specific location: Where does it hurt (or where is the problem)? Can you put your finger on where it hurts the most? Does it hurt anywhere else?

Quality of pain: What does it feel like? Sharp, stabbing pain? Dull ache? Throbbing pain? How severe is it? Mild, moderate, severe? (Some like to use a pain scale of 0 to 5 or 0 to 10, with 0 being no pain at all and the highest number representing the worst pain the patient can imagine.) Does it wake you up at night?

What aggravates: When is it worse? What seems to aggravate it? Is it worse after meals (at night, when you walk)?

What alleviates: What has helped in the past? Does that still help? What seems to help now? Does the time of day (amount of rest or change in position) make a difference?

Tact and caution are required when obtaining a history. Anxious patients may read too much into your questions. Information regarding such serious matters as cancer, surgery, or heart attacks is best elicited in a general way rather than through blunt questions. "Do you know why your doctor ordered this examination?" is less threatening than "Is your doctor checking for cancer?" Victims of accidents for which legal liability is in question may be reluctant to provide information that could increase their liability or jeopardize a legal settlement. Minors may be hesitant to reveal personal information in the presence of their parents. When information is difficult to obtain, it is usually wise for the physician to take the complete history.

At this point the process of taking a history may seem complex and confusing. This is a skill that improves with practice. Role-playing with other students, including a critical observer, will improve your ability to take a history with sensitivity and confidence. As clinical practice provides additional knowledge and experience, you will find that your observation and history-taking skills become increasingly accurate and pertinent.

ASSESSING CURRENT PHYSICAL STATUS

Establishing a Baseline

You may be the first and primary observer of a significant change in the patient's current condition. To accurately assess change, you must first establish a baseline for your observations.

Before you begin a radiographic procedure it is important to review the requisition. Unfortunately, the requisition may not have enough specific information, and this is a place where your skill in history taking will prove valuable. If you have access to the medical record, read the diagnosis and the most recent chart notes. An order for the x-ray study should be there. Some notations have special significance. It is important to note any allergies, as a patient with a history of allergies is more likely to have an adverse reaction to medications, especially when administered by injection.

Physical Evaluation

In the context of this chapter, evaluation is an ongoing process of observation, assessment, and measurement to note and evaluate changes in patient condition. How do you know when the condition of a patient is changing for the worse? What do you look for?

The most important process is sometimes called *eyeballing the patient*, a skill of acute observation that compares the actions and appearance of *this* patient with those of similar patients you have seen. You also use this skill to compare the appearance of this patient *now* with the way he or she appeared earlier. Although this may seem intuitive, you are actually responding to subtle changes in the overall appearance of the patient.

One of the easiest signs to recognize is a change in skin color. Individual complexions vary, but when pale skin becomes **cyanotic** or olive skin becomes pale and waxen, the change is usually quite apparent. The term *cyanotic* denotes a bluish coloration in the skin and indicates a lack of sufficient oxygen (O_2) in the tissues. This is most easily seen on the mucous membranes, such as the lips or the lining of the mouth. Nail beds may also show a bluish tinge. For some patients with heart or lung conditions, this may be a chronic or usual state, but the patient who *becomes* cyanotic needs oxygen and immediate medical attention. Any patient who looks pale and anxious and does not feel well is subject to fainting and needs to sit or lie down immediately. Do not leave the patient! A patient who loses consciousness and falls to the floor may suffer injuries far more serious than the cause of the fainting.

We have discussed the importance of touch as a form of communication and reassurance, but contact with your hands also allows you to make physical observations. The acutely ill patient in pain may be pale, cool, and **diaphoretic** (perspiring) in what is frequently called a *cold sweat*. Hot, dry skin may indicate a fever, whereas warm, moist skin may only be a response to the weather or the room temperature. Cool, moist skin may indicate acute anxiety. Wet palms and shaking hands are typical of the apprehensive individual who will need an unusual amount of reassurance. These patients may find it difficult to concentrate. They often need more frequent instructions during the procedure and should receive written directions for any required follow-up care.

If you note any of these signs, it is important to determine whether this is a new symptom. Has the patient just received any new medication? If so, notify your supervisor or the physician immediately. You may be observing the first signs of an impending allergic reaction.

Vital Signs

The next four procedures used for assessment are usually referred to as *vital signs*. They involve the measurement of temperature, pulse rate, respiratory rate, and blood pressure. The ability to take vital signs is a valuable clinical skill. Even if taking vital signs is not a part of your usual job description, you may need to assess them in an emergency. If you do not take vital signs routinely, keep your skills sharp by reviewing your technique frequently. When time allows, check your co-workers. We should all be aware of our own baseline vital signs, so your practice will benefit you, the person on whom you practice, and the patient who may need your skill in an emergency. Know the location of equipment for measuring vital signs and other items that might be needed in an emergency. Even before you are proficient in their use, you may be asked to obtain them for a nurse or physician. Table 22-2

provides a reference to normal vital sign measurements by age.

Temperature

The first of the vital signs is temperature. Taking a temperature is a basic clinical skill that can also be used in your own home. An accurate temperature reading measures the body's basic metabolic state, the rate at which it uses energy.

Body temperatures vary during the day, being lowest in the morning and highest in the evening. Normal oral temperatures vary from 96.8° to 99.6° F (36° to 37.6° C). Rectal temperatures range from 0.5° to 1.0° F (0.28° to 0.56° C) higher than oral temperatures; axillary temperatures range from 0.5° to 1.0° F lower. In addition, normal temperatures vary slightly from person to person. A tense, quick-moving individual is likely to have a higher basal temperature than a placid, slow-moving person, all else being equal.

Fever, also termed *pyrexia* or *hyperthermia*, is a sign of an increase in body metabolism, usually in response to an infectious process. For adults, fever commonly refers to any temperature of 100.4° F (38° C) or higher when taken orally, or 101.4° F (38.6° C) taken rectally.

Temperatures may be obtained by the oral, rectal, axillary, temporal artery, or tympanic routes. Alert, cooperative patients usually prefer the familiar oral route. It has long been held that the oral method is less accurate than the rectal method, but research does not confirm this belief. The oral route provides an accurate measure of changes in body core temperature when taken correctly with the probe of the thermometer well under the base of the tongue.

The oral method is *not* appropriate when the patient has recently had a hot or cold beverage, is receiving oxygen, or breathes through the mouth. In these situations, the rectal or axillary method may be used. The rectal temperature is both more accurate and faster to take than the axillary temperature; however, the axillary method is

Table 22-2

A Quick Reference for Normal Vital Signs by Age

Age	Temperature (Oral)	Temperature (Rectal, Tympanic, and Temporal)	Pulse	Respirations	Blood Pressure (Systolic)
Premature newborn		99.6° F (37.5° C)	140	<60	50-60
Full-term newborn		99.6° F (37.5° C)	125	<60	70
6 months		99.6° F (37.5° C)	120	24-36	90
1 year		99.6° F (37.5° C)	120	22-30	96
3 years		99.6° F (37.5° C)	110	20-26	100
5 years	98.6° F (37° C)	99.6° F (37.5° C)	100	20-24	100
6 years	98.6° F (37° C)	99.6° F (37.5° C)	100	20-24	100
8 years	98.6° F (37° C)	99.6° F (37.5° C)	90	18-22	105
12 years	98.6° F (37° C)	99.6° F (37.5° C)	85-90	16-22	115
16 years	98.6° F (37° C)	99.6° F (37.5° C)	75-80	14-20	Below 120
Adult female	98.6° F (37° C)	99.6° F (37.5° C)	60-100	12-20	Below 120
Adult male	98.6° F (37° C)	99.6° F (37.5° C)	60-100	12-20	Below 120

sometimes preferred because it is less invasive. Taking the rectal temperature may be contraindicated to avoid stimulating the vagus nerve, the tenth cranial nerve, which has connections to the sympathetic nervous system throughout the thoracic, abdominal, and pelvic cavities, and within the rectum. Stimulation of this nerve produces physiologic changes called the *vasovagal response:* relaxation of the muscles in the walls of the blood vessels, slowing of the heart rate, lowering of blood pressure, and sometimes fainting. A vasovagal response can cause serious problems for certain patients with cardiac conditions.

You are probably familiar with the use of glass thermometers. They are no longer recommended for clinical use because they contain mercury, a toxic substance, and it is the goal of the Occupational Safety and Health Administration (OSHA) to remove mercury from the workplace when the same result can be obtained with products that do not involve mercury. Most health care facilities now use digital electronic thermometers with interchangeable oral and rectal probes (Fig. 22-2). These instruments can be read in 1 minute or less. They emit a short beep when the highest temperature is recorded. The temperature is read from a digital display on the thermometer itself or on a handheld display unit. Disposable sleeves are used to cover the probes, which avoids the need to disinfect the thermometer after each use.

Digital tympanic thermometers (Fig. 22-3) are also used, primarily with pediatric patients. They measure temperature at the tympanic membrane (eardrum) in the ear.

Disposable thermometers that consist of a strip of temperature-sensitive paper are available in two forms,

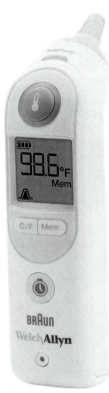

Fig. 22-3 Tympanic thermometer probe is inserted into external auditory canal.

one for oral use and one with adhesive backing that may be attached to the forehead.

Temporal artery–scanning thermometers (Fig. 22-4) contain an infrared sensor that measures the temperature over the temporal artery in the region of the forehead and predicts the body core temperature based on this reading. The gentle scan across the forehead and temporal region is easily and quickly accomplished and is not objectionable to patients. Research indicates that this method is more consistently accurate than the tympanic method.

Temporal artery or tympanic routes are best for children under the age of 6 years and for anyone who is confused or unable to follow directions. A general

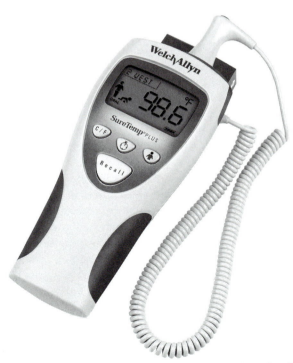

Fig. 22-2 Digital thermometer used for oral, rectal, and axillary temperature measurements.

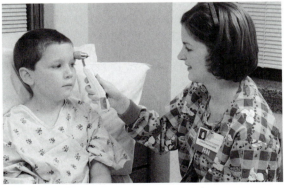

Fig. 22-4 Temporal artery scanning thermometer.

Box 22-2

Measuring Temperature With a Digital Thermometer

Oral Route
- Perform hand hygiene.
- Cover the oral probe with a clean plastic sleeve.
- Turn on the thermometer.
- Insert the probe under the patient's tongue. Instruct the patient to keep lips closed.
- Remove the probe when the audible tone or flashing number indicates that the maximum temperature has been reached (about 1 minute).
- Note the temperature reading.
- Remove and discard the plastic sleeve.
- Repeat hand hygiene.
- Make sure the thermometer is off and return it to storage.
- Record the temperature.

Axillary Route
- Perform hand hygiene.
- Cover the probe with a clean plastic sleeve.
- Turn on the thermometer.
- Place the probe in the axilla so that the skin folds are in direct contact with the probe. Instruct the patient to hold the upper arm firmly against the chest wall.
- Remove the probe when the audible tone or flashing number indicates that the maximum temperature has been reached (about 1 minute).

- Note the temperature reading.
- Remove and discard the plastic sleeve.
- Perform hand hygiene.
- Make sure the thermometer is off and return it to storage.
- Record the temperature.

Rectal Route
- Perform hand hygiene and don disposable gloves.
- Cover the rectal probe with a clean plastic sleeve.
- With the patient in a lateral recumbent position, cover the patient and expose the anus by raising the top fold of the buttocks.
- Slowly insert the probe until the anal sphincter is passed. Hold the probe in place.
- When the audible tone or flashing number indicates that the maximum temperature has been reached (about 1 minute), remove the probe slowly.
- Note the temperature reading.
- Remove and discard the plastic sleeve.
- Remove and discard the gloves.
- Repeat hand hygiene.
- Make sure the thermometer is off and return it to storage.
- Record the temperature.

procedure for obtaining accurate temperature readings for each common route is found in Box 22-2. Remember to tell your patient what you are about to do. When taking an oral temperature, remind the patient not to bite down and to keep the lips closed. *Never leave a patient alone with a rectal or axillary thermometer in place.*

Pulse

A pulse is the advancing pressure wave in an artery caused by the expulsion of blood when the left ventricle of the heart contracts. Because this wave occurs with each contraction, it provides an easy and effective way to measure the rate at which the heart is beating.

Average normal pulse rates in adults vary between 60 and 100 beats per minute (bpm). The tense, nervous individual is more likely to be in the upper range, whereas athletes tend to have a slower rate. A rapid pulse, called **tachycardia,** occurs when the heart rate is greater than 100 bpm. This may be a temporary state, as after exertion or when the person is nervous or excited, or it may be constant, caused by a damaged heart or an endocrine disorder. A rapid pulse rate may also result from interference with oxygen supply or from significant blood loss. In these cases, the heart must beat faster to circulate the remaining blood and to supply oxygen to the cells of the body. In addition to rate, the pulse volume or quality may vary. A weak, rapid pulse is described as *thready*. A **thready pulse** may indicate that the heart is not pumping enough blood.

Common pulse points are shown in Fig. 22-5. The most common site for palpation of the pulse is the radial artery on the lateral aspect of the wrist at the base of the first metacarpal. Because your own thumb has a pulse, you cannot take an accurate pulse using your thumb. Place your fingers over the artery with your thumb on the back of the wrist. Compress gently but firmly. When the artery is compressed against the radius, the pulse is easy to feel, especially if the patient's wrist is held palm down (Fig. 22-6).

If the pulse is weak or difficult to count, you can use the carotid artery. Place your fingers against the neck below the angle of the mandible (Fig. 22-7). This site is easily accessible and is particularly important if a patient loses consciousness. If the pulse is not palpable at this site, the heart is not beating effectively and emergency measures are necessary. These measures are discussed later in this chapter.

The *dorsalis pedis* or pedal pulse is taken over the instep of the foot (Fig. 22-8). This pulse may be significant when there is a question of compromise in the peripheral circulation. For example, you may be requested to check the pedal pulse following the application of a cast to the lower extremity. Because inability to feel this pulse may be an important diagnostic sign, you must practice until you are certain that you can detect the pulse when it is present.

If the pulse is slow or irregular, it may be important to use a stethoscope to take an apical pulse. Look at the stethoscope carefully and become familiar with its use. It may have a bell and a diaphragm; less expensive models

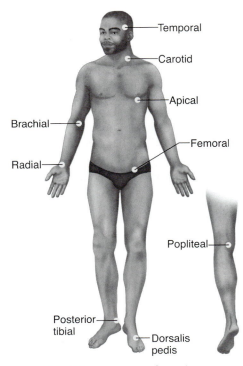

Fig. 22-5 Common pulse points.

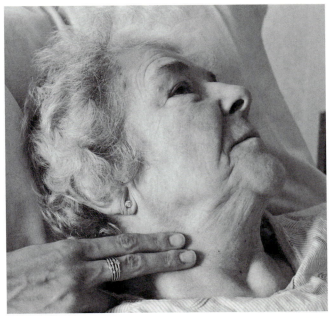

Fig. 22-7 Palpate for the carotid pulse below the angle of the mandible.

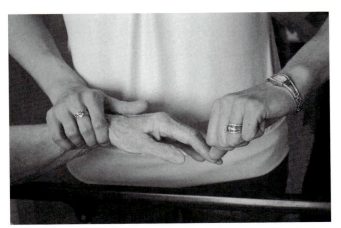

Fig. 22-6 Taking a radial pulse with the palm down.

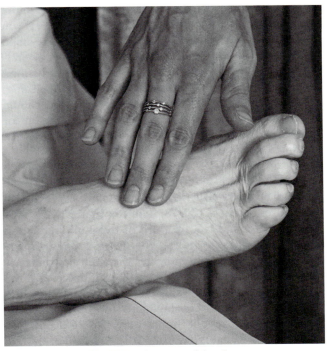

Fig. 22-8 Taking a pedal pulse.

may have a diaphragm only. On the bimodal stethoscope, you can switch from bell to diaphragm. For most purposes, however, the diaphragm is preferred.

When you hold the earpieces of the stethoscope horizontally in front of you, the ear tips should point up slightly (Fig. 22-9). Insert the tips in your ears and then tap the diaphragm gently with your finger to be sure you can hear. Now press the diaphragm firmly over the **apex** or tip of the heart. This is normally found in the fifth anterior intercostal space at the left midclavicular line. Count the pulse for a full minute and record the rate, noting any irregularities.

When the radial pulse rate is taken routinely, it is common to count for 15 seconds and multiply the count by 4 to obtain a measurement of the total bpm. Whenever there is an irregular rate or rhythm, count for a full

60 seconds. If the apical rate is faster than the radial rate, the heart is not beating efficiently. This should be recorded on the chart or requisition. If the patient also shows signs of distress, report them to the physician immediately.

Respirations

When a patient shows evidence of respiratory distress, a measurement of respiratory rate will help in making an

emergency is over, check to be sure that you have cleaned or replaced the receptacle and replaced the disposable tip and tubing so that the suction unit will be ready for use when needed.

In the event that you must suction the patient yourself, call for help while you unwrap the catheter and turn on the suction. After you have cleared the mouth, pull the chin down and forward while inserting the suction catheter tip over the tongue in the midline. Do not insert the catheter forcibly, because you may injure the larynx (voice box). Any suctioning beyond the nasopharynx (back of the throat) should be done by a physician or someone trained in this procedure.

Respiratory Emergencies

Reactive Airway Disease

The term *reactive airway disease* is not a specific diagnosis; it is a general term used to describe conditions characterized by coughing, wheezing, or shortness of breath with an undetermined cause. When these symptoms are present, asthma is one of the possible causes. Some doctors use the terms "reactive airway disease" and "asthma" interchangeably, but they are not necessarily the same thing.

Asthma is difficulty in breathing caused by bronchospasm, which restricts the patient's ability to take in a sufficient volume of air. Asthmatic attacks are sometimes related to allergies and are frequently precipitated by stress. If the radiologic procedure is new or frightening, dyspnea may result. Most chronic asthmatic individuals carry a metered dose inhaler with a bronchodilating medication. Patients with asthma should take their medication into the examining room.

In the event of an acute episode of reactive airway disease, call for assistance. The usual treatment is to administer oxygen to keep the O_2 saturation level above 92%. The administration of albuterol by inhaler or nebulizer and parenteral administration of corticosteroids may be ordered by the responding physician. Subcutaneous injections of epinephrine or terbutaline (Brethine, a bronchodilating medication) may be ordered in cases of a severe attack. Although it is frightening for both the patient and the limited operator, a single attack is seldom fatal.

Airway Obstruction

Blockage of a patient's airway is a life-threatening situation that can cause respiratory arrest if not successfully treated immediately. The obstruction may be caused by a solid object but is more likely to involve liquid or semiliquid material. This may be mucus, blood, or vomitus that cannot be expelled by a patient who is unconscious or semiconscious. If your facility has emergency response codes, call the code for a respiratory emergency. If a code system is not in place, call for a physician and

prepare suction for use. The use of suction is discussed earlier in this chapter.

Cardiac Emergencies

Angina Pectoris

Angina pectoris, often simply called **angina,** is the term for chest pain that occurs when the coronary arteries are unable to supply the heart with sufficient O_2 to meet current needs. Episodes of chest pain are precipitated by exertion or stress and are usually relieved by rest or nitroglycerin tablets administered under the tongue. The discomfort caused by angina often presents as pain under the sternum and may vary from a vague ache to an intense crushing sensation. Sometimes it resembles the distress of severe indigestion. Most patients who are known to suffer from angina carry their medication with them at all times. An emergency supply of nitroglycerin is usually stocked in medical health care facilities.

Heart Attack

Patients experiencing the early onset of a heart attack sometimes seek immediate care in physicians' offices or clinics. If at any time a patient suddenly develops an irregular pulse; appears diaphoretic and pale and is feeling short of breath, faint, weak, or nauseated; or has a sudden onset of pain in the chest, shoulder, or jaw, *a physician must be notified immediately* regarding the possible onset of a heart attack. Patients experiencing a heart attack may complain of sudden, intense chest pain, often described as a crushing pain, but pain may not be present at all. Because the symptoms are caused when a portion of the heart wall becomes ischemic (lacking O_2), you must prevent further damage by minimizing patient exertion. Patients may underestimate the importance of this type of pain and assume instead that it is caused by heartburn or indigestion. These patients often appear diaphoretic and pale. They may feel nauseated and short of breath and may have an irregular heartbeat. Assist the patient to a comfortable position, obtain help, and stay with the patient. If the patient has shortness of breath, raise the head and administer O_2 at a rate of 3 to 5 L/min.

Cardiac Arrest

One of the most anxiety-producing situations encountered by health care workers is the discovery of an unconscious patient or observation of a patient suddenly losing consciousness. When this occurs, it is important to initiate the "shake and shout" maneuver. Most patients who have simply fainted will respond if you call out their name and give them a gentle shake. If there is no response, feel for the carotid pulse and observe for respiration. If the patient has stopped breathing or no pulse is detected, the attention of a specially trained medical team is required. Summon help using the procedure prescribed by your facility for this type of emergency. You must be familiar with this protocol. If no protocol exists, call 911 and then summon the physician, telling him or her that emergency medical services are on the way.

Time is vital, because lack of effective circulation to the central nervous system can cause irreparable brain damage in 3 to 5 minutes. While awaiting the emergency medical team, you should proceed with cardiopulmonary resuscitation (CPR) only if you are trained and certified in this procedure.

CPR is the basic life support system that is used to ventilate the lungs and circulate the blood in the event of respiratory or cardiac arrest. Correct instruction and certification in CPR is important for all health care personnel. Your class should be taught by a certified instructor, and you should take responsibility for updating your CPR card every 2 years. CPR instruction is not provided in this text, because recommendations are updated frequently and printed materials are easily obtained from the American Heart Association or the American Red Cross. Practice on a resuscitation mannequin is essential. Your local college, fire department, and hospital may also offer courses taught by certified instructors that include lecture, video, practice time, and review and testing sessions.

Even if you are certified in adult CPR, do not attempt CPR on infants or children unless you are currently certified specifically in pediatrics as well. Courses for health care personnel usually include the techniques for infants and children.

Once the emergency medical team has arrived, you may no longer feel needed, but you still can perform several important tasks. Record-keeping is essential. Write down the time the attack started and when the emergency team responded. You may be asked to record times and amounts of medications. It may be necessary to obtain equipment, call for other personnel, or monitor a telephone.

During cardiac arrest and/or resuscitation, a rapid, weak, and ineffective heartbeat may be present. This state is called **fibrillation** and is caused by interruption of the electric signals that control the heart muscle. An electric shock to the chest from a defibrillator can stimulate the heart to return to a normal rhythm. One development in treating cardiac arrest is the use of automatic external defibrillators (AEDs). These devices are very effective when used by personnel with only a limited amount of training. They are often part of a clinic's emergency equipment. Learning to use an AED is much easier than learning to use a conventional defibrillator or to perform CPR. Some of these defibrillators are completely automatic and have the ability to analyze cardiac rhythm, identify the need for defibrillation, and automatically deliver a shock. A semiautomatic version also exists in which the operator presses a button to start rhythm analysis. If the AED identifies the need for defibrillation, an indicator signal is given, instructing the operator to press the shock control.

The use of AEDs has been reduced to four simple steps:
1. Turn on the power.
2. Attach the adhesive pads to the victim's chest.
3. Turn on rhythm analysis.
4. Press the shock control to deliver the shock, if indicated.

While different brands and models have a variety of features, including different monitors, paper strip readouts, and instructions to the operator, application of the device is simple. If your facility has an AED, periodic instruction should be provided. Your participation in both CPR and AED classes can help you to be both prepared and effective in cardiac emergencies.

Trauma

Head Injuries

Patients who have received a blow to the head may have sustained serious injury, even when no external signs of trauma are present. Damage may occur with or without a skull fracture. The brain is soft, has a rich blood supply, and is suspended in cerebrospinal fluid within the skull. A blow to the head may cause a concussion or contrecoup damage as discussed in Chapter 17. If bleeding or swelling occurs inside the skull, a rise in intracranial pressure (ICP, pressure within the skull) may cause seizures, loss of consciousness, or respiratory arrest. Brain tumors can also result in increased intracranial pressure, causing patients to exhibit similar symptoms.

Sometimes the signs and symptoms of serious head injuries develop slowly. A patient might seek treatment at an outpatient facility following a fall or a minor car crash because of other less severe injuries. If there has been a blow to the head, be alert for any change in the patient's level of consciousness that could signal a head injury.

Four levels of consciousness (LOCs) are generally recognized and may be described as follows:
1. Alert and conscious
2. Drowsy but responsive
3. Unconscious but reactive to painful stimuli
4. Comatose

The patient who is alert and oriented on arrival and then becomes increasingly incoherent and drowsy may be showing signs of ICP. The earliest signs of increasing pressure may be irritability and lethargy, often associated with a slowing pulse and slow respirations. Notify the physician immediately if you suspect a change in LOC.

Extremity Fractures

Trauma involving the long bones of the body may be classified into two categories: (1) compound fractures, in which the splintered ends of bone are forced through the skin, and (2) closed fractures. Compound fractures are usually partially reduced and have a dressing applied to them before radiographic examination. They are more commonly treated in trauma centers. Some common fracture types are described and illustrated in Chapters 12 and 13.

There are many ways to temporarily immobilize extremity fractures. The two legs may be fastened together for stability during transportation (self-splinting) or a stiff object, such as a board or rolled-up magazine, may serve as a splint. Splinting devices should not be removed except under the physician's direct supervision.

It is important to minimize motion of the fracture fragments. This helps avoid unnecessary pain and, more importantly, the initiation of a muscle spasm that could interfere with the physician's attempt to reduce (realign) and immobilize the fracture more permanently. Movement of fracture fragments may tear surrounding soft tissues, nerves, and blood vessels, seriously complicating the patient's condition. When you must position a fractured extremity that is not supported by a splint, maintain a *gentle* traction (pull) while supporting and moving the arm or leg. Traction helps prevent the fracture fragments from rubbing against each other. Two people may be required to support and position a patient with a potential long bone fracture because the extremity must be supported at sites both proximal and distal to the injury.

Special care is required when positioning extremities following application of a plaster cast. Undue pressure against a fresh (wet) cast may cause it to change shape. Lift the casted extremity by placing your open hands underneath it; never grasp it from above. Observe the patient's fingers or toes for evidence of impaired circulation. They should be warm, pink, and sensitive to touch and pressure. Coldness, numbness, or lack of normal coloration should be reported to the physician at once. Swelling within the cast and subsequent pressure can cause permanent nerve and tissue damage if not relieved promptly.

Wounds

Patients with open wounds have usually been treated before you see them in the radiology suite. Bleeding has been controlled, and a dressing has been applied. Your primary responsibility regarding open wounds is to maintain the dressings and to report promptly any significant amount of fresh bleeding. This is usually considered to be the amount of bright red blood sufficient to soak through a fresh dressing. If a laceration or incision opens, causing severe **hemorrhage** (continuous abnormal blood flow), apply direct pressure to the site of bleeding while summoning immediate assistance.

Medical Emergencies

Drug Reactions

The administration of any medication has the potential to cause a medical emergency. The reaction can range

in severity from a sudden bout of nausea and vomiting to cardiac arrest. The nature of the symptoms will determine the appropriate treatment. Treatments for the various conditions seen in response to drug administration are found throughout this chapter. Individuals who have been sensitized to an over-the-counter medication may be just as prone to an allergic reaction as those who are receiving prescription medications. Reactions may occur to medications administered orally or by injection. When drugs are administered intravenously (directly into a vein), the effects will appear more rapidly.

A moderate allergic reaction is characterized by **erythema** (redness of the skin), **urticaria** (hives), and/or dyspnea. In the event of such a reaction, the physician should be notified while you remain with the patient. The treatment for these patients is administration of an antihistamine medication, such as diphenhydramine, intravenously or intramuscularly, depending on the severity of the reaction. Some physicians prefer to give epinephrine at this point.

A severe allergic reaction is called **anaphylaxis** or *anaphylactic shock*. This life-threatening condition may result in respiratory or cardiac arrest and less often in seizures. The earliest symptoms of anaphylaxis include a sense of warmth, tingling, and itching of palms and soles. Within seconds or minutes, the patient experiences difficulty swallowing, constriction in the throat, a feeling of doom, an expiratory wheeze, and then progression into laryngeal and bronchial edema (swelling) that can block the airway completely. In addition to the administration of epinephrine, the treatments for shock, respiratory arrest, and cardiac arrest are appropriate and are discussed elsewhere in this chapter. At the onset of anaphylaxis, you should maintain the patient's airway, alert the physician, and call 911.

Diabetic Emergencies

Patients who have diabetes mellitus (DM) are seen in clinics for diabetic monitoring and care as well as for the same variety of problems that bring other patients to the physician. The diabetic patient can often be identified by means of a pendant or bracelet with a medical alert message. Persons with medical conditions that may require emergency treatment often wear this type of identification, which can be a great help in rapidly diagnosing urgent conditions and providing an appropriate emergency response.

Diabetes is a disease characterized by the body's inability to metabolize blood glucose. Insulin is an enzyme normally produced in the pancreas in response to food intake. Insufficient insulin prevents the use of glucose by the muscles. When the muscles cannot use glucose, excess ketone bodies appear in the blood, causing ketoacidosis, a change in the pH of the blood. The body attempts to compensate for the acidosis by

hyperventilation (air hunger with rapid respirations) and excretion of minerals and water into the urine. When the blood glucose level is very high, glucose also "spills over" into the urine. The individual who is terribly thirsty, urinates copious amounts frequently, and has fruity-smelling breath (because of ketones excreted via the respiratory tract) may be approaching **diabetic coma.** This condition is characterized by a relatively slow onset. Diabetes is diagnosed through blood and urine tests and treated with diet, exercise, and medication, such as insulin or oral hypoglycemic agents.

The diabetic patient who has taken insulin but no food may develop **hypoglycemia,** a low blood glucose level. Unlike the slow onset of diabetic coma, hypoglycemia is characterized by a *sudden* onset of weakness, sweating, tremors, hunger, and finally loss of consciousness. While the patient is still alert and cooperative, hypoglycemia can be quickly remedied by administration of a small amount of candy or sweet fruit juice. Squeeze tubes containing a measured amount of glucose may be stored with the emergency medications. These prepackaged tubes are useful because the gel-like material can be placed inside the patient's cheek. This decreases the chance that a semiconscious or confused patient will aspirate it, as might be the case with candy or juice.

Report the occurrence of hypoglycemia to the physician. You must help these patients to sit or lie down until the sugar takes effect. Occasionally individuals with the same symptoms do not have diabetes. They may have hypoglycemia without diabetes; the treatment is the same.

There are two major classifications of DM: type I and type II. Type I, or insulin-dependent diabetes, may be characterized by a lean individual under age 25 who produces little or no insulin and may develop circulatory impairment of vision, the kidneys, or the extremities. Blood glucose levels must be closely monitored, and insulin is administered by injection. Diabetic coma is more likely to occur with type I DM.

Type II DM, on the other hand, occurs most commonly in the obese individual over the age of 40 with a marked family tendency. This type of diabetes usually responds to oral hypoglycemic medications and to changes in diet and lifestyle.

Table 22-3 summarizes the physical findings associated with both high blood glucose level, which is indicative of approaching diabetic coma and low blood glucose level, which may signify an impending insulin reaction.

Cerebrovascular Accidents

A **cerebrovascular accident (CVA),** also called a *stroke*, is caused by lack of adequate blood circulation to the brain. This occurs most frequently in the elderly, but can occur at any age. Rupture of a cerebral artery can cause a hemorrhage into the brain tissue, or an artery may become occluded (blocked) and cause an interruption in the blood supply to the area beyond the occlusion.

A patient who is beginning to suffer a stroke may stumble or complain of a headache or of feeling faint. The symptoms may occur very suddenly or may develop over a period of hours, and may include extreme dizziness, severe headache, muscle weakness on one or both sides, difficulty in vision or deviation in one eye, slurred or difficult speech, and temporary loss of consciousness.

The American Stroke Association reports that widespread awareness could result in prompt diagnosis and treatment of strokes and the prevention of brain damage. This organization recommends that the acronym FAST be used to help remember and identify the warning signs of a stroke:

- **F**—Face drooping: Does one side of the face droop or is it numb? Ask the person to smile. Is the smile uneven?
- **A**—Arm weakness: Is one arm weak or numb? Ask the person to raise both arms. Does one arm drift downward?

Table 22-3

Diabetic Crises

Crisis	Cause	Symptoms	Treatment
Hyperglycemia; impending diabetic coma	Food consumption over dietary allowance; fever, infection, stress; insufficient insulin	Increased thirst; increased urinary output; decreased appetite; nausea, vomiting; weakness; confusion; coma	Inform physician immediately; administer sugar-free liquids if conscious
Hypoglycemia; insulin reaction	Insufficient food; excessive exercise	Headache; hunger; diaphoresis; tremors; tachycardia; impaired vision; personality change; loss of consciousness	Administer food or juice with high sugar content if conscious; glucose gel may be placed inside the cheek; inform physician immediately. Glucagon may be ordered.

- **S**—Speech difficulty: Is speech slurred? Is the person unable to speak or hard to understand? Ask the person to repeat a simple sentence, like "The sky is blue." Is the sentence repeated correctly?
- **T**—Time to call 9-1-1: If someone shows any of these symptoms, even if the symptoms go away, call 9-1-1 and get the person to a hospital immediately. Check the time so you will know when symptoms first appeared.

In the event of a suspected stroke, report the situation to a physician. If this occurs outside a health care facility, call 9-1-1 and describe the symptoms to the dispatcher. These symptoms may be only temporary, but should be reported immediately. The patient should be helped to a recumbent position with the head elevated. Do not leave the patient but summon assistance and have the emergency supplies and O₂ at hand. Monitor vital signs every 5 minutes or as ordered by the physician.

A **transient ischemic attack (TIA)** presents similar symptoms but usually lasts only minutes or, at most, a few hours. These temporary attacks should not be ignored, because they are frequently precursors to more permanent damage.

Seizure Disorders

A seizure occurs as a result of a focal or generalized disturbance of brain function and is accompanied by a change in the LOC. A major motor (grand mal or tonic-clonic) seizure may be preceded by an aura, or premonitory sign. The patient may say, "I'm going to have a spell" and should be assisted to a supine position as rapidly as possible. Often a seizure is signaled by a hoarse cry when air is forced past the vocal cords by a sudden contraction of all the abdominal and chest muscles. In the event of a patient seizure, your first duty is to keep the patient as safe as possible. Notify the physician immediately, request assistance, and *do not leave the patient.* If the patient is on the x-ray table, your first concern is to prevent a fall. Remove any objects that might be hazardous and place padding under the patient's head. Do not attempt to restrain the patient and do not attempt to force objects into the patient's mouth. If a padded tongue blade is available and can be easily inserted, it may help avoid a laceration of the tongue.

Loss of consciousness and a rigid arching of the back are followed by alternate relaxation and rigidity of the muscles until the seizure passes and the patient slowly regains consciousness. Have emergency medication (diazepam) ready for administration in the event of prolonged or repeated seizures *(status epilepticus)*. While the patient is unconscious, involuntary voiding and defecation may occur. As the seizure passes, turn the patient to a lateral recumbent position to prevent aspiration of secretions and remain with the patient to provide reassurance and assistance. In the period immediately after the seizure (postictal period), the patient may be somewhat irritable or confused and wish only to sleep.

Less intense partial (focal) seizures may cause severe, uncontrollable tremors. This condition often produces extreme anxiety and hyperventilation in a conscious patient. These seizures are exhausting to the patient and may persist for more than an hour unless treatment is given. Instruct the patient to breathe slowly and place a paper bag over the nose and mouth if hyperventilation is otherwise uncontrollable.

Another type of seizure is characterized by a brief loss of consciousness (absence) during which the patient stares or may lose balance and fall. Many patients are not aware that they undergo this loss of consciousness.

Patients taking anticonvulsant medication may not have seizures for long periods. Most of these medications have a relatively slow excretion rate, which allows the patient to miss a dose or two without precipitating an attack. On the other hand, fatigue, stress, or apprehension may initiate a seizure in a previously stable patient.

Realize that the seizure will run its course. The most important actions you can take are to protect the patient from harm and to be an accurate observer. Note when the seizure began and how long it lasted. Did it involve both sides of the body equally, and did the contractions start in one area and progress from one extremity to another? These observations can be helpful to the physician in reaching an accurate diagnosis.

Not all seizure-prone individuals have the same diagnosis. Seizures may be a response to drug sensitivity, infection, epilepsy, tumor, or fever. Only in recent years have the old superstitions and myths about seizure disorders begun to be dispelled. No direct, consistent correlation exists between seizures and mental acuity, emotional instability, or heredity.

Hyperventilation

The anxious patient who breathes too deeply or too often (hyperventilates) may complain of feeling faint or dizzy and note tingling and numbness in the extremities. These patients have breathed in too much O₂ and have exhaled too much carbon dioxide, which disturbs the chemical balance of the blood. Try to persuade them to breathe more slowly or to breathe into a paper bag, which will help to return their carbon dioxide level to normal.

Vertigo and Postural Hypotension

A lightheaded or dizzy sensation is not unusual when patients sit up suddenly from a recumbent position. This is especially common after prolonged periods of bed rest. This condition is called *postural hypotension* or *orthostatic hypotension* and results from the same basic mechanism that causes syncope, or fainting, which is discussed later in this chapter. Blood pools in the extremities when the torso is elevated and causes momentary cerebral **anoxia,** a lack of O_2 to the brain. This condition can usually be avoided by having the patient sit up gradually. This sensation frequently affects elderly patients, so remain close to them and provide support when a change in position is necessary.

Vertigo is a sensation of dizziness with a different cause. The patient does not feel lightheaded but feels as if the room is moving or whirling. Such patients frequently cling to the furniture and will fall if not assisted to lie down. They may experience violent nausea. This sensation is usually attributed either to a middle ear disturbance or to a lesion in the brain or spinal cord. Vertigo may also be associated with a TIA or CVA, and alcohol or the administration of certain drugs may affect individuals in a similar manner. A sudden onset of vertigo in a patient who does not have a history of it should be reported immediately to the physician.

Epistaxis

A nosebleed, or **epistaxis,** can be rather frightening to the patient but is usually not serious. Remove eyeglasses when necessary and provide an ample supply of tissues. Instruct the patient to breathe through the mouth and to squeeze firmly against the nasal septum for 10 minutes. The patient should not lie down, blow the nose, or talk. Provide an emesis basin, instructing the patient to spit out blood that runs down the nasopharynx rather than swallow it. If bleeding lasts more than a few minutes, inform the physician, who may want to apply more direct treatment.

Nausea and Vomiting

Nausea and vomiting are not uncommon in health care settings, and a well-prepared health care worker learns to cope easily with this situation. Vomiting can often be prevented by your reassuring presence and by specific breathing instructions. "Breathe through your mouth, taking short, rapid, panting breaths" and "Take some long, slow, deep breaths through your mouth" are both effective instructions, and each has strong adherents. In both cases, the purpose is to focus the patient's attention on a physical function that is controllable. On the other hand, if a patient expresses a need for an emesis basin or bag, offer it immediately and bring the patient a clean one before removing the soiled one. Provide tissues and water to rinse the mouth. It is especially important to support the patient in a sitting or lateral recumbent position to avoid aspiration of vomitus. If the patient loses consciousness, turn the head to the side and clear the airway.

Shock

Shock is a general term used to describe a failure of circulation in which BP is inadequate to support O_2 perfusion of vital tissues and to remove the byproducts of metabolism.

Fainting, also called **syncope,** is a very mild form of shock that sometimes occurs when fright, pain, or unpleasant events are beyond the coping ability of the patient's nervous system. The BP falls as the diameter of the blood vessels increases and the heart rate slows. When the BP is too low to supply the brain with O_2, the patient faints. Placing the patient in a dorsal recumbent position with the feet elevated usually relieves this type of shock. Patients who have not eaten for an extended period and are feeling anxious and stressed may undergo syncope. Patients who feel faint should be assisted into a sitting or recumbent position. If a chair is not within reach, ease the patient to the floor. If the patient does not rouse immediately, spirits of ammonia held under the nose usually produce a rapid return to consciousness. Small, crushable vials of ammonia are usually stocked with the emergency supplies. A physician's order is not required for their use. Anyone who has more than a momentary loss of consciousness should be evaluated by a physician before the examination is resumed.

Shock other than syncope is a dangerous, potentially fatal condition. It may be caused by blood loss, severe infection, head trauma, heart failure, or a severe allergic response. Early signs of shock are pallor, increased heart rate and respiration rate, and restlessness or confusion.

The following symptoms, in any or all combinations, indicate some degree of shock:

- Restlessness and a sense of apprehension
- Increased pulse rate
- Pallor accompanied by weakness or a change in thinking ability
- Cool, clammy skin
- A fall in BP of 30 mm Hg below the baseline systolic pressure or a drop in diastolic pressure below 50 mm Hg

Your responsibility with regard to patients with any type of shock is to recognize its symptoms, to know the location of emergency medical supplies, and to be thoroughly familiar with the emergency protocols of your facility. The physician may call on your knowledge of medications and your medication administration skills during treatment. Your role in suspected shock is as follows:

- Stop the procedure.
- Assist the patient to a supine position to avoid a fall.
- Obtain help. Notify the physician. If in doubt, call 9-1-1. It is much better to be mistaken than to have a patient die because of inadequate treatment.
- Check BP.
- Assist the dyspneic patient with O_2.
- Be ready to perform CPR.
- Assist the physician or emergency medical team as necessary.
- Chart the occurrence, the treatment administered, and the patient's response on an incident report form or in the medical record.

SUMMARY

Quality patient care requires assessment and response to patients' needs, both emotional and physiologic. Assessment of physical status involves trained observation and touch. In addition, physical condition is evaluated by taking vital signs: temperature, pulse, respiration rate, and BP. When you can take accurate vital signs and recognize abnormal readings, you can use these skills to assist with routine patient evaluation and to identify changes in patient status in an emergency.

Shock, respiratory arrest, heart attack, and cardiac arrest are life-threatening emergencies. You must recognize the signs of these conditions and be capable of responding quickly and appropriately. Other medical emergencies, such as syncope, vomiting, hypoglycemia, and epistaxis, require appropriate responses as well. When you are alert and well prepared, any emergency is more likely to have a positive outcome.

Chapter 23

Medications and Their Administration

Learning Objectives

Learning Objectives

At the conclusion of this chapter, you will be able to:

- Explain the role of the limited operator with respect to medication administration in outpatient facilities
- Differentiate between chemical, generic, and trade names for medications
- Look up medication information in standard references, on medication package inserts, and on the Internet
- List and state the classification of six medications commonly used in outpatient imaging facilities
- List and describe common routes of medication administration
- Name medications commonly needed in emergencies and describe their effects
- Demonstrate the steps used in the administration of oral medication
- List the routes of parenteral medication administration and explain the reason why each route may be desirable
- Identify the equipment and supplies used for parenteral injections and select appropriate supplies for each route of administration
- Demonstrate the steps used in the parenteral administration of medication
- Identify appropriate sites for intramuscular and subcutaneous injections
- Describe the precautions required to ensure safety when injecting medications
- Chart medications accurately
- Assist the physician to initiate intravenous injections and monitor infusions

Key Terms

agonist
allergen
antagonists
antidote
antihistamines
benzodiazepines
dehydration
efficacy
enteral
extravasation
generic
hematoma
hydration
idiosyncratic

infiltration
intradermal
intramuscular (IM)
intravenous (IV)
opiate
opioids
parenteral
potency
proprietary
standing order
subcutaneous (SC)
synergistic
topical
toxic

THE LIMITED OPERATOR'S ROLE IN MEDICATION ADMINISTRATION

Each state has regulations regarding the qualifications of individuals who are permitted to administer medications. You must be familiar with the rules governing medication administration in your state and in your facility. As stated in Chapter 21, health care facilities use written policies and procedures to ensure patient safety and to reduce the risk of liability for errors. Medication administration is an area of patient care with a high potential for both error and medicolegal problems. For this reason, there will be an established policy with respect to who may administer medication in the facility. There may also be standard procedures for medication administration. *Never administer any medication unless you are certain beyond doubt that you are authorized to do so.*

If regulations and established policies allow it, your job description may involve medical assisting duties that include medication administration. Even if you are not permitted to administer medications, your duties may include checking the allergy history of patients, preparing medication for administration, verifying patient identification, assisting the physician, and monitoring the patient after the medication has been given.

Even when your job description is limited primarily to radiography, knowledge of medications and their administration is valuable in an emergency. You should be familiar with the location of medications that might be required if there is a sudden change in a patient's status. As discussed in Chapter 22, acute attacks of angina, sudden asthmatic episodes, and insulin reactions are typical of the types of emergencies seen in radiography departments for which prompt administration of medication may be essential.

Whenever medications are given in a physician's office or clinic, the physician selects the drug, determines the route of administration, and prescribes the exact dosage. *No medication is ever given without a physician's order.* Orders may be verbal or written. Verbal orders should be written or countersigned by the physician before he or she leaves the area or within the following 24-hour period. In some states, only registered nurses are allowed to accept medication orders by telephone. These matters should also be addressed in the policy and procedures manual.

A **standing order** consists of written directions for a specific medication or procedure, signed by a physician, and used only under the specific conditions stated in the order. For example, a standing order might allow a nurse to administer a specific dose of nitroglycerin to a patient experiencing angina when the physician is not present to issue a specific order. These orders are found in a policy and procedures or standing orders book available for immediate reference.

Although a comprehensive knowledge of drugs is not usually essential for a limited operator, you should become familiar with the names, dosages, and routes of administration for medications frequently used and those most likely to be needed in emergencies. If this seems intimidating, be reassured that only a limited number of drugs, in a few standard dosages, are used with any regularity. Knowledge of these medications greatly facilitates the task of assisting the physician and also aids in determining whether departmental stocks of medications and medication supplies are adequate and up to date. Checking expiration dates on medication supplies is especially important when such supplies are used infrequently. Medication knowledge also enables you to prevent errors by questioning and double-checking any medication orders or records that seem unusual or inappropriate.

Any drug may produce side effects in certain patients. You can use this knowledge to anticipate possible adverse drug reactions and to recognize and report signs and symptoms of side effects as they occur. This awareness is very important because you may be the first to observe the onset of medication responses that could have serious consequences.

MEDICATION NOMENCLATURE AND INFORMATION RESOURCES

The terms *drugs* and *medications* are often used interchangeably. As a working definition, *medications* are substances that are prescribed for treatment and that produce therapeutically useful effects. Some medications, such as digitalis, are made from plants; others, like heparin, come from animal sources; and some, such as penicillin, are produced by microorganisms. The more general term *drugs* denotes substances used in diagnosis, treatment, or prevention of disease or as a component of a medication. Drugs may replace a missing substance in the body, such as estrogen or insulin. This term is sometimes confusing because it is also used to denote chemicals, such as narcotics or hallucinogens, that affect the central nervous system (CNS), causing behavioral changes and possible addiction. Many drugs today are manufactured from synthetic materials. Drug synthesis and the rapidly expanding application of genetic engineering promise vast possibilities for the future.

Each medication has a **generic** name that identifies its specific composition. If the drug consists principally of one chemical, it may also be referred to by its chemical name. For example, *acetylsalicylic acid* is the chemical name for the generic drug aspirin. Manufacturers give their products brand names that are also called **proprietary** or *trade names*. The same generic substance may be manufactured by several different companies and given a different trade name by each. For example, a synthetic antibacterial medication containing the chemicals trimethoprim and sulfamethoxazole is generically named *co-trimoxazole*. It is produced by Roche in the United States under the name *Bactrim* and by GlaxoSmithKline as

Septra. The generic and trade names of some drugs are used interchangeably. For instance, the generic term *epinephrine* is used just as frequently as the trade name *Adrenalin* for this common emergency drug. Because medications may be ordered by either generic or trade names, you should be familiar with both terms. When the physician calls for epinephrine, it is important to immediately identify the Adrenalin without having to read the small print on each container in the emergency drug box.

Setting the standards for control of drugs is part of the role of the U.S. Food and Drug Administration (FDA). This role includes establishing strict rules concerning **efficacy** (effectiveness), purity, **potency** (strength), safety, and toxicity (the degree to which a drug may have a poisonous effect) of both prescription and nonprescription over-the-counter (OTC) medications.

The study of drugs is an ongoing process, because new medications are constantly being made available. No single textbook can provide information to cover all situations. For these reasons, you should be acquainted with other methods of obtaining medication facts on a continuing basis. One useful resource is the information sheet enclosed in each drug package. The FDA requires that all drug packages include the trade name, generic name, chemical composition, chemical strength, usual dosage, indications, contraindications, and reported side effects. Package inserts from frequently used drugs may be kept on file to avoid the necessity of opening a package when this information is needed. If you collect and study inserts from these drugs, you will soon develop a working knowledge and useful base of information about medications that are important in your clinical setting.

Another useful resource is a reference work of medication information, such as the *Physicians' Desk Reference (PDR)*. Drugs are listed alphabetically by their generic names and their trade names and according to their uses. A separate section indexes the products made by each manufacturer. In the product description, you will find information similar to that found in the package inserts. Several companies publish drug guides especially for nurses. These references may be especially useful to you because they tend to emphasize the most common side effects and can help you recognize physical changes that may be significant. The libraries of most health care facilities include a drug reference manual, and you should become familiar with its use. Drug reference manuals are published annually, and some include a CD-ROM and/or a subscription to an online website for easy reference via computer. For example, *Clinical Pharmacology* (available at www.clinicalpharmacology.com) is a comprehensive medication reference that provides instant access via the Internet to the most current medical information and updates. In addition, in-service classes and college courses may also provide useful information on medications. Formal instruction may be especially important to you if your state law and job description permit you to administer medications.

ROUTES OF MEDICATION ADMINISTRATION

The most common routes for medication administration are enteral, topical, and parenteral.

Enteral medications are those that are placed directly into the gastrointestinal tract. Although enteral medications may be given rectally or by means of a nasogastric tube, the oral route of administration is the most common. Oral medications are swallowed. They are dissolved or digested in the stomach and then pass into the small intestine, where the majority of the absorption takes place.

With the **topical** route of administration, a drug is applied to the surface of the skin. This route may be used for a local effect, such as application of calamine lotion to relieve the itch of poison ivy. Some topical medications are used for a systemic effect. These medications are absorbed through the skin into the bloodstream and are applied to the skin in a paste form or on small adhesive disks (patches). One such topical drug is nifedipine, used by patients with heart conditions to increase vascular dilation. Another example is scopolamine, which is applied on adhesive disks to treat vertigo and to help prevent motion sickness.

Some medications are applied to the mucous membrane of the mouth and may be classified as oral and/or topical medications. They are placed under the tongue (sublingual) or inside the cheek (buccal) and are absorbed directly into the blood through the mucous membrane. Sublingual or buccal administration makes certain drugs work rapidly because they are immediately available without having to be digested and absorbed through the stomach or intestine. Examples of these medications are nitroglycerin, which is administered sublingually for angina pectoris, and glucose paste, which is administered by buccal application to treat hypoglycemia (see Chapter 22).

Although patients may prefer to take medications orally, some drugs cause irritation of the gastrointestinal tract, cannot be absorbed by this route, or must be given by a route that will produce a more rapid response. The **parenteral** route is the term for any administration that involves injecting a medication directly into the body. Parenteral injections may be given in several ways and are classified according to the depth and/or location of injection: **intradermal** injections are shallow injections between the skin layers; **subcutaneous (SC)** injections are deeper, beneath the skin; the **intramuscular (IM)** route involves injection into muscle tissue; and **intravenous (IV)** injections are made directly into a vein. IV administration is the parenteral route that provides the most immediate effect. The medication is dispersed by the bloodstream, so the time needed to reach the site of action is very short. IV administration is outside the scope of practice for limited operators in most circumstances and is beyond the scope of this text.

Procedures for both oral and parenteral medication administration are discussed later in this chapter.

MEDICATION PROPERTIES

Drugs differ in the ways they enter the body, are absorbed, reach their site of action, are metabolized, and exit the body. The study of these properties is called *pharmacokinetics*. These processes are important because they affect the ways in which individuals respond to medications. Individual response can vary greatly depending on age, physical condition, sex, weight, or immune status. Response may also depend on the body's state of **hydration,** that is, the water content of the tissues. Insufficient fluid intake causes a state of **dehydration,** which has a negative effect on the body's general condition and may alter the effects of medications.

Absorption

Absorption is the process by which the drug enters the systemic circulation to produce a desired effect. The method of absorption varies with the route of administration. Oral medications are absorbed through the mucosal lining of the gastrointestinal tract. Other medications are injected and absorbed through the blood vessels in the muscles, subcutaneous tissues, or skin layers. When medications are injected directly into a vein or artery, no absorption is needed.

Distribution

Distribution is the means by which drugs travel from the site of absorption to the site of action, usually through the bloodstream. This process depends on adequate circulation. Drugs act most rapidly in organs that have an abundant blood supply, such as the liver, heart, brain, and kidneys.

Metabolism

Metabolism is the process by which the body transforms drugs into an inactive form that can be eliminated from the body. Most drug metabolism occurs in the liver, where enzymes transform drugs into substances that can be excreted by way of the intestinal tract or the kidneys.

Excretion

Excretion refers to the elimination of drugs from the body after they have been metabolized. Drugs may be excreted by way of the kidneys, intestines, lungs, or exocrine glands, such as the sweat glands. The kidneys are the chief organs of excretion, but the route depends largely on the chemical makeup of the drug. Portions of some drugs may escape metabolism and be excreted unchanged in the urine. Volatile substances, such as alcohol and certain anesthetics, are excreted through the lungs. For this reason, postoperative patients are encouraged to cough and breathe deeply to help clear their bodies of the anesthetic agent. Other drugs are metabolized in the liver, excreted into the bile, and then routed through the intestines for elimination. Some medications are metabolized in the liver and their metabolites (substances produced in the process of metabolism) are transported by the bloodstream to the kidneys for excretion. If kidney function is impaired or if the patient is dehydrated, drugs can be retained in the body and a toxic effect can occur. Therefore, adequate fluid intake is very important for most patients taking medication.

MEDICATION EFFECTS

The study of the effects of drugs on the normal physiologic functions of the body is called *pharmacodynamics*. After a drug reaches the site of action, it exerts specific effects on the cells. The effect of a drug on specific cells is called the *therapeutic action*. Therapeutic action results in anticipated outcomes, such as diuresis (fluid elimination), increased cardiac output, or relief from pain.

The most common mechanism of drug action is the binding of drugs to receptor sites on cells. The drugs and receptors fit together much as a key fits a lock. When receptors and drugs lock together, the therapeutic effects occur. Each cell in the body contains specific, unique receptors. For example, diphenhydramine blocks the receptor sites of histamine cells and reduces the itching and swelling caused by an allergic reaction.

A drug that produces such a specific action and promotes the desired result is referred to as an **agonist.** Analgesics, for example, are agonists. An **antagonist** is a drug that attaches itself to the receptor, preventing the agonist from acting. Common antagonists include those used to reverse the effects of certain drugs, such as opioids and benzopdiazepines, as discussed in the section that follows.

Drugs are administered to produce a predictable physiologic response, the therapeutic effect. In addition to the desired outcome, side effects may occur that may or may not be harmless. If the side effects are severe enough to outweigh the benefits of the medication, the physician may choose to discontinue the drug.

Knowing the effects of common medications helps you evaluate changes in the condition of patients in your care. Reference to the medication record in the patient's chart may help you determine whether a change in status is caused by medication or by deterioration in the patient's condition. For example, an anticholinergic medication, such as atropine, may cause a dry mouth. This is a specific side effect that has nothing to do with the patient's state of hydration. Opiates may slow the respiratory rate, and vasodilators may cause blood pressure to drop. Such effects are the usual consequence of the specific medication and are taken into account when the drug is prescribed.

Adverse effects are negative side effects that are not expected as a usual consequence of prescribed medications. They may range from mild nausea, flushing, or diarrhea to critical situations, including cardiac arrest or other life-threatening states. An allergic reaction is an adverse side effect that occurs when a patient has been sensitized to the initial dose of a medication and develops an allergic response to the **allergen** (allergy-causing substance) and related drugs. Drug allergies may be slight or severe, and the extent of the reaction is unpredictable. Urticaria, respiratory distress, and abrupt changes in blood pressure are all symptoms demanding a physician's immediate intervention. Chapter 22 provides information on appropriate responses to acute allergic reactions and other changes in patient condition that may occur as adverse effects of medications.

Toxic effects are poisonous consequences that develop when a drug accumulates in the body because of inadequate excretion, impaired metabolism, overdose, or sensitivity to the drug. Elderly patients are more likely to have poor heart, kidney, or liver function. These conditions increase the possibility that toxic effects might occur. A specific drug that treats a toxic effect is called an **antidote.**

An **idiosyncratic** (unusual or peculiar) reaction occurs when a patient overreacts or underreacts to a drug or has an unusual reaction. For example, when phenobarbital (a sedative) is administered, some individuals become very agitated rather than sedated.

There are many occasions when drugs taken together have a **synergistic** (interactive) effect that may go far beyond the desired outcome. For example, a patient who is taking a prescribed medication for high blood pressure and then takes an OTC diuretic may become hypotensive and feel weak and faint. Because many drugs interact when taken together, the physician who orders a new drug should have the patient's chart and should question the patient about taking OTC medications or drugs prescribed by a different physician.

FREQUENTLY USED MEDICATIONS

The medications described in the following subsections are used regularly in many outpatient health care facilities. The general descriptions provided illustrate how such medications are used but are not meant to be comprehensive. The specific drugs used in your facility may be different while meeting the same needs. See Table 23-1

Table 23-1

A Categorized Table of Some Common Medications

Category	Effect	Example	Common Side Effects
Adrenergics (vasoconstrictors)	Stimulate the sympathetic nervous system, causing relaxation of smooth muscles of bronchi (bronchodilation) Vasoconstriction Cardiac stimulation	Epinephrine (Adrenalin), ephedrine, isoproterenol (Isuprel), metaraminol bitartrate (Aramine), phenylephrine hydrochloride (Neo-Synephrine), norepinephrine bitartrate (Levophed)	Dry mouth
Adrenergic blocking agents	Block the production of epinephrine in the body, causing dilation of blood vessels and decreased cardiac output; used as antihypertensives	Methyldopa (Aldomet), clonidine (Catapres), prazosin (Minipress)	Fatigue, light-headedness
Analgesics	Relieve pain	Acetaminophen (Tylenol) Aspirin, ibuprofen (Advil), Hydrocodone (Vicodin), oxycodone (Percocet), codeine, hydromorphone hydrochloride (Dilaudid), meperidine (Demerol), methadone, morphine	Negligible Anticoagulant effects Respiratory depression
Anesthetics	Promote loss of feeling or sensation	*General:* thiopental sodium (Pentothal), halothane (Fluothane), nitrous oxide *Local:* lidocaine (Xylocaine)	Nausea
Antiarrhythmics	Prevent or relieve cardiac arrhythmias (dysrhythmias)	Quinidine, verapamil, propranolol, amiodarone, lidocaine	Bradycardia, congestive heart failure
Anticholinergics	Depress the parasympathetic nervous system and act as antispasmodics of smooth muscle tissue; decrease contractions, saliva, bronchial mucus, digestive secretions, and perspiration; used as preparation for surgery and endoscopy to suppress secretions	Atropine, belladonna, propantheline bromide (Pro-Banthine), scopolamine (hyoscine)	Dry mouth

Continued

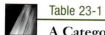

Table 23-1

A Categorized Table of Some Common Medications—cont'd

Category	Effect	Example	Common Side Effects
Anticoagulants	Inhibit the clotting mechanism of the blood; used to keep intravenous lines and arterial catheters open during diagnostic procedures Prevent blood clots following heart attack or stroke	Heparin, warfarin (Coumadin), clopidogrel bisulfate (Plavix), apixaban (Eliquis), dabigatran (Pradaxa), and rivaroxaban (Xarelto)	Bruising, spontaneous bleeding
Anticonvulsants	Inhibit convulsions	Phenytoin (Dilantin) Carbamazepine (Tegretol) Lorazepam (Ativan) Fosphenytoin (Cerebyx) Divalproex sodium (Depakote)	Rash, slurred speech Rash, itch, sun sensitivity Sedation, dizziness, weakness, unsteadiness
Antidepressants	Relieve or prevent depression	Amitriptyline (Elavil), imipramine (Tofranil) Fluoxetine (Prozac)	Drowsiness, dizziness, weight gain Nervousness, diarrhea
Antiemetics	Relieve or prevent vomiting	Trimethobenzamide hydrochloride (Tigan), prochlorperazine (Compazine), dolasetron mesylate (Anzemet)	Drowsiness, dry mouth, blurred vision
Antifungals	Treat or prevent fungal infections	*Systemic:* griseofulvin *Topical:* tolnaftate (Tinactin) *Mucosal:* nystatin (Mycostatin)	Negligible
Antihistamines	Relieve the symptoms of allergic reactions	Diphenhydramine (Benadryl), chlorpheniramine maleate (Chlor-Trimeton)	Drowsiness
		Cetirizine hydrochloride (Zyrtec), loratadine (Claritin), fexofenadine hydrochloride (Allegra)	Negligible
Antihypertensives	Lower blood pressure	ACE inhibitors: captopril (Capoten), enalapril (Vasotec), lisinopril (Prinivil) Beta blockers: propranolol (Inderal), metoprolol (Lopressor, Toprol XL)	Dizziness, headache, drowsiness, weakness
Antimicrobials	Suppress the growth of microorganisms	*Systemic:* penicillin, tetracyclines, sulfadiazine, erythromycin, cephalosporins (Keflex, Keflin, Rocephin, Cefazolin)	Diarrhea, yeast infections
		Topical: Sulfonamides, thimerosal (Merthiolate), povidone-iodine (Betadine)	Allergic reactions
Antiperistaltics	Slow peristalsis of the gastrointestinal tract	Tincture of opium (paregoric), loperamide (Imodium)	Constipation
Antipsychotics	Treat psychoses, schizophrenia	Haloperidol (Haldol)	Nausea, decreased sweating, dry mouth, stiffness
		Fluphenazine (Prolixin), risperidone (Risperdal)	Constipation, shaking
Antipyretics	Reduce fever	Aspirin Acetaminophen (Tylenol)	Bruising Negligible
Antitussives	Reduce coughing	Dextromethorphan (Romilar) Codeine	Negligible Nausea
Antivirals	Prevent or treat viral diseases	Acyclovir (Zovirax), amantadine (Symadine), zidovudine (AZT)	Nausea, vomiting, diarrhea, and headache
Barbiturates	Depress the central nervous system, respirations, and blood pressure; induce sleep	Pentobarbital sodium (Nembutal), secobarbital (Seconal)	Nausea, itching, constipation

Table 23-1

A Categorized Table of Some Common Medications—cont'd

Category	Effect	Example	Common Side Effects
Bronchodilators	Relax smooth muscle; used to treat asthmatic attacks and some allergic reactions	Theophylline (Theo-Dur), aminophylline	Insomnia, decreased appetite, irritability
		Albuterol (Proventil), albuterol inhaled (Xopenex), metaproterenol sulfate (Alupent)	Hypertension, angina, vomiting, vertigo
Cardiac depressants	Restrain or slow heart activity	Quinidine, procainamide (Pronestyl)	Nausea, diarrhea, heartburn
Cardiac stimulants	Strengthen and tone the heart; increase cardiac output	Digitalis, gitalin (Gitaligin), lanatoside C (Cedilanid)	Weakness, blurred vision
Cathartics	Stimulate peristalsis; promote defecation	Bisacodyl (Dulcolax), magnesium citrate, polyethylene-glycol (Miralax)	Dehydration, weight loss, abdominal cramping
Diuretics	Stimulate the flow of urine	Chlorothiazide (Diuril), furosemide (Lasix)	Potassium depletion, diarrhea, cramps
		Acetazolamide (Diamox)	Fatigue, metallic taste
Emetics	Induce vomiting	Ipecac	Potential dehydration
Hypoglycemics	Lower blood sugar level	Insulin	Cold sweat, anxiety, headache, confusion
		Tolbutamide (Orinase), glyburide (Micronase), liraglutide (Victoza), sitagliptin (Januvia)	Hypoglycemia
		Metformin (Glucophage)	Risk of severe acidosis in cases of kidney failure. Contraindicated with iodine contrast media until normal kidney function has been confirmed
Opioids (narcotics)	Analgesic sedatives with a potential for addiction; classified as controlled substances under the Harrison Act	Injectable: morphine, meperidine (Demerol) Oral: hydrocodone (Vicodin), oxycodone (Percocet), codeine	Respiratory depression Drowsiness
Opioid antagonists	Prevent or counteract respiratory depression and depressive effects of morphine and related drugs	Naloxone hydrochloride (Narcan), nalorphine (Nalline), naltrexone (Trexan)	Nausea, vomiting, tachycardia, hypertension
Radioisotopes	Radioactive forms of elements used for diagnosis and treatment	Iodine (I^{131}), cobalt (Co^{60}), Technetium (Tc^{99m})	Negligible
Sedatives	Depress and relax the central nervous system and reduce mental activity	Barbiturates, paraldehyde, chloral hydrate	Clumsiness, dizziness, drowsiness
Skeletal muscle relaxants	Relax skeletal and striated muscle tissue	Succinylcholine chloride (Anectine), pancuronium bromide (Pavulon)	Respiratory depression
Stimulants	Stimulate the central nervous system	Caffeine, sodium benzoate, amphetamines (e.g., dextroamphetamine, [Dexedrine])	Insomnia, restlessness
Tranquilizers	Reduce anxiety	*Minor:* diazepam (Valium), lorazepam (Ativan), chlordiazepoxide (Librium)	Drowsiness, decreased coordination, slurred speech
		Major: chlorpromazine (Thorazine), trifluoperazine (Stelazine)	
Vasodilators	Relax the walls of blood vessels, permitting a greater flow of blood	Isosorbide dinitrate (Sorbitrate)	Dizziness, headache, flushing, tachycardia
		Nitroglycerin	Headache, hypotension
		Hydralazine (Apresoline)	Headache, anorexia, vomiting, diarrhea, palpitations

ACE, Angiotensin-converting-enzyme.

for a more extensive list of medications that you may encounter.

Antiallergic Medications

Antihistamines are drugs used to treat mild to moderate allergic reactions. Diphenhydramine (Benadryl) is the most frequently used antihistamine. It also has sedative (calming) and anticholinergic (drying) side effects. Diphenhydramine may be given orally, IM, or IV. Cortisone (Solu-Cortef) is a corticosteroid medication that is also prescribed for these purposes.

For a patient with an acute allergic reaction, epinephrine (Adrenalin) is administered SC, IM, or IV. To control hives, shock, or respiratory distress, the physician administers a small dose of epinephrine and increases the dose if required.

When patients with a severe or incapacitating allergic response do not respond to antihistamine or epinephrine, methylprednisolone (Solu-Medrol) may be administered IV. This is a corticosteroid that acts as an antiinflammatory agent, preventing or reducing swelling of the trachea and bronchi. This treatment reduces the likelihood of respiratory arrest. Methylprednisolone is provided in a two-compartment vial with the diluting fluid and soluble powder separated by a plunger/stopper. The directions for mixing are provided, but you should become familiar with the preparation of this and all common medications before the need arises.

Antimicrobial Medications

Antimicrobial medications include disinfectants such as alcohol and povidone-iodine (Betadine), a compound commonly used for skin preparation before sterile procedures.

Also classified as antimicrobials are *antibiotics*. Given to treat wound infections and infectious diseases, antibiotics can be subclassified as antibacterial, antiviral, or antifungal according to the type of organisms against which they are most effective. Some antibiotics treat a very narrow range of microorganisms. Co-trimoxazole, for example, is used to treat specific infections of the urinary tract. Other antimicrobials are referred to as *broad-spectrum* antibiotics and are effective against a wide variety of pathogens.

Analgesics

Analgesics are defined as drugs that can relieve pain without causing loss of consciousness. As a group, **opioids** are the most effective analgesics. The term *opioid* describes any drug, natural or synthetic, whose actions are similar to the actions of morphine. The opioid family, whose name derives from opium, includes morphine, codeine, and meperidine (Demerol). **Opiate** is the more specific term applied only to natural opium derivatives. The term

narcotic is no longer used with precision as a synonym for *analgesic* because it has also come to stand for those analgesic CNS depressants that may lead to addiction. In a *legal* sense, cocaine, marijuana, and lysergic acid diethylamide (LSD) are classed with opiates as narcotics.

Controlled substances are drugs whose availability is outlawed or strictly regulated because of their potential for abuse or addiction. Opioids and other controlled drugs that can be legally prescribed are kept in a locked container and must be counted daily. The administration of any controlled medication must be recorded on forms that list the date, the patient's name, the dose, and the name and title of the person administering the medication. Use of these drugs is monitored by the U.S. Drug Enforcement Administration (DEA), and they can be prescribed only by persons who hold a DEA license.

Opioids act by depressing the CNS, relieving pain, and producing drowsiness. Excessive doses, however, can result in depressed respirations, coma, and possibly death. They may be given orally or injected. Common oral opioid analgesics include hydrocodone (Vicodin) and oxycodone (Percocet). Among the most frequently prescribed injectable opioids are morphine sulfate (MS) and meperidine (Demerol). Fentanyl (Sublimaze), another highly potent opioid analgesic, is given to patients who are sensitive to other analgesics or who are not responding to such medications with adequate pain relief. The action of fentanyl is almost immediate and lasts 30 to 60 minutes after IV administration. Respiratory depression peaks 5 to 10 minutes after injection and may last for several hours, depending on the dose.

Patients who have received any CNS depressant must be monitored closely. Respiratory depression is a life-threatening side effect. Resuscitation equipment and emergency drugs to counteract this effect should be immediately available. Because patients may be some distance away, a pulse oximeter is attached to the patient's finger, toe, or earlobe (see Fig. 22-11). A digital readout of the pulse and the oxygen saturation of the blood can be viewed on a monitor. If the oxygen saturation drops below 95%, the patient is asked to respond and take a few deep breaths, then is observed closely. If the oxygen saturation continues to drop or the patient does not respond adequately, a physician is notified immediately.

Analgesics may be given to help patients cope with painful procedures or to lessen preexisting pain. Analgesics with a low potential for side effects, such as aspirin, ibuprofen (Advil), acetaminophen (Tylenol), and naproxen sodium (Aleve), are frequently used to alleviate discomfort. With the exception of acetaminophen, these products are all categorized as nonsteroidal antiinflammatory drugs (NSAIDs). Although they are all analgesics, these drugs are not controlled substances. All are available without prescription. Self-medication with OTC analgesics is very common, especially in the elderly. Patients should be encouraged to keep a record of these medications and the frequency of use so that physicians can identify possible incompatibilities among patients' medications. As a general rule, patients should not be given OTC medications except under a physician's order or under standing orders. At home, children should be given analgesics other than acetaminophen only under the direct instruction of a physician. Even acetaminophen may be hazardous if recommended dosages are not followed.

Sedatives and Tranquilizers

Sedatives and tranquilizers exert a quieting effect, often inducing sleep. They are not analgesics but may provide relief from pain by promoting muscle relaxation.

Phenobarbital and other barbiturates are sedatives and were formerly used as preoperative medications and as sleeping aids. Their use for these purposes has been largely supplanted by other drugs. Phenobarbital is still used with other medications to treat patients with seizures.

Tranquilizers reduce anxiety and mental tension more effectively than sedatives and often provide some sedation as well. At low doses tranquilizers do not impair mental acuity, but as the dosage increases patients tend to feel drowsy, and speech may become slow and slurred. Some patients experience a brief loss of inhibition, similar to the effect of alcohol, which causes them to talk and act inappropriately. Individuals taking tranquilizers may have slowed reaction times and thus should not drive or operate machinery.

Diazepam (Valium) and midazolam (Versed) are tranquilizers that belong to the drug class of **benzodiazepines**. Diazepam is prescribed for oral administration to patients with anxiety, and this tranquilizer is commonly ordered as premedication for various diagnostic and therapeutic procedures. When diazepam is injected IV, it is administered slowly, with at least 1 minute taken for each 5 mg (1 ml) given. The small veins of the hand and wrist should not be used because diazepam is irritating to blood vessels and may cause phlebitis and damage to the vein. **Extravasation** of diazepam (infiltration into surrounding tissues) causes irritation and swelling and can be quite painful. Midazolam is sometimes given when a previous administration of an analgesic or diazepam has not achieved the desired state of pain relief and relaxation.

Benzodiazepines may be given with morphine to patients who are highly anxious and uncomfortable. Very large doses are sometimes given to control grand mal seizures.

Antagonists

Antagonists are drugs that counteract the effects of other drugs. The antagonists most likely to be encountered are those formulated to counteract the effects of sedatives and analgesics.

Diazepam and midazolam are benzodiazepine drugs that may be given to produce relaxation and/or sedation, as described earlier. An overdose produces respiratory depression and loss of psychomotor function as a toxic (poisonous) effect. Flumazenil (Mazicon) is a medication developed to counteract the effects of these drugs. Flumazenil can antagonize the sedation and reverse the impairment of recall and psychomotor function produced by benzodiazepines. Patients who receive flumazenil should be monitored for resedation, respiratory depression, and other residual effects for up to 2 hours, based on the dose and duration of the benzodiazepine used. If the desired level of consciousness is not obtained within a minute after starting the initial dose, additional doses may be given to a maximum of 1 mg (10 ml) until the desired effect is achieved. To minimize the possibility of pain or inflammation, flumazenil should be administered through a freely flowing IV line into a large vein. The use of flumazenil is known to be associated with seizures in some patients who have been taking benzodiazepines over a long period.

Naloxone (Narcan) counteracts the effects of opiates such as morphine, and prevents or reverses respiratory depression, sedation, and hypotension. A rapid reversal of opiate depression can cause nausea, vomiting, tachycardia, and nervousness. Although naloxone can be administered SC or IM, the most rapid onset of action is obtained with a dilution of naloxone in saline or 5% dextrose in water administered IV.

Local Anesthetics

Lidocaine (Xylocaine) is a local anesthetic used to eliminate sensation in a specific area before a painful procedure. You may have received such an injection before having dental work or when having stitches placed to close a wound. Lidocaine is provided in a variety of strengths and is available both with and without epinephrine. The addition of epinephrine causes constriction of adjacent blood vessels, preventing bleeding and localizing the anesthetic effect to the immediate area. If your facility stocks more than one type, be sure you understand clearly which one the physician requires.

Hypoglycemic Agents

Hypoglycemic agents are drugs used to control the level of glucose in the blood, primarily as a treatment for diabetes mellitus (see Chapter 22). Type 1 diabetes mellitus is treated with insulin, whereas type 2, or non–insulin-dependent diabetes mellitus, is often treated with oral agents: a sulfonylurea (Amaryl or Glucotrol), tolbutamide (Orinase), chlorpropamide (Diabinese), rosiglitazone (Avandia), or metformin (Glucophage). It is helpful to recognize these agents in a drug list, because they will alert you and the physician to the diabetes diagnosis.

Antihypertensives

There are two principal types of medications for the control of high blood pressure: angiotensin-converting enzyme (ACE) inhibitors and beta blockers. ACE is a body chemical that is part of a complex system of enzymes that increase blood pressure. ACE inhibitors such as captopril (Capoten), enalapril (Vasotec), and lisinopril (Prinivil) lower blood pressure by interrupting this cycle. Common side effects include dizziness because of hypotension, headache, drowsiness, and weakness.

Beta blockers, also called beta adrenergic blocking agents, suppress the action of the sympathetic nervous system, blocking the catecholamines, epinephrine and norepinephrine. In addition to treating hypertension, these drugs are prescribed to treat a number of cardiac conditions, including irregular heart rhythm and the occurrence of angina (see Chapter 22). Common beta blockers include propranolol (Inderal) and metoprolol (Lopressor, Toprol XL).

MEDICATION ADMINISTRATION

The information in this section provides a basis for assisting the physician in medication administration but is not intended as a substitute for directions from the physician.

Preparation

In preparation for medication administration, the first step is to check both the order and the patient's identification. Current recommendations require two separate means of patient identification. This is usually accomplished by having the patient state his or her full name and birth date. If you have questions about dosage or method of administration, check with the physician or your supervisor. Second, make certain that you have the correct medication in the correct strength and check the expiration date. The medication label indicates not only the name of the medication and the strength (amount per milliliter) but also gives an expiration date past which the drug should not be used. Third, check for allergies in the chart or obtain an allergy history from the patient. Finally, remember to perform hand hygiene before preparing the medication.

A common rule of thumb is to read the label three times: first when selecting the container, second while preparing the dose, and a third time just before administration. This is essential to be absolutely certain that you have the correct drug and the proper strength. Be sure to keep the container until the medication has been charted.

When medications are not used frequently (as in an emergency kit), they should be checked often and out-of-date supplies discarded and replaced. When you prepare medications, the memory device in Box 23-1 will help you to avoid errors.

Box 23-1

Six Rights of Medication Administration

- The right dose
- Of the right medication
- To the right patient
- At the right time
- By the right route
- With the right documentation

Dose

The usual dosage or dosage range for each medication is included in the information on the package insert and is also available in the *PDR* or other suitable drug reference. Physicians are not required to prescribe the usual dosage and may specify a different dosage for very good reasons, but when an order specifies a much higher dosage than usual, be sure to verify the accuracy of the order before proceeding.

Some textbooks provide formulas for calculating pediatric drug dose based on the child's age and the usual adult dose. No formula is provided here because of the risk of serious error. Some drugs are not approved for pediatric use. Others require a higher or lower dose than such formulas would indicate. When a medication is approved for pediatric use, the recommended pediatric dose according to the child's age and/or weight will be stated in the package insert and in medication references.

The metric system is used for measuring patients' weight when calculating dosage and is also used for measuring medications. To convert a patient's weight from pounds to the kilogram (kg) unit used in the metric system, divide the weight in pounds by 2.2, the number of pounds in a kilogram.

$$\text{Pounds (lb)} \div 2.2 = \text{kilograms (kg)}$$

Example: What is the metric weight of a child weighing 46 lb?

$$46 \text{ lb} \div 2.2 \text{ lb/kg} = 20.9 \text{ kg}$$

Liquid medications are measured in units from liters (L, slightly more than a quart) down to milliliters (ml), which are thousandths of a liter. One milliliter is equal to 1 cubic centimeter (cc), and 1 ounce equals 30 ml.

Because liquid agents are often diluted for use, the strength is expressed as a ratio of the amount of the drug to the total volume of solution. For example, 1:1000 indicates a dilution of 1 part drug to 1000 parts of water or other solvent.

If the active ingredient is a solid, it is measured by weight in grams (g), milligrams (mg), or micrograms (mcg or μg). The strength of solids dissolved in a liquid is designated in terms of weight per volume, often milligrams per milliliter. You will often need to determine how much liquid will provide a given dose of a solid:

$$\frac{\text{Dose}}{\text{Strength}} = \text{Volume}$$

Example: If the drug is supplied in a strength of 4 mg/ml, and you want to administer 10 mg, you will need 2.5 ml:

$$\frac{10 \text{ mg}}{4 \text{ mg/ml}} = 2.5 \text{ ml}$$

Conversely, you may need to know how much of a solid is delivered in a given volume of liquid:

$$\text{Strength} \times \text{Volume} = \text{Dose}$$

Example: If 2 ml of solution is given and the strength is 4 mg/ml, the dose would be 8 mg:

$$4 \text{ mg/ml} \times 2 \text{ ml} = 8 \text{ mg}$$

Practice these calculations so that you can do them quickly without error whenever you are required to prepare a parenteral medication. Additional examples and practice problems are included in Chapter 3.

Oral Administration

The oral route of medication administration is the easiest and most familiar. The charting abbreviation for oral administration is *PO* for *per os*, by mouth. When medication is taken orally, it must be swallowed, dissolve in the stomach, and then pass into the small intestine where the majority of the absorption takes place.

Oral medications are supplied in a variety of forms, including tablets, capsules, granules, and liquids. Some oral medications are irritating to the stomach and are provided in a coated form that allows tablets to pass through the stomach before dissolving. These medications should not be chewed or broken because this would negate the action of the enteric coating. Some tablets are chewable, but almost all medication should be swallowed with varying amounts of liquid, usually water. Liquid medications are usually taken with water as well. Granules are mixed with a specified amount of liquid. Follow the directions on the package insert.

One way to minimize errors in the administration of drugs is to establish a set routine and follow it unfailingly. The steps in Box 23-2 serve as a guide to establish a procedure for the administration of oral medications.

Parenteral Administration

Parenteral Equipment

Needles for injections are supplied in various diameters and lengths. The gauge of a needle indicates its diameter, and the gauge increases as the diameter of the bore decreases.

Box 23-2

Procedure for Oral Medication Administration

- Perform hand hygiene.
- Obtain the proper medication and read the label. Check the medication name, strength, and expiration date.
- Prepare the medication tray with a medicine cup and a glass of water (if appropriate). Read the label again.
- If the physician is present, show the physician the label.
- Pour the correct amount of medication directly into the medicine cup. When pouring liquids, hold the label against the palm of your hand so that it will stay clean and legible.
- If requested by the physician to administer the medication, check the patient's identification using two identifiers, stay with the patient while the medication is swallowed, and offer water if permitted.
- Return the tray and discard the remaining water and medicine cup.
- Repeat hand hygiene.
- Chart the medication.
- Discard packaging from single-dose packages or return medication container to storage.

For example, an 18-gauge needle is larger around than a 22-gauge needle and delivers a given volume of fluid more rapidly. A 22-gauge needle can be used for much smaller veins, because it makes a smaller hole and **hematoma** (bleeding under the skin) is less likely when it is removed. This size is also used for IM injections; smaller gauges are needed for SC and intradermal administration.

The length of hypodermic needles is measured in inches and may vary from ½ inch, used for accessing IV line ports and for intradermal injections, to 4½ inches, needed for intrathecal (spinal canal) injections. A length of ⅝ inch to 1½ inches is typical for parenteral injections, and the usual gauge ranges from 18 to 25 for adults. As stated in Chapter 21, the widespread incidence of blood-borne infection has placed increasing emphasis on the prevention of accidental needle sticks. Regulations of the Occupational Safety and Health Administration (OSHA) now require the use of engineering controls to decrease the risk to health care workers from contaminated needle sticks, and these regulations have led to the development of new devices. These engineering controls include two basic types of devices: needleless systems for accessing established IV lines and sharps with a built-in safety feature or mechanism that effectively reduces the risk of an exposure incident. These sharps are called *sharps with engineered sharps injury protection* (SESIPs). Some examples are illustrated in Fig. 23-1.

Disposable plastic syringes are supplied in individual sterile paper wraps, sometimes with a needle attached. Syringes consist of a barrel with a measurement scale on the outside and a plunger to force the contents through

of air equal to the amount of fluid you wish to remove. Remove the needle cover and pull down the plunger of the syringe to the desired reading. Insert the needle through the stopper and inject the air into the bottle.

thetic are sometimes used repeatedly for the same patient during a radiographic procedure. When using a vial after the first time, clean the stopper with an alcohol wipe. (Alcohol is not needed for the first injection because the

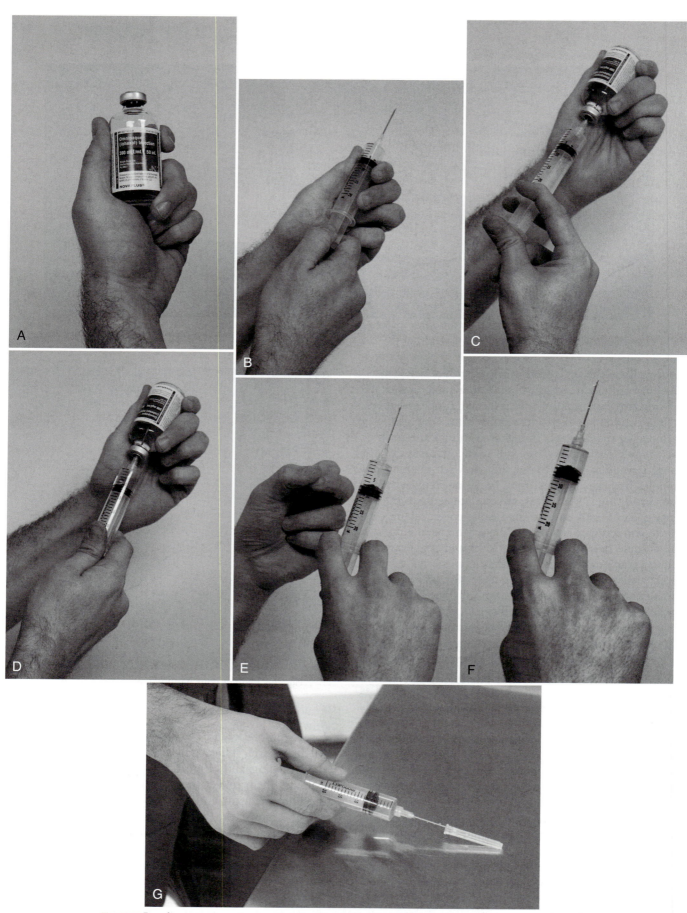

Fig. 23-5 Loading a syringe from a vial. **A,** Check the label for drug name, correct strength, and expiration date. **B,** Pull back on the plunger to the desired dose reading. **C,** Inject air into the air space in the vial. **D,** Tip vial downward to withdraw the solution. **E,** Tap syringe to dislodge bubbles. **F,** Eject remaining air and check that the dosage is accurate. **G,** Recap needle using one hand only. Label the syringe. Note: Only sterile needles may be recapped.

stopper is sterile on opening the vial.) When the procedure is complete, discard the vial and any remaining medication. Some vials are not meant for multiple use and are so marked.

Parenteral Injection Procedure

Injection techniques are practical skills that cannot be learned through study alone. You will want to observe these techniques performed competently and have an experienced observer present when you perform injections until you gain confidence.

The basic procedure for intradermal, SC, and IM injections is stated in Box 23-3. The loading of the syringe is the same for all injections and is illustrated in Fig. 23-5. The injection sites, the equipment used, and the injections themselves are different for each of these three routes, and these variations are summarized in Table 23-2. The injection depths and angles are illustrated in Fig. 23-6.

Intradermal injections involve a shallow puncture between the layers of the skin. The anterior surface of the forearm is a typical site for intradermal injections. Only very small quantities may be injected intradermally. A tuberculin syringe is used; it is finely calibrated and comes with a very small (26-gauge) needle. The tuberculin skin test discussed in Chapter 21 involves an intradermal injection to the anterior forearm. This route is also sometimes used to test allergic sensitivity.

For SC injections, a 23- to 25-gauge needle with a ⅝-inch length is used. It is directed through the skin at a 45-degree angle. Syringes used for SC injections are usually 2 ml or smaller because it is painful to inject a large quantity beneath the skin. The most convenient areas for SC injections are on the upper arm and on the outer aspect of the thigh.

IM injections are sometimes given in larger amounts. The syringe may be larger than that used for SC injection (up to 5 ml), and the needle size is also larger, usually 22 gauge. The injection is given into the deltoid muscle of the upper arm (Fig. 23-7), the gluteal muscles in the hip area (Fig. 23-8), or the vastus lateralis muscle of the lateral thigh (Fig. 23-9). For children under 5 years of age, the vastus lateralis site is preferred to the gluteus site because the gluteus maximus muscle is not fully developed and there is risk of damage to the sciatic nerve. Injections are not usually given into the anterior thigh because injection into this site is extremely painful and the discomfort may persist for several days.

Assisting With Intravenous Injections and the Establishment of Intravenous Lines

IV fluids and medications are administered to meet specific needs. Patients respond rapidly to medication administration via this route. The IV injection is used for delivering most emergency medications when an immediate response is critical. The IV route may serve to transport medications, parenteral nutrition, or chemotherapy. Dehydrated patients may need fluid and electrolyte replacement by means of IV infusion. This is also the route used to inject contrast media for radiographic examinations of the urinary tract and for some computed tomographic studies, and to provide sedation during invasive procedures and magnetic resonance imaging examinations.

Box 23-3

Procedure for Parenteral Administration (Intradermal, Subcutaneous, and Intramuscular)

- Explain to the patient what you are about to do.
- Perform hand hygiene and don clean gloves.
- Select the appropriate site.
- Cleanse the selected area with an alcohol wipe.
- Hold the skin taut with your nondominant hand.
- Insert the needle at the correct angle and pull back slightly on the plunger.
- If no blood is drawn into the syringe, inject the medication.
- Withdraw the needle quickly and wipe the injection site.
- Dispose of the needle and syringe.
- See to the patient's comfort.
- Remove your gloves and repeat hand hygiene.
- Chart the medication.
- Dispose of the medication container, syringe, and needle.

Table 23-2

Parenteral Injection Summary

Injection Route	Injection Volume	Needle Length	Needle Gauge	Injection Site(s)	Angle of Injection
Intradermal	<1 ml	½ to ⅝ inch	25-26 gauge	Anterior forearm	15 degrees
Subcutaneous (SC)	<2 ml	⅝ inch	23-25 gauge	Upper arm, outer aspect of thigh	45 degrees
Intramuscular (IM)	<5 ml	1 to 1½ inches	22 gauge	Deltoid muscle, vastus lateralis muscle, gluteal muscle (over age 5)	90 degrees

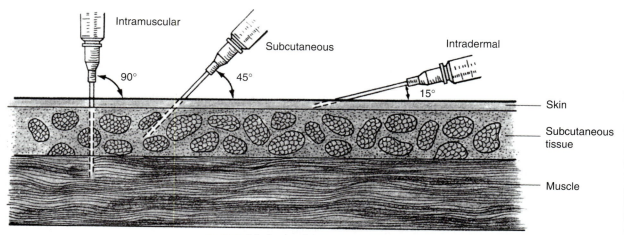

Fig. 23-6 Methods of parenteral injection.

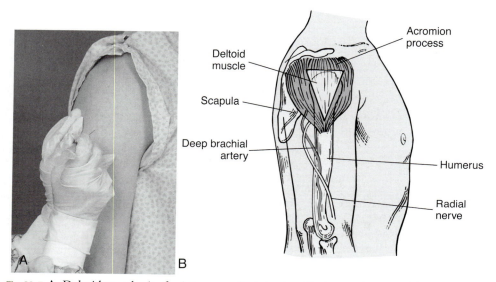

Fig. 23-7 A, Deltoid muscle site for intramuscular injection. **B,** Anatomic view of deltoid muscle injection site.

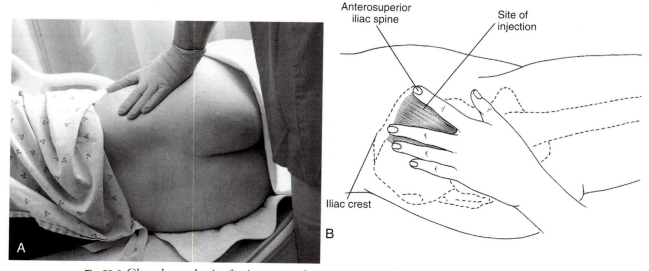

Fig. 23-8 Gluteal muscle site for intramuscular injection. **A,** The injection site into the ventro-gluteal muscle avoids major nerves and blood vessels. **B,** Anatomic view of ventrogluteal muscle injection site.

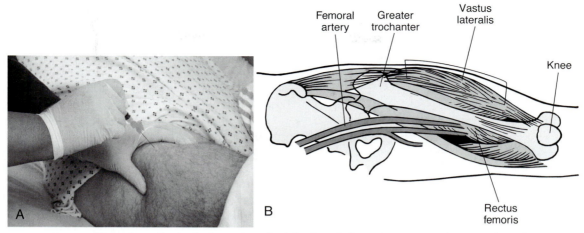

Fig. 23-9 Vastus lateralis site for intramuscular injection. **A,** Injection site into the vastus lateralis muscle. **B,** Anatomic view of vastus lateralis muscle injection site.

As stated earlier, starting IV lines and administering medication by the IV route are procedures beyond the limited operator's scope of practice, but you may need to assist the physician with these procedures or monitor the infusion of IV fluids after an IV line has been established. If your work involves the IV administration of medication or contrast media, consult other resources that provide specific information on these products and the procedures and precautions for their use.

Venipuncture may be accomplished with a hypodermic needle, a butterfly set, or an IV catheter. The use of hypodermic needles is generally restricted to phlebotomy for obtaining laboratory samples (see Chapter 24) and for single, small injections. A butterfly set (Fig. 23-10) is preferable to a conventional hypodermic needle for most IV injections and is often used for direct injections with a syringe. This apparatus consists of a needle with plastic projections on either side that aid in holding the needle during venipuncture and may be taped to the patient's skin after the needle is in place. This prevents movement of the needle in the vein. Attached to the needle is a short length of tubing with a hub that connects to a syringe. The syringe is filled from a vial or ampule with a needle, as in preparation for other parenteral injections. The needle is then discarded, and the syringe is attached to the butterfly tubing. Before the butterfly needle is inserted into the vein, the tubing is filled with liquid from the syringe to avoid injecting air into the vein.

IV catheters are used instead of needles or butterfly sets when repeated or continuous IV injections or infusions are administered. The IV catheter is a two-part system consisting of a needle that fits inside a flexible plastic tube (Fig. 23-11). The catheter hub has wing-shaped plastic projections similar to those in the butterfly set. Once the catheter is properly situated in the vein, it is connected to the syringe or supply system. Fluid can be administered by syringe or through tubing from a

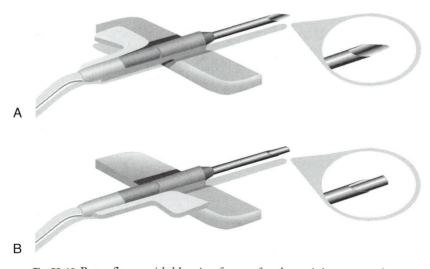

Fig. 23-10 Butterfly set with blunting feature for sharps injury protection.

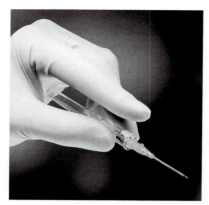

Fig. 23-11 Intravenous catheter set.

hanging bottle or bag. Medication can also be injected from a syringe into an injection port on the IV fluid tubing. OSHA-compliant versions of safety-engineered IV catheters and butterfly sets are available.

Large volumes of solution are administered intravenously by IV infusion. The most common replacement fluids are normal saline (NS, a solution of 0.9% saltwater that has the same ion concentration as the fluid in normal body tissue) or a 5% solution of dextrose in water (D5W). These IV solutions are provided in bottles and plastic bags. They may be stocked with the emergency supplies or may be stocked for general use if your facility regularly performs procedures that require an IV line. If you are assisting with the starting or replacing of IV fluids, *be certain that the solution is correct.* Less common solutions, including some that contain medication, may be stocked for special purposes. Checking labels for IV fluids is just as important as checking other medication labels.

The setup for IV fluid administration requires the bottle or bag of fluid, an infusion set, and an IV pole. The infusion set consists of a drip chamber that attaches to the bag or bottle with tubing that attaches to the needle or catheter. It includes an injection port for adding medication to the infusion.

The bags have a cap over the sterile port through which the drip chamber is inserted. The drip chamber is removed from its wrappings and inserted into the sterile port. Care must be taken not to contaminate either component or else the contaminated item must be discarded. Solutions supplied in bottles have a removable cap and sometimes a rubber diaphragm covering a rubber stopper. The cap is removed and the diaphragm is pulled off without touching the stopper. The drip chamber is then inserted through the stopper, with the physician taking care that the clamp on the IV tubing is closed. The bottle or bag is then inverted and hung on the IV pole. When it is in place, the cover at the other end of the IV tubing is removed, the clamp is opened, and the fluid is allowed to run into a basin until the tubing is free of bubbles. The clamp is then closed and the tip covered to keep it sterile. The procedure for setting up an IV infusion is illustrated

in Fig. 23-12. The physician or nurse will attach the tubing to the needle or catheter and adjust the fluid flow rate.

Monitoring Infusions

If you are caring for a patient who is receiving an IV infusion, it is your duty to monitor the flow rate and the condition of the injection site.

The flow rate is measured in units of drops per minute. Note the flow rate when you first encounter the patient and then check at regular intervals to ensure that this rate is maintained. Most patients easily tolerate 15 to 20 drops/min from a standard IV set. At this rate the patient receives approximately 60 ml/hr. The drip rate is controlled by a clamp below the drip meter, which can be opened or closed to adjust the rate of flow.

If an IV infusion runs too fast, a patient with a condition such as chronic obstructive pulmonary disease or congestive heart failure may receive more fluid than can be readily assimilated, which causes fluid to accumulate in the lungs (pulmonary edema). Because an IV infusion may also contain medication, the patient could suffer a toxic effect or an overdose. On the other hand, too slow a flow rate might prevent effective treatment.

The height of the bottle or bag affects the flow rate and should always be 18 to 20 inches above the level of the vein. If the bottle is inadvertently placed lower than the vein, blood will flow back into the catheter or tubing and may clot, causing the fluid to stop flowing. This frequently necessitates restarting the IV line at a new site. On the other hand, if the IV solution is too high, fluid may infiltrate into the surrounding tissue because of the increased pressure.

Occasionally, IV fluids or medications may leak or be accidentally injected into the tissue surrounding a vein. This extravasation, also called **infiltration,** can be both painful and dangerous. The patient is likely to complain of discomfort, and you may observe swelling at the site. Remember to check the area around the injection site frequently. If it is cool, swollen, and boggy, these are signs that the IV solution has infiltrated.

When extravasation occurs, shut off the flow of fluid immediately and notify a nurse or the physician. The needle must be removed and the problem attended to before proceeding with an injection at another site. When the needle or catheter has been removed and the bleeding has stopped, a cold pack is applied to the affected area to help alleviate the pain. This will also cause constriction of the blood vessels in the area and help to keep the infiltration localized. If cold packs are not readily available, a terry towel can be wrapped around ice cubes, or ice in a plastic bag can be applied. A dry towel may be wrapped around the bag to hold it in place. Replace the cold pack with another as soon as it melts. Ice packs are applied to the extravasation site for 20 to 60 minutes until swelling is diminished. If the patient is allowed to leave before the swelling has

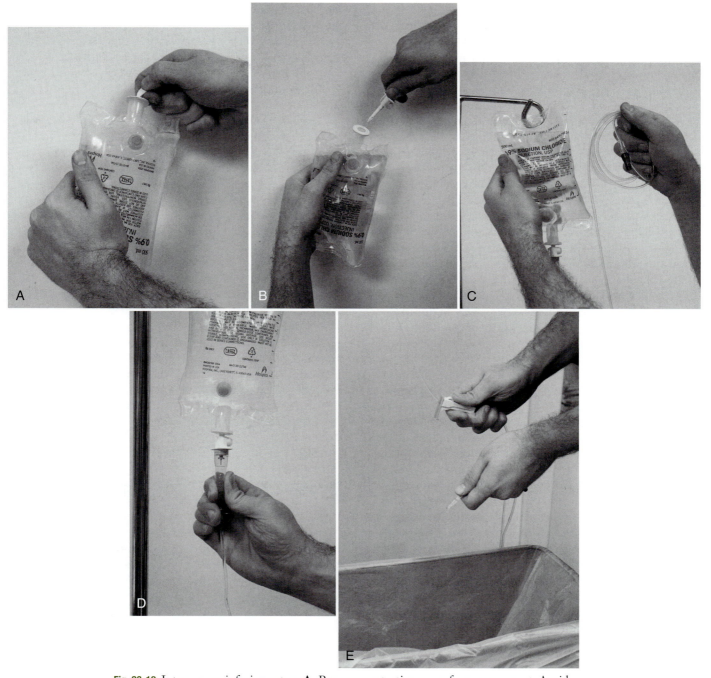

Fig. 23-12 Intravenous infusion setup. **A,** Remove protective cover from access port. Avoid contamination. **B,** With tubing clamped off, insert drip chamber firmly into access port. **C,** Invert bag or bottle and suspend from pole. **D,** Pinch drip chamber to draw fluid into chamber. Fill chamber about half full. **E,** Unclamp to fill tubing and reclamp once air has been removed from the line. Setup is ready for attachment to IV catheter.

completely disappeared, the physician may order continued cold pack treatments at home and instruct the patient to return or go to the emergency room if inflammation or discomfort persists. It is recommended that an incident report be completed for any extravasation involving a potentially irritating medication or contrast medium.

Previously, hot packs were recommended for the treatment of IV infiltration in the belief that the increased circulation that occurs with heat would result in the body's absorbing the extravasated fluid more rapidly. Recent research confirms that the safest and most effective treatment is the cold pack.

Discontinuing Infusions

When you must discontinue an IV line, you will need a sterile adhesive bandage, bandage scissors, and cotton balls or gauze sponges. Perform hand hygiene, and explain the procedure to the patient. Wearing protective gloves, close the drip control, and gently remove the adhesive tape holding the catheter. If it is necessary to cut the tape, take care not to cut the catheter, which may be doubled back under the tape. With the site exposed where the catheter enters the vein, remove the catheter with a long, smooth pull, and check that the catheter tip is intact when removed. Apply pressure to the site with a dry cotton ball or sponge. A dry contact is preferred to an alcohol wipe so that the adhesive bandage will stick to the skin. Maintain the pressure for one minute or until the bleeding stops, and then cover the site with a sterile adhesive bandage or secure the cotton ball to the site with tape. Discontinuation of the IV must be documented in the medical record. With the patient in a safe, comfortable position, dispose of the equipment in the proper container, remove your gloves, and repeat hand hygiene.

Precautions for All Injections

As discussed in Chapter 21, following Standard Precautions is essential. Most needles and syringes are provided in sterile wraps, used once, and then destroyed. Use safety equipment and safe procedures to avoid accidental skin puncture by a contaminated needle and adhere to the following rules to ensure your safety and that of the patient:

- Wear protective gloves when performing injections or when dealing with any object contaminated by blood.
- Dispose of all syringes and needles without recapping, placing them directly into a puncture-proof sharps container.
- Always follow established rules of aseptic technique.
- Read the label three times: before drawing up the medication, after drawing it up, and before administration.
- Check patient identification using two identifiers before administration.
- Monitor the patient carefully for side effects.

CHARTING OF MEDICATIONS

When a medication is given by a physician or under the physician's supervision, it is always recorded in the patient's medical record. The notation should include the time of day, the name of the drug, the dose, and the route of administration. A typical entry in the medication record might read, "6/21/16, 14:50 (time on a 24-hour clock), diphenhydramine, 50 mg, PO." Each entry must include the identification of the person who charted it. Initials alone are not considered to be adequate identification. If a medication record calls for initials, there is another place in the chart (often on the same page) where each set of initials is identified with the signer's full name. For legal reasons, all who chart medication must use the exact procedure established by the health care facility.

If an emergency prevents the charting of medications at the time they are given, make a written notation of the time, drug, and dose so that accurate information will be available when the charting is completed. If this is not done, the pressure of the situation may lead to confusion of the facts, and the time, sequence, and doses of several medications may be forgotten or charted incorrectly. Any medication prescribed or administered by a physician should be charted by the physician; if it is charted by someone else, the entry should be countersigned by the physician. The legal significance of complete accountability in such situations cannot be overemphasized.

Physicians enter an account of the procedure and any medications given in the patient's medical record. When you are involved in medication administration, you are responsible for checking that the drug, time, dose, and route of administration are noted and clearly expressed. This avoids the possibility of duplication or omission. Charting routines vary. Familiarize yourself with the routine of your facility. Charting is discussed in greater detail in Chapter 20.

SUMMARY

Depending on the facility and the job description, you may be called upon to play an important role in the administration of medications. Knowledge of common medications and their proper administration will enable you to fulfill this role.

Medications are commonly administered by the oral, topical, or parenteral route, and each route requires specialized knowledge and equipment. IV access systems may also be used in your facility, depending on the procedures performed. The monitoring of these systems requires that you have a high degree of knowledge and awareness. Supervised clinical practice and familiarity with institutional procedures are required to implement this knowledge.

The charting of medication and the monitoring of patients are significant aspects of medication administration and must not be overlooked. You must recognize the potential harm and legal complications that could result from medication administration errors and strive for error-free performance.

Chapter 24

Medical Laboratory Skills

At the conclusion of this chapter, you will be able to:

- Demonstrate general knowledge of laboratory safety (Standard Precautions)
- Identify basic venipuncture equipment, state its purpose, and demonstrate its correct use
- Provide appropriate patient instructions for venipuncture
- Identify an appropriate puncture site for venipuncture
- Demonstrate correct procedures for handling blood specimens
- Dispose of contaminated items correctly and safely
- Solve common problems encountered when collecting blood specimens
- Identify basic equipment for urinalysis, state its purpose, and demonstrate its correct use
- Provide appropriate patient instructions for urine specimen collection
- Explain correct timing and technique of urine specimen collection
- Demonstrate correct step-by-step performance of macroscopic and chemical urinalysis
- Accurately record urinalysis test results
- List urinalysis findings that indicate the need for microscopic evaluation
- Demonstrate proper disposal of urine and contaminated items
- Solve common problems encountered with urinalysis

Key Terms

analyte
antecubital fossa
biohazardous waste
centrifuge
clean-catch midstream specimen (CCMS)
glans penis
hematuria

hemolysis
reagent strips
sharps
tourniquet
urethral meatus
urinalysis
venipuncture

Limited x-ray machine operators who work in a clinic or medical office may be expected to perform basic laboratory procedures in addition to their work in the radiology department. The purpose of this chapter is to provide basic information regarding the skills of collecting specimens of both blood and urine and performing simple urine tests. On-the-job instruction and supervision, followed by clinical practice, are necessary parts of the learning process to become proficient in these skills.

STANDARD PRECAUTIONS

As stated in Chapter 21, Standard Precautions were developed to protect the health care worker from infection with blood-borne pathogens, such as hepatitis B virus, hepatitis C virus, and human immunodeficiency virus. The essence of Standard Precautions is embodied in the statement that *all patients' body fluids are potentially infectious.* The basics of Standard Precautions as they relate to handling blood and urine are discussed in the sections that follow. They include hand hygiene, barrier techniques, and proper disposal of biohazardous waste.

Hand Hygiene

Hand hygiene (see Chapter 21) should always be carried out before and after all patient care and after removing protective gloves. Hand-washing is always an acceptable form of hand hygiene, but use of alcohol-based hand rubs is also acceptable as long as the hands are not visibly soiled or contaminated with blood or body fluids.

Barrier Techniques

Protective gloves should be worn when body fluids are handled, when mucous membranes or open wounds are touched, or when there is contact with contaminated skin, equipment, or counter surfaces. Protective gloves are usually made of latex, but vinyl gloves may be used if the worker or the patient has a latex allergy. Liquid-resistant gowns or laboratory coats with knit cuffs are required if there is a risk of splashing. These must be properly laundered on a daily basis and removed when soiled with blood or other body fluids. Disposable gowns are also available. Masks and protective eyewear or face shields are needed when splashing is anticipated.

Biohazardous Waste Disposal

Biohazardous waste is any refuse that is poisonous or dangerous to living creatures. **Sharps** is a term that refers to any objects that can puncture the skin, such as needles, glass tubes, glass slides, and finger lancets. Sharps must be discarded into an appropriate sharps container that is puncture-proof and marked with the biohazard symbol (Fig. 24-1). Contaminated nonsharps (items that cannot

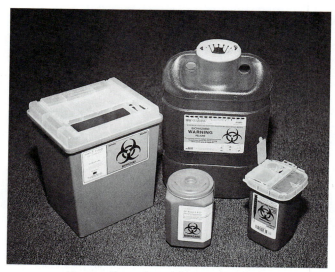

Fig. 24-1 Examples of sharps containers.

puncture the skin, such as a gauze sponge) must be disposed of into a biohazard bag. When full, the containers and bags should be autoclaved or taken away by a commercial biohazard waste company. Be sure not to fill containers beyond the line indicated by the manufacturer and never try to remove any item that has been placed in a biohazardous waste container.

VENIPUNCTURE

Venipuncture is the technique of entering a vein with a needle to withdraw a blood sample and is the most common method of blood collection. Although many different veins can be used for venipuncture, the veins in the **antecubital fossa** (the front side of the elbow) are most commonly used and are the sites discussed in this chapter.

Equipment and Supplies

Evacuated Blood Collection Tubes

The evacuated tube system is most commonly used in routine venipuncture. Tubes are made of plastic and come in a variety of sizes to accommodate the amount of specimen required (Fig. 24-2). Specimen tube volumes commonly range from 2 to 15 ml. The tube stoppers may be entirely made of rubber or may consist of rubber inserted into a protective plastic cap. The stoppers are color coded to indicate the presence or absence of specific additives. Table 24-1 summarizes the most commonly used stopper colors, additives, types of specimens, and associated tests. The colors of the stoppers are universal for all manufacturers. However, a tube with a protective plastic cap may have a different color than its counterpart with a plain rubber stopper.

Tubes with additives must be gently inverted after filling to ensure adequate mixing. Tubes without additives must be filled before tubes with additives. The vacuum in

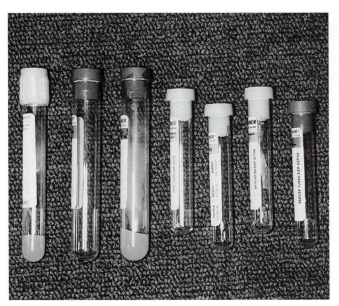

Fig. 24-2 Evacuated blood collection tubes.

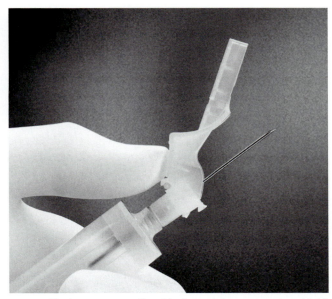

Fig. 24-3 Venipuncture needle with sharps injury protection shield.

the tube is expended once the stopper is punctured. For this reason, a tube cannot be used a second time following an unsuccessful venipuncture. Tubes are marked with expiration dates, and outdated tubes must not be used. The laboratory facility that does your testing can provide information regarding tubes and specimen requirements.

Needles

Standard venipuncture needles are 21 gauge and are either 1 or 1½ inches long. One-inch-long needles are adequate for most patients. Smaller-gauge needles are available for patients with thinner-than-average veins. Needles are sterile when purchased and can be used only once. They are packaged in protective plastic containers that are closed with a paper seal. A needle should be discarded if the seal appears broken.

A standard venipuncture needle is actually two needles attached to a threaded plastic hub. The needle mounted to the threaded side of the hub is designed to puncture the stopper of the evacuated collection tube. The other

needle, mounted to the nonthreaded end of the hub, is for puncturing the skin. The threaded hub screws into the needle holder.

The U.S. Occupational Safety and Health Administration (OSHA) establishes standards for safety in the workplace and provides specific recommendations for the protection of health care workers in situations where exposure to bloodborne pathogens is a possibility. Needles for venipuncture that are compliant with OSHA standards have protective shields or blunting features. A needle with a sharps injury protection shield is illustrated in Fig. 24-3. A blunt-tipped blood-drawing needle has a dull, rounded tip that moves forward through the needle and past the sharp point with a push on the collection tube. The blunt tip of this needle can be activated before it is removed from the vein.

Needle Holder

The needle holder, sometimes called a *barrel*, is a plastic tube designed to grip the venipuncture needle and support the vacuum tube during specimen collection.

Table 24-1

Guide to Commonly Used Evacuated Blood Specimen Tubes

Stopper Color	Additive	Type of Specimen	Common Use
Red	None	Serum	Chemistry, serology
Red/gray mottled	Clot activator	Serum	Chemistry, serology
Gold	Clot activator	Serum	Chemistry, serology
Green*	Heparin	Plasma	Chemistry
Gray*	Sodium fluoride	Serum	Glucose
Lavender*	EDTA	Whole blood	Hematology
Light blue*	Sodium citrate	Plasma	Coagulation

*Same color for plain rubber stopper and plastic protective cap.
Italics indicate tube with plastic protective cap.
EDTA, Ethylenediaminetetraacetic acid.

Holders come in different sizes to accommodate different sizes of collection tubes. The needle is screwed into the holder and gently tightened without excessive force (Fig. 24-4).

Until recently, needle holders were considered to be reusable items; however, because they frequently become contaminated by blood, the U.S. Environmental Protection Agency (EPA) now recommends the use of disposable needle holders. Disposable holders may be discarded directly into the sharps container without removing the needle.

Needles and butterfly sets with preattached needle holders are now available with sharps injury protection features (Fig. 24-5). These blood collection sets eliminate the need to handle the needle and attach it to the barrel. The entire unit can be discarded into a sharps container.

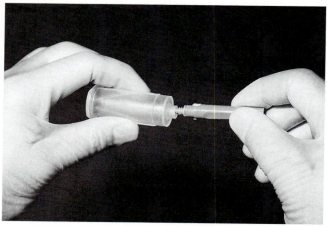

Fig. 24-4 Attaching a venipuncture needle to a needle holder.

Tourniquet

A **tourniquet** is a tight band placed around the arm to facilitate distention of the vein. Types of tourniquets include simple rubber straps, 1-inch-wide latex strips, and Penrose tubing. These tourniquets must be applied with a slip loop for easy one-handed release. Latex tourniquets should not be used on patients with a latex allergy. Rubber strap tourniquets with Velcro closures are also available. For venipuncture in the antecubital fossa, the tourniquet is applied approximately one hand-width above the elbow crease. The tourniquet should be applied tightly enough to cause distention of the veins without causing discomfort or turning the skin white around the tourniquet. Additional information about tourniquet application and removal is provided later in this chapter.

Alcohol Wipes

Alcohol wipes are used to cleanse the venipuncture site. Because routine venipuncture is not a sterile procedure, 70% isopropyl alcohol prep wipes are adequate. Antiseptic wipes containing povidone-iodine (Betadine) instead of alcohol must be used if the specimen is being collected for blood cultures or for blood alcohol testing. Cleansing should begin at the proposed puncture site and move outward with a circular motion. Once cleansed, the puncture site must not be touched again.

Gauze or Cotton Balls

After the puncture site is cleansed, the alcohol should be allowed to dry completely, or it can be wiped with a dry gauze sponge or cotton ball. Residual alcohol on the skin can cause discomfort during the puncture. Alcohol can

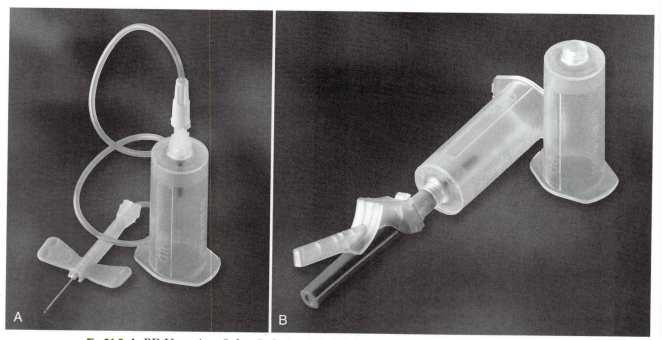

Fig. 24-5 A, BD Vacutainer Safety-Lok (BD, Franklin Lakes, NJ) butterfly-type blood collection set with preattached holder. **B,** BD Vacutainer Eclipse (BD, Franklin Lakes, NJ) blood collection needle with preattached holder.

also enter the needle and can lead to **hemolysis** (rupture of red blood cells). The dry gauze or cotton ball can also be used to cover the puncture site after the needle is removed from the arm following completion of the venipuncture.

Bandage

An adhesive strip bandage is used to cover the puncture. Alternatively, the gauze or cotton ball can be used as a bandage by taping it in place. When patients are allergic to tape, gauze may be wrapped around the arm and secured with tape so that the bandage is secure but the tape is not in contact with the skin. A pressure bandage may be needed if the patient is taking anticoagulant medications such as warfarin (Coumadin), heparin, or Plavix.

Biohazard Waste Receptacles

The used needle is disposed of into a sharps container, together with the disposable needle holder. There are various types of sharps containers (see Fig. 24-1). Contaminated nonsharp items are disposed of into a biohazard bag.

Splash Shield

Use of a splash shield is required when uncapping filled evacuated tubes. Even when the tube is fully filled, a small amount of vacuum pressure remains in the tube. As the cap is removed and air rushes into the tube, an aerosol or fine spray of blood is created. The splash shield provides a protective barrier between the tube and the face when the tube is uncapped. Usually a simple plastic shield or face mask is used. As mentioned earlier, some manufacturers produce evacuated tubes with a stopper covered by a plastic cap. The plastic cap acts to minimize aerosol production but does not eliminate the need for a shield. Under most circumstances, you will not be required to open evacuated blood tubes. They will be sent to the laboratory without opening.

Patient and Equipment Preparation

The first step is to appropriately identify the patient and provide a basic explanation of the procedure. As with medication administration, two identifiers are essential for proper patient identification. Ask the patient to state his or her full name and birth date. Any foreign materials in the mouth, such as candy or chewing gum, should be removed. Most ambulatory patients comfortably tolerate routine venipuncture in a seated position. Standard phlebotomy chairs are best for this purpose. The patient should lie supine if fainting or light-headedness was experienced during previous venipunctures. Perform hand hygiene and apply protective gloves. Examine both arms to identify a suitable venipuncture site. Do not perform venipuncture above the site where intravenous fluids are being infused. Avoid sites where excess scarring is evident near the proposed puncture site and do not use the arm on the side of a mastectomy. Patients often know which arm has the best veins. The arm should be fully extended at the elbow and supported. The tourniquet is then applied, and the veins palpated.

In the antecubital fossa, the median cubital vein is most commonly used. However, the cephalic or basilic vein also can be used (Fig. 24-6). Choice of a vein is based

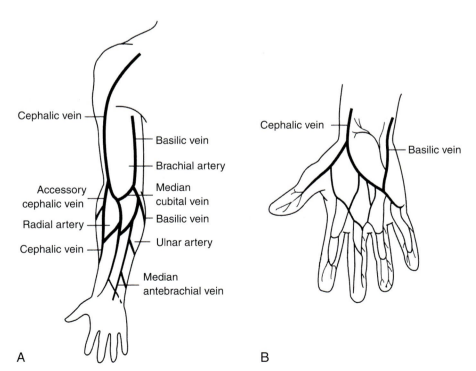

Fig. 24-6 Veins used for venipuncture. **A,** Veins of anterior aspect of forearm. **B,** Superficial veins of dorsal aspect of hand.

on palpation, not visualization. Veins do not pulsate; they palpate with a spongy feel, whereas tendons are hard. Locate the vein best anchored within the subcutaneous tissues. Palpation assesses the depth and course of the vein.

Venipuncture is performed from an ergonomically safe standing position with all of the equipment organized and within easy reach. Open the needle by breaking the paper seal with a twist and pulling it apart. Screw the needle into the holder and discard the empty cap. The first tube can be placed into the holder, but do not engage the stopper onto the internal needle.

Step-by-step Venipuncture Procedure

1. Double-check the requisition and prepare the necessary specimen tubes. Attach the needle to the needle holder.
2. Greet and identify the patient and provide a simple explanation of the procedure.
3. Perform hand hygiene and don protective gloves.
4. Apply the tourniquet; it should not be applied for more than 1 minute; if more time is needed, the tourniquet should be released for at least 3 minutes before continuing.
5. With the arm extended at the elbow, have the patient clench the fist.
6. Palpate the veins and determine the puncture site.
7. Cleanse the site with alcohol and wipe dry or allow to air dry; do not touch the site after cleansing.
8. Grasp the holder with the thumb on top and the second and third fingers below.
9. Uncap the needle by pulling the cap straight off without twisting; the beveled edge of the needle should point upward.
10. With the other hand, anchor the vein by placing the second finger above and the thumb below the puncture site, stretch the skin, and apply gentle downward pressure (Fig. 24-7).

11. Tell the patient to expect a "stick"; allow the patient to watch if desired.
12. Puncture the skin at an angle of approximately 40 degrees; use a shallower angle if the vein is superficial.
13. Thread approximately half of the needle into the vein.
14. Anchor the holder and needle in place by applying gentle downward pressure; the fifth finger can be wrapped around the elbow.
15. Engage the first tube onto the internal needle, taking care to not allow the needle in the arm to move; the tube should begin to fill (Fig. 24-8).
16. Remove the tourniquet and instruct the patient to relax the fist; the tube will fill until the vacuum is expended.
17. Remove the filled tube, still taking care that the needle does not move in the arm. If the tube contains an additive, it can be gently inverted at this time or as the next tube fills.
18. Fill additional tubes (if required) in the same manner. Fill tubes without additives first, then fill tubes with additives.
19. Remove the last tube from the holder before removing the needle from the arm.
20. If using needles with blunt tip technology, activate the safety feature at this point.
21. Quickly withdraw the needle from the arm and immediately place gauze or a cotton ball over the puncture site. Apply pressure. Do not allow the patient to bend the arm; the patient can be asked to apply the pressure.
22. Immediately dispose of the needle in the appropriate sharps container. Warning: *Never* recap used needles.
23. Label the tubes according to the standards of the laboratory.
24. After 5 minutes, check the puncture site to ensure that bleeding has stopped.
25. Apply a bandage. Provide appropriate instructions to be followed in case the puncture site starts to bleed after the patient is dismissed.

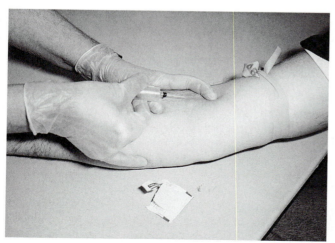

Fig. 24-7 Vein anchored with needle about to puncture.

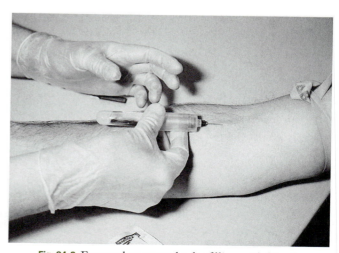

Fig. 24-8 Engaged evacuated tube filling with blood.

26. Dismiss the patient.
27. Appropriately dispose of biohazardous material.
28. Clean the work area.
29. Remove gloves and repeat hand hygiene.
30. Initiate transport of the specimens to the laboratory.

Common Problems

Tube Does Not Fill With Blood

When a tube fails to fill with blood, the needle is not properly situated in the lumen (channel) of the vein. The needle may be under the skin but not within the vein. The needle may have gone too deep and passed all the way through the vein, but more commonly the needle lies on one side of the vein under the skin. When this occurs, gently palpate the position of the tip of the needle. The vein can be anchored again, and the needle redirected into the vein. Withdraw the needle slightly if it is determined that the initial puncture went too deep. This skill takes practice and experience. Always be sensitive to the patient. Some individuals will not tolerate this procedure. The venipuncture may need to be discontinued and attempted again on the other arm.

Patient Feels Faint

Some patients become faint during a routine venipuncture. The complexion may turn pale, and the person may appear slightly sweaty. At this point the patient may not be able to respond verbally to questions. If the patient is seated, it is best to discontinue the procedure and assist the patient to lie down. Once the patient has recovered, retry the procedure, preferably using the other arm, while the patient is still lying supine. See Chapter 22 for further discussion of syncope and appropriate response to this condition.

URINALYSIS

Urinalysis is the physical, microscopic, and/or chemical examination of urine. A routine urinalysis consists of three components: (1) macroscopic examination of physical characteristics, (2) chemical analysis performed with a urine reagent strip, and (3) microscopic examination of the urine sediment.

Equipment and Supplies

Reagent Strips

Urine **reagent strips,** sometimes referred to as *dipsticks* (Fig. 24-9), are used to perform from 1 to 10 tests. Small pads of an absorbent material are impregnated with chemical reagents and attached to plastic strips. Once dipped into urine, a pad will change color. The intensity of the color is proportional to the concentration of the **analyte** (substance being tested). Essential information is

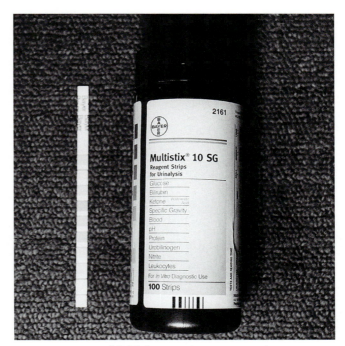

Fig. 24-9 Multiple test urine reagent strips.

provided with each bottle of reagent strips, and you should be thoroughly familiar with the manufacturer's instructions and recommendations. Containers are marked with expiration dates, and the strips should be discarded if they are outdated because they will not produce accurate results. To protect the strips from moisture and light, the bottle should be capped immediately after a strip is removed; the bottle should be stored at room temperature.

Quality assurance that involves periodic testing using commercially prepared urine controls should be a part of the facility's standard quality control procedure. Control testing supplies should be available from the laboratory that provides clinical testing for your facility. Instructions will accompany the supplies.

Collection Containers (Cups)

A variety of collection containers is available (Fig. 24-10). Some have caps that should be used if the specimen will not be analyzed immediately following collection. Some have pour spouts that facilitate filling the urinalysis tubes. The containers should be clean and dry and are used only once.

Urinalysis Tubes

Urinalysis tubes are generally made of plastic and must be clear (see Fig. 24-10). They can hold up to 15 ml of urine. Tubes may come with optional caps that should be used if the specimen will not be analyzed immediately.

Gauze Sponges and Cleansing Solution

Gauze sponges moistened with an appropriate cleansing solution are used to cleanse the patient before urine collection. Standard 2 × 2–inch gauze sponges are adequate.

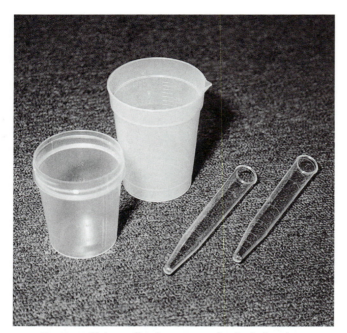

Fig. 24-10 Urine collection cups and urinalysis tubes.

A variety of appropriate cleansing solutions is available. Towelettes premoistened with cleansing solution are also available in individual packets and can be used in place of gauze sponges.

Specimen Collection

Because urine collection is such a simple procedure, proper care is not always taken. Improperly collected urine may yield incorrect test results.

Timing

The greatest amount of diagnostic information is obtained when a first morning specimen is collected. This urine has incubated in the bladder during the night and is collected as soon as the patient awakens in the morning. However, it is often not practical to obtain a first morning specimen. Urine collected regardless of the time of day is termed a *random specimen*. Some diagnostic information may be sacrificed when a random specimen is obtained. The ordering physician must determine which specimen best meets clinical requirements.

Technique of Collection

Urine should always be collected via the **clean-catch midstream specimen (CCMS)** technique. The tissues adjacent to the **urethral meatus** (the external opening of the urethra) are cleansed with an appropriate cleansing solution. The initial portion of the urine stream is discarded, the middle portion of the stream is collected for analysis, and the last portion of the urine stream is also discarded.

The precollection cleansing technique varies according to gender. A female patient spreads the labia and

cleanses in an anterior to posterior direction with three separate gauze sponges moistened with cleansing solution or with premoistened towelettes. Separate sponges are used to cleanse each side of the urinary opening, and a third sponge is wiped directly over the urethral meatus. A dry sponge is then wiped directly over the meatus. The labia are kept spread, and a small amount of urine is passed into the toilet. At least 15 ml of urine is collected into an appropriate collection container. The remaining urine in the bladder is then passed into the toilet.

A circumcised male simply cleanses the **glans penis,** the conical tip of the penis. Using sponges moistened with cleansing solution, he wipes with a circular motion from the center outward. An uncircumcised male must first retract the foreskin and keep it retracted during the cleansing and collection. A dry sponge is used to wipe directly over the meatus. As described previously for the female patient, at least 15 ml of urine is passed into a collection cup from the middle portion of the urine stream.

Specimen Testing

The urine should be analyzed as quickly as possible, within 1 hour at most after collection, because some analytes deteriorate if analysis is delayed. If a delay is unavoidable, the specimen should be capped, protected from the light, and refrigerated until the analysis is performed. Refrigerated urine should be allowed to warm to room temperature before analysis. After being gently remixed, the urine is transferred into a clear plastic urinalysis tube.

Macroscopic Examination

Color and appearance (clarity) are judged by visual examination of urine in a clear plastic urinalysis tube. These characteristics should not be assessed with the urine in the collection cup. Urine color normally ranges from colorless to yellow. Shades of yellow should be reported with modifiers, such as *light yellow* or *dark yellow*. Appearance of urine normally ranges from clear to slightly hazy. Degrees of haziness are reported as *slightly hazy, moderately hazy, markedly hazy, cloudy,* or *turbid.* Haziness greater than slight may indicate the need for a microscopic examination of the urine sediment. See the following guidelines for contacting the physician in such an instance.

Chemical Analysis

Chemical analysis is performed using a urine reagent strip. Typical reagent strips test for 10 different components or characteristics of urine: glucose, ketones, blood, bilirubin, protein, nitrite, leucocyte esterase, urobilinogen, specific gravity, and pH.

Timing is critical, and the test result must be read at the time indicated by the manufacturer. The end-point color of each pad on the strip is compared with a color

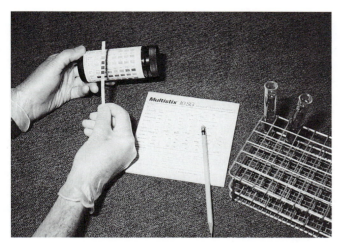

Fig. 24-11 Reading reagent strip and recording results.

chart attached to the reagent strip bottle, and the result is recorded. Some manufacturers provide report forms that correlate directly with the strip (Fig. 24-11). Most test results are reported as *negative* (normal, or none detected), *trace*, *1+*, *2+*, *3+*, or *4+*. Alternatively, test results may be recorded as negative, trace, small, moderate, or large. Specific gravity and pH are recorded as specific numerical values. Physicians are trained to interpret the results regardless of the reporting system employed.

Step-by-step Reagent Strip Urinalysis

1. Wear protective gloves.
2. Check the expiration date on the reagent strip container to be sure the strips are not outdated.
3. Remove a strip and immediately recap the bottle. Do not touch the test pads.
4. Immerse the strip in the urine specimen, taking care that all pads contact the urine. Timing begins when the strip is immersed.
5. Immediately remove the strip and blot the edge of the strip on a paper towel to remove excess urine.
6. Carefully time the test.
7. Read and record the results.
8. Flush the remaining urine down the toilet or wash it down a sink drain with cold water.
9. Discard the used reagent strip, contaminated paper towel, urinalysis tube, and collection cup into a biohazard bag.
10. Remove gloves and perform hand hygiene.

Common Problems

Collection and Handling Problems

The most common problems encountered in routine urinalysis are associated with specimen collection and handling. Failure to use the CCMS technique may result in bacterial contamination of the specimen. Analysis of urine longer than 1 hour after collection, especially if the urine is not refrigerated, may produce erroneous results.

Unmatchable End-point Color

Sometimes an end-point color not matching the reference chart cannot be explained. It may be because of a faulty strip. The specimen should be retested. If the problem persists, try a different bottle of strips. If this does not resolve the problem, the urine may contain a substance that interferes with the determination of a specific analyte. The specimen should be sent to the laboratory for analysis by a different method.

Occasionally the urine color is abnormal, most often because of a medication. The abnormal urine color may interfere with appropriate color development on the strip. An alternative method of analyzing the chemical analytes is required in this situation.

Multiple End-point Colors

Multiple end-point colors may occur if excess urine on the strip is not properly blotted (see step 5 earlier). This allows reagents from one test pad to run into another.

An unusual result of multiple end-point colors sometimes occurs within the test area for blood. It may occasionally reveal a green speckled pattern overlying an orange background caused by the presence of intact red blood cells in the urine. This is reported as "positive for nonhemolyzed blood."

Menstrual Blood Contamination

One of the most common causes of **hematuria** (blood in the urine) is urine collection from females during menstruation. Often a routine urinalysis can be delayed until the menstrual bleeding has stopped. If it is necessary to perform a urinalysis during the menstrual period, the CCMS technique is employed immediately following the insertion of a fresh tampon.

Indications for Microscopic Examination

Microscopic examination of urine sediment is beyond the scope of this text. This analysis should be performed by a trained medical technologist or experienced physician. However, if you are performing the first two components of the routine urinalysis, you need to be aware that the urine sediment should be examined when there are certain abnormal results from the assessment of physical characteristics or from the chemical analyses. Most commonly the following test results, either individually or in combination, should be brought to the physician's attention *before discarding the urine specimen* so an appropriate decision can be made about performing a sediment examination:

- Hazy urine (more than slightly hazy)
- Positive result for glucose, protein, blood, nitrite, or leukocyte esterase

When a microscopic analysis of sediment is indicated, the urine will be centrifuged while still in the urinalysis tube. A **centrifuge** is a special electric device that spins the tubes rapidly to separate solids from liquid. The sediment that accumulates at the bottom of the tube is then examined under a microscope by an appropriately qualified technologist or physician.

Miscellaneous Laboratory Tests

Many simple laboratory test kits are available for use in the diagnosis of various specific conditions, including pregnancy, infectious mononucleosis, rheumatoid arthritis, and colorectal cancer (stool guaiac test for occult blood). You may be expected to perform some of these procedures and to instruct patients regarding specimen collection. The manufacturers of these kits provide detailed instructions regarding required specimens, essential equipment, testing procedure, expected test result parameters, and safety precautions. Read these instructions carefully and follow them exactly. Consult with clinical laboratory personnel if you have any questions.

SUMMARY

Laboratory skills involve contact with potentially infectious body fluids, so Standard Precautions are employed for safety.

Venipuncture is used to obtain blood specimens for a variety of tests. After the procedure has been explained to the patient and the equipment has been prepared, a suitable vein is selected and the vein is entered using a sterile needle attached to a needle holder. One or more evacuated tubes are then filled with blood. It is important that the correct tubes be selected and that the tubes are correctly handled for accurate test results.

Urinalysis involves proper specimen collection technique, prompt and correct specimen handling, and accurate evaluation. The limited operator or medical assistant may perform macroscopic and chemical analyses. When microscopic analysis is required, qualified personnel perform it. You must identify the need for this procedure and provide appropriate notification.

Chapter 25

Additional Procedures for Assessment and Diagnosis

Learning Objectives

At the conclusion of this chapter, you will be able to:

- Demonstrate the correct procedure for weighing and measuring a patient
- Conduct a Snellen test for far-distance visual acuity and properly record the results
- Conduct a reading test for near-distance visual acuity and properly record the results
- Conduct an Ishihara test for color perception and record the results
- Instruct and prepare a patient for electrocardiography and perform the test
- List the leads recorded for a standard 12-lead electrocardiogram and code them correctly
- Recognize common artifacts seen on electrocardiograms and list steps to be taken to correct each
- State the purpose of forced expiration spirometry and two significant measurements involved in this test
- Instruct and prepare the patient for a forced expiration spirometry test and conduct the test
- Discriminate between acceptable and unacceptable forced expiration maneuvers

Key Terms

cardiac ischemia
ECG leads
electrocardiogram (ECG, EKG)
electrocardiograph
electrodes
exercise tolerance test (stress test)
forced expiration test
forced expiratory volume (FEV)
forced vital capacity (FVC)
glottic closure
hemoptysis
hyperopia

Ishihara test
myopia
presbyopia
Snellen alphabet chart
Snellen E chart
spirogram
spirometer
spirometry
standardization mark
stylus
visual acuity

In small clinics and physicians' offices, it is often the case that x-ray personnel must perform other functions when there is not enough radiography to keep them occupied. In these circumstances, it is common for personnel to be cross-trained in a number of diagnostic procedures and patient assessment skills. Some patient assessment skills have been described in other chapters. Vital signs, for example, are explained in Chapter 22 and the techniques for obtaining blood and urine samples are covered in Chapter 24. This chapter provides an introduction to additional skills that will enhance your value in the clinical setting, including weighing and measuring patients, performing vision screening tests, recording electrocardiograms, and conducting forced expiration spirometry examinations.

These procedures are not difficult to learn and are often taught in the employment setting without formal instruction. You will need a clinical orientation to the equipment used in your facility, practical instruction in its use, and a degree of supervised clinical practice to become competent. Additional information about these procedures, including variations for pediatric patients, may be found in nursing and medical assisting texts. Texts devoted to electrocardiography and pulmonary functioning testing, including spirometry, are also available.

MEASURING WEIGHT AND HEIGHT

Measuring patients' weight is an important aspect of patient assessment. Weight is sometimes used to determine medication dosage. In addition, any sudden weight gain or weight loss may be a significant diagnostic sign. Patients whose treatment involves a dietary regimen for weight loss or weight gain will be monitored to determine the effectiveness of the treatment. Infants and children are weighed and measured to monitor their growth and development. For these reasons, many facilities routinely weigh patients on each visit.

Because the height of adult patients is not subject to sudden change, height is usually measured only on the first visit or as part of a comprehensive physical examination.

Measuring Weight

Some facilities use upright balance scales to obtain weight measurements. These scales have two calibration bars: upper and lower. The calibration bars are connected on the ends to form a rectangle and mounted on each bar is a sliding weight (Fig. 25-1). This rectangle tips when the scale is not in balance. An indicator on the right end shows when the rectangle is level and the scale is balanced. The lower calibration bar is divided into 50-lb increments, with grooves for placement of the

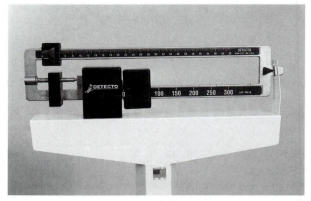

Fig. 25-1 Balance scale has two calibration bars. Lower weight is set in grooves indicating 50-lb increments. Upper weight slides smoothly over 50-lb range in ¼-lb increments.

weight at each setting. The upper calibration bar is divided into pounds and quarter pounds with a range of 0 to 50. The upper calibration bar has no grooves and the weight slides smoothly along it. The patient's weight is determined by adding the weight measurements from the two calibration scales.

Patients are usually weighed in their normal clothing. Any heavy outer clothing, such as a jacket, is removed, as are the patient's shoes. Paper may be placed on the scale platform to prevent transmission of disease. The scale should be located in a nonpublic area because many patients are self-conscious about their weight. For this reason, take care not to make any comments that might embarrass or upset patients who are sensitive about their weight.

Before the patient steps onto the scale, check to see that the weights on both bars are set exactly at 0 and that the scale is in balance. If the scale is not in balance, adjust the screw at the left end until balance is achieved. The scale platform moves slightly, so the patient may feel insecure while stepping onto it. Assist the patient onto the platform and ensure that the patient's position is stable. The patient must not touch or lean on you or on any object to maintain balance during weight measurement because this will result in an inaccurate reading. All of the patient's weight must be centered over the scale. Instruct the patient to stand very still because it is not possible to balance the scale when the platform is in motion.

To obtain the weight measurement, move the weight on the lower calibration bar to the highest groove on the bar that does not cause the scale to tip. Be certain that the weight is properly situated in the groove. Then, slowly move the upper weight until the scale is in balance (Fig. 25-2). Note the readings on both calibration bars and add them together. For example, if the lower weight is set at 150 lb and the upper weight is at 11½ lb, the patient's weight is 161½ pounds. Record the patient's weight to the nearest quarter pound.

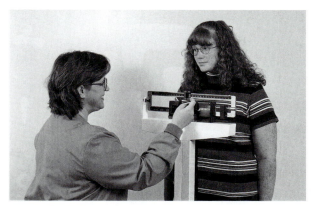

Fig. 25-2 Weighing patient on balance scale.

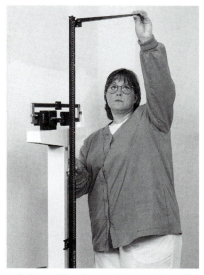

Fig. 25-3 Extend the calibration rod upward until its top is well above the height of the patient's head, and unfold the measuring bar so that it is horizontal.

Some facilities use a digital electronic scale. These battery-powered scales consist of a platform with a digital readout and a foot lever that activates the scale. When the patient is ready to be weighed, activate the scale with your foot. The scale should read 000.0. A dial on the bottom of the scale is used to calibrate the scale to zero, when necessary. Assist the patient onto the scale. Within a few seconds, the scale will indicate the patient's weight. If the reading keeps changing or does not appear promptly, the cause may be patient motion. The procedure must be repeated. Assist the patient in stepping off the scale and provide instruction to hold very still after stepping onto the scale. Reactivate the scale and weigh the patient again.

Measuring Height

Most upright balance scales include a calibration rod for measuring height. The calibration rod extends for height adjustment and has a measuring bar hinged to the top that unfolds into a horizontal position. Use caution and perform the steps of the procedure in the proper order so that movement of the measuring bar does not injure the patient.

Extend the calibration rod upward until its top is well above the patient's head and unfold the measuring bar so that it is horizontal (Fig. 25-3). Instruct the patient to step onto the platform with his or her back to the scale. Assist the patient into this position, if required. Instruct the patient to stand erect and to look straight ahead. Then, slowly lower the measuring bar until it rests gently on top of the patient's head (Fig. 25-4). Hold the bar in position while the patient steps off the scale.

After the patient has stepped down, read the height measurement. This measurement is read at the junction of the movable and stationary portions of the calibration rod (Fig. 25-5) unless the patient is shorter than the stationary portion, in which case it is read directly from the stationary portion. Record the patient's height to the nearest quarter inch.

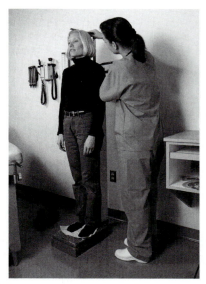

Fig. 25-4 Measuring patient height on balance scale.

VISION SCREENING TESTS

Vision tests to determine the correction needed for eyeglasses or contact lenses are usually performed by an optometrist. Screening tests, however, may be performed in the physician's office and are commonly used to determine whether **visual acuity** (sharpness of perception) is normal or whether a referral to an optometrist is necessary. These tests are usually included in a complete physical examination. Conditions identified by simple screening tests include myopia, hyperopia, presbyopia, and defects in color perception.

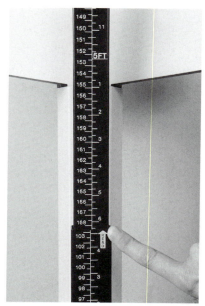

Fig. 25-5 Height measurement is noted at junction of stationary and extending calibration rods.

Myopia is a condition in which the patient is unable to see normally at a distance and is referred to in lay terms as *nearsightedness.* **Hyperopia,** or *farsightedness,* on the other hand, refers to a vision defect that prevents focus at close range. **Presbyopia** is a type of farsightedness that occurs with advancing age, starting between the ages of 40 and 45. Although few people are totally "colorblind," or completely unable to perceive colors, defects in color perception are not uncommon, especially in males.

Distance Vision Assessment

Distance vision is usually evaluated using a **Snellen alphabet chart,** which has various letters of the alphabet arranged in numbered lines by size (Fig. 25-6). For children who have not learned the alphabet or patients who are unfamiliar with the English alphabet, the **Snellen E chart** may be used. This chart contains the block letter E in various positions on numbered lines by size (Fig. 25-7).

When the E chart is used, the patient must first be instructed in how to indicate to the examiner the position of the E. The patient may state the direction of the open end of the letter—left, right, up, or down. For some patients, especially children, it is best to have the patient extend the three middle fingers to demonstrate the position of the E. Before starting the test, instruct the patient and practice using a card with a large E held in various positions at close range (Fig. 25-8). This will ensure that the accuracy of the test is not compromised by confusion in reporting.

Distance vision assessment is usually done with the patient positioned 20 feet from the eye chart. This distance

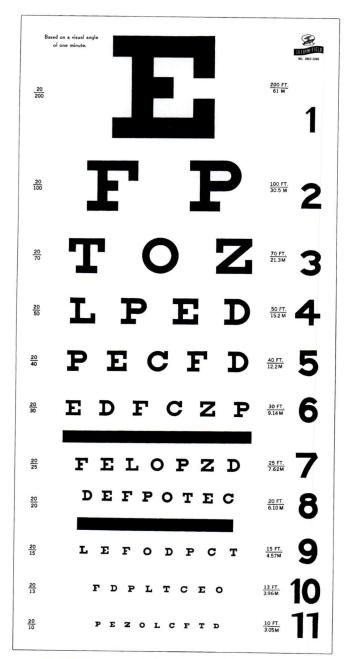

Fig. 25-6 Snellen alphabet distance vision eye chart.

may be marked on the floor with paint or tape to avoid the need to measure it for each test. The chart should be at eye level in a well-lit area. The patient may be standing or seated for the test.

Each eye is examined separately while the opposite eye is covered. An optical occluder that resembles a plastic cup with a straight handle may be used to cover the eye, or the patient may cover the eye with one hand. The same standard procedure should always be followed to minimize error. The right eye is examined first.

The examiner stands near the chart and points to each line, starting at the top (Fig. 25-9). The patient is instructed to read the indicated line without squinting. The

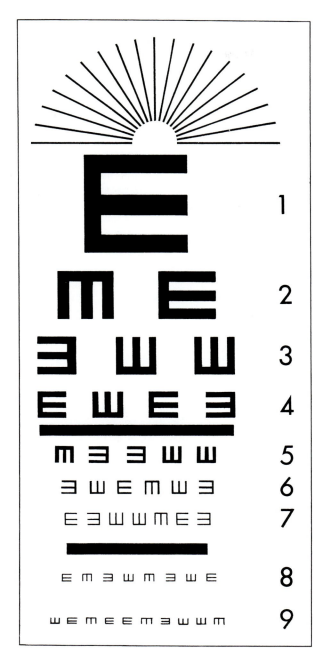

Fig. 25-7 Snellen E distance vision chart.

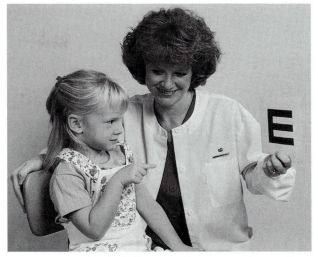

Fig. 25-8 A preschool child is taught to use the Snellen E chart.

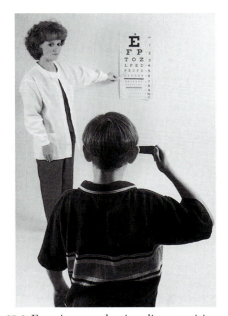

Fig. 25-9 Examiner conducting distance vision test.

examiner notes the lowest line on the chart that the patient can read. If one or two errors are made in any line, the errors are noted and the patient is asked to continue. If more than two errors are made, the previous line is recorded as the lowest line read.

Beside each row of letters on the chart are two numbers with a line between them. The upper number indicates the distance in feet at which the test is conducted, usually 20. The lower number indicates the distance in feet at which a person with normal visual acuity can read the line. This format is used to record measurements of visual acuity. When a patient can read the line marked 20/20, this means that the patient can read at 20 feet what

a person with normal vision can read at 20 feet. This indicates normal distance visual acuity, or 20/20 vision. If the smallest line the patient can read is marked 20/40, this indicates that the patient can read at 20 feet what a person with normal acuity can read at 40 feet and therefore indicates that the patient has less than normal distance acuity.

To chart the test results, state the date and time, the name of the test, and the visual acuity measurement for the smallest line the patient was able to read with each eye. If there were errors in the reading of this line, the measurement is followed by a minus sign and the number of errors. Because distance vision is sometimes tested both with and without corrective lenses, the record must indicate how the test was done by adding the abbreviation *sc* (without correction) or *cc* (with correction). If the patient squinted or blinked excessively or the eyes watered during the test, these observations should also be noted. An example of a record of a distance visual acuity test is: "4/21/2016, 10:30 AM, Snellen test: OD 20/20−1. OS 20/30, sc. Exhibited squinting while reading 20/25 line OD." The abbreviation *OD* indicates the right eye and *OS* refers to the left eye.

Near Vision Assessment

Several different types of cards are available for the assessment of near vision, but the method for using them is similar in each case. The patient holds a card with lines or paragraphs of print that range in size from the height of newspaper headlines to the type used in telephone books or on roadmaps. An example is shown in Fig. 25-10. Cards using pictures and Es are also available for testing patients who do not read English well. The card is held at eye level at a distance of 14 to 16 inches.

The test is conducted in a quiet, well-lit room. The eyes are tested separately, right eye first. The patient may cover one eye during the test or simply close it. If the patient normally wears reading glasses, they are usually also worn for the near vision test.

This test may be scored in several different ways, depending on the chart used. A common method is similar to that used with the Snellen chart, with 14/14 indicating normal vision when the test is conducted at a reading distance of 14 inches. Results of near vision tests are charted in the same manner as those of the Snellen test.

Color Perception Assessment

The classic method of evaluating color perception is the **Ishihara test.** It uses a special book with a multicolor plate on each page. Each plate shows a circle containing dots of various sizes that are arranged to form a number. The background also consists of dots, but the background color is in contrast to the dots that form the number. The number is clearly visible to those with

---

No. 1.
.37M

In the second century of the Christian era, the empire of Rome comprehended the fairest part of the earth, and the most civilized portion of mankind. The frontiers of that extensive monarchy were guarded by ancient renown and disciplined valor. The gentle but powerful influence of laws and manners had gradually cemented the union of the provinces. Their peaceful inhabitants enjoyed and abused the advantages of wealth.

No. 2.
.50M

fourscore years, the public administration was conducted by the virtue and abilities of Nerva, Trajan, Hadrian, and the two Antonines. It is the design of this, and of the two succeeding chapters, to describe the prosperous condition of their empire; and afterwards, from the death of Marcus Antoninus, to deduce the most important circumstances of its decline and fall; a revolution which will ever be remembered, and is still felt by

No. 3.
.62M

the nations of the earth. The principal conquests of the Romans were achieved under the republic; and the emperors, for the most part, were satisfied with preserving those dominions which had been acquired by the policy of the senate, the active emulations of the consuls, and the martial enthusiasm of the people. The seven first centuries were filled with a rapid succession of triumphs; but it was

No. 4.
.75M

reserved for Augustus to relinquish the ambitious design of subduing the whole earth, and to introduce a spirit of moderation into the public councils. Inclined to peace by his temper and situation, it was very easy for him to discover that Rome, in her present exalted situation, had much less to hope than to fear from the chance of arms; and that, in the prosecution of

No. 5.
1.00M

the undertaking became every day more difficult, the event more doubtful, and the possession more precarious, and less beneficial. The experience of Augustus added weight to these salutary reflections, and effectually convinced him that, by the prudent vigor of

No. 6.
1.25M

his counsels, it would be easy to secure every concession which the safety or the dignity of Rome might require from the most formidable barbarians. Instead of exposing his person or his legions to the arrows of the Parthians, he obtained, by an honor-

No. 7.
1.50M

able treaty, the restitution of the standards and prisoners which had been taken in the defeat of Crassus. His generals, in the early part of his reign, attempted the reduction of Ethiopia and Arabia Felix. They marched near a thou-

No. 8.
1.75M

sand miles to the south of the tropic; but the heat of the climate soon repelled the invaders, and protected the unwarlike natives of those sequestered regions

No. 9.
2.00M

The northern countries of Europe scarcely deserved the expense and labor of conquest. The forests and morasses of Germany were

No. 10.
2.25M

filled with a hardy race of barbarians who despised life when it was separated from freedom; and though, on the first

No. 11.
2.50M

attack, they seemed to yield to the weight of the Roman power, they soon, by a signal

Fig. 25-10 Near vision acuity chart.

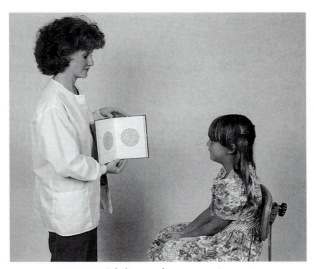

Fig. 25-11 Ishihara color perception test.

normal color perception. The first plate in the book is similar to the others, but the number can be read by anyone, even patients who are totally unable to perceive color. This plate is used as a teaching tool to explain the test to the patient.

It is best to conduct this test in a quiet room, well-lit by daylight, because color is perceived most accurately in natural light. The book is held approximately 30 inches from the patient. It should be at the patient's eye level and perpendicular to the line of sight. Show the patient the first plate and explain the test (Fig. 25-11). The patient should understand that he or she will have 3 seconds to identify each number.

As the patient identifies the number on each plate, record the response and display the next page. If the patient is unable to identify the number in 3 seconds, record an *X* for that plate and continue to the next page. The most commonly used Ishihara test books consist of 14 plates, although some books contain more to provide a more comprehensive and sensitive test. In the usual test book, plates 1 through 11 constitute the basic test. Plates 12, 13, and 14 are used to further evaluate the perception of patients who exhibit red-green color deficiency. If the patient reads 10 plates correctly, color perception is considered normal. If the patient provides normal responses to the first 11 plates, the final 3 plates may be omitted from the test. If the patient can read only 7 or fewer of the plates, the patient is identified as having a color vision deficiency. The test is so structured that a score of 8 or 9 is unlikely. The test is charted by recording the date and time, the test name (Ishihara test), and the patient's response to each plate presented. Any unusual signs exhibited during the test are also recorded. It is helpful to have a special form for recording the results of the Ishihara test. A simple page with spaces for the name of the test, date, patient name, and any other identifying information constitutes the header.

The recording section consists of numbered lines for each plate with space following each number to record the response for the corresponding plate and to note any unusual signs.

ELECTROCARDIOGRAPHY

Electrocardiography is one of the diagnostic tools commonly used in the assessment of heart disease. It provides a graphic representation of tiny electric currents generated within the heart that cause the heart muscle to contract. A machine called an **electrocardiograph** is attached to the patient with cables and **electrodes** (contacts that receive electric signals). Electric impulses from the patient are transmitted to the machine, where they are amplified and translated into signals that cause movement of a balanced tracing pen called a **stylus.** The pattern of these electric impulses is traced by the stylus on graph paper. The resulting tracing is called an **electrocardiogram,** abbreviated **ECG** or **EKG.**

The Cardiac Impulse

It may help your understanding of this section if you first review the basic anatomy and physiology of the heart as described in Chapter 16. The myocardium (heart muscle tissue) is of two types: contracting tissue and conducting tissue.

The cardiac impulse is a tiny electric current that originates at the junction of the vena cava and the right atrium in conducting myocardium called the *sinoatrial (SA) node.* It spreads in circular waves over the atrial walls, causing the atria to contract. The impulse then passes through the *atrioventricular (AV) node,* a second area of conducting myocardium. From this node, it passes through a band of conducting muscle that connects the atria to the ventricles and is called the *bundle of His.* The bundle of His divides into the left and right bundle branches, conducting the cardiac impulse to the left and right ventricles. The bundle branches further divide into *Purkinje fibers,* fine strands of conducting muscle that transmit the impulse to the contracting muscle of the ventricles. The electric conduction system of the heart is illustrated in Fig. 25-12.

The normal cardiac cycle includes atrial contraction, ventricular contraction, and rest. The transmission of the electric wave causing contraction of the chamber walls is called *depolarization.* Each contraction is followed by repolarization, an electric recovery period. Following ventricular repolarization, the heart rests for a moment in a state of polarization, and then the cycle begins again. With normal heart function, this cycle is repeated 60 to 100 times per minute at a regular rate.

The ECG tracing records the electric impulses as deflections above or below a baseline. These deflections

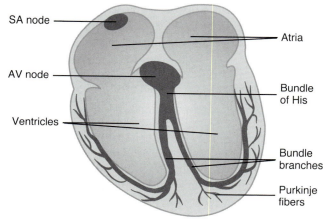

Fig. 25-12 Diagram of the heart identifying the structures involved with the conduction of electric impulses through the heart.

are referred to as *waves* and are labeled P, Q, R, S, and T (Fig. 25-13). Together, the Q, R, and S waves are called the *QRS complex*. The P wave indicates contraction of the atria, the beginning of depolarization. The space between the P wave and the R wave is called the *P-R interval* and represents the time from the beginning of the atrial contraction to the beginning of the ventricular contraction. The QRS complex represents ventricular contraction. The S-T segment indicates the time between ventricular contraction and the beginning of ventricular recovery. The T wave represents ventricular recovery (repolarization). After the T wave, the tracing

shows a straight line, indicating the period of heart rest. On rare occasions, you may observe a small U wave following the T wave. This is an abnormal wave that indicates a low serum potassium level or other metabolic disturbance that affects the conduction of the heart impulses.

The physician observes the morphology (shape), amplitude (height), and duration (graph width) of each wave in relation to the baseline and the other waves. Taken together, these findings enable the physician to detect disturbances in heart rhythm and to identify different types of cardiac disorders.

Electrocardiography Leads

A standard ECG study includes 12 separate recordings from electrode combinations called **ECG leads.** Each lead represents cardiac activity as recorded from a different angle and provides somewhat different information about the heart to the physician. To obtain these various recordings, electrodes are placed in 10 locations: one on each arm and each leg, and six on the chest. The tracing for each lead must be marked or coded so that the physician will know which angle is represented. The resulting 12 leads are described in the following paragraphs and are categorized as standard (limb) leads, augmented leads, and precordial (chest) leads.

There are three limb or standard leads, sometimes referred to as *bipolar leads*. They are designated by Roman numerals I, II, and III. Each uses two limb

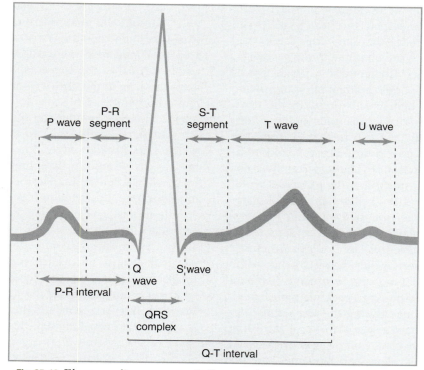

Fig. 25-13 Electrocardiogram waves indicate each portion of the cardiac cycle.

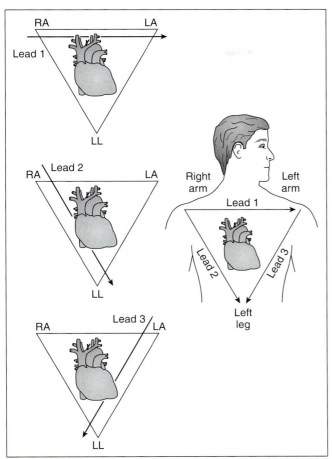

Fig. 25-14 Standard limb leads are recordings of activity of the heart from three angles. *LA*, Left arm; *LL*, left leg; *RA*, right arm.

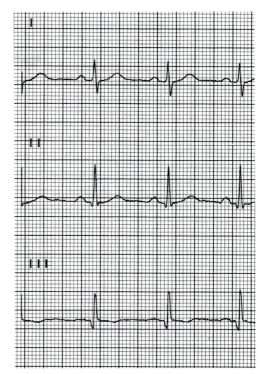

Fig. 25-15 Electrocardiogram leads I, II, and III.

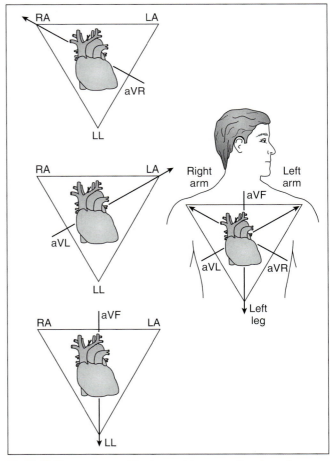

Fig. 25-16 For augmented leads, machine records voltage between one point and the midpoint of two others. *LA*, Left arm; *LL*, left leg; *RA*, right arm.

electrodes to record the electric activity (Fig. 25-14). Lead I records the electric potential (voltage) between the right arm and the left arm. Lead II records the voltage between the right arm and the left leg. Lead III records the voltage between the left arm and the left leg. For all leads, the right leg provides an electric ground. Normal recordings of leads I, II, and III are illustrated in Fig. 25-15.

The three augmented leads are termed *aVR, aVL,* and *aVF.* The *aV* portion of these terms stands for "augmented voltage." *R* indicates the right arm, *L* indicates the left arm, and *F* stands for foot, indicating the left leg. Each of these leads represents the voltage from one limb electrode to the midpoint between two others (Fig. 25-16). Lead aVR represents the voltage measured from the midpoint between the left arm and left leg to the right arm. Lead aVL represents the voltage measured from the midpoint between the right arm and left leg to the left arm. Lead aVF represents voltage measured from the midpoint between the right arm and the left arm to the left leg. Again, the right leg serves as a ground. Normal recordings of the augmented leads are seen in Fig. 25-17.

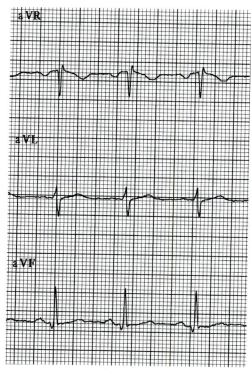

Fig. 25-17 Electrocardiogram leads aVR, aVL, and aVF.

The six precordial or chest leads are designated *V1* through *V6*, each representing a specific location on the chest. These leads record the voltage between the chest wall and a point within the heart. Normal recordings of leads V1 through V6 are seen in Fig. 25-18.

Electrocardiograph Paper and Standardization

ECG paper is divided into squares to facilitate measurement of the waves, intervals, and segments by the physician. Each square measures 1 mm in each dimension and every fifth square is indicated with a bold line (Fig. 25-19). The bold lines form large squares that measure 5 mm × 5 mm.

International agreements have established standards for ECGs to ensure that tracings read anywhere in the world will be interpreted in the same way. When the machine is properly calibrated, 1 mV of electric potential difference will cause the stylus to move vertically 10 mm. This standard ensures that voltage will be interpreted accurately when the graph is read.

To check the calibration of the machine, depress the standardization button using a quick, pecking motion of the finger. Depression of the standardization button generates a 1-mV signal that produces a **standardization mark** on the tracing. The mark should be 10 mm high, approximately 2 mm wide, and rectangular in shape. The operation manual for the machine will provide instructions for making adjustments when the standard mark is not accurate.

Most machines have three standard (STD) position settings: 1 STD, ½ STD, and 2 STD. The 1 STD setting is usually used. If the amplitude of the QRS complex is so great that it causes the stylus to move off the paper, the ½ STD setting should be used. When recording is done at the ½ STD setting, 1 mV causes the stylus to deflect only 5 mm. If the amplitude of the QRS complex is very low, the 2 STD setting may be used to increase the readability of the tracing. At the 2 STD setting, the standard mark will be the height of four large squares (20 mm). Fig. 25-20 shows standardization marks for each STD setting. A standardization mark is usually placed at the beginning of the first lead recording.

The speed of the paper feed must also be standardized for the tracing to be interpreted accurately. The universal recording speed is 25 mm/sec. When the patient's heart rate is very rapid or when certain parts of the complex are too close together for accurate assessment, it may be desirable to adjust the machine so that the paper runs at double speed, 50 mm/sec. This change in setting will extend the recording to twice its normal length and must be noted on the tracing. The difference in appearance of the recording between normal and double speed is illustrated in Fig. 25-21.

Types of Electrocardiography Machines

Electrocardiography machines vary depending on age, manufacturer, and level of technical sophistication. An operator's manual should accompany the machine. Those who perform ECGs should be familiar with the features of the equipment and the guidelines provided in the manual.

The least sophisticated electrocardiographs are single-channel machines that record one lead at a time. The operator selects the lead to be recorded and starts and stops the recording manually. There are six lead wires (machine connections) for the chest. The operator may need to enter a code to identify each lead. The standard marking codes are listed in Table 25-1.

Multichannel machines are available that can record three or six leads at once. A multichannel electrocardiogram is illustrated in Fig. 25-22.

Modern machines, both single-channel and multichannel, are equipped with automatic sequencing capability. Once started, these units proceed automatically from one lead to the next without input from the operator. These machines also identify each lead and place a standardization mark on the tracing. Machines with automatic sequencing usually have a manual option, which permits longer tracings when necessary.

Interpretive electrocardiographs incorporate a computer that analyzes the tracing as it is made and prints the

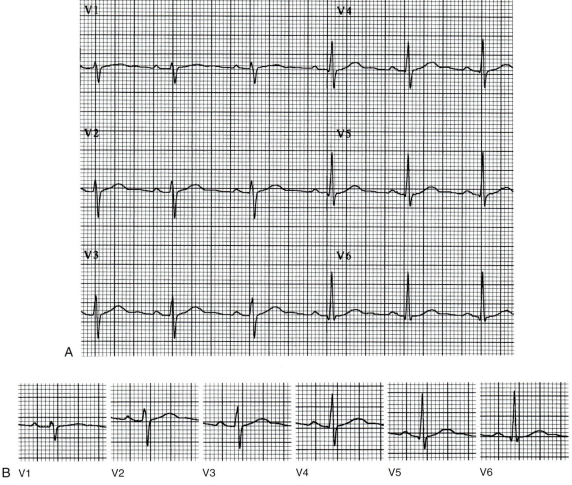

Fig. 25-18 Electrocardiogram chest leads. **A,** Normal recording. **B,** Sequence of individual heart-beats from each of the precordial leads demonstrates progression of electric signal from the sinoatrial node to the left ventricle.

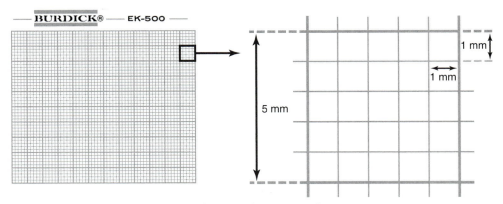

Fig. 25-19 Electrocardiogram graph paper.

ECG interpretation and the specific reason(s) for the interpretation on the tracing. Patient data are entered into the computer before recording begins, and these data are also printed on the ECG.

Telephone transmission equipment is available for sending ECGs to remote locations for interpretation.

Preparation for Electrocardiography

At the time of scheduling, patients should be informed of what to expect and instructed not to apply any lotion or oil to the arms, legs, or chest. They should be advised that they will need to expose their arms, legs, and chest for the application of the electrodes so that they can dress for

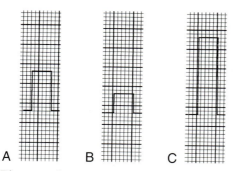

Fig. 25-20 Electrocardiogram standardization marks. **A,** 1 STD. Normal standardization mark is 10 mm high. **B,** ½ STD. One half standardization mark is 5 mm high. **C,** 2 STD. Double standardization mark is 20 mm high.

Table 25-1		
Standard Electrocardiogram Lead Codes		
Leads	**Electrodes Connected**	**Marking Code**
Standard Limb Leads		
Lead I	LA and RA	.
Lead II	LL and RA	. .
Lead III	LL and LA	. . .
Augmented Limb Leads		
aVR	RA and LA-LL	–
aVL	LA and RA-LL	– –
aVF	LL and RA-LA	– – –
Precordial (Chest) Leads		
V_1	C and LA-RA-LL	– .
V_2	C and LA-RA-LL	– . .
V_3	C and LA-RA-LL	– . . .
V_4	C and LA-RA-LL	– . . . .
V_5	C and LA-RA-LL	– . . . . .
V_6	C and LA-RA-LL	– . . . . . .

C, Chest; *LA,* left arm; *LL,* left leg; *RA,* right arm.

convenience in this regard. Patients who have not had an ECG before may assume from the name of the test that electricity will be applied to their bodies. Explain that the test is painless and that only electricity *from* their bodies is being measured. Some facilities provide patient brochures that answer common questions and list instructions.

The room should be quiet and warm, with a table for the patient to lie on. The table should be padded and wide enough for the patient to relax comfortably with both arms and legs fully supported. If the table has metal parts, there must be insulation between these parts and the patient. Small pillows under the patient's head and knees will add comfort and make it easier for the patient to lie still for the duration of the test. It is most convenient to position the table so that the operator is on the patient's left side. The ECG machine should be placed as far from other electric equipment as possible. The power cord should point away from the patient and should not pass under the table.

The patient should disrobe to the waist and wear a gown. Shoes and stockings must be removed and the lower legs exposed. The patient is instructed to lie supine with the legs separated from each other. Any tight clothing should be loosened. Arrange the gown so that the

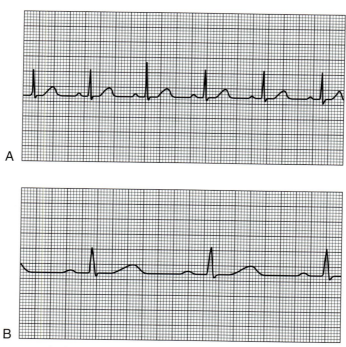

Fig. 25-21 Paper run speed. **A,** Normal recording speed is 28 mm/sec. **B,** Double speed is 50 mm/sec.

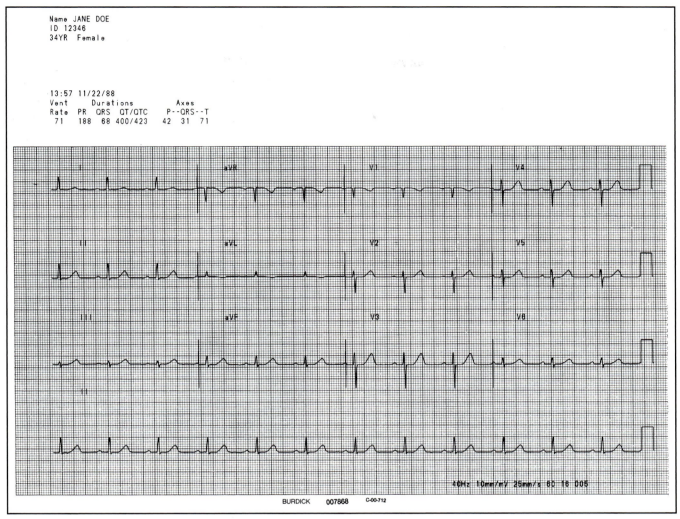

Name JANE DOE
ID 12346
34YR Female

13:57 11/22/88

Vent	Durations			Axes		
Rate	PR	QRS	QT/QTC	P--	QRS--	T
71	188	68	400/423	42	31	71

40Hz 10mm/mV 25mm/s 8O 16 005

BURDICK 007868 C-00-712

Fig. 25-22 Multichannel electrocardiogram.

chest is accessible for electrode placement but modestly covered for the patient's comfort. For the best test results, the patient should rest in this position for about 10 minutes before the start of the test. Some physicians may want you to record any medications that the patient is taking. Explain that the patient should remain in a relaxed position and must not move during the recording of the ECG. Talking during recording is usually not a problem as long as the patient remains still and relaxed.

Turn on the machine's power switch and allow it to warm up. The operation manual will state the time needed for this process.

The next step is to attach the electrodes to the patient. The skin in the areas to which electrodes are applied must be clean, dry, and oil free. If the patient did not have an opportunity to prepare for the examination, you may have to remove oil or lotion from the skin before applying the electrodes. This can be accomplished by rubbing the area briskly with an alcohol pad and wiping it with gauze or a tissue. Disposable adhesive electrodes are most commonly used. They adhere to the patient's skin and have attachments for the cable ends. Because skin does not

conduct electricity well, an electrolyte compound is applied between the skin and the electrode to enhance the electric contact and help ensure a reliable tracing. Electrolytes are incorporated into disposable electrodes.

Attach one electrode firmly to the fleshy, outer surface of each upper arm (Fig. 25-23) and to the inner surface

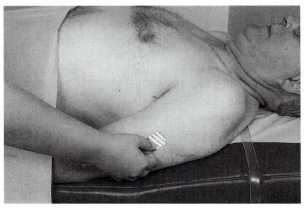

Fig. 25-23 Attach one electrode firmly to the fleshy, outer surface of each upper arm.

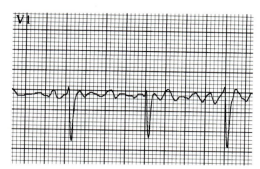

Fig. 25-30 Subtle wandering baseline.

sources when this occurs. If these measures do not solve the problem, try moving the patient table to another location at a greater distance from the walls.

Subtle wandering baseline (Fig. 25-30) is an indication of poor electric contact. This artifact is seen when electrodes are not in firm contact with the skin or when the contacts between the electrodes and the lead wires are loose. Wandering baseline may also result when oily skin has not been properly cleansed or when there is insufficient electrolyte between the electrodes and the skin. It is important to identify and correct this artifact because it can sometimes be mistaken for evidence of pathology.

Major wandering baseline (Fig. 25-31) is caused by patient movement or by electric interference from activity

within the room. People moving about near the patient may cause this artifact.

Interrupted baseline (Fig. 25-32) is an artifact that occurs when there is an intermittent interruption of electric transmission. This may be caused by the detachment of a lead wire or by a broken wire. When a broken wire is determined to be the cause, the patient cable must be repaired or replaced.

Preparing the Tracing for Interpretation and Storage

The electrocardiogram is part of the patient's permanent record. It must be accurately identified with the patient's name and an identifying number, such as the birth date or file number. Data should also include the patient's age and sex, the testing date, and any variations from the usual stylus deflection (STD setting) or recording speed. If required by the physician, also note any medications taken by the patient before the test.

Some types of ECG paper are delicate and subject to damage when folded or scratched. Paper clips and staples must not be used to secure ECGs. If clear tape is used, it must be a high-quality tape that will not deteriorate or yellow with age. There are four basic types of graph paper: chemical thermal, wax coated, plain paper, and

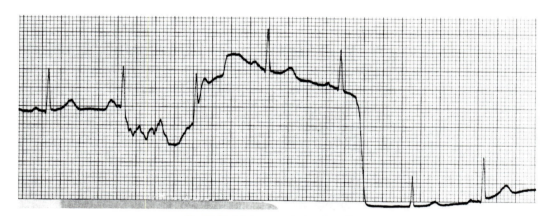

Fig. 25-31 Major wandering baseline.

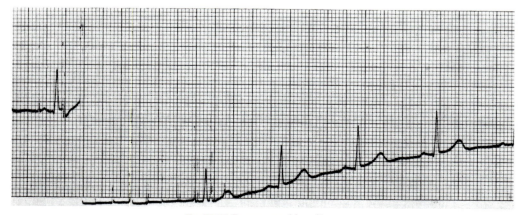

Fig. 25-32 Interrupted baseline.

glossy paper. Tape should not be used on chemical thermal paper because chemicals in the adhesive will darken the tracing.

Depending on the format of the ECG, your facility's protocol may require that it be photocopied and/or mounted in a special mounting folder. Convenient mounts are commercially available that display the entire study on a single surface. When it is mounted, the tracing is edited to eliminate excess recording and portions that contain artifacts. Select the best portion of each lead when editing. Take care to match each lead to its correct location in the mount and to mount each tracing right side up.

After being correctly identified, edited, and prepared, the ECG is presented to the physician for interpretation, together with the patient's chart and any previous ECG studies for comparison.

Exercise Tolerance Testing

An **exercise tolerance test,** also called an *ECG stress test,* is used to detect and/or evaluate **cardiac ischemia,** inadequate blood supply to the heart muscle. The ECG is monitored and recorded while the patient performs exercise. The exercise is usually performed on a treadmill, but a stationary bicycle or stair-step machine is sometimes used. The patient's blood pressure and pulse are also monitored during the test. Resting ECGs are usually performed both before and after the exercise portion of the test.

Exercise tolerance testing is performed only in facilities that have trained staff and special equipment to respond to a cardiac emergency, which could arise as a result of the test.

Various protocols are used for stress testing. If your duties involve assisting with exercise tolerance ECG tests, you will be instructed in the specific protocols observed in your facility and the procedure for patient instruction and preparation.

SPIROMETRY

The term **spirometry** refers to the measurement of lung airflow using a machine called a **spirometer.** Although several types of tests may be performed using a spirometer, this discussion covers only the **forced expiration test,** which is the principal test for most purposes. Forced expiration spirometry is a simple and extremely useful form of pulmonary function test (PFT) and is sometimes referred to by that name. It is used to evaluate ventilation in patients for a number of reasons. As a screening test, it may alert the physician to early signs of pulmonary disease. This is especially true when the tests are taken periodically and the results compared over time. Spirometry is also used to evaluate the effectiveness of treatment for pulmonary conditions. It is particularly

helpful in monitoring patients with asthma, cystic fibrosis, and chronic obstructive pulmonary disease (COPD, specifically emphysema and/or chronic bronchitis). Spirometry may be used to assess the risk associated with surgical procedures that are known to affect lung function, such as those requiring a general anesthetic.

In work situations in which air quality or inhalation of irritants may cause occupational disease, workers may be required to have a baseline spirometry test when they are hired and may be monitored with spirometry for signs of pulmonary problems over the course of their work. If your facility serves as a provider of occupational health care, spirometry may be performed as a part of routine preemployment physical examinations and/or occupational health evaluations. When there is a legal need to establish pulmonary impairment or disability, spirometry provides an objective measurement.

During this test the patient takes a deep breath and exhales forcefully into the spirometer tube. The spirometer measures the air flow, recording how much air is forced out of the lungs and how rapidly this is accomplished. The spirometer provides measurements and mathematical data and also produces a graph of the exhalation, which is called a **spirogram.** Depending on the equipment, data recorded for the test may include a number of parameters and calculations of the relationships between the measurements. All spirometers record at least two significant measurements: FVC and FEV_1. **FVC** stands for **forced vital capacity,** the total amount of air the lungs can hold. **FEV** stands for **forced expiratory volume,** and *FEV*1 indicates the quantity of air that can be forcefully exhaled during the first second of the test.

The patient's cooperation and effort are essential to the success of the test, so proper patient instruction is necessary. Enthusiastic coaching during the test is equally important.

Equipment

There are two commonly used types of spirometers: the volume-displacement type and the flow-sensing type. Many variations and models of each type exist. Most provide measurements, mathematical data, and a spirogram. An operator's manual should accompany the machine. Those who perform spirometry should be familiar with the features of the equipment and the guidelines provided in the manual.

Recent advances in electronics and microprocessor technology have led to the development of portable spirometers of the flow-sensing type that are ideal for use in physicians' offices and clinics. These units automatically calculate a range of ventilation indices that assist the physician in interpreting the results and eliminate the need for mathematical calculations by the technician.

There are two types of spirograms. One plots flow according to the volume of air and is called a *flow-volume*

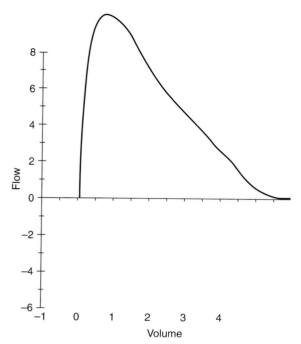

Fig. 25-33 Flow-volume spirogram.

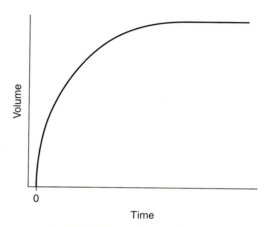

Fig. 25-34 Time-volume spirogram.

graph (Fig. 25-33). The other is a *time-volume graph* in which the volume of air is plotted over the time of the exhalation (Fig. 25-34).

The calibration of equipment is very important. Calibration procedures vary greatly depending on the equipment and are explained in the operation manual.

Flow-sensing spirometers may have disposable or nondisposable flow sensors. Disposable flow sensors are discarded and replaced after each use, and each new sensor must be calibrated. Nondisposable sensors must be disinfected after each use to prevent the spread of disease from patient to patient. The operation manual for the equipment will detail these procedures.

Patient Preparation and Testing

It would be unusual for a physician to order a spirometry test for a patient for which the test is contraindicated. Even

so, personnel who perform these tests should be aware of the principal contraindications. The test should not be performed on patients who have had recent abdominal surgery, thoracic surgery, or eye surgery, including cataract operations. **Hemoptysis** (coughing up blood) from an unknown cause and pneumothorax (collapsed lung) are also contraindications. Certain cardiovascular conditions may prevent the use of this test. For example, patients with angina or unstable blood pressure may experience aggravation of their conditions.

Patients taking bronchodilating medications should discontinue their use before the test. The physician will specify when the medication should be stopped, depending on the specific drug and the duration of its effectiveness. The effect of bronchodilating medications on the patient's condition is sometimes evaluated with spirometry. A baseline test is given, followed by the administration of bronchodilating medication. After a set interval (usually less than 15 minutes), the test is repeated. The physician will prescribe the medication and the exact procedure for postbronchodilator testing.

To prepare for a spirometry test, the patient should loosen any tight clothing about the throat and the waist. Any clothing that could restrict the patient's ability to breathe should be loosened or removed.

Explain the purpose of the test in simple terms. For example, say, "This test measures how much air your lungs can hold and how fast you can blow all the air out." Then explain how the patient should perform the test. When instructed to do so, the patient will seal his or her lips around the mouthpiece, take the deepest possible breath, and blow the air out as fast as possible until the lungs are completely empty. It may be helpful for you to demonstrate the maneuver using a disposable mouthpiece that is not connected to the spirometer. The chin should be lifted enough so as not to crowd the throat. The patient should stand or sit erect and should not bend forward during the test (Fig. 25-35). A standing posture is preferred. The lips must seal tightly around the mouthpiece. Disposable nose clamps are not required, but they are sometimes used to ensure that no air escapes from the nose. After taking a deep breath, the patient must make a vigorous effort *from the start* to breathe out hard and fast and must continue to breathe out smoothly until absolutely no more air can be exhaled.

When the equipment and the patient are ready, check the patient's posture and instruct the patient to seal the lips around the mouthpiece and inhale through the nose, taking the deepest possible breath. As the patient inhales, encourage deeper and deeper inhalation to obtain a maximum breath. When maximum inhalation is achieved, instruct the patient to blow. During this maneuver it is very important that you coach the patient, as this will result in a better effort. Raise your voice somewhat and in an urgent tone say, "BLOW, blow hard, keep blowing, keep blowing, don't stop blowing." Continue coaching until the patient has expelled all of the air. At the conclusion of the maneuver,

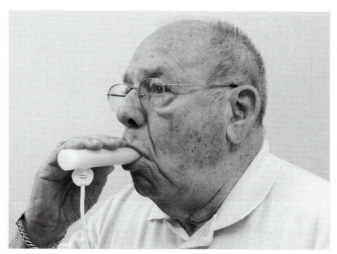

Fig. 25-35 Instruct patient to place the mouthpiece in the mouth and seal the lips around it.

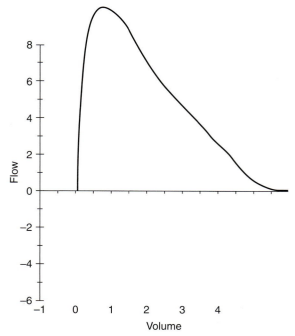

Fig. 25-36 Good effort.

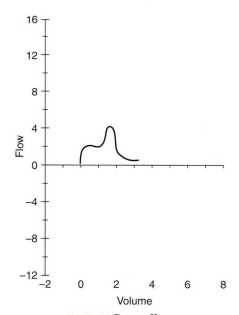

Fig. 25-37 Poor effort.

the patient should remove the mouthpiece before taking another breath unless the equipment is designed for measuring inhaled air.

After each maneuver, check the graph and discuss the patient's performance. Point out any aspect of the patient's effort that can be improved and praise the good points. For example, you might say, "That was a great start, but you stopped too soon. Next time, try to keep blowing longer until *all* of the air is exhaled."

The maneuver is repeated until you have obtained three recordings that represent the patient's best effort and are consistent with one another. If this is not accomplished after eight repetitions of the maneuver, stop the test and notify the physician. It is usually not helpful to continue the test beyond this point because fatigue will negatively affect the result.

A satisfactory test is characterized by an immediate forceful start, a maximum effort, and a smooth, continuous exhalation that does not end abruptly (Fig. 25-36). The most common patient-related problems when performing the forced expiration maneuver are as follows:

- Less than maximum effort (Fig. 25-37)
- Air leaks between the lips and the mouthpiece
- Incomplete inspiration or expiration
- Hesitation at the start of the expiration (Fig. 25-38)
- Coughing, especially during the early part of the expiration (Fig. 25-39)
- **Glottic closure** (sudden cessation of exhalation because of closure of the opening to the trachea) (Fig. 25-40)
- Obstruction of the mouthpiece by the tongue
- Vocalization (voice sounds) during the maneuver
- Poor posture

During the test, be alert for any sign of patient distress. Although this is a very safe test, patients may occasionally experience dizziness, syncope, chest pain, fits of coughing, or difficulty breathing. If any of these symptoms is seen or reported, stop the test and provide appropriate assistance to the patient (see Chapter 22). If the problem does not resolve immediately, notify the physician.

Infection Control

There is an obvious and significant danger of infection transmission from body fluids on mouthpieces. Modern spirometers are designed to minimize the possibility of spreading infection, and disposable mouthpieces are usually used. When nondisposable mouthpieces are used,

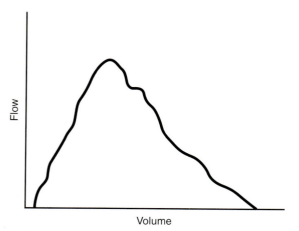

Fig. 25-38 Poor start. Initial exhalation is not forceful enough.

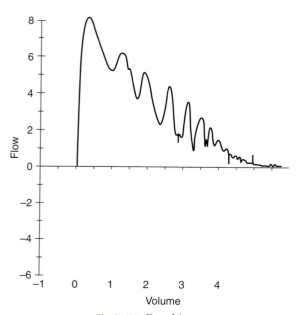

Fig. 25-39 Coughing.

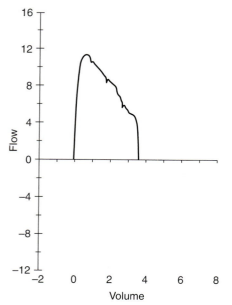

Fig. 25-40 Glottic closure.

they must be disinfected with a high-level disinfectant after each use. Unless the spirometer is specifically designed to permit both inhalation and exhalation, the patient should not inhale through the mouthpiece.

Other specific infection control measures vary greatly, depending on the design of the equipment. The operation manual will explain the required procedures, which should be followed explicitly. As with any patient procedure, you should carry out hand hygiene before and after the procedure for the patient's safety and for your own health.

SUMMARY

Diagnostic assessment skills not directly related to radiography may be a significant asset to the limited x-ray equipment operator. This is particularly true when he or she is part of the health care team in a small facility. Weighing and measuring patients and conducting vision screening tests are common practices in physicians' offices and clinics, and the procedures for carrying out these activities are easily learned. Electrocardiography and spirometry are more technical and require a higher level of learning for accurate performance. The background knowledge and technical skills obtained in radiography are good starting points for learning these complex procedures.

Height and weight may be measured using a balance scale, but electronic scales are also commonly used. Vision screening tests include distance vision acuity measurement using a Snellen chart at a 20-foot distance, near vision evaluation using a reading chart at a distance of 14 to 16 inches, and color perception assessment using the Ishihara color plate test. All these tests must be conducted in a quiet setting with appropriate lighting. Correct recording of results is essential.

Electrocardiography is a heart function test that measures the electric impulses that cause the heart to beat. The patient is connected to the electrocardiograph machine by electrodes and cables, and a tracing is made on graph paper. Those who perform this test must be thoroughly familiar with the equipment used and the procedures for preparing the patient for the test. They must recognize the characteristics of a high-quality tracing and be able to correct artifact problems when they occur.

Forced expiration spirometry is a very useful test for evaluating pulmonary health and for monitoring various conditions affecting lung function. To perform this test, the patient blows into the mouthpiece of the spirometer, and the machine measures airflow, calculates data, and produces a graph. Those who administer this test should be thoroughly familiar with the equipment, including procedures for its calibration and disinfection. Effective patient teaching and coaching are essential to the success of this test.

Chapter 26

Bone Densitometry

At the conclusion of this chapter, you will be able to:

- Define the types of osteoporosis and risk factors
- State the diagnostic criteria for osteoporosis as defined by the World Health Organization (WHO)
- Understand the function and types of bone
- Summarize the bone remodeling cycle
- List the standards for bone health
- Understand the basic statistical concepts of densitometry
- Apply the concepts of measuring bone mineral density (BMD) and reporting patient results as it relates to a T-score and Z-score
- Understand the properties of the x-ray beam, including quality (kilovolts peak), quantity (milliamperes), and time (seconds)
- Perform daily computer operation and electronic file management
- Describe the various types of dual-energy x-ray absorptiometry (DXA) systems, including pencil beam and fan (array) beam
- Perform equipment quality control procedures using calibration and phantom methods, and troubleshoot problems
- Determine quality in bone mineral densitometry using precision and accuracy
- Describe the concept of FRAX and vertebral fracture assessment (VFA)
- Apply the fundamentals of radiation safety for the patient and the operator using the principle of ALARA (As Low As Reasonably Achievable)
- Describe the units used to measure absorbed dose (gray) and effective dose (sievert)
- Utilize the correct anatomy, positioning, acquisition, and analysis for spine, proximal femur, and forearm scanning; identify the common problems of serial scans as described

Key Terms

ALARA
array-beam system
bone densitometry
bone mass
bone mineral content (BMC)
bone mineral density (BMD)
compare feature
cortical bone
discordance
dual-energy x-ray absorptiometry (DXA)
fragility fractures
FRAX
mean
osteoblasts
osteoclasts
osteopenia

osteoporosis
pencil-beam collimation system
percent coefficient of variation (%CV)
primary osteoporosis
precision assessment
reference population
regions of interest (ROIs)
secondary osteoporosis
serial scans
standard deviation (SD)
T-score
trabecular bone
type I osteoporosis
type II osteoporosis
vertebral fracture assessment
Z-score

Bone densitometry encompasses the art and science of measuring the bone mineral content and density of specific skeletal sites or the whole body. The bone measurement values are used to assess bone strength, diagnose diseases associated with low bone density (especially osteoporosis), monitor the effects of therapy for such diseases, and predict the risk of future fractures.

The most versatile and widely used method of performing bone densitometry is **dual-energy x-ray absorptiometry (DXA).** This technique, considered the gold standard, has the advantages of low radiation dose, wide availability, ease of use, short scan time, high-resolution images, good precision, and stable calibration.

All bone densitometry operators must possess, utilize, and maintain knowledge in the core competency areas of radiation protection, patient care, history taking, basic computer operation, scanner quality control, patient positioning, scan acquisition, scan analysis, and proper record keeping and documentation. Consistent positioning and scan acquisition along with proper analysis are the fundamentals of precise and accurate results, which can affect the treatment plan for the patient.

DXA VERSUS CONVENTIONAL RADIOGRAPHY

X-ray machines from different manufacturers are operated in essentially the same manner and produce identical images. This is not the case with DXA equipment. There are three major DXA manufacturers in the United States: GE Lunar Corp., Hologic Inc., and Norland Swissray Corp. (Fig. 26-1). The operator must be educated to operate the specific scanner model in his or her facility. The numeric bone density results obtained on machines from different manufacturers cannot be compared without proper standardization. This chapter presents general information on scan positioning and analysis, but the manufacturer's specific procedures must be used when actual scans are performed.

DXA can be conceptualized as a subtraction technique. To quantitate **bone mineral density (BMD),** it is necessary to eliminate the contributions of soft tissue and measure the x-ray attenuation of bone alone. This is accomplished by scanning at two different x-ray photon energies (thus the term *dual-energy x-ray*) and mathematically manipulating the recorded signal to take advantage of the differing attenuation properties of soft tissue and bone at the two energies (Fig. 26-2). The density of the isolated bone is calculated based on the principle that denser, more mineralized bone attenuates (absorbs) more x-rays. It is essential to have adequate amounts of artifact-free soft tissue to help ensure the reliability of the bone density results.

Bone densitometry results are computed by proprietary software from the x-ray attenuation pattern striking the detector, not from the scan image. DXA scans provide images only for the purpose of confirming correct positioning of the patient and correct placement of the **regions of interest (ROIs).** Therefore, the images may not be used for diagnosis, and any medical conditions apparent on the image must be followed up by appropriate diagnostic tests. The interpreting physicians must be skilled in interpreting the clinical and statistical aspects of the numeric density results and relating them to the specific patient history obtained by the operator.

Bone densitometry differs from diagnostic radiology in that good image quality, which can tolerate variability in technique, is not the ultimate goal. The goal is accurate and precise quantitative measurement by the scanner software, which requires stable equipment and careful, consistent work from the operator.

OSTEOPOROSIS

Osteoporosis is a systemic skeletal disease characterized by low **bone mass** and microarchitectural deterioration of bone tissue. As a result, the bones are at increased risk for **fragility fractures.** It is estimated that 10 million Americans have osteoporosis, with 80% (8 million) of those being women. Another 34 million Americans have **osteopenia** or low bone mass, which puts them at risk of developing osteoporosis in the future (Fig. 26-3). Persons with osteoporosis may experience decreased quality of life from the pain, deformity, and disability of fragility fractures (especially at the hip and spine) and increased risk of morbidity and mortality, especially from hip fractures. In the United States, annual medical costs for osteoporosis, including hospitalization for osteoporotic hip fractures, were $19 billion in 2005, and the cost is increasing. By 2025, it is expected to be $25.3 billion. Controllable and uncontrollable risk factors are shown in Box 26-1. Patients with a normal rate of bone loss may still develop osteoporosis if their peak bone mass is low.

Primary and Secondary Osteoporosis

Primary osteoporosis can be **type I** (postmenopausal) and/or **type II** (senile or age-related). Type I osteoporosis arises when bone resorption exceeds bone formation because of estrogen deprivation in women. Type II osteoporosis occurs in aging men and women because of a decreased ability to build bone.

Secondary osteoporosis is osteoporosis caused by other conditions. Common causes of secondary osteoporosis include hyperparathyroidism, gonadal insufficiency (including estrogen deficiency in women and hypogonadism in men), osteomalacia (rickets in children), rheumatoid arthritis, anorexia nervosa, gastrectomy, adult sprue (hypersensitivity to gluten [wheat protein]), multiple myeloma, and use of corticosteroids, heparin, or anticonvulsants or excessive thyroid hormone treatment.

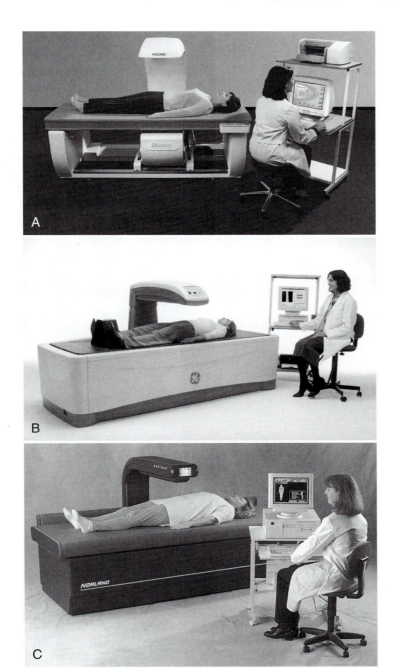

Fig. 26-1 A, DXA spine scan being performed on a Hologic Discovery scanner. **B,** DXA spine scan being performed on a GE Lunar Advance scanner. **C,** DXA whole-body scan being performed on a Norland Swissray XR-46 scanner.

Several prescription medications arrest bone loss and may increase bone mass. These include traditional estrogen or hormone replacement therapies and bisphosphonates (which have antiresorptive properties), as well as selective estrogen receptor modulators (SERMs), salmon calcitonin, and parathyroid hormone (which stimulate bone formation). Another newer therapy is a RANK ligand (RANKL) inhibitor.

Laboratory tests for *biochemical markers* of bone turnover may be used in conjunction with DXA to determine the need for or the effectiveness of therapy.

Bone Biology and Remodeling

The skeleton serves several purposes. It supports the body and protects vital organs so that movement, communication, and life processes can be carried on. It also manufactures red blood cells, and it stores the minerals that are necessary for life, including calcium and phosphate.

The two basic types of bone are cortical (or compact) and trabecular (or cancellous). **Cortical bone** forms the dense, compact outer shell of all bones, as well as the

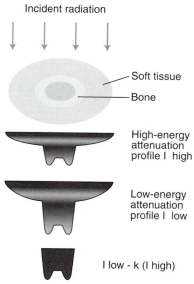

Incident radiation

Soft tissue

Bone

High-energy attenuation profile I high

Low-energy attenuation profile I low

I low - k (I high)

Fig. 26-2 Soft tissue compensation using DXA. Because data are obtained at two energies, the soft tissue attenuation can be mathematically eliminated. The remaining attenuation is because of the amount of bone present.

Box 26-1

Risk Factors for Developing Osteoporosis

Uncontrollable Risk Factors
- Advanced age
- Female gender—women are at higher risk
- Family and personal history of fractures as an adult
- White or Asian race—women in these groups are at highest risk
- Small bones and body weight under 127 lb
- Menopause—loss of estrogen protection for the bone
- Menstrual history that includes cessation of menses before menopause because of eating disorders
- Excessive physical exercise
- Some medications/chronic diseases—use of certain medications to treat disorders such as rheumatoid arthritis, endocrine disorders, seizure disorders, and gastrointestinal disorders; glucocorticoids are the class of drugs with particularly damaging effects

Controllable Risk Factors
- Low calcium intake
- Low vitamin D intake
- Estrogen deficiency
- Smoking
- Excessive alcohol intake
- Sedentary lifestyle

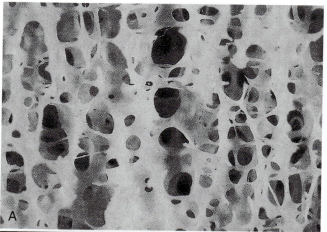

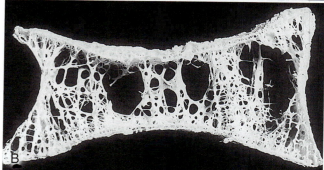

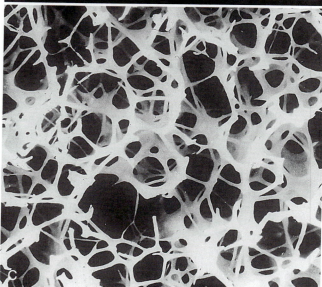

Fig. 26-3 Trabecular bone obtained from vertebrae. **A,** Micrograph of normal bone. **B,** Vertebral body demonstrating osteoporosis. **C,** Micrograph of osteoporotic bone. Note loss of trabecular continuity resulting from resorptive perforations in the osteoporotic specimen.

shafts of the long bones. It supports weight, resists bending and twisting, and accounts for about 80% of the skeletal mass. **Trabecular bone** is the delicate, latticework structure within bones that adds strength without excessive weight and accounts for 20% of the skeletal mass. It supports compressive loading in the spine, hip, and os calcis. It is also found at the ends of long bones, such as the distal radius.

Bone is constantly going through a remodeling process in which old bone is replaced with new bone. Bone-destroying cells called **osteoclasts** break down and remove old bone, leaving pits. This part of the process is

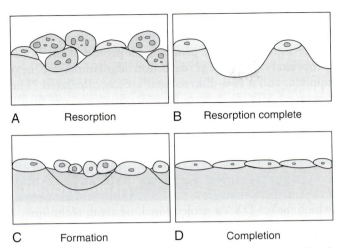

Fig. 26-4 The bone remodeling process. **A,** Osteoclasts break down bone in the process of resorption. **B,** Pits develop in the bone. **C,** Osteoblasts form new bone. **D,** With equal amounts of resorption and formation, the bone mass is stable.

called *resorption.* Bone-building cells called **osteoblasts** fill the pits with new bone. This process is called *formation* (Fig. 26-4).

Bone mass increases in youth until peak bone mass is reached at about 30 to 35 years of age. This is followed by a stable period in middle age. A decrease in bone mass becomes pronounced in women at menopause because of the loss of bone-preserving estrogen during this time; this decrease occurs at a somewhat later age in men (after 70 years).

Bone health requires adequate calcium and vitamin D intake and absorption. Calcium is a mineral that is essential for life, yet the majority of Americans do not get adequate calcium on a daily basis. Calcium plays an important role in building stronger, denser bones early in life and keeping bones strong and healthy later in life. About 99% of the calcium in our bodies is found in our bones and teeth. In addition to building and maintaining healthy bones, calcium allows blood to clot, nerves to send messages, muscles to contract, and other body functions to occur. Each day, our bodies lose calcium through skin, nails, hair, sweat, urine, and feces. The human body cannot produce calcium on its own. That is why it is important to obtain enough calcium through the foods we eat. When the diet does not provide enough calcium for the body's needs, calcium is taken from the bones.

Vitamin D plays an important role in protecting bones. The body requires vitamin D to absorb calcium. Children need vitamin D to build strong bones, and adults need it to keep bones strong and healthy. Studies show that patients with low levels of vitamin D have lower bone density or bone mass and are more likely to break bones when they are older. Vitamin D deficiency is becoming more widespread nationally and internationally. It can cause a disease known as *osteomalacia* in which the bones become soft. In children, this condition is known as *rickets.*

Building and Maintaining Bone

Two types of exercise are important for building and maintaining bone mass and density: weight-bearing exercise and muscle-strengthening exercise. Weight-bearing exercise is exercise in which bones and muscles work against gravity. This includes any exercise in which the feet and legs are bearing weight. Jogging, walking, stair climbing, dancing, and soccer are examples of weight-bearing exercise with different degrees of impact. Swimming and bicycling are not weight bearing.

The second type of exercise is muscle strengthening or activities that use muscular strength to improve muscle mass and strengthen bone. One example of this activity is weight lifting, such as the use of free weights and weight machines found at gyms and health clubs.

PHYSICAL AND MATHEMATICAL PRINCIPLES OF DXA

X-rays are produced in a vacuum tube when high-speed electrons suddenly decelerate at the tube target. The electrons are liberated by heating the tungsten filament and are accelerated by high voltage from a step-up transformer.

The properties of the x-ray beam are described by three measures:
- *Quality*—Voltage is measured at the peak of the electric cycle. When the voltage across the x-ray tube is measured, the units are often stated as *kilovolts peak*, abbreviated *kVp*. The terms *kV* and *kVp* are used interchangeably in radiography, with kVp being the preferred term. The voltage applied to the x-ray tube controls the speed of the electrons and the penetrating power of the x-ray photons produced.
- *Quantity*—Milliamperage (mA) is a measure of the rate of current flow across the x-ray tube, that is, the number of electrons flowing from filament to target each second. Milliamperage controls the volume of x-ray production and thus also the rate of exposure. It controls the intensity of the x-ray beam.
- *Duration or time*—Exposure time refers to the length of time that the x-rays are turned on. It is the duration of the x-ray exposure. Exposure time is measured in units of seconds.

The measurement of bone density requires separation of the x-ray attenuating effects of soft tissue and bone. The mass attenuation coefficients of soft tissue and bone differ and also depend on the energy of the x-ray photons. The use of two different photon energies (as in a dual-energy x-ray) optimizes the difference between soft tissue and bone. GE Lunar and Norland Swissray

least 100 patient scans. If a new DXA system is installed, a repeat precision assessment should be done. A repeat assessment should also be done if an operator's skill level has changed.

Procedure to Determine Precision Error for Each Operator

Measure 15 patients 3 times or 30 patients 2 times, repositioning the patient after each scan. Use the International Society for Clinical Densitometry (ISCD) Precision Assessment tool at www.ISCD.org to calculate precision. Calculate LSC for the group at 95% confidence interval. This information is then used by the clinician to interpret all serial scans.

The minimum acceptable precision for an individual technologist is:
Lumbar spine: 1.9% (LSC = 5.3%)
Total hip: 1.8% (LSC = 5.0%)
Femoral neck: 2.5% (LSC = 6.9%)

Retraining is required if an operator's precision is worse than these values. Precision assessment should be standard clinical practice. It is not research and may potentially benefit patients. Therefore, it should not require approval from an institutional review board. Adherence to any local or state radiologic safety regulations is necessary. A precision assessment requires the consent of participating patients (ISCD 2007 Position Statements).

BMD Comparison Between Facilities

It is not possible to quantitatively compare BMD or to calculate LSC between facilities or different machines without cross-calibration of the machines. See ISCD Position Statements for further instructions at www. ISCD.org.

T-scores and Z-scores

A BMD measurement from a patient is most useful when it can be compared statistically with an appropriate sex-matched **reference population.** The three DXA equipment manufacturers have separately collected reference population databases. These reference databases vary because different populations, entrance criteria, and statistical methods were used. To correct this problem, the third National Health and Nutrition Examination Survey (NHANES III) DXA total hip database was adapted to provide a standardized hip reference database for all manufacturers. All reference databases are separated by gender and provide the BMD mean and SD at each age.

To compare a patient's BMD with the reference population BMD, two standardized scores have been developed called the *Z-score* and *T-score.* In older adults, the Z-score will be higher than the T-score.

The **T-score** indicates the number of SDs by which the patient's BMD differs from the average BMD of young, normal, sex-matched individuals with peak bone mass. The T-score is used to assess fracture risk, diagnose osteoporosis and osteopenia, and determine if therapy is recommended. It is calculated as follows:

$$\text{T-score} = \text{Measured BMD} - \text{Young adult mean BMD}/\text{Young adult SD}$$

The **Z-score** indicates the number of SDs by which the patient's BMD differs from the average BMD for the patient's respective age and sex group. The Z-score is used to determine if the measured BMD is reasonable and if evaluation for secondary osteoporosis is warranted. It is calculated as follows:

$$\text{Z-score} = (\text{Measure BMD} - \text{Age-matched mean BMD})/\text{Age-matched SD}$$

Bone mass is normally distributed (i.e., described by a bell-shaped curve) in the population, and no one exact cut point exists below which a person has osteoporosis. However, with the widespread availability of DXA scanning and T-scores, there was pressure to declare such a cut point. In 1994, the World Health Organization (WHO) recommended that the classifications presented in Table 26-1 be used in DXA studies of postmenopausal white women.

Discordance refers to the fact that T-scores may vary for different anatomic sites in a given patient, different individuals within populations, and different measurement modalities. It makes the diagnosis of osteoporosis more complicated than simply applying T-score criteria, and the problems are being researched to find more standardized diagnostic criteria. For example, a patient may be found to have a low T-score at the hip but not at the spine.

Table 26-1

World Health Organization Definitions of Osteoporosis Based on Bone Density Levels

Normal	Bone density is within 1 SD of the young adult mean (T-score of +1 to −1).
Low Bone Mass	Bone density is 1 to 2.5 SD below the young adult mean (T-score of −1 to −2.5).
Osteoporosis	Bone density is 2.5 SD or more below the young adult mean (T-score below −2.5).
Severe (Established) Osteoporosis	Bone density is 2.5 SD or more below the young adult mean and there has been one or more osteoporotic fractures (T-score −2.5 or lower plus fragility fracture).

SD, Standard deviation.

Vertebral fracture assessment (VFA) is the term that encompasses looking at the spine "morphometrically" in the lateral projection, which means visualizing the shapes of the vertebral bodies of both the lumbar and thoracic spine to determine if there has been some deformity with resultant compression of the vertebral bodies. Dual-energy vertebral assessment (DVA), lateral vertebral assessment (LVA), instant vertebral analysis (IVA), and radiologic vertebral assessment (RVA) are synonymous for this process. The manufacturers of bone densitometers have devised their own way of either enhancing the image or improving the scan acquisition and analysis. Images are obtained in both dual-energy acquisition and the single-energy method. Both methods are comparable. VFA is used for the sole purpose of detecting vertebral fractures not measuring bone density.

Unlike traditional lateral spine x-rays, VFA has the capability of visualizing both the lumbar and thoracic spine as one continuous image. This capability aids the interpreting physician in identifying the vertebral level where abnormalities are present. PA views can also be incorporated into a VFA study. For an accurate representation of the vertebral bodies, the patient's spine must be as straight as possible.

The PA view can help identify artifacts and deformities, such as scoliosis. Scoliosis is the one condition that can cause the greatest challenge in VFA and possibly make a study "unreadable." VFA also exposes the patient to about one one-hundredth the radiation dose of just a single lateral x-ray image. VFA is an adjunct to DXA scanning in cases when a patient might not have been x-rayed for vertebral fracture beforehand. General spine x-ray is still the gold standard for visualizing abnormalities in the spine.

VFA uses single x-ray absorptiometry, SXA (for image only) or DXA (for image and BMD) lateral scans of the thoracic and lumbar spines from the level of about T4 to L5 (Fig. 26-7). The images are used to determine vertebral shape abnormalities that may indicate vertebral fragility fractures, which are a strong risk factor for future vertebral fractures. Fig. 26-8, *A*, shows the Genant grading system. The three columns show the types of fracture, and the rows show the grades of severity. Seeing a severe fracture is easy, and seeing a moderate fracture is relatively easy, but it is difficult to determine if a mild deformity is normal for the patient or the beginning of a problem.

VFA should be interpreted by a trained physician by viewing the images on the scan monitor (Fig. 26-8, *B*).

RADIATION SAFETY AND PROTECTION

Following proper radiation protection practices and achieving the goal of **ALARA** (*As Low As Reasonably Achievable*) in radiation exposure is relatively simple for

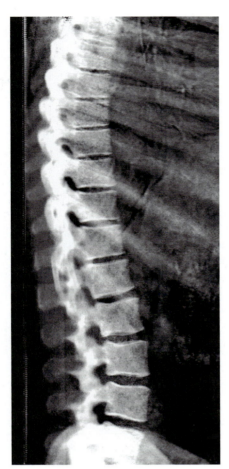

Fig. 26-7 Morphometric x-ray absorptiometry to detect vertebral shape abnormality.

DXA. The radiation dose for DXA scans is very low compared with conventional radiography doses and similar to natural background radiation (Table 26-2). If the positioning or acquisition parameters of a scan are questionable, the scan should be repeated because the risk from the additional radiation dose is negligible compared with the risk of an incorrect medical diagnosis. Accuracy will be determined by the quality of the baseline scan.

Radiation Measurement

Several units are used to measure radiation exposure. X-ray output is expressed in coulombs per kilogram or roentgens. This measure is used to describe the amount of radiation reaching the patient's skin. Absorbed dose is expressed as gray (Gy) or rad. One gray is equal to 100 rad. This measure describes the radiation that interacts with a substance such as tissue. Dose equivalent is expressed as sievert (Sv) or rem. One sievert is equal to 100 rem. This unit expresses the relative biologic effect of radiation on human tissue and is encountered in radiation-monitoring reports. Fractions of these units are used in bone densitometry because a typical DXA scan

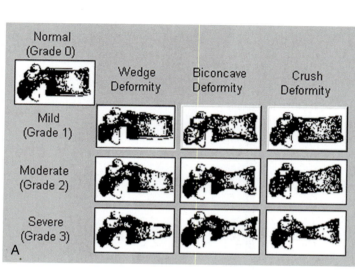

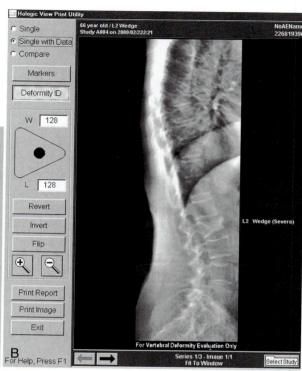

Fig. 26-8 **A** and **B,** Dual VFA.

Table 26-2

Bone Densitometry Radiation Doses Compared With Other Commonly Acquired Doses

Type of Radiation Exposure	Effect Dose (mcSv)
Daily natural background radiation	5-8
Round-trip air flight across the United States	60
Lateral lumbar spine radiograph	700
Posteroanterior chest radiograph	50
QCT with localizer scan (from scanner offering low kilovoltage and milliampere-seconds; may be up to 10 times higher for other scanners)	60
DXA scan (range allows for different anatomic sites; GE Lunar Expert-XL may be higher)	1-5
SXA scan	<1
Quantitative ultrasound	0

DXA, Dual-energy x-ray absorptiometry; *QCT,* quantitative computed tomography; *SXA,* single x-ray absorptiometry.

results in a dose between 1 and 5 mcSv. For more complete information, see Chapter 11.

Radiation Protection Concepts Related to DXA Scanning

The primary factors in radiation protection for both operators and patients are time, distance, and shielding.

These factors relate to DXA scanning in the following ways:
- Scan time is determined by the mode or array.
- The distance from the x-ray tube to the patient is fixed. Distance is the best form of protection from x-ray exposure for scanner operators. The computer console should be at least 3 feet (1 m) from the scanner for pencil-beam scanners and up to 9 feet (3 m) for frequently utilized array-beam scanners. Operators may further protect themselves with a mobile radiation shield if time and distance are concerns.
- Shielding is built into the scanner via collimation. Additional lead shielding does not have to be used on patients undergoing DXA scanning.

Other practical measures that the operator should use to minimize unnecessary radiation exposure include the following:
- The operator should wear an individual dosimetry device (film badge, thermoluminescent dosimeter, or optically stimulated luminescence device) at the collar on the side adjacent to the scanner. Another monitor may be placed outside the scan room.
- The operator should monitor the dosimetry records.
- A radiation warning sign should be posted and highly visible.
- The operator should remain in the room during the scan and monitor the acquisition image.
- The operator should have adequate instruction and experience to minimize repositioning and repetition of scans.

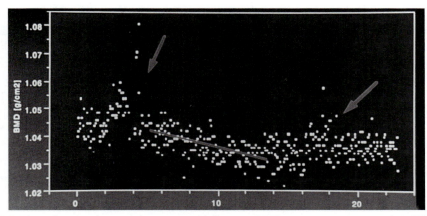

Fig. 26-9 Plot of spine phantom bone mineral density (BMD) over time (in months). The two *arrows* show abrupt shifts in BMD. The *straight line* shows a slow drift downward in BMD. These indicate changes in scanner calibration.

- The operator should follow proper procedures to avoid scanning a pregnant patient and place documentation in the permanent record.
- Patients should be screened at scheduling for problems that require postponement of scanning, such as pregnancy and recent barium or nuclear medicine examinations, to avoid unnecessary radiation exposure.

Computer Competency

DXA scan acquisition, analysis, and archiving are controlled with a personal computer (PC). Therefore, DXA operators must be familiar with the basic PC components and how they work, such as the disk drives and storage media; keyboard; monitor; printer; and mouse.

Digital networking allows a scan to be performed at one location and then be sent electronically to a remote location for reading or review by an interpreting or referring physician.

An operator must be able to back up, archive, locate, and restore patient scan files. Daily backup and archiving are recommended to preserve patient scan files and data. A third copy of data should be stored offsite to ensure retrieval of patient data, as well as to be able to rebuild databases, if there is a computer failure, fire, flood, or theft.

Manufacturers frequently upgrade software versions, and the operator is responsible for performing this task. Records of upgrades and software installation should be maintained. Current software media should be accessible to service engineers at the time of preventive maintenance and repairs.

Computers consist of software and hardware. Software consists of programs written in code that instruct the computer how to perform tasks. The DXA manufacturer's software controls many aspects of DXA scanning from starting the scan to calculating and reporting the results. Hardware comprises the physical components for central processing, input, output, and storage.

Scanner Quality Control

Daily calibration must be performed on all scanners. Daily calibration is accomplished by imaging an anthropomorphic phantom. Each scanner is supplied with a phantom that has been calibrated to the individual scanner. It has known values that were verified in the factory. This allows monitoring of scanner stability by detecting shifts or drifts. Daily quality assurance testing:
- May be an automated or manual procedure
- Calibrates and performs a functional test *before* patient scanning
- Provides simple pass/fail evaluations
- Is internal or external depending on the manufacturer of the scanner

If the daily calibration procedure fails, repeat the procedure. Make a notation as to the nature of the failure (e.g., operator error, electric failure). If the procedure fails a second time, cancel patient appointments and call the manufacturer's applications department or help desk. The goal of this procedure is to ensure that patients are scanned on properly functioning equipment with stable calibration. Unstable calibration can be manifested as abrupt shifts or slow drifts in BMD, as seen on plots of phantom scan results (Fig. 26-9). These shifts can cause the patient's BMD values to be too high or too low, which prevents a valid comparison between the results of baseline and follow-up scans.

Records of all quality control tests and results must be maintained. A current list of software upgrades, service performance, and preventive maintenance must also be kept. This information may be requested by state radiation inspectors.

FRACTURE RISK MODELS

The **FRAX** tool has been developed by the WHO to evaluate fracture risk in patients. It is based on individual patient models that integrate the risks associated with clinical risk factors as well as bone mineral density at the femoral neck. The FRAX algorithm gives the 10-year probability of fracture. It is designed to be used on patients between the ages of 40 and 90 of both genders. FRAX cannot be calculated on patients who are on pharmacological treatment. The FRAX tool and other fracture risk models may assist physicians in making decisions about who to treat, especially patients with low bone mass. Fracture prediction models should be used judiciously in managing individual patients (www.shef.ac.uk/FRAX/).

BASELINE AND SERIAL SCANNING

DXA scanning requires knowledge of relevant anatomy, which directly relates to proper positioning of the patient for scanning and the placement of the ROI for scan image analysis. The information presented in this section generally applies to all DXA scanners. However, instruction from the particular scanner's manufacturer is recommended before the scanner is used. The operator's manual that accompanies the equipment is the ultimate authority.

Like all technologies, DXA has operating limits. Accuracy and precision may be adversely affected if the bone mass is very low, the patient is too thick or too thin, the anatomy is abnormal, or there have been significant changes in soft tissue between **serial scans.** The benefit provided by experienced DXA operators is that they can recognize and adapt to abnormal situations. They also have knowledge of the limits of the technology. All abnormalities that might compromise the scan results in an individual patient must be noted by the operator. This information is taken into consideration by the interpreting physician.

Baseline Scans

The baseline scan is the first DXA scan that a patient has ever had, or has had on your scanner. The baseline scan determines the patient's BMD value, because it measures the true bone density compared with that of young adult normal (T-score) and age-matched individuals (Z-score). A high-quality baseline scan will be the foundation for all serial scans.

Serial Scans

The BMD of a patient may be monitored over time. Direct comparisons of BMD results are valid only if serial scans are performed on the same scanner that was used for the baseline scans.

It is imperative that the patient positioning be exactly the same for the baseline and all serial scans. The same scan settings must be used (e.g., field size, mode, speed, current), and the ROIs must be placed identically on the images. The baseline printouts or a software feature that allows side-by-side viewing at the time of the scan acquisition is required for proper serial scan acquisition. An additional tool, the software's **compare feature,** can be used if recommended by the manufacturer. If it is not recommended for analysis, it can still be used for positioning comparison. All extraordinary measures taken for positioning and analysis for the baseline must be documented and available to the operator when performing serial scans.

SKELETAL SITES TO MEASURE

- Measure BMD at both the PA spine and hip in all patients.
- Forearm BMD should be measured under the following circumstances:
  - Hip and/or spine cannot be measured or interpreted
  - Hyperparathyroidism
  - Very obese patients (over the weight limit for DXA table)
- Spine ROI
  - Use PA L1-L4 for spine BMD measurement.
  - Use all evaluable vertebrae and only exclude vertebrae that are affected by local structural change or artifact. Use three vertebrae if four cannot be used and two if three cannot be used.
  - BMD-based diagnostic classification should not be made using a single vertebra.
  - If only one evaluable vertebra remains after excluding other vertebrae, diagnosis should be based on a different valid skeletal site.
  - Anatomically abnormal vertebrae may be excluded from analysis if:
    - They are clearly abnormal and nonassessable within the resolution of the system.
    - There is more than a 1.0 T-score difference between the vertebra in question and adjacent vertebrae.
  - When vertebrae are excluded, the BMD of the remaining vertebrae is used to derive the T-score.
  - The lateral spine should not be used for diagnosis, but may have a role in monitoring.
- Hip ROI
  - Use femoral neck or total proximal femur, whichever is lowest.
  - BMD may be measured at either hip.
  - There are insufficient data to determine whether mean T-scores for bilateral hip BMD can be used for diagnosis.
  - The mean hip BMD can be used for monitoring, with total hip being preferred.

- Forearm ROI
  - Use 33% radius (sometimes called one-third radius) of the nondominant forearm for diagnosis. Other forearm ROIs are not recommended.

DXA SCAN ACQUISITION, IMAGE CRITIQUE, AND ANALYSIS

DXA Scanning of the Lumbar Spine

Lumbar spine scans are most appropriate for predicting vertebral fracture risk in patients younger than 65 years of age. Degenerative changes in the elderly elevate spinal BMD, resulting in an underestimation of increased fracture risks. Degenerative changes in the spine such as osteophytosis, scoliosis of greater than 15 degrees, overlying calcification, and compression fractures falsely elevate the BMD. Artifacts in the vertebral bodies or very dense artifacts in the soft tissue also affect the BMD. The supervising physician should develop policies for consistent procedures for dealing with such issues.

Routine Examination

The routine examination of the lumbar spine includes the middle of L5 through the middle of T12. The patient position is supine, but the view is called PA because of the location of the x-ray tube in relation to the image receptor.

Preparation

1. Select existing or new patient function.
2. Enter patient demographics.
3. Select the Spine Measure or Measure Patient function. Ensure that the proper scan or array mode has been chosen by the software. Make any changes before proceeding.
4. Instruct the patient to remove all external or heavily attenuating materials (e.g., belts, buttons, snaps, bra hook) from the lumbar spine scan region. If possible, have the patient change into a gown to ensure that there are no external artifacts and to provide consistency in serial scanning.

Positioning Aids

The positioning aids vary depending on the specific manufacturer. Typically, a positioning leg block is used for the PA lumbar spine. The leg block is positioned so that the front edge aligns with the bend of the knees. The placement of the leg block positioner varies based on the length of the patient's femur (i.e., 45-, 60-, or 90-degree angle between the tabletop and the patient's legs). The One Scan technique (GE Lunar) does not require a leg block positioner.

Use a minimal sponge or pillow for head comfort, making sure not to lift the shoulders from the table pad.

Positioning and Procedure Details: PA Lumbar Spine Scan

Body Position:

- Patient is supine and centered on scan table and scan table pad. Check that patient is lying straight on the table by viewing from the head and foot end of the table.
- Arms and hands are parallel to table pad and on the table pad.

Part Position:

- Body is centered to the midline of the table pad.
- Body is centered within the table pad length and parameters.
- Shoulders and pelvic girdle are squared to the table pad.
- Legs are bent at a 60- to 90-degree angle on positioner block or not (based on technique).

Central Ray/Laser Light Placement:

- Varies according to manufacturer
- Perpendicular to midlevel of L5 or 1 to 2 cm below the iliac crest
  or
- Perpendicular to the xiphoid junction

Scan Field:

Once the scan field is determined, the automated scan field is set (based on manufacturer) by entering height and weight or by manual adjustments. The scanning program will acquire the necessary data from the scan field, which must then be analyzed.

Shielding:

None required

Patient Instruction:

Do not move.

Completing the Procedure:

- Review the scan acquisition before removing the patient from the scan table. If all the required anatomy is not visualized, repeat the scan to acquire the necessary body parts.
- The PA spine scan image displays primarily the vertebral posterior elements, which have characteristic shapes. These shapes can be used to place the intervertebral markers and label the vertebral levels when degenerative disease has obscured the intervertebral spaces. L1, L2, and L3 have a Y shape; L4 has an H or X shape and appears to have "feet"; and L5 looks like a sideways I or "dog bone" (Fig. 26-10). L3 commonly has the widest transverse processes; L1, L2, and L3 are approximately the same height, and L4 is a little taller than the others; and the iliac crest usually lies at the level of the L4-L5 intervertebral space.

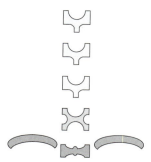

Fig. 26-10 Characteristic shapes of L1 through L5 and their relationship to the iliac crests as seen on a DXA anteroposterior spine scan.

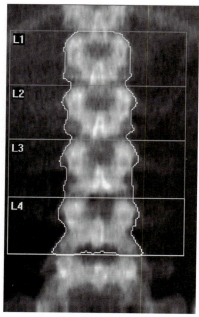

Fig. 26-11 Properly acquired and analyzed lumbar spine DXA scan.

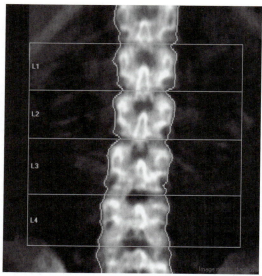

Fig. 26-12 Six lumbar vertebrae. Note that the vertebral labeling is done from the bottom to the top according to the shape of the vertebrae. This is an atypical case.

Image Analysis: PA Lumbar Spine Scan

Automated manufacturer's software is sensitive and accurate most of the time. The least amount of operator intervention will allow for precise and reliable serial scanning, which is crucial in monitoring a patient's percentage change in BMD over time.

1. Select the image to be analyzed.
2. Select Analyze or Analyze Patient from the toolbar.
3. Select and adjust the image contrast when needed.
4. Verify the ROIs.
   a. Intervertebral markers
   b. Vertebral labels
5. Use the standard analysis or manual analysis tools to modify placement of the ROI and vertebral labels.
6. Verify that the bone edges are correct. Accept the program's placement of edges unless they are obviously incorrect.
7. Select Results and save the image analysis.

Helpful Hints:

- The iliac crest is an excellent landmark for consistent placement of the intervertebral markers at baseline and follow-up scanning.
- A small percentage of patients appear to have four or six lumbar vertebrae rather than five, which is most commonly seen. The vertebrae can be labeled by locating L5 and L4 based on their characteristic shapes and then counting up (Fig. 26-12). The procedure of counting from the bottom superiorly biases toward a higher BMD and avoids including T12 without a rib, which significantly lowers the BMD. This procedure ensures a conservative diagnosis of low BMD.

Structures Seen:

- All five lumbar vertebrae and midsection of T12, intervertebral disk spaces, iliac crests, superior portion of the sacroiliac joints.
- This projection demonstrates the bodies, disk spaces, and transverse processes of the lumbar spine and T12.

Image Critique (Fig. 26-11):

- The spine is straight and centered in the scan field.
- Note that patients with scoliosis should have relatively equal amounts of soft tissue on either side of the spine.
- The scan contains a portion of the iliac crest and half of T12; the last set of ribs is shown.
- The entire scan field is free of external artifacts.
- The intervertebral markers are properly placed, and vertebrae are properly labeled.
- The bone edges are reasonably placed.

- Only if absolutely necessary should the bone edges be adjusted or the intervertebral markers angled. If used, these techniques should be performed in a manner that will be easy to reproduce at follow-up scanning.

Scan Results:

- The results can be sent electronically to the referring physician using a picture archiving and communication system (PACS), email address, or fax number directly from the densitometry computer. If desired, a hard copy can also be printed.
- Results are expressed as BMD, T-score, and Z-score.

DXA Scanning of the Proximal Femur

The proximal femur scan is perhaps the most important skeletal scan in bone densitometry because its results are the best predictor of future hip fracture, which is the most devastating of the fragility fractures. The proximal femur scan is more difficult to perform properly and precisely because of variations in anatomy and the small ROIs. Degenerative changes, scoliosis, paralysis, avascular necrosis, and polio can influence the proximal femur BMD results. Thorough history-taking by the operator is important to relate disease processes that may influence BMD outcome and understanding to the interpreting physician. All scanners come with positioning aids that should be used according to the manufacturer's instructions.

Routine Examination

The routine examination of the proximal femur(s) includes the area from 3 to 4 cm below the greater trochanter to 2 to 3 cm above the greater trochanter.

Preparation

1. Select existing or new patient function.
2. Enter patient demographics.
3. Select the Femur Measure or Measure Patient function. Ensure that the proper scan or array mode has been chosen by the software. Make any changes before proceeding.
4. Instruct the patient to remove all external or heavily attenuating materials (e.g., belts, buttons, snaps, wallets, rivets) from the proximal femur region. If possible, have the patient change into a gown to ensure that there are no external artifacts and to provide consistency in serial scanning.

Positioning Aids

The positioning aids will vary depending on the specific manufacturer. Typically, a femur positioner device is used. Follow the specific manufacturer's recommendation.

Use a sponge or pillow for head comfort. A rice bag or sandbag can be used to stabilize the nonscanned femur. If the position is challenging for the patient, rolled towels or radiographic sponges can be used under the knee of the nonscanned leg to provide comfort.

Positioning and Procedure Details: Proximal Femur Scan

Body Position:

- Patient is supine and centered on scan table and scan table pad.
- Arms are flexed at the elbow and rested across the abdomen or clear of the scan region.

Part Position:

- Body is centered to the midline of the table pad.
- Body is centered within the table pad length and parameters.
- The femoral neck is parallel with the tabletop.
- Correct positioning requires that the femoral shaft be slightly abducted from the natural position to achieve a straight femoral shaft.
- Shoulders and pelvic girdle are squared to the table pad.
- The femoral shaft is internally rotated (15 to 25 degrees).
- Ensure proper rotation from the knee to the trochanter.
- Rotate and attach the foot to the femur positioning device.

Central Ray/Laser Light Placement:

- Varies according to manufacturer
- Place the central ray or laser light approximately 7 to 8 cm below the greater trochanter *or*
- 2 to 3 cm below the symphysis pubis

Scan Field:

Once the scan site is selected, the automated scan field is determined (based on manufacturer) by entering height and weight or by manual adjustments. The scanning program will acquire the necessary data from the scan field, which must then be analyzed.

Shielding:

None required

Patient Instruction:

Do not move.

Completing the Procedure:

- Review the scan acquisition before removing the patient from the scan table. If all the required anatomy is not visualized, repeat the scan to acquire the necessary body parts.
- A few patients have little or no space between the ischium and the femoral neck. In some cases, part of the ischium lies under the neck, which elevates the BMC and thus falsely elevates the femoral neck BMD (Fig. 26-13, *A*). This might be caused by the

femoral neck. In cases of unilateral disease, scan the less affected hip. A fractured or replaced hip with orthopedic hardware should not be scanned.

The limits of the technology are taxed by patients with extreme thinness or thickness and/or very low bone mass. These problems are revealed by poor bone edge detection and/or a mottled or "moth-eaten" appearance of the image. Use the fastest speed for thin patients and the slowest speed for thick patients. Some images show the bone edges, and it is obvious when the proper edge cannot be detected. For images that do not show the bone edges, the area values must be checked and compared. A very large Ward's triangle area or a very small trochanter area is a clue that the bone edges are not being properly detected. The operator's manual may not adequately cover these problems. It is the responsibility of the operator to recognize the problems and query the manufacturer's applications department about the best ways to handle such difficulties. If a patient is deemed unsuitable for a DXA hip scan, consider scanning the nondominant forearm as an alternate site.

DXA Scanning of the Forearm

The preferred ROI of the DXA forearm scan is the one-third (33%) region, which measures an area that is primarily cortical bone near the mid-forearm. Although the ulna is available for analysis, only the radius results are usually reported. The following information can help in positioning patients for forearm DXA scans, analyzing the scan results, and evaluating the validity of the scans.

Positioning and Procedure Details: Forearm

- The nondominant forearm is generally scanned because it is expected to have slightly lower BMD than the dominant arm. In patients with a history of wrist fracture, internal hardware, or severe deformity resulting from arthritis, the affected forearm should not be scanned. If both forearms are unsuitable for scanning, other anatomic sites should be considered.
- At the time of the initial scan, the forearm should be measured according to the manufacturer's instructions. Usually the ulna is measured from the ulna styloid to the olecranon process. The distal one-third of this measurement is used to place the one-third or 33% ROI. The baseline measurement should be noted and then used again for follow-up scans to ensure that the one-third region is placed at the same anatomic point on every scan. The directions for determining the starting and ending locations of the scan must be followed exactly. Follow the manufacturers' guidelines.
- The forearm must be straight and centered in the scan field. Soft tissue must surround the ulna and radius, and several lines of air must be present on the ulnar

side. If the forearm is very wide, the scan must be set manually for a wider scan region so that adequate air is included.

- Motion is a common problem. The patient should be seated in a chair in a comfortable position so that the arm does not move during the scan. Avoid unnecessary conversation during the scan to minimize movement. The same chair should be used for all patients to ensure consistency over time. The chair should have a back but no wheels or arms.
- Historically, the placement of the ultradistal ROI has varied according to several different protocols. One popular method is to manually place the distal end of the ROI just below the radial endplate. This placement is easy to replicate on follow-up scans. The ultradistal ROI is subject to low BMD, which creates bone edge detection problems. The bone edge should be carefully checked and manually adjusted if needed. Baseline and follow-up bone edges must match to avoid changes in BMD solely because of area changes caused by inconsistent bone edge detection.

Image Critique (Fig. 26-16):

- The forearm is straight and centered in the scan field.
- Adequate amounts of soft tissue and air are included.
- No motion blurring is present.

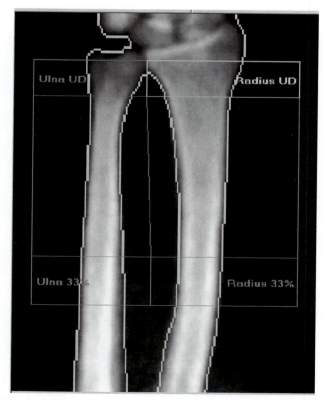

Fig. 26-16 Properly acquired and analyzed distal forearm DXA scan.

- The proximal and distal ends of the scan field are properly placed.
- Bone edges are properly and consistently placed.
- No artifacts, such as watches or bracelets, are present in the scan field.

Scan Results:

- The results can also be sent electronically to a PACS, DICOM functions, email address, or fax number directly from the densitometry computer. If desired, a hard copy can also be printed.
- Results are expressed as BMD, T-score, and Z-score.

SUMMARY

The main purpose of bone densitometry is to facilitate the diagnosis of osteoporosis by detecting low bone mass before fractures occur. DXA is the gold standard for diagnosis and longitudinal monitoring of metabolic bone changes over time. DXA scans of the proximal femur (hip) and lumbar spine are the most widely performed. However, the forearm is also scanned for osteoporosis evaluation.

Regardless of the type of scanner, the operator performing the scans must be properly trained by the manufacturer in equipment operation and scanner quality control, as well as patient positioning, scan acquisition, and analysis. This will ensure accurate and precise bone density results. History taking and data input are essential tasks for completion of the examination. Knowledge of the current treatments and expected outcomes is important to perform complete technical evaluation of the scan results and to answer patient questions. Quality assurance is essential to ensure accurate and precise DXA scan acquisition and analysis. Operators must stay current to have the knowledge to properly maintain and update their equipment.

State Licensure Information

Information regarding licensure for limited x-ray machine operators (LXMO) in each state is frequently updated. To find the most current information for your state, we suggest you consult the website of the American Society of Radiologic Technologists (ASRT) at www.asrt.org. The information can be found in the *Legislative & Regulatory* section of the website. Select the link for *Individual State Licensure Information.*

As of the publication of this book, according to the ASRT website, 32 states license LXMO as follows:

Arizona	New Mexico
Arkansas	North Dakota
California	Ohio
Colorado	Oregon
Delaware	Pennsylvania
Florida *(fluoroscopy under direct MD supervision)*	Rhode Island
	South Carolina
Illinois	Tennessee
Indiana	Texas
Iowa *(must pass hospital fluoroscopy exam)*	Utah
	Vermont
Kentucky	Virginia
Maine	Washington
Minnesota	West Virginia *(podiatry only)*
Mississippi	Wisconsin
Montana	Wyoming
Nebraska	
New Jersey	

As of the publication of this book, according to the American Registry of Radiologic Technologists (ARRT) website at www.arrt.org, the ARRT contracts with more than 25 states for administering ARRT exams to state license/permit candidates. For this reason, *Radiography Essentials for Limited Practice* and the accompanying Workbook and Licensure Exam Prep are designed to prepare the LXMO student to successfully pass the ARRT Examination for the Limited Scope of Practice in Radiography and the Bone Densitometry Equipment Operators Examination.

The authors of *Radiography Essentials for Limited Practice* use the name limited x-ray machine operator (LXMO) throughout the book because this is the name adopted by the ASRT. However, the licensure laws of many states contain other names for these licensees. The following is a list of the name used in each state, as of the publication of this book.

Limited X-ray Machine Operator Titles by State

State	Title
Arizona	Practical Technologist in Radiology
Arkansas	Limited Licensed Technologist
California	(Limited Permit) X-ray Technician
Colorado	Limited (X-ray Machine) Operator
Delaware	Radiation Technician
Florida	Basic X-ray Machine Operator
Illinois	Limited Radiographer
Indiana	Limited Radiographer
Iowa	Limited Diagnostic Radiographer
Kentucky	Limited X-ray Machine Operator

Continued

Limited X-ray Machine Operator Titles by State—cont'd

State	Title
*Louisiana	"Private" Radiologic Technologist
Maine	Limited Radiographer
*Massachusetts	Limited (Scope) Radiographer
Minnesota	Limited X-ray Machine Operator
Mississippi	Limited X-ray (Machine) Operator
Montana	Limited Permit Radiologic Technologist
Nebraska	Limited Radiographer
New Jersey	Limited Radiologic Technologist
New Mexico	Limited X-ray Machine Operator
North Dakota	Limited Scope X-ray Operator
Ohio	General X-ray Machine Operator
Oregon	Limited X-ray Machine Operator
Pennsylvania	Limited Radiographer
Rhode Island	Limited License Radiographer
South Carolina	Limited (General) Radiographer
Tennessee	X-ray Operator
Texas	Limited Medical Radiologic Technologist
Utah	Radiology Practical Technician
Vermont	Limited Radiographer
Virginia	Limited Radiologic Technologist
Washington	Registered X-ray Technician
Wisconsin	Limited X-ray Machine Operator
Wyoming	(Restricted License) Radiologic Technician

*Conflicting data regarding status as a limited license state or category.

The American Registry of Radiologic Technologists Rules of Ethics[n]

The Rules of Ethics form the second part of the Standards of Ethics. They are mandatory standards of minimally acceptable professional conduct for all Certificate Holders and Candidates. Certification and Registration are methods of assuring the medical community and the public that an individual is qualified to practice within the profession. Because the public relies on certificates and registrations issued by ARRT, it is essential that Certificate Holders and Candidates act consistently with these Rules of Ethics. These Rules of Ethics are intended to promote the protection, safety, and comfort of patients. The Rules of Ethics are enforceable. Certificate Holders and Candidates engaging in any of the following conduct or activities, or who permit the occurrence of the following conduct or activities with respect to them, have violated the Rules of Ethics and are subject to sanctions as described hereunder:

1. Employing fraud or deceit in procuring or attempting to procure, maintain, renew, or obtain or reinstate certification and registration as issued by ARRT; employment in radiologic technology; or a state permit, license, or registration certificate to practice radiologic technology. This includes altering in any respect any document issued by the ARRT or any state or federal agency, or by indicating in writing certification and registration with the ARRT when that is not the case.

2. Subverting or attempting to subvert ARRT's examination process, and/or the structured self-assessments that are part of the Continuing Qualifications Requirements (CQR) process. Conduct that subverts or attempts to subvert ARRT's examination and/or CQR assessment process includes, but is not limited to:

   (i) disclosing examination and/or CQR assessment information using language that is substantially similar to that used in questions and/or answers from ARRT examinations and/or CQR assessments when such information is gained as a direct result of having been an examinee or a participant in a CQR assessment or having communicated with an examinee or a CQR participant; this includes, but is not limited to, disclosures to students in educational programs, graduates of educational programs, educators, anyone else involved in the preparation of Candidates to sit for the examinations, or CQR participants; and/or

   (ii) soliciting and/or receiving examination and/or CQR assessment information that uses language that is substantially similar to that used in questions and/or answers on ARRT examinations or CQR assessments from an examinee, or a CQR participant, whether requested or not; and/or

   (iii) copying, publishing, reconstructing (whether by memory or otherwise), reproducing or transmitting any portion of examination and/or CQR assessment materials by any means, verbal or written, electronic or mechanical, without the prior express written permission of ARRT or using professional, paid or repeat examination takers and/or CQR assessment participants, or any other individual for the purpose of reconstructing any portion of examination and/or CQR assessment materials; and/or

   (iv) using or purporting to use any portion of examination and/or CQR assessment materials that were obtained improperly or without authorization for the purpose of instructing or preparing any Candidate for examination or participant for CQR assessment; and/or

   (v) selling or offering to sell, buying or offering to buy, or distributing or offering to distribute any portion of examination and/or CQR assessment materials without authorization; and/or

   (vi) removing or attempting to remove examination and/or CQR assessment materials from an examination or assessment room; and/or

(vii) having unauthorized possession of any portion of or information concerning a future, current, or previously administered examination or CQR assessment of ARRT; *and/or*

(viii) disclosing what purports to be, or what you claim to be, or under all circumstances is likely to be understood by the recipient as, any portion of or "inside" information concerning any portion of a future, current, or previously administered examination or CQR assessment of ARRT; *and/or*

(ix) communicating with another individual during administration of the examination or CQR assessment for the purpose of giving or receiving help in answering examination or CQR assessment questions, copying another Candidate's, or CQR participant's answers, permitting another Candidate or a CQR participant to copy one's answers, or possessing unauthorized materials including, but not limited to, notes; *and/or*

(x) impersonating a Candidate, or a CQR participant, or permitting an impersonator to take or attempt to take the examination or CQR assessment on one's own behalf; *and/or*

(xi) using any other means that potentially alters the results of the examination or CQR assessment such that the results may not accurately represent the professional knowledge base of a Candidate, or a CQR participant.

3. Convictions, criminal proceedings, or military courts-martial as described below:

   (i) conviction of a crime, including a felony, a gross misdemeanor, or a misdemeanor, with the sole exception of speeding and parking violations. All alcohol and/or drug related violations must be reported; *and/or*

   (ii) criminal proceeding where a finding or verdict of guilt is made or returned but the adjudication of guilt is either withheld, deferred, or not entered or the sentence is suspended or stayed; or a criminal proceeding where the individual enters an Alford plea, a plea of guilty or nolo contendere (no contest); or where the individual enters into a pre- trial diversion activity; *or*

   (iii) military courts-martial related to any offense identified in these Rules of Ethics.

4. Violating a rule adopted by a state or federal regulatory authority or certification board resulting in the individual's professional license, permit, registration or certification being denied, revoked, suspended, placed on probation or a consent agreement or order, voluntarily surrendered, subjected to any conditions, or failing to report to ARRT any of the violations or actions identified in this Rule.

5. Performing procedures which the individual is not competent to perform through appropriate training and/or education or experience unless assisted or personally supervised by someone who is competent (through training and/or education or experience).

6. Engaging in unprofessional conduct, including, but not limited to:

   (i) a departure from or failure to conform to applicable federal, state, or local governmental rules regarding radiologic technology practice or scope of practice; or, if no such rule exists, to the minimal standards of acceptable and prevailing radiologic technology practice;

   (ii) any radiologic technology practice that may create unnecessary danger to a patient's life, health, or safety.

   Actual injury to a patient or the public need not be established under this clause.

7. Delegating or accepting the delegation of a radiologic technology function or any other prescribed health-care function when the delegation or acceptance could reasonably be expected to create an unnecessary danger to a patient's life, health, or safety. Actual injury to a patient need not be established under this clause.

8. Actual or potential inability to practice radiologic technology with reasonable skill and safety to patients by reason of illness; use of alcohol, drugs, chemicals, or any other material; or as a result of any mental or physical condition.

9. Adjudication as mentally incompetent, mentally ill, chemically dependent, or dangerous to the public, by a court of competent jurisdiction.

10. Engaging in any unethical conduct, including, but not limited to, conduct likely to deceive, defraud, or harm the public; or demonstrating a willful or careless disregard for the health, welfare, or safety of a patient. Actual injury need not be established under this clause.

11. Engaging in conduct with a patient that is sexual or may reasonably be interpreted by the patient as sexual, or in any verbal behavior that is seductive or sexually demeaning to a patient; or engaging in sexual exploitation of a patient or former patient. This also applies to any unwanted sexual behavior, verbal or otherwise.

12. Revealing a privileged communication from or relating to a former or current patient, except when otherwise required or permitted by law, or viewing, using, releasing, or otherwise failing to adequately protect the security or privacy of confidential patient information.

13. Knowingly engaging or assisting any person to engage in, or otherwise participating in, abusive or fraudulent billing practices, including violations of federal Medicare and Medicaid laws or state medical assistance laws.

14. Improper management of patient records, including failure to maintain adequate patient records or to furnish a patient record or report required by law; or

making, causing, or permitting anyone to make false, deceptive, or misleading entry in any patient record.

15. Knowingly assisting, advising, or allowing a person without a current and appropriate state permit, license, registration, or an ARRT registered certificate to engage in the practice of radiologic technology, in a jurisdiction that mandates such requirements.

16. Violating a state or federal narcotics or controlled-substance law.

17. Knowingly providing false or misleading information that is directly related to the care of a former or current patient.

18. Subverting, attempting to subvert, or aiding others to subvert or attempt to subvert ARRT's Continuing Education (CE) Requirements, and/or ARRT's Continuing Qualifications Requirements (CQR). Conduct that subverts or attempts to subvert ARRT's CE or CQR Requirements includes, but is not limited to:

    (i) providing false, inaccurate, altered, or deceptive information related to CE or CQR activities to ARRT or an ARRT recognized recordkeeper; *and/or*

    (ii) assisting others to provide false, inaccurate, altered, or deceptive information related to CE or CQR activities to ARRT or an ARRT recognized recordkeeper; *and/or*

    (iii) conduct that results or could result in a false or deceptive report of CE or CQR completion; *and/or*

    (iv) conduct that in any way compromises the integrity of the CE or CQR Requirements such as

sharing answers to the post-tests or self-learning activities, providing or using false certificates of participation, or verifying credits that were not earned.

19. Subverting or attempting to subvert the ARRT certification and registration processes by:

    (i) making a false statement or knowingly providing false information to ARRT; or

    (ii) failing to cooperate with any investigation by the ARRT.

20. Engaging in false, fraudulent, deceptive, or misleading communications to any person regarding the individual's education, training, credentials, experience, or qualifications, or the status of the individual's state permit, license, or registration certificate in radiologic technology or certificate of registration with ARRT.

21. Knowing of a violation or a probable violation of any Rule of Ethics by any Certificate Holder or Candidate and failing to promptly report in writing the same to the ARRT.

22. Failing to immediately report to his or her supervisor information concerning an error made in connection with imaging, treating, or caring for a patient. For purposes of this rule, errors include any departure from the standard of care that reasonably may be considered to be potentially harmful, unethical, or improper (commission). Errors also include behavior that is negligent or should have occurred in connection with a patient's care, but did not (omission). The duty to report under this rule exists whether or not the patient suffered any injury.

3. Performing calculations involving percentages.
   a. $37\% + 33\% = 70\%$
   b. $100\% + 65\% = 165\%$
   c. $25\% - 13\% = 12\%$
   d. $20\% \times 80\% \rightarrow 0.2 \times 0.8 = 0.16 = 16\%$
   e. $150\% \div 30\% \rightarrow 1.5 \div 0.3 = 5 = 500\%$
   f. $\frac{1}{2} \times 40\% \rightarrow 0.5 \times 0.4 = 0.2 = 20\%$
   g. $1.10 \times 80\% \rightarrow 0.1 \times 0.8 = 0.08 = 8\%$
   h. $80\% - 10\% = 70\%$
4. Calculating the value of percentages.
   a. 20% of $88 \rightarrow 0.2 \times 88 = 17.6$
   b. 90% of $200 \rightarrow 0.9 \times 200 = 180$
   c. 50% of $61 \rightarrow 0.5 \times 61 = 30.5$
   d. 130% of $40 \rightarrow 1.3 \times 40 = 52$
   e. 300% of $12 \rightarrow 3 \times 12 = 36$
   f. $3\% \times 50 \rightarrow 0.03 \times 50 = 1.5$
   g. $29\% \times 1000 \rightarrow 0.29 \times 1000 = 290$
   h. $15\% \times 90 \rightarrow 0.15 \times 90 = 13.5$
5. Determining percentages.
   a. $13 \div 63 = 0.206 = 20.6\%$
   b. $29 \div 80 = 0.363 = 36.3\%$
   c. $43 \div 200 = 0.215 = 21.5\%$
   d. $40 \div 160 = 0.25 = 25\%$
   e. $50 \div 35 = 1.429 = 142.9\%$
   f. $20 \div 2 = 10 = 1000\%$
   g. $100 \div 25 = 4 = 400\%$
   h. $25 \div 1000 = 0.025 = 2.5\%$
6. Calculating the increase or decrease of numbers by a percentage.
   a. $100\% + 15\% = 115\% = 1.15$ $100 \times 1.15 = 115$
   b. $100\% + 250\% = 350\% = 3.5$ $30 \times 3.5 = 105$
   c. $100\% + 25\% = 125\% = 1.25$ $150 \times 1.25 = 187.5$
   d. $100\% - 10\% = 90\% = 0.9$ $85 \times 0.9 = 76.5$
   e. $100\% - 12\% = 88\% = 0.88$ $20 \times 0.88 = 17.6$
   f. $100\% + 40\% = 140\% = 1.4$ $15 \times 1.4 = 21$
   g. $100\% + 100\% = 200\% = 2.0$ $2.0 \times 46 = 92$
   h. $100\% - 50\% = 50\% = 0.5$ $0.5 \times 200 = 100$

PRACTICE SOLVING EQUATIONS

1. $3x + 6 = 10 + 2$
   Perform calculation: $3x + 6 = 12$
   Subtract 6 from both sides: $3x = 12 - 6$
   $3x = 6$
   Divide both sides by 3: $x = 2$
2. $\frac{21}{x} = 8 - 1$
   Perform calculation: $\frac{21}{x} = 7$
   Multiply both sides by x: $21 = 7x$
   Divide both sides by 7: $\frac{21}{7} = x$ $3 = x$ $x = 3$
3. $x - 17 = 13$
   Add 17 to both sides: $x - 17 + 17 = 13 + 17$
   Perform calculations: $x = 30$
4. $20 = 3x - 4$
   Add 4 to both sides: $20 + 4 = 3x - 4 + 4$
   Perform calculations: $24 = 3x$
   Divide both sides by 3: $24/3 = x$ $8 = x$ $x = 8$

5. $2x = \frac{18}{2}$
   Perform calculation: $2x = 9$
   Divide both sides by 2: $x = \frac{9}{2}$
   Perform calculation: $x = 4\frac{1}{2}$ (4.5)
6. $45 = 9x$
   Divide both sides by 9: $\frac{45}{9} = x$
   Perform calculation: $5 = x$ $x = 5$
7. $\frac{30}{x} = \frac{6}{2}$
   Perform calculation: $\frac{30}{x} = 3$
   Multiply both sides by x: $30 = 3x$
   Divide both sides by 3: $10 = x$ $x = 10$
8. $\frac{x}{7} = \frac{36}{6}$
   Cross multiply: $6x = 36 \times 7$
   Perform calculation: $6x = 252$
   Divide both sizes by 6: $x = 42$
9. $\frac{56}{8} = \frac{49}{x}$
   Cross multiply: $56x = 49 \times 8$
   Perform calculation: $56x = 392$
   Divide both sides by 56: $x = 7$
10. $\frac{12}{4} = \frac{x}{15}$
    Cross multiply: $4x = 12 \times 15$
    Perform calculation: $4x = 180$
    Divide both sides by 4: $x = 45$

PRACTICE PROBLEMS INVOLVING EXPONENTS AND SQUARE ROOTS

1. Calculating the value of exponential terms.
   a. 5 cubed $= 5^3 = 5 \times 5 \times 5 = 125$
   b. $2^4 = 2 \times 2 \times 2 \times 2 = 16$
   c. $9^2 = 9 \times 9 = 81$
   d. $10^4 = 10 \times 10 \times 10 \times 10 = 10,000$
   e. $4^3 = 4 \times 4 \times 4 = 64$
2. Determining square roots.
   a. $\sqrt{49} = 7$
   b. $\sqrt{36} = 6$
   c. $\sqrt{64} = 8$
   d. $\sqrt{400} = 20$

PRACTICE PROBLEMS USING MEASUREMENT UNITS

1. Conversions from one metric unit to another.
   a. $75\ V \times 1000\ V/kilovolt = 75,000\ V$
   b. $3\ cm/x\ cm = 1\ m/100\ cm$ per m $= 300\ cm$
   c. $10\ ml/x\ L = 0.1000\ ml/1\ L = 0.01\ L$
   d. $20\ gm/x\ kg = 1000\ gm/1\ kg = 0.02\ kg$
   e. $15\ cg/x\ gm = 100\ cg/1\ gm = 0.15\ gm$
2. Conversions from one English unit to another.
   a. $16\ in \div 36\ in/yard = 0.4444\ yd$
   b. $\frac{1}{2}\ pt \times 16\ oz/pt = 8\ oz$
   c. $84\ in \div 12\ in/ft = 7\ ft$
   d. $18\ qt \div 4\ qt/gal = 4.5\ gal$
   e. $4.8\ lb \times 16\ oz/lb = 76.8\ oz$

3. Conversions between English and metric units.
   a. 3 oz × 30 ml/oz = 90 ml
   b. 0.25 lb ÷ 2.2 lb/kg = 0.1136 kg
      0.1136 kg × 1000 gm/kg = 113.6 gm
   c. 5 in × 2.54 cm/in = 12.7 cm
      12.7 cm ÷ 100 cm/m = 0.127 m
   d. 30 mm ÷ 10 mm/cm = 3 cm
      3 cm ÷ 2.54 cm/in = 1.18 in
   e. 40 gm ÷ 1000 gm/kg = 0.04 kg
      0.04 kg × 2.2 lb/kg = 0.088 lb
      0.088 lb × 16 oz/lb = 1.408 oz
4. Time and temperature conversions.
   a. $\frac{1}{20}$ sec × 1000 msec/sec = 50 msec
   b. 330 sec ÷ 60 sec/min = 5.5 min
      5.5 min ÷ 60 min/hr = 0.0917 hr
   c. 3.4 days × 24 hr/day = 81.6 hr
   d. (19° C × 1.8) + 32 = 34.2 + 32 = 66.2° F
   e. 50° F − 32 ÷ 1.8 = 18 ÷ 1.8 = 10° C

SOLVING MILLIAMPERE-SECOND PROBLEMS

1. Calculating mAs, given mA and time.
   a. 200 mA × $\frac{1}{40}$ sec = 5 mAs
   b. 300 mA × $\frac{1}{20}$ sec = 15 mAs
   c. 100 mA × $\frac{2}{15}$ sec = 13.33 mAs
   d. 500 mA × 0.02 sec = 10 mAs
   e. 50 mA × 0.3 sec = 15 mAs
   f. 150 mA × 1¼ sec = 150 × 1.25 sec = 187.5 mAs
   g. 400 mA × 2 msec = 400 × 0.002 sec = 0.8 mAs
   h. 300 mA × $\frac{1}{120}$ sec = 2.5 mAs
   i. 1200 mA × 0.005 sec = 6 mAs
   j. 600 mA × 0.04 sec = 24 mAs
   k. 750 mA × 0.1 sec = 75 mAs
   l. 300 mA × 0.3 sec = 90 mAs
   m. 200 mA × 0.4 sec = 80 mAs
2. Calculating exposure time, given the mA and mAs.
   a. 40 mAs ÷ 50 mA = 0.8 sec or $\frac{4}{5}$ sec
   b. 25 mAs ÷ 200 mA = 0.125 sec or $\frac{1}{8}$ sec
   c. 10 mAs ÷ 300 mA = 0.033 sec
   d. 1 mAs ÷ 100 mA = 0.01 sec
   e. 8 mAs ÷ 400 mA = 0.02 sec
   f. 50 mAs ÷ 500 mA = 0.1 sec or $\frac{1}{10}$ sec
   g. 20 mAs ÷ 800 mA = 0.025 sec or 25 milliseconds
   h. 300 mAs ÷ 150 mA = 2 sec
   i. 150 mAs ÷ 25 mA = 6 sec
   j. 5 mAs ÷ 1000 mA = 0.005 or 5 milliseconds
3. Calculating mA, given mAs and time.
   a. 10 mAs ÷ $\frac{1}{30}$ sec = 10 mAs × 30 = 300 mA
   b. 25 mAs ÷ ½ sec = 25 mAs × 2 = 50 mA
   c. 40 mAs ÷ $\frac{2}{15}$ sec = 40 × $\frac{15}{2}$ = $\frac{600}{2}$ = 300 mA
   d. 5 mAs ÷ 0.01 sec = 500 mA
   e. 8 mAs ÷ 0.02 sec = 400 mA
   f. 100 mAs ÷ 0.5 sec = 200 mA
   g. 20 mAs ÷ 0.2 sec = 100 mA
   h. 3 mAs ÷ 0.01 sec = 300 mA
   i. 60 mAs ÷ 0.3 sec = 200 mA

PRACTICE PROBLEMS INVOLVING DISTANCE CHANGES

1. $\frac{1}{x}=\frac{30^2}{40^2}$ $\frac{1}{x}=\frac{3^2}{4^2}$ $\frac{1}{x}=\frac{9}{16}$ $9x=16$
   $x=16/9=1\frac{7}{9}(1.77)\times I_1$

2. $\frac{1}{x}=\frac{40^2}{72^2}$ $\frac{1}{x}=\frac{5^2}{9^2}$ $\frac{1}{x}=\frac{25}{81}$ $25x=81$
   $x=81/25=3.24\times I_1$

3. $\frac{15}{x}=\frac{40^2}{48^2}$ $\frac{15}{x}=\frac{5^2}{6^2}$ $\frac{15}{x}=\frac{25}{36}$ $25x=15\times36$
   $25x=540$ $x=21.6$ mAs

4. $\frac{40}{x}=\frac{72^2}{84^2}$ $\frac{40}{x}=\frac{6^2}{7^2}$ $\frac{40}{x}=\frac{36}{49}$ $36x=40\times49$
   $36x=1960$
   $x=1969/36=54.44$ mAs

5. $\frac{10}{x}=\frac{40^2}{72^2}$ $\frac{10}{x}=\frac{5^2}{9^2}$ $\frac{10}{x}=\frac{25}{81}$ $25x=10\times81$
   $25x=810$ $x=32.4$ mAs

6. $\frac{1}{x}=\frac{40^2}{72^2}$ $\frac{1}{x}=\frac{5^2}{9^2}$ $\frac{1}{x}=\frac{25}{81}$ $25x=81$
   $x=\frac{81}{25}=3.24\times I_1$

7. $\frac{25}{x}=\frac{40^2}{60^2}$ $\frac{25}{x}=\frac{2^2}{3^2}$ $\frac{25}{x}=\frac{4}{9}$ $4x=225$
   $x=\frac{225}{4}=56.25$ mAs

8. $\frac{100}{x}=\frac{72^2}{60^2}$ $\frac{100}{x}=\frac{6^2}{5^2}$ $\frac{100}{x}=\frac{36}{25}$ $36x=25\times100$
   $36x=2500$ $x=69.4$ mAs

9. $\frac{20}{x}=\frac{60^2}{48^2}$ $\frac{20}{x}=\frac{5^2}{4^2}$ $\frac{20}{x}=\frac{25}{16}$ $25x=20\times16$
   $25x=320$ $x=12.8$ mAs

10. $\frac{8}{x}=\frac{72^2}{40^2}$ $\frac{8}{x}=\frac{9^2}{5^2}$ $\frac{8}{x}=\frac{81}{25}$ $81x=8\times25$
    $81x=200$ $x=2.45$ mAs

PRACTICE PROBLEMS INVOLVING PATIENT PART SIZE CHANGES

1. 3 kVp/cm × 3 cm = 9 kVp change
   96 kVp − 9 kVp = 85 kVp for 27 cm
2. 2 kVp/cm × 2 cm = 4 kVp change
   74 kVp + 4 kVp = 78 kVp for 18 cm
3. 50 mAs × 0.8 = 40 mAs for 22 cm
   40 mAs × 0.8 = 32 mAs for 20 cm
   32 mAs × 0.8 = 25.6 mAs for 18 cm
4. 30 mAs × 1.3 = 39 mAs for 21 cm
   39 mAs × 1.3 = 50.7 mAs for 23 cm
   50.7 mAs × 1.3 = 65.9 mAs for 25 cm

5. 10 mAs × 1.3 = 13 mAs for 14 cm
   13 mAs × 1.3 = 16.9 mAs for 16 cm
6. 2 kVp × 3 cm = 6 kVp change
   55 kVp + 6 kVp = 61 kVp for 7 cm
7. 100 mAs × 0.8 = 80 mAs for 34 cm
   80 mAs × 0.8 = 64 mAs for 32 cm
   64 mAs × 0.8 = 51.2 mAs for 30 cm
8. 4 mAs × 1.3 = 5.2 mAs for 21 cm
9. 40 mAs × 1.3 = 52 mAs for 22 cm
   52 mAs × 1.3 = 67.6 mAs for 24 cm

PRACTICE PROBLEMS USING THE 15% RULE

1. 86 kVp × 0.85 = 73 kVp
   25 mAs × 2 = 50 mAs
2. 80 kVp × 1.15 = 92 kVp
   100 mAs ÷ 2 = 50 mAs
3. 66 kVp × 1.15 = 76 kVp
   10 mAs ÷ 2 = 5 mAs
4. 94 kVp × 0.85 = 80 kVp
   40 mAs × 2 = 80 mAs
5. 72 kVp × 1.15 = 83 kVp
   60 mAs ÷ 2 = 30 mAs
6. 96 kVp × 0.85 = 82 kVp
   80 mAs × 2 = 160 mAs
7. 70 kVp × 1.15 = 81 kVp
   20 mAs ÷ 2 = 10 mAs
8. 54 kVp × 1.15 = 62 kVp
   5 mAs ÷ 2 = 2.5 mAs
9. 120 kVp × 0.85 = 102 kVp
   30 mAs × 2 = 60 mAs
10. 68 kVp × 1.15 = 78 kVp
    50 mAs ÷ 2 = 25 mAs

PRACTICE PROBLEMS CALCULATING MEDICATION DOSAGE

1. 100 mg/25 mg/tablet = 4 tablets
2. 250 mg/50 mg/ml = 5 ml
3. 40 mcg/80 mcg/tablet = ½ tablet
4. 5 mg/1 mg/ml = 5 ml
5. 200 mg/tablet × 8 tablets = 1600 mg/day (1.6 g/day)

Sample Manual X-ray Technique Charts

	Extremities								
	Small Hand, Wrist, Foot 40 SID, NONGRID			Medium Elbow, Ankle, Leg 40 SID, NONGRID			Large Shoulder, Knee 40 SID, 12:1 GRID		
cm	mA	sec	kVp	mA	sec	kVp	mA	sec	kVp
2	100	.02	56						
3	100	.03	56						
4	100	.04	56						
5	100	.05	56						
6	100	.06	56	100	.35	62			
7	100	.07	56	100	.04	62			
8	100	.08	56	100	.05	62	100	.04	76
9				100	.06	62	100	.05	76
10				100	.07	62	100	.06	76
11				100	.08	62	100	.07	76
12				100	.10	62	100	.08	76
13				100	.11	62	100	.09	76
14				100	.12	62	100	.1	76
15							100	.11	76
16							100	.12	76
17							100	.13	76
18							100	.15	76
19							100	.16	76
20							100	.18	76

Note: Shield gonads.

SID, Source–image receptor distance.

	Cervical Spine								
	Lateral Flexion, Extension, Nongrid Oblique 72 SID, NONGRID			AP Cervical Oblique, Grid 40 SID, 12:1 GRID			AP Upper Cervical (Open Mouth) 40 SID, 12:1 G RID		
cm	mA	sec	kVp	mA	sec	kVp	mA	sec	kVp
8	100	.35	76	200	.04	76	200	.04	80
9	100	.04	76	200	.05	76	200	.05	80
10	100	.05	76	200	.06	76	200	.06	80
11	100	.06	76	200	.07	76	200	.07	80
12	100	.07	76	200	.08	76	200	.08	80
13	100	.08	76	200	.1	76	200	.1	80
14	100	.1	76	200	.11	76	200	.11	80
15	100	.11	76	200	.12	76	200	.12	80
16	100	.12	76	200	.15	76	200	.15	80

Note: Shield gonads on all views. Shield thyroid on all views except AP lower cervical. Measure through path of central ray, except for AP open-mouth. For AP open-mouth, measure as for AP lower cervical.
AP, Anteroposterior; *SID,* source–image receptor distance.

	Thoracic Spine					
	AP 40 SID, 12:1 GRID			Lateral 40 SID, 12:1 GRID		
cm	mA	sec	kVp	mA	sec	kVp
16	200	.04	86			
17	200	.05	86			
18	200	.05	86			
19	200	.06	86			
20	200	.07	86			
21	200	.08	86			
22	200	.1	86			
23	200	.11	86			
24	200	.12	86	25	.6	86
25	200	.13	86	25	.7	86
26	200	.15	86	25	.8	86
27	200	.18	86	25	.8	86
28	200	.2	86	25	.9	86
29	200	.22	86	25	1.	86
30	200	.25	86	25	1.2	86
31	200	.27	86	25	1.2	86
32	200	.3	86	25	1.5	86
33	200	.3	86	25	1.8	86
34	200	.35	86	25	2.	86
35	200	.4	86	25	2.	86
36	200	.5	86	50	1.2	86
37				50	1.5	86
38				50	1.8	86
39				50	2.	86
40				50	2.2	86

Note: Shield gonads.
AP, Anteroposterior; *SID,* source–image receptor distance.

	Lumbar Spine					
	AP 40 SID, 12:1 GRID			Lateral 40 SID, 12:1 GRID		
cm	**mA**	**sec**	**kVp**	**mA**	**sec**	**kVp**
16	200	.06	82			
17	200	.07	82			
18	200	.08	82			
19	200	.1	82			
20	200	.12	82			
21	200	.15	82			
22	200	.18	82			
23	200	.2	82			
24	200	.25	82	200	.22	90
25	200	.3	82	200	.25	90
26	200	.35	82	200	.27	90
27	200	.4	82	200	.3	90
28	200	.5	82	200	.35	90
29	200	.6	82	200	.35	90
30	200	.7	82	200	.4	90
31	200	.8	82	200	.4	90
32	200	.9	82	200	.5	90
33	200	1	82	200	.5	90
34	200	1.2	82	200	.6	90
35	200	1.5	82	200	.7	90
36	200	1.7	82	200	.8	90
37		1.7	82	200	1	90
38		2	82	200	1.2	90
39		2	82	200	1.2	90
40		2.2	82	200	1.5	90

Note: Shield gonads.
AP, Anteroposterior; *SID,* source–image receptor distance.

| | Chest | | | | | | Ribs | | | | | |
| | PA and Oblique 72 SID, 10:1 GRID | | | Lateral 72 SID, 10:1 GRID | | | Above Diaphragm AP, PA, Oblique 40 SID, 12:1 GRID | | | Below Diaphragm AP, PA, Oblique 40 SID, 12:1 GRID | | |
cm	mA	sec	kVp	mA	sec	kVp	mA	sec	kVp	mA	sec	kVp
16	300	.004	120				200	.04	72	200	.08	78
17	300	.005	120				200	.05	72	200	.09	78
18	300	.005	120				200	.05	72	200	.1	78
19	300	.006	120				200	.06	72	200	.12	78
20	300	.007	120				200	.06	72	200	.13	78
21	300	.008	120				200	.07	72	200	.15	78
22	300	.008	120				200	.07	72	200	.18	78
23	300	.01	120				200	.08	72	200	.18	78
24	300	.01	120	300	.015	120	200	.08	72	200	.2	78
25	300	.012	120	300	.018	120	200	.1	72	200	.25	78
26	300	.012	120	300	.018	120	200	.1	72	200	.27	78
27	300	.015	120	300	.02	120	200	.12	72	200	.3	78
28	300	.018	120	300	.022	120	200	.12	72	200	.35	78
29	300	.02	120	300	.025	120	200	.15	72	200	.4	78
30	300	.02	120	300	.03	120	200	.15	72	200	.45	78
31	300	.022	120	300	.035	120	200	.18	72	200	.5	78
32	300	.025	120	300	.035	120	200	.18	72	200	.6	78
33	300	.027	120	300	.04	120	200	.2	72	200	.7	78
34	300	.03	120	300	.04	120	200	.2	72	200	.75	78
35	300	.035	120	300	.05	120	200	.22	72	200	.8	78
36	300	.04	120	300	.05	120	200	.25	72	200	.9	78
37	300	.04	120	300	.06	120	200	.27	72	200	1	78
38	300	.05	120	300	.07	120	200	.3	72	200	1.2	78
39	300	.06	120	300	.08	120	200	.33	72	200	1.2	78
40	300	.07	120	300	.1	120	200	.25	72	200	1.5	78
41				300	.12	120	200	.37	72	200	1.5	78
42				300	.05	120	200	.4	72	200	1.7	78

Note: Shield gonads. Measure through path of central ray.

AP, Anteroposterior; *PA,* posteroanterior; *SID,* source–image receptor distance.

Abdomen			
AP, Oblique (Upright or Recumbent) 40 SID, 12:1 GRID			
cm	mA	sec	kVp
16	200	.1	70
17	200	.12	70
18	200	.15	70
19	200	.2	70
20	200	.25	70
21	200	.3	70
22	200	.35	70
23	200	.4	70
24	200	.5	70
25	200	.6	70
26	200	.7	70
27	200	.8	70
28	200	1	70
29	200	1.2	70
30	200	1.5	70
31	200	1.7	70
32	200	2	70
33	200	2	70
34	200	2.2	70
35	200	2.5	70
36	200	2.7	70
37	200	3	70
38	200	2.5	76
39	200	3	76
40	200	3	78

AP, Anteroposterior; *SID*, source–image receptor distance.

	AP, PA PA Axial (Caldwell) 40 SID, 12:1 GRID			Skull									
				Lateral 40 SID, 12:1 GRID			AP Axial (Towne) Submentovertical (SMV) 40 SID, 12:1 GRID			40 SID, 12:1 GRID			
cm	**mA**	**sec**	**kVp**	**mA**	**sec**	**kVp**	**mA**	**sec**	**kVp**	**mA**	**sec**	**kVp**	
10				200	.018	80				100	.06	70	
11				200	.022	80				100	.07	70	
12				200	.03	80				100	.1	70	
13				200	.035	80				100	.11	70	
14				200	.045	80				100	.12	70	
15	200	.05	80	200	.05	80				100	.15	70	
16	200	.07	80	200	.06	80	200	.07	86	100	.18	70	
17	200	.08	80	200	.07	80	200	.08	86	100	.2	70	
18	200	.09	80	200	.08	80	200	.08	86	100	.25	70	
19	200	.1	80	200	.09	80	200	.1	86	100	.3	70	
20	200	.12	80	200	.1	80	200	.12	86	100	.35	70	
21	200	.15	80	200	.11	80	200	.15	86	100	.4	70	
22	200	.18	80	200	.12	80	200	.15	86	100	.4	70	
23	200	.18	80				200	.18	86	100	.5	70	
24	200	.2	80				200	.18	86	100	.6	70	
25	200	.2	80				200	.2	86	100	.7	70	
26	200	.22	80				200	.2	86	100	.8	70	
27							200	.25	86				
28							200	.25	86				

AP, Anteroposterior; *PA*, posteroanterior; *SID*, source–image receptor distance.

Sample Automatic Exposure Control Technique Chart

	Pelvis and Upper Femora							
Part	**cm**	**kVp***	**sec**	**mA**	**mAs**	**AEC**	**SID**	**IR**
Pelvis and upper femurs—AP†	19	70		200s		⬤⬤	40″	14 × 17 cm
Femoral necks—AP oblique†	19	70		200s		⬤⬤	40″	14 × 17 cm
Hip—AP†	18	65		200s		⬤⬤	40″	10 × 12 cm
Hip—lateral (Lauenstein-Hickey)†	18	65		200s		⬤⬤	40″	10 × 12 cm
Hip—axiolateral (Danelius-Miller)‡	24	80	.80	200s	160		40″	10 × 12 cm

*Kilovoltage peak values are for a three-phase, 12-pulse generator.
†Bucky, 16:1 grid.
‡Tabletop, 8:1 grid.
AEC, Automatic exposure control; *AP*, anteroposterior; *s*, small focal spot; *SID*, source–image receptor distance.

Optimum Kilovoltage (kVp) Ranges

NONGRID/NON-BUCKY

Limbs

Small (fingers, hand, wrist, toes, foot)	50 to 60 kVp
Medium (forearm, elbow, ankle)	55 to 65 kVp
Large (lower leg, knee,° humerus, shoulder°)	60 to 70 kVp

Chest

PA° (heart, lungs, mediastinum)	75 to 90 kVp
Lateral° (heart, lungs, mediastinum)	80 to 90 kVp
Ribs,° PA, AP	60 to 68 kVp

Spine

Cervical, lateral	75 to 85 kVp

Skull

Sinuses° (all views)	60 to 70 kVp
Facial bones° (Waters method, Caldwell method, lateral, tangential)	65 to 75 kVp
Nasal bones (axial, lateral)	52 to 60 kVp

WITH GRID/BUCKY

Extremities

Humerus, shoulder	72 to 82 kVp
Knee	70 to 84 kVp

Chest

PA, lateral (heart, lungs, mediastinum)	100 to 130 kVp
Ribs (above diaphragm)	66 to 74 kVp
Ribs (below diaphragm)	70 to 78 kVp
Sternum, oblique	60 to 72 kVp

Spine

Cervical, AP lower	70 to 80 kVp
Cervical, AP upper (open-mouth)	74 to 86 kVp
Cervical, lateral, oblique	70 to 80 kVp
Thoracic, AP	85 to 95 kVp
Thoracic, lateral	82 to 92 kVp
Thoracic, swimmer's technique	80 to 90 kVp
Lumbar, AP	80 to 95 kVp
Lumbar, oblique	85 to 95 kVp
Lumbar, lateral	90 to 105 kVp
Lumbar, lateral spot, L5 to S1	95 to 115 kVp
Sacrum, AP	80 to 90 kVp
Sacrum, lateral	95 to 110 kVp
Coccyx, AP	70 to 82 kVp
Lateral	78 to 89 kVp

Pelvis/Hips

AP	78 to 88 kVp
Frog-leg lateral	72 to 82 kVp
Cross-table lateral	80 to 90 kVp

Skull

AP, PA, Caldwell method, Waters method	74 to 86 kVp
Occipital (Towne method), axial (SMV/VSM)	80 to 90 kVp
Sinuses, Caldwell method, PA	70 to 80 kVp
Facial bones, all views except lateral	66 to 76 kVp
Sinuses/facial bones, lateral	60 to 70 kVp

°Grid/Bucky techniques preferred.
AP, Anteroposterior; *PA,* posteroanterior; *SMV,* submentovertical; *VSM,* verticosubmental.

Milliampere-seconds (mAs) Table

Time		Milliampere-seconds (mAs)							
	sec	25	50	100	150	200	300	400	500
0.008	0.008	0.21	0.42	0.83	1.25	1.67	2.5	3.33	4.17
0.017	0.016	0.42	0.83	1.67	2.5	3.33	5	6.67	8.33
0.025	0.025	0.625	1.25	2.5	3.75	5	7.5	10	12.5
0.033	0.033	0.83	1.67	3.33	5	6.67	10	13.33	16.67
0.042	0.042	1.04	2.08	4.17	6.25	8.33	12.5	16.67	20.83
0.05	0.05	1.25	2.5	5	7.5	10	15	20	25
0.067	0.066	1.67	3.33	6.67	10	13.33	20	26.67	33.33
0.083	0.083	2.08	4.17	8.33	12.5	16.67	25	33.33	41.67
0.1	0.10	2.5	5	10	15	20	30	40	50
0.133	0.13	3.33	6.67	13.33	20	26.67	40	53.33	66.67
0.2	0.20	5	10	20	30	40	60	80	100
0.25	0.25	6.25	12.5	25	37.5	50	75	100	125
0.3	0.30	7.5	15	30	45	60	90	120	150
0.333	0.33	8.33	16.67	33.33	50	66.67	100	133.33	166.67
0.4	0.40	10	20	40	60	80	120	160	200
0.5	0.50	12.5	25	50	75	100	150	200	250
0.6	0.60	15	30	60	90	120	180	240	300
0.8	0.80	20	40	80	120	160	240	320	400
1	1.00	25	50	100	150	200	300	400	500
1.25	1.25	31.25	62.5	125	187.5	250	375	500	625
1.5	1.50	37.5	75	150	225	300	450	600	750
1.75	1.75	43.75	87.5	175	262.5	350	525	700	875
2	2.00	50	100	200	300	400	600	800	1000
2.5	2.50	62.5	125	250	375	500	750	1000	1250
3	3.00	75	150	300	450	600	900	1200	1500
3.5	3.50	87.5	175	350	525	700	1050	1400	1750
4	4.00	100	200	400	600	800	1200	1600	2000
5	5.00	125	250	500	750	1000	1500	2000	2500

Nomogram for Determining Patient Skin Dose from X-ray Exposure[p]

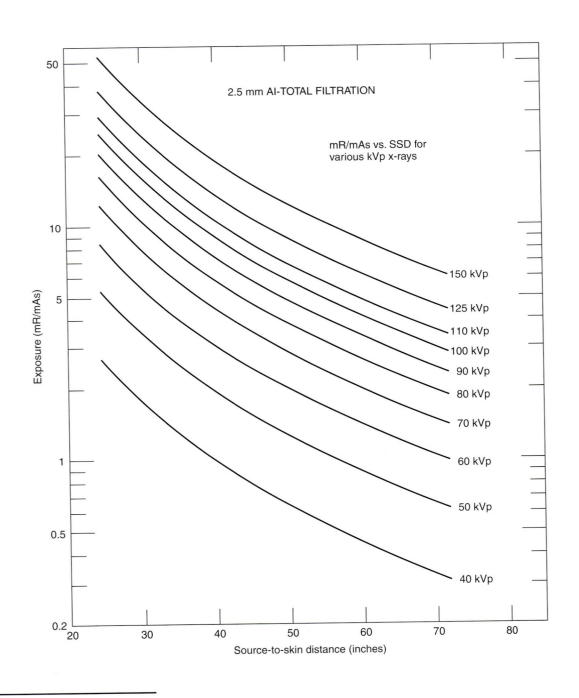

2.5 mm AI-TOTAL FILTRATION

mR/mAs vs. SSD for various kVp x-rays

150 kVp
125 kVp
110 kVp
100 kVp
90 kVp
80 kVp
70 kVp
60 kVp
50 kVp
40 kVp

Exposure (mR/mAs)

Source-to-skin distance (inches)

[p]Courtesy Edward McCullough.

573

Note: To calculate skin dose, intersect the source-to-skin distance (SSD) on the horizontal line with the kVp graph in the chart. Read the dose on the left vertical column. This number is the dose for each mAs. Multiply the number for each mAs to determine the total dose. For example, if you intersect an SSD of 30 inches with a kVp of 90, you see the dose on the vertical column is 12 mR per mAs. If the mAs for the exposure is 10, the total dose is 120 mR. When referencing this chart, please convert the exposure value (in mR) you determine into the new unit of exposure, Air Kerma. See Chapter 11 to make this conversion. The air kerma value will be 1/100th of the mR value.

Screen/Film Image Receptor Systems[q]

Key Terms

artifacts
backscatter
film-screen contact
fluorescence
latitude
phosphors

radiolucent
rare earth phosphors
screen speed
silver halide
spectral emission
spectral sensitivity

---

[q]The material in this appendix was formerly Chapter 8 in the third edition of this text. Screens and film are declining in use because of the expanded use of digital imaging. The chapter is included here for reference purposes.

This chapter is about imaging systems: cassettes, intensifying screens, and film. Although filmless imaging systems (digital radiography) are being installed in large institutions at an expanding rate, it will be some time before these systems will be available to the vast majority of limited operators. When this time comes, there will be technologic advances in these systems that will make any detailed discussion in this writing obsolete. For these reasons, this text focuses on imaging systems that involve the use of film.

Proper care and handling of cassettes and film are essential to radiographic quality and are skills needed by radiographers on a continuing basis. An understanding of the image receptor system will aid in the formation of good work habits for the production of quality radiographic images.

CASSETTES

Radiographic film holders, called *cassettes*, were first described in Chapter 2. Common sizes are listed in Table 2-1. Cassettes serve three important functions:

1. They protect the film from exposure to light during use.
2. Their rigid structure protects the delicate film from bending and scratching during use.
3. They contain intensifying screens and keep them in close contact with the film during exposure.

The exposure side of the cassette (Fig. H-1) is considered to be its "front." A label on the front indicates the position of an area on the film that is protected from exposure. This area is often called the *ID (identification) blocker* because radiation is blocked from exposing the film in this location. The ID blocker reserves this area for the printing of patient identification at the time of processing. Some specialized cassettes may be purchased with the ID blocker at another corner and on either margin; however, the standard location is the one illustrated.

The cassette "back" is the access side of the cassette (Fig. H-2). When you are unloading and reloading the cassette, this side faces up. Note that this position usually places the ID blocker in the upper left corner.

The structure of the cassette is diagrammed in Fig. H-3. The front is made of a **radiolucent** material, that is, a substance that is easily penetrated by the x-ray beam. It may be a very lightweight metal alloy or a plastic material made of a durable resin. Mounted to the inside of the cassette front is the front intensifying screen.

The back of the cassette may also be made of metal or plastic. Inside the back is a layer of lead foil. The purpose of this layer is to prevent **backscatter**. Backscatter is radiation from the cassette back and the cassette tray that is scattered back toward the film. Backscatter would cause fog on the film if not absorbed by the lead foil layer.

Inside the foil layer is a layer of padding, usually a plastic foam. The purpose of this layer is to keep the intensifying screens pressed tightly against the film when the cassette is closed, so as to maintain good **film-screen contact**. The importance of good film-screen contact is discussed later in this chapter.

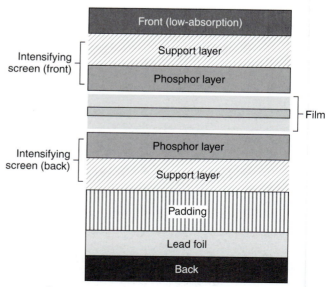

Fig. H-2 Cassette back, access side. Properly positioned, the cassette opens like a book. *ID*, Identification.

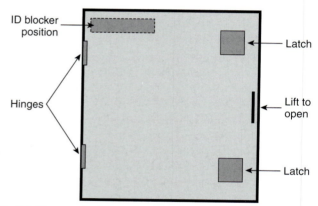

Fig. H-3 Cross-section of cassette with film between the two screens.

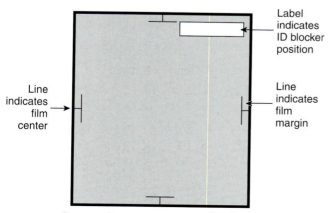

Fig. H-1 Cassette front, exposure side. *ID*, Identification.

The back intensifying screen is mounted on the padding layer. The intensifying screens cover the inside surfaces of the cassette. When the film is placed in the cassette, it is sandwiched between the intensifying screens.

Special cassettes are used with some phototiming systems. These cassettes must allow remnant radiation to pass readily through the cassette back to the detector. For this reason, they have a radiolucent back and no lead foil layer. Each is usually clearly marked "phototiming cassette" and should be used only for this purpose.

INTENSIFYING SCREENS

An intensifying screen is a flat surface coated with fluorescent crystals called **phosphors.** These phosphors give off light when exposed to x-rays. This is called **fluorescence.** The phosphors absorb x-ray energy and emit the energy in the form of light. Direct x-rays expose the film to some degree; however, the greatest amount of exposure on radiographs is from the light of the intensifying screens. More than 99% of the x-ray image is formed by the screen light.

The purpose of intensifying screens is to reduce the amount of exposure required to produce an image. They enhance the efficiency of the exposure process. Direct x-ray exposure can produce an image on film; however, this would require 25 to 400 times more milliampere-seconds (mAs) than to produce the same images with intensifying screens. The use of intensifying screens greatly reduces both exposure time and patient dose because of the reduction in mAs. Screen use also reduces the generator size and x-ray tube capacity required for radiography.

Screen Construction

The structure of an intensifying screen is illustrated in Fig. H-4. It consists of a polyester base, or support layer, with an adhesive coat that holds the phosphors in a thin, smooth layer. A clear protective coating helps to prevent stains and wear to the crystal layer. The thickness of the screen is very thin, with the base about 1 mm thick. The screen must be flexible to permit good contact with the film.

Screen Speed

The efficiency of a screen in converting x-rays to light is called **screen speed.** A screen with greater efficiency requires less exposure, so the screen is said to be "faster." The industry uses a relative speed (RS) of 100 as the standard against which the speeds of screens are measured. A screen with a speed of 200 would be twice as fast as a 100-speed screen and would require only half as much exposure. Typical screen RSs are 50, 100, 200, 400, 600, and 800. In the radiology department, one will usually find, at a minimum, a screen with an RS of about 300 to 400 for general-purpose radiography. For the limbs (fingers, hand/wrist, toes, and foot), a slower screen with an RS of 50 to 100 will typically be used for greater recorded detail.

Screen Speed Versus Recorded Detail

Intensifying screen phosphors glow when struck by the energy of the x-ray photons. When a phosphor absorbs sufficient energy, the entire phosphor will glow, not just the portion that was exposed. This results in an area of exposure on the film that is greater in size than the original area of exposure to the phosphor. For this reason, the use of intensifying screens produces images with less recorded detail than images produced by direct exposure to x-rays.

Large crystals and a thick phosphor layer produce more film exposure from a given amount of x-ray exposure (greater speed) but also provide less radiographic detail (Fig. H-5). Larger crystals produce a larger image of a "point" of exposure. Light rays diverge from within the screen until they reach the film, creating an exposure area on the film that is larger than the phosphor size. When the phosphor layer is thick, there is more light divergence from deep within the screen, which enlarges the film area exposed and decreases image sharpness.

Screens in the range of RS 200 to 600 are used for routine radiography. These screens are referred to as *regular* screens. Most screens may be used either on the tabletop or in the Bucky. Some screens also have a reflective layer between the base and the phosphors. This layer increases the efficiency of the screen by reflecting the majority of the screen light toward the film.

Fine phosphors in a thin layer provide greater radiographic detail but require more exposure. Speed values of 50 or 100 are slower than regular screens and provide high-detail images for small anatomic parts and the smaller parts of the limbs. They may be referred to as *extremity* or *detail* screens and are generally used only on the tabletop.

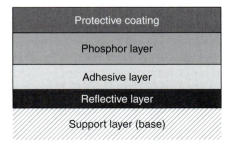

Fig. H-4 Screen composition.

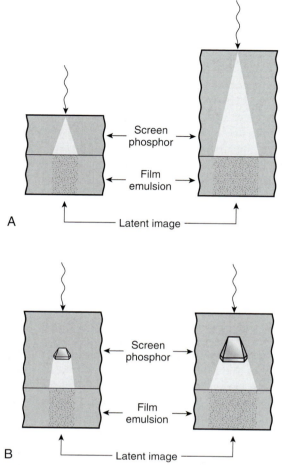

Fig. H-5 Crystal size and phosphor layer thickness affect recorded detail. **A,** Thick phosphor *(right)* produces less detail. **B,** Larger crystal *(right)* produces less detail.

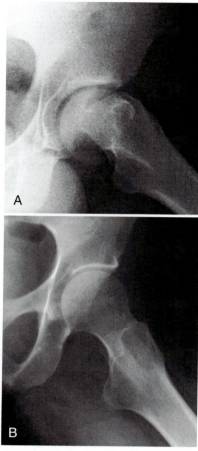

Fig. H-6 A, Radiograph of the hip showing quantum mottle (grainy) appearance typical of a fast radiograph screen. **B,** Greater recorded detail is shown on a hip radiograph using a slower speed. No quantum mottle is seen.

Quantum mottle (described in Chapter 7) will become more pronounced as the speed of the screen increases. The grainy-appearing mottle will become noticeable in screens with speeds higher than RS 400 (Fig. H-6). Box H-1 lists the basic screen design characteristics that enhance either speed or detail.

Extremely fast screens in the 1000- to 1200-speed class are available, but these screens do not provide sufficient image quality for general work and are used only when very high speed is required. Hospitals may have extra-fast screens for very large patients or for special applications.

Screen Phosphors

For several decades, the conventional screen phosphor was calcium tungstate, which is now obsolete. During the 1970s, new screen technology was introduced using **rare earth phosphors.** These are phosphors containing one of the rare earth elements gadolinium, lanthanum, or yttrium. Screens using rare earth phosphors are about four times more efficient than the old calcium tungstate

 Box H-1

Typical Modern Screen Characteristics

Regular	Detail
Rare earth phosphors	Rare earth phosphors
Moderate crystal size	Small crystal size
Medium phosphor thickness	Thin phosphor thickness
Reflective layer	Reflective layer
Relative speed: 200-600	Relative speed: 50-100

screens, reducing exposure to approximately one fourth of the amount previously required, with no negative consequences in terms of film quality.

Spectral emission refers to the color of light emitted by a phosphor. Typical colors of light emitted by rare earth phosphors are green or yellow-green and blue or blue-violet. The light of the screen must be matched with the spectral sensitivity of the film. A green-emitting screen must be matched with a green-sensitive film.

Screen Care and Cleaning

Intensifying screens tend to build up a static electric charge. The static charge on the screens attracts dust and dirt. A discharge of this static electricity may expose the film, creating black static **artifacts** (unwanted marks or images) on the radiograph. These marks and their prevention are discussed in Appendix I.

Cleaning Intensifying Screens

1. Remove dust with pressurized air or a very soft brush.
2. Using a recommended commercial screen cleaner that contains an antistatic ingredient and a very soft, lint-free applicator, apply screen cleaner sparingly (never pour liquid on screen).
3. Stand open cassette on edge to dry before reloading.

Dirt on screens prevents the screen light from reaching the film, causing unexposed (white) areas on the film image. To prevent these artifacts, intensifying screens must be kept clean. The frequency of cleaning is determined by the frequency of use and by the amount of dust in the environment. All screens should be inspected and cleaned at least every 3 months. Screens may be marked in one corner so that an identifying number or letter is evident on all the films in the cassette. The outside of the cassette carries the same identifying mark. When a film exhibits evidence of screen dirt, it is easy to locate the offending cassette for cleaning without inspecting all cassettes of that size.

Dust and dry dirt may be removed with a *soft* brush (camel hair or sable) or with a spray of pressurized air from an aerosol can. Pressurized air and suitable brushes are available at camera supply stores. If screen dirt cannot be removed with a soft brush or pressurized air, a liquid cleaner is necessary. In the past, soap and water or grain alcohol was used for cleaning screens. Because modern rare earth phosphor screens may be damaged by these products, a commercial screen cleaner recommended by the screen manufacturer should be used. Commercial screen cleaners have an additional advantage in that they contain an antistatic ingredient. This reduces the static charge buildup on the screen, minimizing the accumulation of screen dirt and helping to prevent artifacts on the film from either screen dirt or static.

When cleaning screens with a liquid cleaner, use a soft, lint-free applicator (Fig. H-7). Pressed cotton squares or nonwoven gauze sponges work well. *Never pour liquid directly onto the screen* because the liquid will be absorbed in the foam pad layer of the cassette and/or the support layer of the screen. This may damage the padding or warp the screen. Moisten the applicator sparingly and use a light touch to wipe the screen clean. Do not pick, scratch, or scrape at screen dirt; this practice damages the screen and worsens the problem.

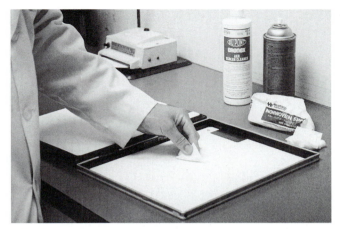

Fig. H-7 Radiographer cleaning a screen with liquid cleaner.

White or light-colored "dirt" may be difficult to detect on screens in ordinary light, but it can be easily seen when the screen is illuminated with an ultraviolet light in a darkened room. Scanning with an ultraviolet light will also reveal areas where the screen crystals have been worn away or lost because of damage. Loss of screen crystals will produce artifacts similar to those caused by specks of dirt.

When the screens are clean, stand the cassette on edge to dry completely before reloading it with film.

Cassettes and screens are expensive and damage easily. Proper care and cleaning are essential to ensure that they provide good service for a reasonable period (5 to 8 years). Develop the habit of keeping your hands clean and dry. Remove film from the cassette without completely opening it. Never leave the cassette lying open on the loading bench because it is easy to drop something on the screens or scrape them when working in the dark. In addition, this practice increases wear on the hinges of the cassette. Take care that cassettes are not dropped or bumped, since damage to the cassette frame may cause the screens to fit improperly, leading to poor film-screen contact. Keeping the loading bench clean will reduce screen dirt, minimizing the need to clean the screens.

Film-screen Contact

Poor film-screen contact is a condition that exists when the two screens are not in firm contact with both surfaces of the film. The usual causes are warping of the cassette frame or the screens, dents in screens, deterioration of the padding layer, damaged hinges, or damaged latches. Poor film-screen contact results in poor image quality because the light rays diverge in the space between the film and the screen (Fig. H-8), creating a film image that differs from the precise screen image and appears blurred.

An important component of a quality control program is the test to ensure that the screens have direct contact with the film. Film-screen contact is tested using a special tool called a *screen contact test mesh*. This coarse wire mesh

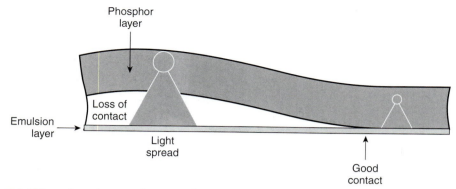

Fig. H-8 When there is space between the screen and the film, divergence of light from the screens causes blurring of the film image.

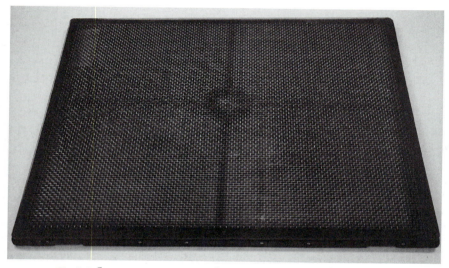

Fig. H-9 Screen contact test mesh positioned on a cassette for test.

is laminated in plastic to keep it flat (Fig. H-9). It is placed on top of the cassette and an exposure is made. A suggested exposure will be provided with the tool. If none is available, try approximately 5 mAs and 50 kVp when using a 400-speed cassette. At a viewing distance of about 9 feet, the radiograph should show a consistent image of the mesh. Dark, unsharp areas on the test film indicate areas of poor film-screen contact (Fig. H-10). All radiology departments should have a screen contact mesh tool.

This test should be performed semiannually on all cassettes and on the offending cassette when unsharp areas are noted on a radiograph.

RADIOGRAPHIC FILM

A processed x-ray film is similar to a photographic negative. The exposed areas appear dark and the unexposed areas are light. Film for general use differs from photographic film, however, in that it is "duplitized," that is, it has a photographic emulsion on both sides. Because x-rays can penetrate film and because each side is in contact with an intensifying screen, the exposure to the film

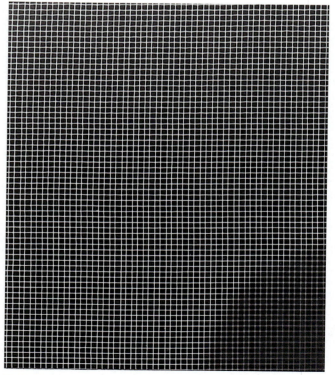

Fig. H-10 Film-screen contact test showing area of poor contact.

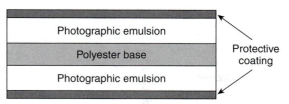

Fig. H-11 Film construction. The thin outer layers are an overcoat that protects the emulsion.

is doubled, decreasing the exposure time and patient dose by half.

Film Construction

The structure of film is illustrated in Fig. H-11. The film base is made of a polyester plastic for strength and to give it flexibility. It must be optically clear, strong, and of consistent thickness. It is tinted a pale blue or blue-gray color. This tint reduces eye strain for the physician when reading the films. The photographic emulsion is coated on both sides of the base. A thin, soluble "overcoat" on both sides protects the emulsion to some degree during film handling.

Film emulsion consists of a mixture of gelatin and **silver halide** crystals. Silver halides are salts of the halogen elements: fluorine, chlorine, bromine, and iodine (class VII in the periodic table of elements).

Composition of Radiographic Film Emulsion

- Gelatin
- Silver halide microcrystals
- Silver bromide: 90%
- Silver iodide: 10%
- Catalyst (sulfur contaminate, usually silver sulfide)

Causes of Film Exposure

Film emulsion readily assumes the "exposed" state. Exposure may be caused by the following:
- Light
- X-rays
- Heat
- Certain chemicals or chemical fumes
- Pressure
- Static electricity discharge
- Age

Most x-ray film emulsions consist mainly of silver bromide, with a small percentage of silver iodide. A tiny amount of sulfur, usually in the form of silver sulfide, is added to the emulsion as a catalyst to enhance the exposure and development process. The sulfur compound forms "sensitivity specks" within the emulsion that attract electrons, providing a focus for chemical changes within the emulsion crystals. Exposure causes the silver halide to assume an exposed state by changing its chemical arrangement, thus forming the latent image.

Film Storage

Unexposed film and film that has been exposed to x-rays are quite vulnerable to additional exposure. The unexposed crystal state is unstable and may be changed to an exposed state by exposure to light, x-rays, chemicals or chemical fumes, pressure, heat, static electricity, and age. For this reason, it is important that unexposed film be properly stored and carefully handled. Improper storage results in a general exposure response, fogging the film. Optimum storage requires a cool, dry place that is protected from x-rays and chemical fumes. Conditions for optimum film storage are listed in Box H-2.

Film boxes should be stored on edge (Fig. H-12) so that the labels and expiration dates are visible. Stacking of boxes should be avoided because fog may be caused by the pressure of the weight of the boxes. Film stock should be rotated so that the oldest boxes are used first to avoid films becoming fogged from age. The expiration date on new film should be at least 1 year after the purchase date. It is false economy to stock more film than can be used within a few months.

Boxes that are opened and in use are kept in a light-proof film bin in the x-ray darkroom for convenience in reloading cassettes. However, the darkroom is not a good place for longer-term film storage, because it tends to be warm, damp, and contaminated with the fumes of processing chemicals.

Film Characteristics and Types

Film is manufactured in a variety of different types, providing different responses to exposure. Inherent film characteristics (those built into the film by the manufacturer) include sensitivity (speed), contrast, and **spectral sensitivity,** the portion of the electromagnetic spectrum to which the film is most sensitive.

 **Box H-2**

Film Storage

- Clean, dry location: 30% to 50% humidity
- Temperature: 50° to 70° F (10° to 21° C)
- Away from chemical fumes
- Safe from radiation exposure
- Standing on edge
- Expiration date clearly visible

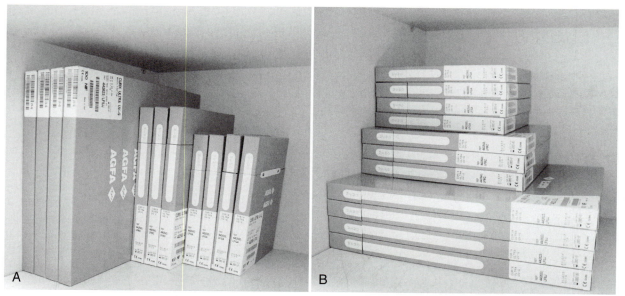

Fig. H-12 Film is placed on edge on the shelf. **A,** Right way. **B,** Wrong way.

The size of the silver halide crystals and the thickness of the emulsion determine both the speed of the film and the degree of recorded detail in the finished radiograph. As with intensifying screens, larger crystals and a thicker crystal layer produce a faster speed. Thinner layers of finer crystals are used to produce greater detail. Film response is also tailored by the manufacturer to vary the amount of radiographic contrast. Radiographic film can be purchased with different contrast properties. Some examinations require a high-contrast film and others a low-contrast film. Some manufacturers also make a medium-contrast film.

The term **latitude** is used to describe radiographic film along with contrast. *Latitude* is the term used when a wide range of densities can be recorded on the film. Latitude and contrast are inversely related. As the contrast of the film decreases, latitude increases. Therefore, a film with "wide latitude" will show many more densities than a film with high contrast. A wide-latitude film will exhibit a more gray appearance because it not only shows black and white areas, but also shows many levels of gray. Whereas intensifying screens are purchased for their speed only, film is purchased with both speed and contrast in mind.

SUMMARY

Cassettes are an integral part of the IR system. They prevent light exposure to the film and keep the intensifying screens in close contact with the film surface. The purpose of the intensifying screens is to reduce the exposure required to produce an image. Rare earth phosphors in the screens emit blue or green light when exposed to x-rays, and this light is primarily responsible for the exposure to the film. Screens are available in a number of speed classes. Fast screens reduce exposure but produce less radiographic resolution; slower screens are used when fine detail is desired. Screens require good care, proper cleaning, periodic inspection, and testing for film-screen contact.

General-purpose radiographic film has a double emulsion coated on a clear, blue polyester base. The spectral sensitivity of the film should be matched to the spectral emission of the screens. The silver halide crystals of the emulsion are unstable in their unexposed state and easily become exposed when subjected to light, x-rays, heat, fumes, pressure, and age. They must therefore be stored properly and handled with care. The inherent characteristics of film include speed, contrast, and spectral sensitivity.

X-ray Darkroom and Film Processing[r]

artifacts
automatic film processors
base + fog
crescent mark
densitometer
film bin

film dryer
film identification printer
pass box
safelights
sensitometer

---

[r]The material in this appendix was formerly Chapter 10 in the third edition of this text. Darkroom processing of film is declining in use because of the expanded use of digital imaging. The chapter is included here for reference purposes.

This chapter introduces the x-ray darkroom and covers the specific information needed for correct film handling and film processing. Both manual and automatic processing methods are presented in detail, as is information about processor maintenance and quality control. This chapter can only be understood when you have mastered the information on film quality in Chapter 7 and have a clear understanding of cassettes and film from Appendix H.

Many problems with radiographic quality are traceable not to the x-ray room but to the darkroom and film processor. An understanding of film handling and film processing will aid in the formation of good work habits for the production of quality radiographic images. This knowledge enables the radiographer to identify and correct problems when they occur.

DARKROOM

An x-ray darkroom is illustrated in Fig. I-1. The essential features include the film processor (automatic) or processing tanks (manual), a loading bench, a film bin, a film identification printer, and one or more safelights. There may be a pass box in the wall, which allows transfer of films to and from the darkroom while ensuring that no light is admitted to the darkroom.

The walls of the darkroom are painted a light color so that the safelight is reflected throughout the room, increasing visibility in the dark. There should be ample ventilation because of the presence of chemical fumes. The doors and any seams in the walls must be effectively sealed so that no white light is admitted during film processing. Foam weather stripping around the door jamb is effective for this purpose and must be replaced as soon as it begins to fail.

Safelights

Safelights are special light fixtures fitted with filters (Fig. I-2). The safelight filter should permit only the passage of light frequencies to which the film is least sensitive. For this reason, the filter must match the spectral sensitivity of the film. GBX filters should be used in the darkroom. They are a deep cherry-red and are safe for use with blue-sensitive, green-sensitive, and x-ray–sensitive films. Even the best safelight emits some white light, so do not leave film in safelight indefinitely. A radiographic film can remain in safelight for about 40 seconds without becoming fogged. Light-emitting diode (LED) safelights are also available for use with both blue- and green-sensitive films.

The safelight is not safe under all conditions. It must be no closer than 3 to 4 feet from the feed tray of the processor and countertops. A distance of 4 feet is preferable. The wattage of safelight bulbs is also important; 7 to 15 W is the maximum, depending on location. If a safelight has to be closer than 4 feet to the film, a 7 W bulb should always be used. Never replace a safelight bulb with a bulb of higher wattage than the one removed. Safelights that are safe for normal use will fog film when the exposure is prolonged. The safety of the safelight should be

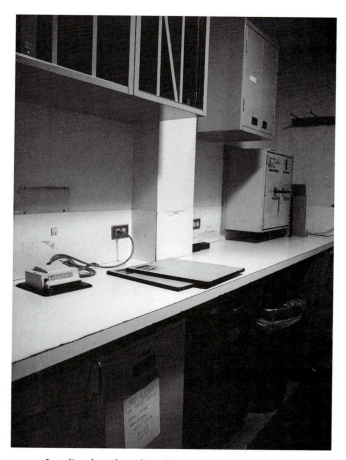

Fig. I-1 Loading bench and work area in typical x-ray darkroom.

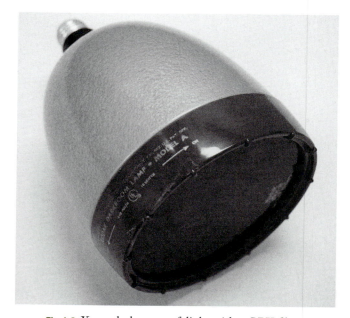

Fig. I-2 X-ray darkroom safelight with a GBX filter.

determined for a period of time that exceeds typical safe-light exposure time, usually 3 minutes. Care should be taken that exposure to safelight illumination does not exceed this period of time.

Darkroom Fog

May be caused by:
- Unsafe safelights
- White light leak
- Excessive developer time, strength, or temperature

May cause:
- Decreased radiographic contrast
- Increased radiographic density

Safelight Testing

A quality control check is performed regularly on the safelight. Safelights are tested using film that has been preexposed to an x-ray exposure of a penetrometer (e.g., about 5 mAs at 70 kVp). Place the penetrometer in the *exact center* of the cassette for the exposure (Fig. I-3). In *total darkness*, the preexposed film is placed on the countertop. Cover one half of the film with an opaque material, such as the cassette or a piece of cardboard. Be sure to bisect the penetrometer by covering exactly half of the film. Turn the safelight on and expose it for *2 minutes*. Turn the safelight off and process the film. Place the film on the illuminator. If no defined line is seen dividing the penetrometer image, then no fog is present. If a fog line is seen, measure the density on each side (Fig. I-4). If the density difference is greater than 0.05 optical density, the safelight needs to be adjusted or replaced. Check the position, light bulb, and filter.

If this test indicates that the safelight is not safe for normal use, check the integrity of the filter (filters tend to crack and peel with age), the wattage of the bulb, and the distance from the safelight to the testing site. Decreasing the bulb wattage or increasing the distance may solve the problem. White light leaks may also result in a positive test result. If the test indicates fog, but the safelight appears to be satisfactory, check the darkroom carefully to ensure that no light is leaking around the door, the vents, or the processor. This is done most effectively after your eyes are well adapted to the dark. When you believe you have solved the problem, be sure to repeat the safelight test to confirm safelight safety.

Film Bin

The **film bin** is a special container in the darkroom that holds film for reloading cassettes. It is usually located under the loading bench. You can open it from the front by pulling its handle toward you. It is light-tight and is divided to hold open boxes of each size of film. *The film bin is opened under safelight illumination only.*

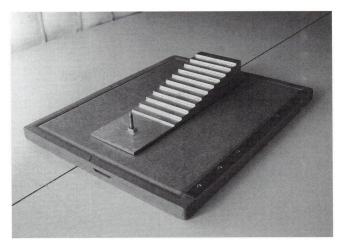

Fig. I-3 The penetrometer should be placed in the exact center of the cassette for the exposure.

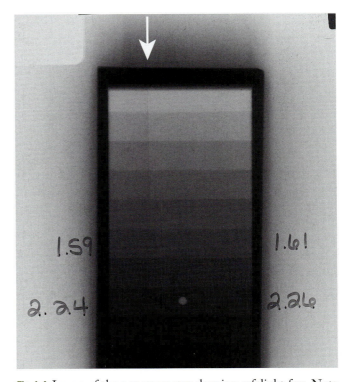

Fig. I-4 Image of the penetrometer showing safelight fog. Note the separation between the side exposed to the safelight and the side covered *(arrow)*.

Film Identification

A **film identification printer** (Fig. I-5), sometimes referred to as a *flasher* or *stamper*, is used to print patient information on each film before processing. A card with the necessary information is inserted into the printer. The corner of the film that was protected by the identification (ID) blocker is then inserted into the printer and the printer is activated. A light in the printer exposes the film through the card, leaving an image of the card data

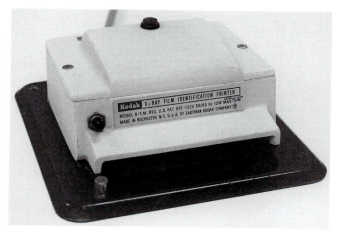

Fig. I-5 Film identification printer is used to identify radiographs before processing.

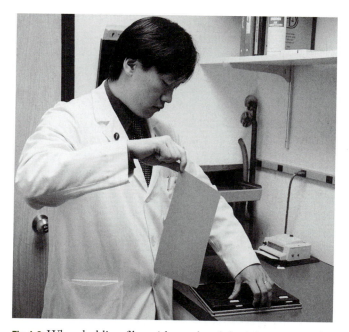

Fig. I-6 When holding film with one hand, let it hang vertically.

on the film. These devices vary in design and are very simple to operate. Become familiar with the film ID printer in your facility before trying to use it in the dark.

Some facilities have a daylight ID system that uses special cassettes. The corner of the cassette is inserted into the printer in the x-ray room so that film can be identified immediately before or after exposure.

Information to be imprinted on the film should include at least the patient's name, an identifying number (file number, chart number, or birth date), the date of the examination, and the name and location of the x-ray facility. Preprinted forms are usually used for this purpose. The patient data may be typed or handwritten. Some x-ray department computer systems generate an ID card along with other patient records when patient data are

entered. If cards are typed or handwritten, do not use correction fluid to fix errors. Because the data are exposed by light passing through the card, the correction fluid will obscure any information on that portion of the card. The ID information will be most legible on the film when the card stock has a smooth, even texture and the printing is as dark as possible.

Pass Box

A **pass box** is a convenient darkroom feature when there is a frequent need to transfer film to and from the darkroom while it is in use. Pass boxes have two compartments, one for exposed film entering the darkroom and one for unexposed film leaving the darkroom after the cassette has been reloaded. Each compartment has two doors, one on the outside of the darkroom and one on the inside. An interlock between the inside and outside doors makes it impossible for both doors to be opened at the same time. Most pass boxes are designed to protect film from exposure to x-rays. When the pass box location is convenient to the x-ray room, the compartment for unexposed film may be used as a storage place for cassettes that are ready for use.

FILM HANDLING

Radiographic film is handled when loading and unloading cassettes and when feeding it into the processing machine or preparing for manual processing. These activities take place in the darkroom under safelight conditions, that is, a very low level of red light with very limited visibility. It will be helpful for you to practice film handling with waste film in the daylight before you need to handle patient films in the darkroom.

Film must be handled with clean, dry hands and touched only on the corners. Dirt or chemical residue on your fingers will cause marks on the film and may also stain the screens. When you are holding a film with one hand, let it hang vertically (Fig. I-6). To place the film horizontal, use both hands, holding it at opposite corners (Fig. I-7). Attempting to hold the film horizontal with one hand causes it to bend, which creates pressure exposure in the form of a "crinkle" or **crescent mark.** Attempting to prevent this by extending your fingers to balance the film will result in finger marks. Crescent marks and finger marks are discussed and illustrated later in this chapter in the section on artifacts.

To unload a cassette, place the cassette on the loading bench with the back side up and the ID blocker positioned in the upper left corner. Release the latches, partially open the cassette, and grasp the film in the lower right corner with your right hand (Fig. I-8). Remove the film, holding it vertically. Grasp the opposite corner with your left hand, holding with both hands to position the film in the ID printer.

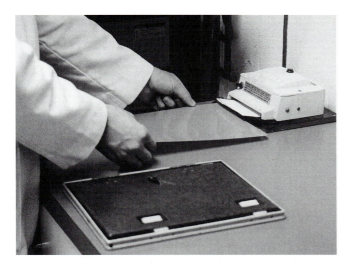

Fig. I-7 To hold film horizontally, use both hands and grasp at opposite corners.

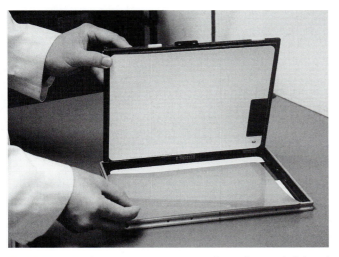

Fig. I-8 To reload cassette, open it partially with your left hand and place the film with your right hand. When film is properly situated, tightly close all latches.

Cassettes are reloaded as soon as possible after unloading. Because it is impossible to tell by looking at a closed cassette whether it is loaded or not and whether the film is exposed or not, follow standard procedures to avoid errors. For this reason, empty cassettes are never completely closed; they are almost closed, but the latches are not fastened. They are reloaded promptly so that they are ready for use when needed. There should be separate standard locations for exposed and unexposed cassettes to avoid the possibility of accidentally reusing an exposed cassette, creating a double exposure.

To reload, open the film bin and select a film of the proper size, grasping it by the upper right corner with your right hand. With your left hand, close the film bin and open the cassette. Place the film in the cassette so that it is properly situated. Because double-emulsion films are identical on both sides, there is no right or wrong side to the film and no top or bottom. Simply place the film so that it fits properly into the cassette. Close the cassette, ensuring that all latches are tightly closed.

It is a good habit to double-check that the film bin is closed and that there are no films out in the darkroom before opening the door or turning on the lights.

AUTOMATIC FILM PROCESSORS

Automatic film processors vary in design according to age and manufacturer. There are large models that stand on the floor and small units that rest on a countertop (Fig. I-9). The essential features of all processors are similar, however, and the specifics of each model are fully explained in the processor operation manual supplied with the unit. This manual is a helpful reference for understanding the operation of and proper settings for the processor.

Compared with a manual processing system, which requires about an hour to process a film "dry to dry," modern automatic processors require 3 minutes or less. Most processors used today in busy departments process film in 90 seconds. This is made possible principally by the increased strength and temperature of solutions, but all aspects of the system are designed to support and enhance this speed.

The operation of an automatic processor may be divided into six parts: transport system, chemistry, replenisher system, recirculation system, water system, and dryer. Processors contain three processing tanks: developer, fixer, and wash (water) tank.

Automatic Film Processor Systems
• Transport system • Chemicals • Replenisher system • Recirculation system • Water system • Dryer system

Transport System

The transport system (Fig. I-10) consists of the drive motor, gear assembly, and a roller assembly or "rack" for each tank. The roller action moves the film through the processor. Roller action also helps to agitate the solution, keeping fresh solution in contact with the film surface. A crossover roller assembly or curved metal "guide shoe" transports the film between the tanks and from the wash tank to the dryer. Turnaround rollers or guide shoes at the bottom of each rack change the direction of film travel when it has reached the

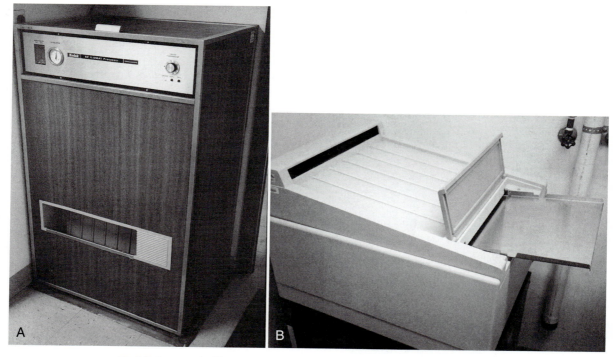

Fig. I-9 Automatic film processors. **A,** Floor model. **B,** Countertop model.

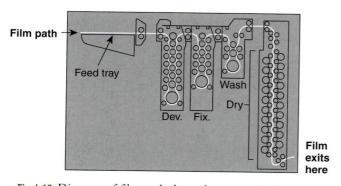

Fig. I-10 Diagram of film path through automatic processor.

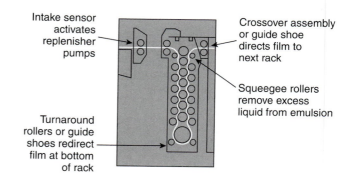

Fig. I-11 Close-up view of developer rack in automatic processor.

bottom of the tank. The exit rollers on each rack provide a squeegee action to remove excess solution from the film before it enters the next rack. A close-up diagram of the developer rack (Fig. I-11) illustrates these features.

The transport mechanism moves at a constant rate and governs the time the film is subjected to each portion of the processing cycle. Broken gear teeth or cogwheels in the transport mechanism may occur as a result of wear or film jams, causing slippage of the film in the area where the damage has occurred. A stopwatch test of cycle time, from the instant the leading film edge enters the processor until it emerges from the dryer, provides a measure of the timing accuracy of the transport mechanism. Actual cycle time varies with the make and model of the processor and is stated in the processor operation manual.

Chemistry Modifications for Automatic Processing

- Stronger preservative decreases deterioration of developer at high temperatures.
- Greater developer strength permits more rapid development.
- Glutaraldehyde, a tanning agent in the developer, prevents overswelling of gelatin.
- Stronger restrainer, called *starter*, prevents chemical fog in new developer.

Automatic Processing Chemistry

The chemicals used in automatic processors are essentially the same as those for manual processing with some modification to accommodate the requirements of higher temperatures and the critical tolerances of the transport system. Greater developer strength promotes rapid development, and stronger preservatives decrease deterioration of the solutions at high temperatures. A stronger restrainer, called *starter*, prevents chemical fog in fresh developer. Starter is used only when fresh developer is put into the processor's developer tank after cleaning or any time after the developer is drained from the tank.

Glutaraldehyde, a hardener, is included in the *developer* to prevent overswelling of the gelatin. Using the correct amount of this chemical is essential. Too little causes the emulsion to become too soft, absorbing too much liquid. This condition results in roller marks on the film from the transport rollers and may also prevent the film from drying completely. In extreme cases, the emulsion becomes so thick and sticky that it cannot pass through the rollers, causing a jam. Too much glutaraldehyde, on the other hand, shrinks the emulsion before sufficient developer has been absorbed, causing under development.

See Box I-1 for suggestions to preserve developer strength.

Replenishment of Automatic Processing Chemicals

Replenisher solutions for the processor are stored in separate holding tanks, connected to the processor by hoses. Replenisher pumps in the processor bring enough fresh solution into the processor tanks for each film as it is processed. As fresh solution is added, the tanks overflow. Developer is allowed to overflow into the drain. Fixer may be pumped through a silver recovery unit before flowing into the drain, or it may flow into a holding container for recycling.

An intake sensor on the processor feed tray, seen in Fig. I-11, activates the replenisher pumps as the film passes over the sensor. The size of the film thus determines the duration of the pumping action and the amount of replenisher added for each film.

The replenishment rates are adjustable and are measured using a 35 × 43 cm film. To measure replenishment rates, the tubes that carry replenisher to the processing tanks are diverted into measuring cups while a test film is fed into the processor. Approximately 60 to 70 mL of replenisher is usually added to the developer and 100 to 110 mL replenisher to the fixer for each 35 × 43 cm film. The replenishment rate must compensate not only for the chemical strength used to process the film but also for strength lost to deterioration when the processor is idle. For this reason, ideal replenisher rates vary according to the volume of film processed. The processor operation manual will state the desired rates for fixer and developer replenishment based on the average number of films processed per week. When film volume changes significantly, replenishment rates must be adjusted accordingly. Higher rates are required when film volume is low, and rates may be reduced when volume is high. Box I-2 lists consequences of incorrect replenishment rates.

Recirculation

When the processor is in operation, recirculation pumps constantly move developer and fixer from the tanks, through a heat exchanger, and back into the tanks. Recirculation through the heat exchanger maintains solution temperature at the desired level, usually between 92° and 96° F (33.3° and 35.6° C) depending on the specific processor type. For example, the temperature of the developer in all 90-second processors is 95° F (35° C). This temperature should be checked daily, first thing in the morning before patient films are processed. This developer temperature cannot vary by more than ±0.5° F. Recirculation also keeps the solution in motion, continuously placing fresh solution in contact with the film surfaces to increase the speed of the chemical action.

Water System

Fresh water runs into the wash tank and overflows into the drain continuously when the processor is in operation. This fresh water flow efficiently washes the film. The water system may also provide cooling when needed in the heat exchanger portion of the recirculation system.

Box I-1

Preservation of Developer Strength

- Do not run processor for prolonged periods when not in use.
- Install a stand-by system that maintains temperature but stops water flow and recirculation when not in use (if not included with processor).
- Use floating lid on developer replenisher tank to reduce deterioration of developer caused by exposure to air. (Observe color: developer should not be darker than light beer.)
- Do not store excess quantities of mixed solutions.

Box I-2

Correct Replenishment Is Essential to Proper Processing

Underreplenishment	Overreplenishment
• Loss of contrast	• Loss of contrast (↑ fog)
• Loss of density	• Decreased D-max
• Inadequate clearing	• Loss of density
• Inadequate hardening	• Waste
• Failure to dry completely	
• Transport failure	

↑, Increased; *D-max*, maximum density.

Depending on the incoming water supply, a filtration system may be necessary to maintain adequate water quality. Filters may be installed on the water line before the water enters the processor. Unlike manual processing systems, modern automatic processors do not require a warm water supply. Cold water only is supplied to the processor and is heated, as needed, within the processor.

Dryer

The dryer section of the processor consists of air tubes with long slits. The air tubes are mounted on both sides of the dryer rack, directing warm air at both sides of the film as it passes through this portion of the roller system. The air is warmed to approximately 110° F (43.3° C) and is filtered to prevent dirt from clogging the tubes or sticking to the film.

The dryer temperature is adjustable but is usually quite stable. When films are damp as they exit the processor, there are several possible causes. Inadequate air supply may be caused by too little space around the processor or clogging of the air filters with dirt. When a small processor is used to process too many films in a short time period, moisture may build up within the dryer, decreasing its effectiveness. The most common cause of damp films, however, is inadequate developer replenishment. Insufficient replenishment causes a decrease in the delicate glutaraldehyde balance, which permits the emulsion to swell with liquid to the point where it cannot dry at standard drying time and temperature.

Processor Operation and Maintenance

Automatic processors are very simple to use. After the film has been identified, it is placed on the processor feed tray and moved into the processor until it is picked up and moved forward by the intake rollers. The width of the feed tray and the recommendations of the manufacturer (see the processor operation manual) will determine whether the film is fed with its long or short dimension parallel to the rollers. Usually the long dimension is parallel to the rollers unless it cannot be accommodated by the feed tray. When the entire film has passed beyond the intake rollers, a tone or a red light, or both, will signal that it is safe to feed the next film or to turn on the lights. Feeding in another film before this signal is given will result in overlap of the two films during processing. This causes incomplete processing of both films and may also cause a jam. White light in the darkroom before the signal will fog the trailing edge of the film. The finished film will drop into a receiving bin 1.5 to 3 minutes after the film enters the processor.

When the processor is first turned on, it takes some time for it to warm to operating temperature. Film processed before the processor is ready will be too light and will lack contrast. Most processors take about 30 minutes to warm up, and most provide an indicator that the desired temperature has been reached. There may be a sound signal or a light indicator. Some processors have digital thermometers that indicate the developer temperature.

The upper portions of the top rollers on each rack are above the level of the solution. When the processor is idle, solutions tend to dry on the exposed rollers. This dried chemical residue is deposited on the first film that is processed after the idle period, leaving undesirable marks. To avoid this problem after the processor has been idle for a long period, or when the processor is first turned on in the morning, four "cleanup" films are fed through the processor before processing patient films. A cleanup film is a 35 × 43 cm film that has not been processed. Film that has aged beyond the expiration date or has been accidentally fogged or exposed may be kept for this purpose. A previously processed throw-away film *should never be used* as a cleanup film because any fixer residue in the emulsion may contaminate the developer.

At the end of the day, the processor and its water supply are turned off. The lid should be partially opened when the processor is turned off. This practice allows chemical fumes to escape, preventing fixer vapor from condensing in the developer and contaminating it. Gelatin residue and warm temperatures in the wash tank may promote the growth of algae. When this occurs, the algae form a scum in the water tank that may cling to the film. Growth of algae can usually be controlled by emptying the wash tank at the end of the day, allowing it to dry out during the night. The three crossover racks must be cleaned each day.

Box I-3 contains a checklist for daily and monthly processor maintenance. Many facilities have a contract for monthly maintenance provided by a processor service company. Every 6 months, a service company should perform a thorough processor cleaning using special system cleaners to clean the insides of the pumps and the recirculation system. This service should include a complete inspection of the processor with replacement of any worn or damaged parts.

PROCESSOR QUALITY CONTROL

Considering the complexity of the automatic processor, it is understandable that variations may occur in temperature, film volume, replenisher rates, and cycle time and that these variations may have a significant impact on film quality. The purpose of processor quality control is to monitor these variations and solve any problems before they become serious. Some state agencies have regulations requiring processor quality control monitoring. These agencies may review quality control records when conducting radiation safety inspections.

Two special pieces of equipment are necessary for monitoring processor performance: a **sensitometer** and a **densitometer.** A sensitometer (Fig. I-12) is a device

Box I-3

Darkroom and Processor Maintenance Checklist

Daily Start-up
- Close wash tank drain.
- Turn on water supply.
- Close processor cover.
- Allow processor to warm to operating temperature.
- Wipe down loading bench.
- Check solution levels in replenisher holding tanks and used fixer overflow container.
- Run four "cleanup" films.
- Expose and process sensitometric test film.
- Evaluate film and graph result. Troubleshoot any problems indicated.

Daily Shutdown
- Turn off processor.
- Turn off water supply.
- Open wash tank drain.
- Clean crossover racks.
- Leave processor cover partially open.

Monthly Processor Maintenance
- Completely drain processing tanks.
- Remove, clean, and inspect roller racks.
- Clean tanks and rinse thoroughly.
- Fill developer and fixer tanks with new solutions; add starter to developer.
- Refill wash tank.
- Turn on processor and warm to operating temperature.
- Check developer temperature with separate, calibrated thermometer.
- Check replenishment rates and adjust, if necessary.
- Measure cycle time with stopwatch.
- Expose and process sensitometric test film and compare to standard.

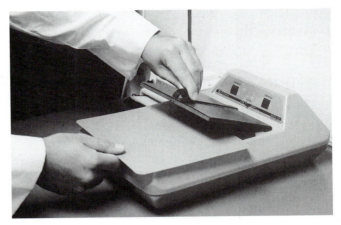

Fig. I-12 Sensitometer uses precisely controlled light source to expose gray scale on film.

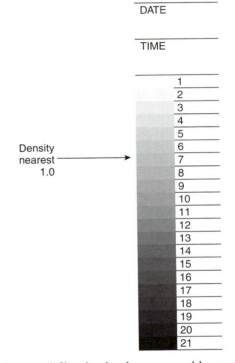

Fig. I-13 Processed film that has been exposed by sensitometer. Note the scale of densities from white to black.

that prints a standard gray scale on film (Fig. I-13). Each tone on the gray scale is called a *step*, and each step is numbered. The exposure is made by a precisely controlled light source, so that the amount of exposure is always exactly the same. A fresh sheet of film is exposed in the darkroom with the sensitometer and is processed. It is a good practice to expose two edges of the film with the sensitometer, one with each side of the emulsion down. The different positions of the two sides of the emulsion with respect to the developer rack sometimes result in slightly different responses to processing. These variations may cause erratic test results unless they are taken into account. The resulting film is evaluated using the densitometer.

A densitometer (Fig. I-14) is used to measure the transmission of light through a tiny area of the film. It is a digital device that measures the optical density of the film. The densitometer is first calibrated to a null (zero) value by engaging it with no film. The test film is then measured, and the optical density value is recorded.

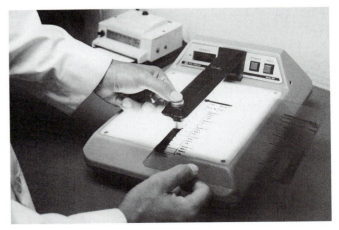

Fig. I-14 Densitometer is used to measure optical density of the gray scale steps on sensitometric film.

When both sides of the emulsion have been exposed, both sides are measured and the results are averaged. *Sensitometers and densitometers should be calibrated annually.*

Setting Up a Quality Control System

Processor performance is monitored by comparing the densities of standardized exposures on the test film with those of a similar film (the control standard or baseline film) that was processed when the processor was performing at an optimal level. The best time to establish this standard is soon after the processor has been cleaned but when sufficient film has been processed to indicate consistent satisfactory performance. It is desirable to do preliminary tests with the sensitometer over a period of several days to be certain that processor performance is stable.

Three or four measurements are compared for each processor test: film density (speed index), contrast, and **base + fog.** Each of these factors is measured on the control standard film to establish baseline measurements for comparison with future tests. These measurements are used to set up a graph on which the results of future tests will be plotted.

To begin, the control film is exposed with the sensitometer and processed when the processor is performing optimally. The density of each step in the gray scale is measured with the densitometer. Comparable steps on the two sides of the film are averaged and the average density recorded.

To establish the speed index, the baseline for film density, the step on the gray scale is chosen that measures closest to an optical density of 1.0 above the base + fog. This density represents a middle gray tone, about halfway between the densities that appear black and white on the view box. The number of this step and its average measurement are recorded on the processor record graph.

For example, if step 7 measures 1.05, it is plotted directly on the graph (Fig. I-15). Note that the actual step number will vary with different sensitometers and different films. Once the step is determined, it is never changed.

Because radiographic contrast is defined as a *difference* in radiographic densities, the contrast index is a measure of the difference between two densities on the gray scale. The step on the gray scale closest to 0.25 above base + fog and the step closest to 2.0 above base + fog are used to measure contrast. The difference between these two steps is plotted. For example, if step 11 is 1.95 and step 3 is 0.40, the contrast is 1.55 (Fig. I-16). The actual value of the contrast index will vary, depending on the inherent contrast of the film and the developer temperature. A value between 1.4 and 1.7 is usual for medium- to high-contrast films at recommended processor temperatures. Note that, as with the speed index, the actual step number will vary with different sensitometers and different films. However, once the three step numbers are determined, they are never changed.

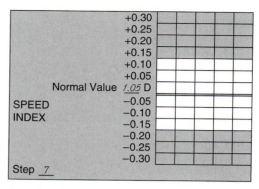

Fig. I-15 Speed index portion of quality control record. The number of the step on the baseline film with an optical density at 1.0 above base + fog is entered at the bottom and its optical density is entered as the normal value. This establishes the value of the center line of the graph.

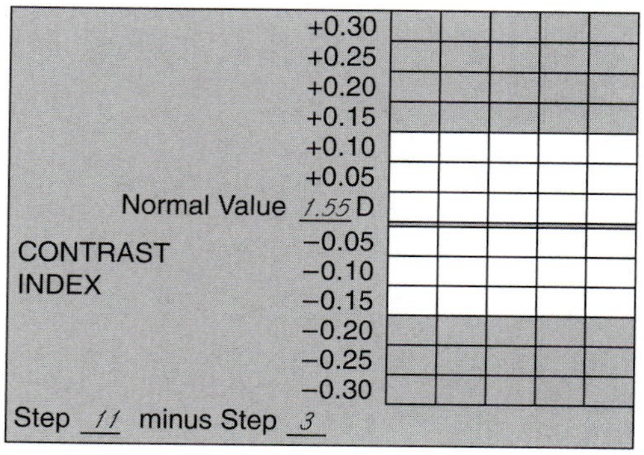

Fig. I-16 Contrast index portion of quality control record is the difference between a high-density step (2.0 above base + fog) and a low-density step (0.25 above base + fog). The difference in optical density between the two steps is entered as the normal value. This establishes the value of the center line of the graph.

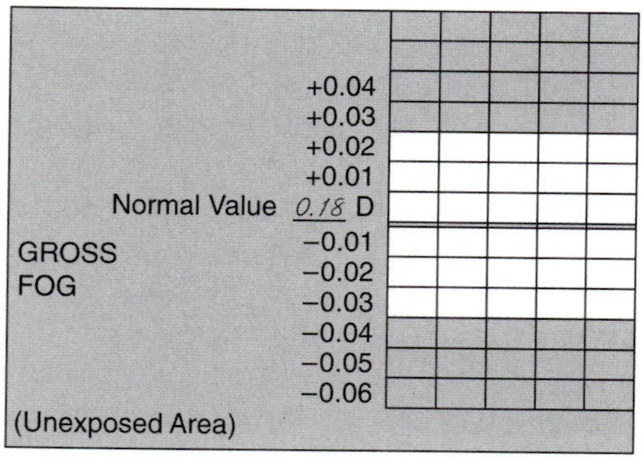

Fig. I-17 Fog index portion of quality control record. The optical density of the unexposed portion of the baseline film is entered as the normal value, establishing the value of the center line of the graph.

The base + fog index is the average measurement of the clear portion of the test film. It can also be measured in any unexposed portion of the film. The value of this step is also entered on the processor record form (Fig. I-17). The usual value for the base + fog index is an optical density between 0.0 and 0.20. This value varies with film speed, with faster films having a higher gross fog index, but it should never exceed 0.25.

The control baseline sensitometric film is kept for reference and is marked to indicate the date and time it was made, the developer temperature, and the replenishment rates for both developer and fixer. If there is a change in the brand or type of film used, a new baseline film must be made to establish a new standard.

An additional way to assess the consistency of processing solutions is to test the pH, that is, the degree of alkalinity of the developer and the acidity of the fixer. Test strips are available for this purpose. These paper strips are dipped into the solutions and their color compared with a standard color strip to obtain a reading. Directions are provided with the strips and should be followed precisely. If pH testing is part of your quality control procedure, the pH of both developer and fixer should be tested when the quality control record is established. The readings are recorded on the baseline film and the processor record form.

Monitoring Processor Performance

Once the baseline indices and the processor performance record have been established, it is easy to maintain a record of processor performance. Box I-4 lists the steps for

sensitometric processor evaluation. A sensitometric film is exposed and processed daily after the processor has reached operating temperature. The densities of the key steps are measured and averaged and their values plotted on the graph (Fig. I-18). Each vertical line on the graph represents one test. The date, time, developer temperature, and

Box I-4

Sensitometric Processor Evaluation

- Expose both sides of a fresh 8- × 10-inch film with sensitometer.
- Process film (be sure processor has reached operating temperature).
- Measure key steps with densitometer and average readings from the two sides.
  - Speed step (step 7 in Fig. I-18, *A*)
  - Contrast step (steps 3 and 11 in Fig. I-18, *B*).
  - Fog level (unexposed area in Fig. I-18, *C*).
- Calculate average density readings for each step measured.
- Calculate contrast index (step 11 minus step 3 in Fig. I-18, *B*).
- Plot readings on graph.
- Troubleshoot for any readings outside acceptable range.

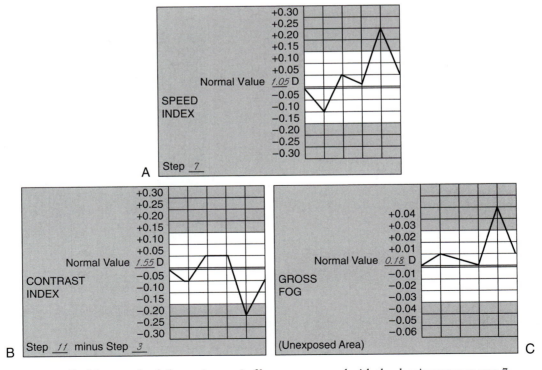

Fig. I-18 In this example, daily sensitometric films are measured with the densitometer at step 7, step 11, and step 3, the unexposed area. Each vertical line represents a separate day and a separate test film. **A,** The graph of speed index is a plotting of the readings of step 7. **B,** Graph of contrast index. **C,** Graph of fog index. Note that on day 5, something happened that caused all three indices to be outside the normal range. Check Table I-1 to determine possible causes.

Table I-1

Troubleshooting Chart

	Developer temperature	Developer depleted	Developer contaminated	Developer overdiluted	No starter in fresh developer	Incorrectly mixed developer	Fixer depleted	Replenishment rates incorrect	Water problems	Dryer problems	Loss of circulation	Dirty rollers	Dirty water	Filter size too small	Misaligned guide shoes	Improper film handling	Safelights	Storage
Increased base fog	1	5	4		2		4	4				3					2	2
Reduced contrast	1	1	2	3	1	1	2	2			4	3					2	2
Increased contrast	1					1		1										
Reduced film speed	1	2	3	3		2		2			5							
Increased film speed	1		1		1	2	2	3			5	3				4	4	3
Wet or damp films	3	2	2	2		2	1	2		3	2	4						
Improper clearing	2	2	2	2	5	3	1				2							
Dirty films	2	2	2	2		2	3		1	3	2	2	2	2		3		
Scratches on films	2	2	3	2		3	2			2			1		1	2		

1, Check first; *2,* check second; *3,* check third; *4,* check fourth; *5,* check last.
From Dupont Diagnostic Imaging and Information Systems.

pH values are also noted. On dates when replenisher rates are measured, these data are recorded on the processor record also. Replenisher rates should be checked at least monthly and whenever the test film indicates a problem that may be related to replenishment.

There will be normal fluctuations in all of the indices, but they should stay within a tolerable range. This range is ±0.15 for the speed and contrast indices and ±0.05 for the gross fog index. Processor record forms are usually marked to indicate clearly when measurements are beyond the acceptable limits. When this occurs, it is important to identify and rectify the problem immediately. Table I-1 is a guide to causes of common processor problems that may be identified in sensitometric quality control tests.

ARTIFACTS

Film **artifacts** are marks, exposures, or images on the radiograph that are not part of the intended image. Artifacts appear dark if they result from unintended exposure and light when caused by interference with exposure or processing.

Cassette and Screen Artifacts

Light leaks in the cassette cause unintended exposure to the film (Fig. I-19). This problem may be caused by wear

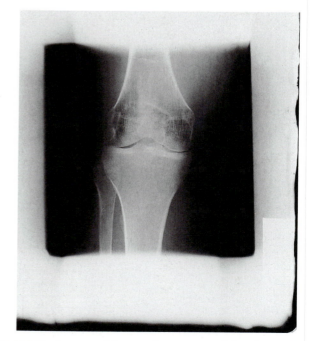

Fig. I-19 Dark areas of fog on the margins of this film indicate that cassette has a light leak. Leaky cassettes should be replaced.

or damage to the cassette. Leaky cassettes usually cannot be repaired. The cassette must be replaced.

A light leak is also caused when the film is not loaded properly and overlaps the cassette edge (Fig. I-20). This results in a black edge on the film and a blurred image

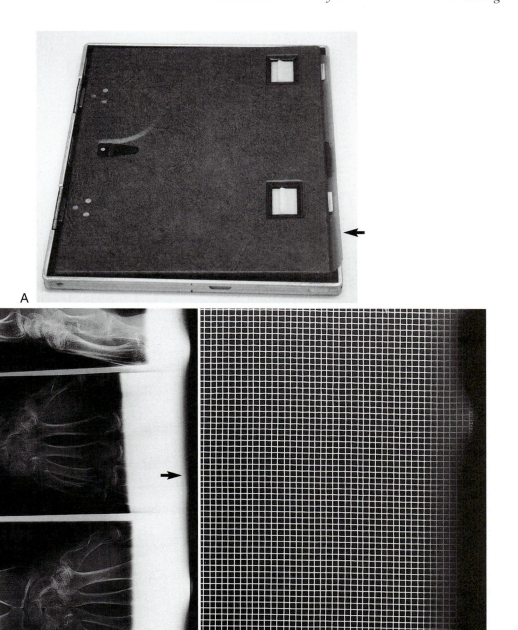

Fig. I-20 A, Cassette is not properly loaded and film extends at the latch edge *(arrow)*. **B,** Film taken in improperly loaded cassette shows light fog on the latch edge *(arrow)*. **C,** Film-screen contact test with cassette improperly loaded shows fog and loss of image sharpness on film margin.

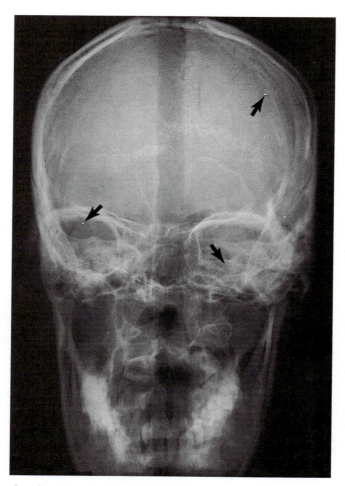

Fig. I-21 Light-colored artifacts on this film *(arrows)* are unexposed areas resulting from dirt on intensifying screens.

adjacent to it, which is caused by poor film-screen contact. This problem is avoided by checking to be certain that the film is properly situated in the cassette during the loading process.

Screen artifacts result when dirt on the screen prevents screen light from exposing the film (Fig. I-21). These artifacts can be minimized by keeping the loading area clean and by cleaning screens with a product that contains an antistatic ingredient. Similar artifacts may occur when the screen is stained or damaged, in which case the screens must be replaced. Even though only one screen is damaged, the pair must be replaced. It is best to have new screens installed by the dealer's local technical representative.

Film-handling Artifacts

Common film-handling artifacts include creases, crescent marks, finger marks, and abrasions. Creases and crescent marks are caused by bending or crimping the film (Fig. I-22). This can be avoided by remembering to let the film hang vertically when holding it with only one hand.

Finger marks (Fig. I-23) are caused whenever the film is touched and are worst when the hands are not clean and dry. These marks are avoided by having clean, dry hands and handling film only at the corners. Finger marks may appear as either dark or light artifacts. Oily skin causes light finger marks by preventing development, whereas developer on fingers causes dark marks.

Abrasions occur when film rubs against any surface, especially if pressure is applied at the same time. Fig. I-24 shows abrasions caused by excess finger pressure on the film against the film tray when feeding the film into the processor. Dropping a film on the floor or placing a cassette on top of it will cause abrasions as well.

Static artifacts result when the discharge of static electricity exposes the film before processing (Fig. I-25). These artifacts may occur as clusters of tiny black dots that have the appearance of smudges. Larger discharges may create the shapes of asterisks ("star static"), clumps of grass ("crown static"), or trees. This can be a particularly difficult problem when the atmosphere is very dry. Static discharge may occur when you are simply touching the film, removing a fresh film from the box, or loading or unloading a cassette, or when the film makes contact

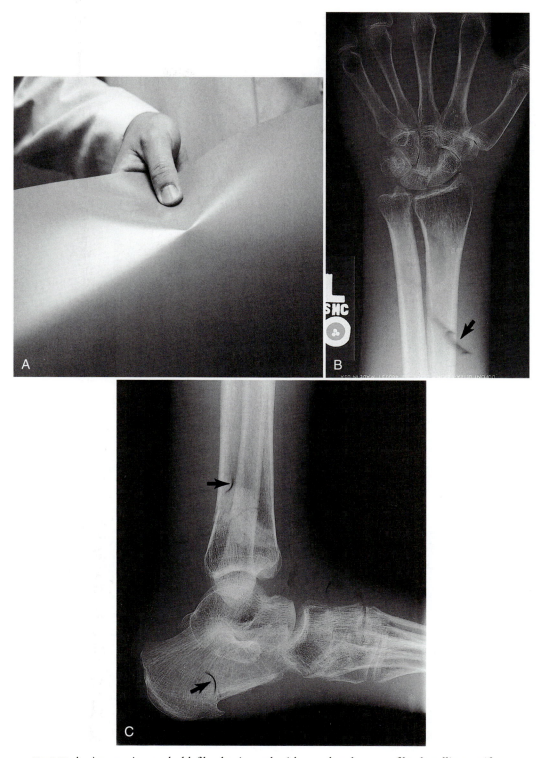

Fig. I-22 A, Attempting to hold film horizontal with one hand causes film-handling artifacts. **B,** Crease mark *(arrow)* is caused by gripping film too tightly. **C,** Crescent marks *(arrow)* on this film are caused by film bending at a crease while operator attempted to hold it horizontal with one hand.

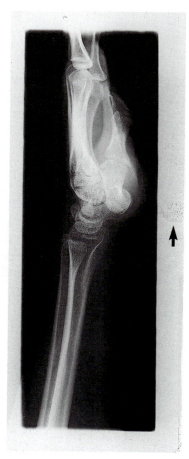

Fig. I-23 Finger marks *(arrow)* seen here can be prevented by handling films by the corners with clean, dry hands.

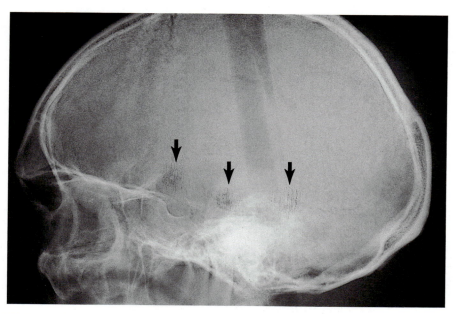

Fig. I-24 Film abrasions *(arrows)* occur when film rubs across a surface. These marks occurred with finger pressure on the film as it moved across the processor feed tray.

with the loading bench or processor feed tray. The most likely event is discharge between the intensifying screens and the film; this is greatly diminished by cleaning the screens with a cleaner that contains an antistatic ingredient. Antistatic solutions can also be purchased for treating the loading bench and the processor feed tray. If these measures do not solve the problem, it may be necessary to install a humidifier to decrease the buildup of static electricity in the environment.

Automatic Processing Artifacts

Chemical marks from uneven development, especially on the leading edge of the film, are usually caused by concentrated chemical residue on the rollers. This can be eliminated by feeding a cleanup film, as discussed earlier.

Roller marks or "pi lines" are artifacts that occur repeatedly at right angles to the direction of film travel. These may be caused by a damaged roller or by an imbalance in glutaraldehyde that permits over softening of the emulsion. If these artifacts occur when the solutions are fresh, the processor racks should be inspected for roller damage and the offending roller(s) replaced. Fig. I-26 shows prominent roller marks that occurred in combination with chemical contamination.

Scratches along the length of film travel (Fig. I-27) may be caused by a sharp point on a guide shoe or by bits of foreign matter lodged in a roller or extending from a dryer tube. These problems are best handled by service personnel.

A brown, "lacy" artifact is the result of algae scum on the film from the wash tank (Fig. I-28). As mentioned earlier, this problem is usually cured by draining the wash tank at night. If the problem persists, it may be necessary to clean the wash tank with a bleach solution and rinse thoroughly to kill the algae spores. Algaecide tablets are available for use in the wash tanks of both

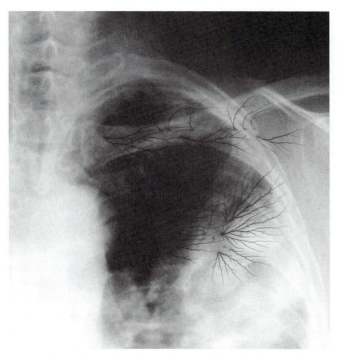

Fig. I-25 Examples of static marks caused by discharge of static electricity.

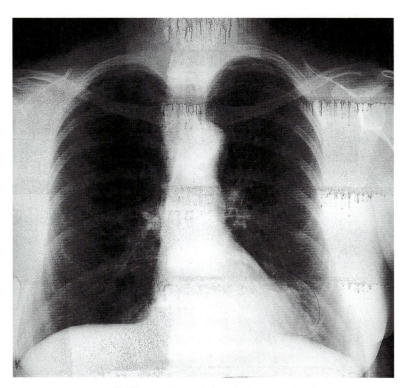

Fig. I-26 Roller marks and chemical contamination.

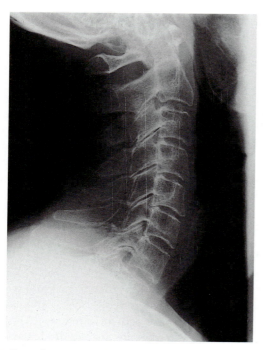

Fig. I-27 Scratches caused by rough projections from corroded guide shoes.

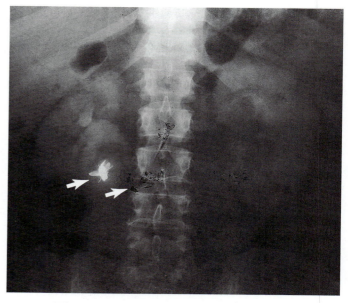

Fig. I-28 The dark, lacy pattern on this film represents algal scum from the automatic processor wash tank. The light artifact is a fly caught in the cassette, actually a "screen dirt" artifact.

processors and manual systems, but these tend to leave a white residue on the film and may create almost as many problems as they solve. They should be used only as a last resort.

SUMMARY

The x-ray darkroom is the place where cassettes are loaded and unloaded and where films are identified and processed. Safelights permit limited visibility in the darkroom during these activities. They may cause fog if they are too bright, too close, or improperly filtered. Periodic testing with presensitized film ensures the safety of safelights.

Careless film handling causes film artifacts. Film should be handled with clean, dry hands and only at the corners. Care must be taken that the film is not creased, bent, scraped, or dropped.

Automatic processors shorten the dry-to-dry processing time to 3 minutes or less by using stronger, warmer solutions in constant motion. These systems require a precise and consistent chemical strength and temperature. Manufacturers' recommendations for operation and maintenance must be followed. To ensure that all conditions are optimal for best radiographic quality, the processor is monitored for quality control using standard exposures from a sensitometer that are measured on the film with a densitometer. A graphic record of these tests is maintained.

Film artifacts may be caused by cassette damage, dirty screens, careless handling, static electricity, and problems within the automatic processor. Improper cassette loading and safelight fog also compromise radiographic quality. Radiographers must be able to recognize the signs of these problems, identify their causes, and take appropriate steps to rectify them.

Usual Projections for Routine Examinations

UPPER LIMB

Hand	PA, PA oblique—lateral rotation, lateral
Finger	PA, PA oblique, lateral
Thumb	AP, PA oblique, lateral
Wrist	PA, PA oblique—lateral rotation, lateral (lateromedial)
Forearm	AP, lateral
Elbow	AP, lateral
Humerus	AP, lateral
Shoulder	AP—external (arm) rotation, AP—internal (arm) rotation
Shoulder (trauma)	AP without rotation, transthoracic lateral or PA oblique (scapular Y)
Clavicle	PA, PA axial
Scapula	AP, lateral
Acromioclavicular joints	Bilateral AP, with and without weight bearing

LOWER LIMB

Foot	AP, AP oblique—medial rotation, lateral
Toe	AP, AP oblique—medial rotation, lateral
Calcaneus	Axial (plantodorsal), lateral
Ankle	AP, AP oblique—medial rotation, lateral
Lower leg	AP, lateral
Knee	AP, lateral
Distal femur	AP, lateral
Proximal femur	AP, lateral
Hip	AP, (frog leg) lateral

SPINE

Cervical	AP axial (lower cervical), AP open mouth (upper cervical), lateral
Thoracic	AP, lateral
Lumbar	AP, lateral
Sacrum	AP axial, lateral
Coccyx	AP axial, lateral
Sacroiliac joints	AP axial, AP oblique

BONY THORAX AND CHEST

Upper posterior ribs	AP, AP oblique
Upper anterior ribs	PA, PA oblique
Lower posterior ribs	AP, AP oblique
Chest	PA, left lateral

ABDOMEN

Abdomen (nonacute)	AP supine (KUB)
Acute abdomen	AP supine (KUB), AP upright, PA chest upright

SKULL, FACIAL BONES, AND PARANASAL SINUSES

Skull	PA axial (Caldwell method), AP axial (Towne method), lateral
Facial bones	PA axial (Caldwell method), parietoacanthial (Waters method), lateral
Paranasal sinuses	PA axial (Caldwell method), parietoacanthial (Waters method), lateral, SMV

AP, Anteroposterior; KUB, kidneys, ureters, and bladder; PA, posteroanterior; RAO, right anterior oblique; SMV, submentovertical.

Evaluation of Sample Images from Chapter 19

REVIEW IMAGE NO. 1, FIG. 19-20

This lateral skull radiograph shows objectionable artifacts in the form of hairpins, which should have been removed. Poor centering resulted in failure to show the contour of the cranium at the skull vertex and position of the identification area over the frontal bone.

REVIEW IMAGE NO. 2, FIG. 19-21

This lateral projection chest radiograph shows rotation out of the lateral position. The posterior portions of the left and right ribs are separated by more than 0.5 inches (1.3 cm). Air in the stomach identifies the left lung, which is posterior to the right lung. A correct lateral position requires the patient's right side to be rotated slightly posterior.

REVIEW IMAGE NO. 3, FIG. 19-22

This lateral projection of the wrist shows rotation out of the lateral position. The radius is anterior to the ulna. To correct this, the wrist should be slightly supinated (rotated laterally).

REVIEW IMAGE NO. 4, FIG. 19-23

This anteroposterior projection of the elbow shows the radius superimposed across the ulna. This is the result of the hand positioned in pronation. The hand should be supinated to correct this positioning error.

REVIEW IMAGE NO. 5, FIG. 19-24

This anteroposterior ankle shows improper rotation. The ankle mortise joint is not open and there is too much super-imposition of the fibula on the talus and tibia. The patient's ankle should be internally rotated to place the plane through the malleoli parallel to the image receptor (IR).

REVIEW IMAGE NO. 6, FIG. 19-25

This lateral projection of the knee shows improper rotation. The medial condyle (closer to the IR so less magnified) is anterior to the lateral condyle. The leg was rotated too much toward the IR. To correct this positioning error, the leg should be rotated away from the IR to place the coronal plane through the patella perpendicular to the IR. The knee is fully extended, but should be flexed approximately 30 degrees.

Charting Terms and Abbreviations

Table L-1

Abbreviations Typically Used in Charting*

Abbreviation	Word or Phrase	Abbreviation	Word or Phrase
abd	abdomen	L	left
ac	before meals	L *or* l	liter
ad lib	freely, as desired	lab	laboratory
AED	automatic external defibrillator	LBP	low back pain
amt	amount	LLQ	left lower quadrant—abdomen
AP	apical pulse, anteroposterior	LP	lumbar puncture
aq	water	LUQ	left upper quadrant—abdomen
bid (2id)	2 times a day	MI	myocardial infarction
BP	blood pressure	mcg	microgram
BRP	bathroom privileges	mg	milligram
C *or* cent	centigrade	ml	milliliter
$\overline{c}$	with	MVC	motor vehicle crash
caps	capsules	NKI	no known injury
CHF	congestive heart failure	noct	at night
cm	centimeter	NPO	nothing by mouth
DC	discontinue	NS	normal saline solution
ECG *or* EKG	electrocardiogram	OB, obs	obstetrics
ED	emergency department	OD	right eye
EEG	electroencephalogram	OJ	orange juice
EENT	eye, ear, nose, and throat	OPC	outpatient clinic
ENT	ear, nose, and throat	OR	operating room
ER	emergency room	OS	left eye
fld	fluid	P *or* $\overline{p}$	after
GB	gallbladder	pc	after meals
GI	gastrointestinal	pH	hydrogen ion concentration
g, Gm, *or* gm	gram	PO	by mouth
gtt	drop, drops	pp	postprandial, after meals
GU	genitourinary	prn	when necessary, as needed
gyn	gynecology	q2h	every 2 hours
(H)	hypodermically	qh	every hour
H *or* hrs	hour, hours	qid (4id)	4 times a day
H_2O	water	qs	sufficient quantity
HA	headache	RBC	red blood cell (count)
Hgb *or* Hb	hemoglobin	RUQ	right upper quadrant—abdomen
HS	bedtime	Rx	therapy
I&O	intake and output	$\overline{s}$	without
IM	intramuscular	SOB	short of breath
IV	intravenous	spec	specimen
Kg *or* kg	kilogram	stat	at once
KUB	kidneys, ureters, and bladder	subcut.	subcutaneous

Continued

603

Table L-1

Abbreviations Typically Used in Charting—cont'd

Abbreviation	Word or Phrase	Abbreviation	Word or Phrase
tid (3id)	3 times a day	WBC	white blood cell (count)
TPR	temperature, pulse, respiration	WC	wheelchair
URI	upper respiratory (tract) infection	wt	weight
UTI	urinary tract infection	x	times

*These abbreviations are consistent with current National Patient Safety Goals and the recommendations of the Institute for Safe Medication Practices (ISMP).

Table L-2

Do Not Use the Following Dangerous Abbreviations and Dose Designations

Abbreviation/Expression	Intended Meaning	Misinterpretation	Correction
D/C	discharge, discontinue	The 2 meanings may be confused	Write "discharge" or "discontinue"
IU	International Unit	Mistaken for IV or the number 10	Write "International Unit"
MS, MSO_4, $MgSO_4$	morphine sulfate or magnesium sulfate	Confused for one another	Write "morphine sulfate" or "magnesium sulfate"
μg	microgram	Mistaken for mg	Use "mcg"
Q.D., QD, q.d., qd	daily	Mistaken for QOD	Write "daily"
Q.O.D., QOD, q.o.d., qod	every other day	Mistaken for QD	Write "every other day"
qhs	nightly at bedtime	Misread as every hour	Write "nightly"
sub q	subcutaneous	"q" is mistaken to mean every	Write "subcut" or "subcutaneous"
SC	subcutaneous	Mistaken for SL (sublingual)	Write "subcut" or "subcutaneous"
U or u	unit or units	May be read as a 0 or a 4	There is no acceptable abbreviation. Write "unit."
cc	cubic centimeters	Misread as "U" (units)	Write "mL" or milliliters
ss	sliding scale (insulin) or 1/2 (apothecary)	Mistaken for 55	Spell out "sliding scale"; use "one-half" or "1/2."
/ (slash mark)	separates 2 doses or indicates "per"	Mistaken for the number 1	Do not use slash mark to separate doses. Write "per."
>	greater than	Mistaken for number 7	Write "greater than"
<	less than	Mistaken for letter L	Write "less than"
@	at	Mistaken for number 2	Write "at"
Zero after decimal point (1.0)	1 mg	Misread as 10 mg if decimal point is not seen	Do not use terminal zeros after whole numbers
No zero before decimal dose (.5 mg)	0.5 mg	Misread as 5 mg if decimal point is not seen	Always use zero before a decimal point when dose amount is less than a whole number

Table L-3

Descriptive Terms Typically Used in Charting

Area of Concern	Factor to Be Charted	Suggested Terms to Use
Abdomen	Hard, boardlike Appears swollen, rounded Soft, flabby, flat Region	Hard, rigid Distended Relaxed, flaccid, flat 1. Right hypochondriac 2. Epigastric 3. Left hypochondriac 4. Right lumbar 5. Umbilical 6. Left lumbar 7. Right iliac 8. Hypogastric 9. Left iliac

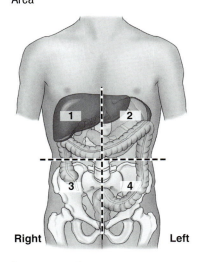

Area of Concern	Factor to Be Charted	Suggested Terms to Use
Abdomen	Area	1. Right upper quadrant 2. Left upper quadrant 3. Right lower quadrant 4. Left lower quadrant
Amounts	Large amount Moderate amount Small amount	Excessive, profuse, copious Moderate, usual Scanty, slight
Appearance, general	Thin and undernourished Fat, greatly overweight Seems very sick	Emaciated Obese Acutely ill
Appetite	Loss of appetite Would not eat	Anorexia Refused food (state reason)
Attitude (mental state)	Has "don't care" attitude Afraid, worried Feeling blue, sad Other characteristic terms:	Apathetic Anxious, apprehensive Depressed Anxiety, defiance, anger, pain, boredom, happiness, dissatisfaction, irritability, worry

Continued

Table L-3

Descriptive Terms Typically Used in Charting—cont'd

Area of Concern	Factor to Be Charted	Suggested Terms to Use
Back regions	Upper back	Thoracic region, dorsal region
	Small of the back	Lumbar region
	Lower spine	Sacral region
	Buttocks	Gluteal area
Bleeding	Very little	Oozing
	Nosebleed	Epistaxis
	Blood in vomitus	Hematemesis
	Blood in urine	Hematuria
	Coughing or spitting up blood	Hemoptysis
	Bleeding stopped	Hemorrhage controlled
Breathing	Breathing	Respiration
	Act of inhaling	Inspiration
	Act of exhaling	Expiration
	Difficulty in breathing	Dyspnea, dyspneic
	Unable to breathe lying down	Orthopnea
	Cessation of breathing for short periods	Apnea
	Rapid breathing	Hyperpnea
	Increasing dyspnea with periods of apnea	Cheyne-Stokes respiration
	Large amount of air inspired or expired	Deep breathing
	Small amount of air inspired or expired	Shallow breathing
	Abnormal variations in rhythm	Irregular respiration
Chill	Blanket applied to keep warm	External heat applied
	Severity (degree of)	Severe, moderate, slight
	Duration	Persistent or short duration
	Came on suddenly	Sudden onset
Level of consciousness	Fully conscious, aware of surroundings	Alert, fully conscious
	Only partly conscious	Stuporous
	Unconscious but can be aroused	Semicomatose
	Unconscious, cannot be aroused	Comatose

From Ehrlich RA, Coakes D: *Patient care in radiography,* ed 9, St Louis, 2016, Elsevier.

Task Inventory for Limited Scope of Practice in Radiography[s]

Activity	Content Categories
1. Confirm patient's identity.	D.2.
2. Evaluate patient's ability to understand and comply with requirements for the requested examination.	D.2.
3. Obtain pertinent medical history.	D.1.B.1., D.2.
4. Examine imaging examination requisition to verify accuracy and completeness of information (e.g., patient history, clinical diagnosis, physician's orders).	D.1.B.
5. Respond as appropriate to imaging study inquiries from patients.	D.2.
6. Assume responsibility for medical equipment attached to patients (e.g., IVs, oxygen) during the imaging procedures.	D.4.B.
7. Follow environmental protection standards for handling and disposing of biohazardous materials (e.g., sharps, blood and body fluids).	D.3.E.
8. Provide for patient safety, comfort, and modesty.	D.1.C., D.4., D.1.A.
9. Notify appropriate personnel of adverse events or incidents (e.g., patient fall, wrong patient imaged).	C.2.A., D.1.B.1., D.4.
10. Communicate scheduling delays to waiting patients.	D.2.
11. Verify or obtain patient consent as necessary.	D.1.A.1.
12. Communicate relevant information to others (e.g., MDs, RNs, other radiology personnel).	D.
13. Explain procedure instructions to patient or patient's family.	D.2.
14. Practice standard precautions.	D.3.B., D.3.C.
15. Follow appropriate procedures when in contact with patient in isolation.	D.3.C., D.3.D.
16. Select immobilization devices, when indicated, to prevent patient's movement and/or ensure patient's safety.	D.1.B.4.
17. Use proper body mechanics and/or mechanical transfer devices when assisting patient.	D.4.A.1.
18. Use sterile or aseptic technique when indicated.	D.3.A.
19. Obtain vital signs.	D.4.C.
20. Recognize and communicate the need for prompt medical attention.	D.5., D.4.C.3.
21. Administer emergency care.	D.5., D.4.C.3.
22. Explain post-procedural instructions to patient or patient's family.	D.2.C.
23. Maintain confidentiality of patient's information.	D.1.A.2., D.1.C.
24. Clean, disinfect, or sterilize facilities and equipment, and dispose of contaminated items in preparation for next examination.	D.3.A., D.3.E.

25. Document required information on patient's medical record (e.g., imaging procedure documentation, images).
  a. On paper
  b. Electronically
	C.2.E., D.1.B.

26. Evaluate the need for and use of protective shielding.	A.2.B.
27. Take appropriate precautions to minimize radiation exposure to patient.	A.1., A.2.
28. Question female patient of child-bearing age about possible pregnancy and take appropriate action (e.g., document response, contact physician).	A.1.D., D.2.

Activity	Content Categories
29. Restrict beam to limit exposure area, improve image quality, and reduce radiation dose.	A.1., A.2.C., C.1.A.1.G., C.1.A.2.G.
30. Prevent all unnecessary persons from remaining in area during x-ray exposure.	A.1., A.4.C.2.
31. Take appropriate precautions to minimize occupational radiation exposure.	A.3.B.
32. Wear a personnel monitoring device while on duty.	A.4.B.
33. Evaluate individual occupational exposure reports to determine if values for the reporting period are within established limits.	A.4.C.
34. Determine appropriate exposure factors using: a. Fixed kVp technique chart b. Variable kVp technique chart c. Calipers (to determine patient thickness for exposure)	C.1.B.2.
35. Select radiographic exposure factors. a. Automatic Exposure Control (AEC)* b. kVp and mAs (manual) c. Pre-programmed techniques (anatomically programmed radiography)	E.1. (focus 4) C.1.A. C.1.B.1.
36. Operate radiographic unit and accessories. a. Fixed unit b. Mobile unit (portable)	B.1., B.2.A., C.1.
37. Operate electronic imaging and record-keeping devices. a. Computed Radiography (CR) b. Direct Radiography (DR) c. Picture Archival and Communication System (PACS) d. Hospital Information System (HIS) e. Radiology Information System (RIS)	C.2.C. B.2.C. B.2.C. C.2.E.2. C.2.E.3. C.2.E.4.
38. Prepare and operate specialized units (chest unit*).	E.1. (focus 4)
39. Remove all radiopaque materials from patient or table that could interfere with the image.	C.3.I.
40. Perform post-processing on digital images in preparation for interpretation (e.g., exposure indicator, brightness/contrast, window width and level).	C.2.C., C.2.D.
41. Use radiopaque markers to indicate anatomical side, position, or other relevant information (e.g., upright, decubitus).	C.2.A., C.3.G.
42. Add electronic annotations on digital images to indicate position, or other relevant information (e.g., upright, decubitus, standing, weight-bearing).	C.2.A., C.3.G.
43. Use film-screen cassettes and automatic film processing.	C.1.E., C.2.B.
44. Select equipment and accessories (e.g., grid, compensating filter, shielding) for the examination requested.	A.2.B., E.1. (focus 4)
45. Explain breathing instructions prior to making the exposure.*	C.1.A.3.H., D.2.C., E.1.E.2.C., E.4. (focus 3)
46. Position patient to demonstrate the desired anatomy using body landmarks.	E., C.3.F.
47. Modify exposure factors for circumstances such as involuntary motion, casts and splints, pathological conditions, or patient's inability to cooperate.	C.1.B.3., C.1.A.
48. Verify accuracy of patient identification on image.	C.2.A., C.3.G.
49. Evaluate images for diagnostic quality.	C.3.
50. Determine corrective measures if image is not of diagnostic quality and take appropriate action.	C.3.
51. Store and handle image receptor in a manner that will reduce the possibility of artifact production.	B.3.C., B.2.C.5., B.2.D.3., C.2., C.3.J., C.3.I.
52. Visually inspect, recognize, and report malfunctions in the imaging unit and accessories.	B.3.B.
53. Recognize the need for basic evaluations of radiographic equipment and accessories. a. Light field to radiation field alignment b. Central-ray alignment c. Shielding accessories (e.g., lead aprons and gloves)	B.3.A.1. B.3.A.2. B.3.D.
54. Perform routine maintenance on digital equipment. a. Perform start-up or shut-down b. Erase CR plate c. Ensure equipment cleanliness (e.g., imaging plates, CR cassettes) d. Recognize and report malfunctions	B.2.C.3. B.2.C.4. B.2.C.5. B.3.B.
55. Chest	E.1.A.
56. Cervical spine	E.4.A.
57. Thoracic spine	E.4.B.

Activity	**Content Categories**
58. Scoliosis series	E.4.C.
59. Lumbar spine	E.4.D.
60. Sacrum and coccyx	E.4.E.
61. Sacroiliac joints	E.4.E.
62. Skull	E.3.A.
63. Facial bones	E.3.C.
64. Nasal bones	E.3.C.
65. Orbits	E.3.C.
66. Paranasal sinuses	E.3.B.
67. Toes	E.2.A., E.5.A.
68. Foot	E.2.A., E.5.A.
69. Calcaneus (os calcis)	E.2.A., E.5.C.
70. Ankle	E.2.A., E.5.B.
71. Tibia, fibula	E.2.A.
72. Knee	E.2.A.
73. Patella	E.2.A.
74. Distal femur	E.2.A.
75. Fingers	E.2.A.
76. Hand	E.2.A.
77. Wrist	E.2.A.
78. Forearm	E.2.A.
79. Elbow	E.2.A.
80. Humerus	E.2.A.
81. Shoulder	E.2.A.
82. Scapula	E.2.A.
83. Clavicle	E.2.A.
84. Acromioclavicular joints	E.2.A.
85. Soft tissue/foreign body	E.2. (focus 3)

*Applies to specific modules
IV, Intravenous; *MD*, medical doctor; *RN*, registered nurse.

Illustration Credits

Adler A, Carlton R: *Introduction to radiologic and imaging sciences and patient care*, ed 6, St Louis, 2016, Saunders.
Fig. 21-16

Atlas RM: *Principles of microbiology*, St Louis, 1999, Mosby.
Fig. 21-18

Ballinger PW, Frank ED: *Merrill's atlas of radiographic positions and radiologic procedures*, ed 10, St Louis, 2003, Mosby.
Figs. 6-17, 7-2, 8-1, 8-2, 8-3A, 8-4A, 8-4C, 8-7, 9-20, 10-2, 10-7 to 10-9, 10-11, 10-12, 11-4, 12-42, 13-8, 13-19, 13-85, 13-87, 14-42, 14-64B, 14-68, 14-84, 15-76, 15-77, 15-79, 15-80, 15-83, 16-38, 16-52, 16-53, 17-9, 17-11, 17-18, 17-23, 17-29, 17-50, 18-16, 18-21, 18-27 to 18-29, 19-1, 26-2, 26-5, 26-6, 26-8 to 26-11, 26-13

Bonewit-West K: *Clinical procedures for medical assistants*, ed 7, Philadelphia, 2008, Saunders.
Fig. 22-3

Bonewit-West K: *Clinical procedures for medical assistants*, ed 9, St Louis, 2015, Saunders.
Figs. 25-1 to 25-3, 25-5 to 25-13, 25-19, 25-23, 25-24

Bontrager KL: *Radiographic positioning and related anatomy*, ed 2, St Louis, 1987, Mosby.
Fig. 13-83

Bushong SC: *Radiologic science for technologists*, ed 10, St Louis, 2013, Mosby.
Figs. 4-2, 4-4, 6-13, 7-5, H-6

Bushong SC: *Radiologic technology*, ed 9, St Louis, 2009, Mosby.
Fig. 11-1

Carter CE, Veale BL: *Digital radiography and PACS*, St Louis, 2010, Mosby.
Figs. 8-6, 8-13B, 8-17, 8-18, 8-21

Carter CE, Veale BL: *Digital radiography and PACS*, ed 2, St Louis, 2014, Mosby.
Figs. 8-3B, 8-13A, 8-20

Cipollaro AC: The earliest roentgen demonstration of a pathological lesion in America, *Radiology* 45:555, 1945.
Fig. 1-3

Deltoff MN: *The portable skeletal x-ray library*, St Louis, 1997, Mosby.
Fig. 18-30

Dibner B: *The new rays of Professor Roentgen*, Norwalk, Conn, 1962, Burndy Library Collection, The Huntington Library, San Marino, Calif.
Fig. 1-1

Dolan K, Jacoby C, Smoker W: The radiology of facial fractures, *Radiographics* 4:576, 1984.
Fig. 17-51

Ehrlich RA, Coakes D: *Patient care in radiography*, ed 8, St Louis, 2012, Mosby.
Figs. 21-1, 21-2, 22-2, 24-6

Ehrlich RA, Coakes D: *Patient care in radiography*, ed 9, St Louis, 2016, Mosby.
Figs. 2-10 to 2-13, 18-3, 18-4, 18-8, 18-11, 18-12, 18-14, 18-18, 20-4, 21-4 to 21-6, 21-11, 21-14, 21-15, 21-22, 21-23, 21-25 to 21-28, 22-1, 22-3, 22-6 to 22-14, 23-4, 23-5, 23-12

Ehrlich RA, Daly JA: *Patient care in radiography*, ed 7, St Louis, 2009, Mosby.
Figs. 3-1, 3-2, 11-7, 11-10, 11-11, 18-34, 18-36, 20-2, 21-3, 21-7, 21-12, 21-17, 21-29, 21-30, 22-15

Eisenberg RL, Dennis CA: *Comprehensive radiographic pathology*, ed 4, St Louis, 2007, Mosby.
Figs. 13-110, 15-84, 15-93, 16-46A

Eisenberg RL, Johnson NM: *Comprehensive radiographic pathology*, ed 6, St Louis, 2016, Mosby.
Figs. 12-40, 13-108, 13-114, 13-115, 13-117, 13-118, 14-85, 14-92, 14-95, 15-81, 15-88, 15-91, 16-42 to 16-45, 16-46B, 16-47, 16-48, 16-50, 17-46, 17-48, 17-49, 17-52 to 17-56

Eriksen E: *Bone histomorphometry*, Philadelphia, 1994, Raven Press.
Fig. 26-3A

Fauber TL: *Radiographic imaging and exposure*, ed 5, St Louis, 2017, Mosby.
Figs. 8-14, 8-15

Frank ED, Long BW, Smith BJ: *Merrill's atlas of radiographic positioning and procedures*, ed 12, St Louis, 2012, Mosby.
Figs. 2-3B, 2-16, 11-5, 17-25

Glasser O: Wilhelm Conrad Roentgen and the early history of the roentgen rays, 1933. In Fauber TL: *Radiographic imaging and exposure*, ed 3, St Louis, 2009, Mosby.
Fig. 1-2

Guebert GM, Yochum TR: *Essentials of diagnostic imaging*, St Louis, 1995, Mosby.
Fig. 2-5

Kleinman PK: *Diagnostic imaging of child abuse*, ed 2, St Louis, 1998, Mosby.
Fig. 18-33

Linn-Watson TL: *Radiographic pathology*, Philadelphia, 1996, Saunders.
Figs. 13-106, 13-109, 14-86, 14-87, 14-91, 14-93, 16-49, 17-47

Long BW, Rollins JH, Smith BJ: *Merrill's atlas of radiographic positioning and procedures*, ed 13, St Louis, 2016, Mosby.
Figs. 2-15, 2-17, 12-15 to 12-17, 12-31, 12-32, 12-36, 12-37, 13-3, 13-6, 13-102, 14-12, 14-16, 14-18, 14-26, 14-30, 14-32, 14-38B, 15-24, 15-55, 15-60, 15-78, 16-13B, 16-18, 17-31, 17-38, 17-40, 17-42, 17-44

Mace J, Kowalczyk N: *Radiographic pathology for technologists*, ed 3, St Louis, 1998, Mosby.
Fig. 18-37

McQuillen Martensen K: *Radiographic image analysis*, ed 4, St Louis, 2015, Saunders.
Figs. 19-21 to 19-25

McQuillen-Martensen K: *Radiographic critique*, Philadelphia, 1996, Saunders.
Fig. I-25

Osborn AG: Head trauma. In Eisenberg RL, Amberg JR, eds: *Critical diagnostic pathways in radiology*, Philadelphia, 1981, Lippincott.
Fig. 15-89

Papp J: *Quality management in the imaging sciences*, ed 3, St Louis, 2006, Mosby.
Fig. I-4

Papp J: *Quality management in the imaging sciences*, ed 5, St Louis, 2015, Mosby.
Figs. 9-22, 9-23

Patton KT, Thibodeau GA: *Structure and function of the body*, ed 15, St Louis, 2016, Mosby.
Figs. 12-3, 12-4, 12-6, 12-7, 12-13, 12-14, 16-7, 16-8, 18-25

Perry AG, Potter PA, Ostendorf WR: *Nursing interventions and clinical skills*, ed 6, St Louis, 2016, Elsevier.
Figs. 22-4, 23-7A, 23-8A, 23-9A

Proctor DB, Adams AP: *Kinn's the medical assistant*, ed 12, St Louis, 2014, Saunders.
Figs. 25-4, 12-35

Rogers LF: *Radiology of skeletal trauma*, New York, 1982, Churchill Livingstone.
Fig. 17-52

Silverman FN, Kuhn JP: *Caffey's pediatric x-ray diagnosis*, ed 9, St Louis, 1993, Mosby.
Fig. 13-107

Taylor JAM, Resnick D: *Skeletal imaging*, Philadelphia, 2000, Saunders.
Figs. 14-88, 14-89, 15-85, 15-86, 16-39, 16-40

Thibodeau GA, Patton KT: *Structure and function of the body*, ed 13, St Louis, 2008, Mosby.
Figs. 12-1, 16-3, 16-4

Thibodeau GA, Patton KT: *Structure and function of the body*, ed 14, St Louis, 2012, Mosby.
Figs. 12-2, 12-5, 12-8 to 12-12, 16-2

Tille P: *Bailey and Scott's diagnostic microbiology*, ed 13, St Louis, 2014, Mosby.
Figs. 21-20, 21-21

Wold LE, et al: *Atlas of orthopedic pathology*, ed 3, Philadelphia, 2008, Saunders.
Figs. 26-3B, 26-3C

Yoost BL, Crawford LR: *Fundamentals of nursing*, St Louis, 2016, Elsevier.
Fig. 22-5

COURTESIES

American College of Radiology, Reston, VA
Fig. 18-37

Andrew Woodard, University of North Carolina
Fig. 8-16

Becton, Dickinson and Company, Franklin Lakes, NJ
Figs. 23-11, 24-3, 24-5

Canon USA, Inc., Melville, NY
Fig. 8-8B

Carestream Health, Inc., Rochester, NY
Figs. 8-11, 8-12

Eastman Kodak, Rochester, NY
Fig. 5-1

Ferlic Filter Company, LLC, White Bear Lake, MN
Fig. 10-10

Fujifilm Medical Systems, Stamford, CT
Fig. 8-5

GE Healthcare, Chicago, IL
Fig. 1-5, 26-1B, 26-14, 26-16

Hologic Systems Division, Bedford, MA
Fig. 2-6, 26-1A, 26-12, 26-15

Natus Medical Incorporated, Pleasanton, CA
Fig. 18-12

Norland Corporation, Fort Atkinson, WI
Fig. 26-1C

Occupational Safety and Health Administration: www.osha.gov
Fig. 23-10

Varian Medical Systems, North Charleston, SC
Fig. 6-8

Welch Allyn, Skaneateles Falls, NY
Figs. 22-2, 22-3

Glossary

abdominal thrust Heimlich maneuver; a technique for dislodging a foreign object from the throat of a person who is choking.

absorbed dose The amount of energy (x-rays) per unit mass absorbed by the irradiated tissue.

absorption The process by which nutrients and drugs enter the systemic circulation.

acanthion The superior prominence formed at the junction of the two maxillary bones; the positioning landmark where the nose meets the upper lip.

acromion process A large, rounded projection that can be felt on the superior surface of the scapula.

acute Having a short and relatively severe course.

AED Automatic external defibrillator.

aggressive Describes an attitude characterized by the angry or hostile and forceful expression of feelings or opinions.

agonist A drug that produces a specific action and promotes a desired result.

AIDS Acquired immunodeficiency syndrome, the disease caused by the human immunodeficiency virus (HIV).

airborne contamination Dust containing either endospores or droplet nuclei circulating through the air.

air gap A space between the patient and the film.

air kerma Represents a measurement of the radiation intensity in the air. Kerma is an acronym for "**k**inetic **e**nergy **r**eleased in **ma**tter."

ALARA A guiding philosophy that means "*As Low As Reasonably Achievable.*" It is the principle of reducing patient radiation exposure and dose to the lowest reasonable amounts. Limited operators should always follow this philosophy when applying radiation to humans.

algebra A mathematical method for determining the value of an unknown quantity that has a specific relationship to one or more known quantities.

allergen An allergy-causing substance.

Alzheimer disease A specific type of brain tissue deterioration that causes memory loss and gradual loss of mental function.

analgesic A drug used to alleviate pain.

analog-to-digital converter (ADC) A device that converts each pixel's value into a digital value.

analyte A chemical substance to be measured or identified when clinical specimens are analyzed.

anaphylaxis A severe allergic reaction.

anatomic position The position in which the patient is standing erect, with the face directed forward, arms extended by the sides with the palms facing forward, and the toes pointing anteriorly.

anesthetic A drug that reduces or eliminates sensation, preventing pain.

angina (angina pectoris) Chest pain that occurs when the coronary arteries are unable to supply the heart with sufficient oxygen to meet current needs.

anoxia Lack of oxygen.

antagonist A drug, such as flumazenil (Mazicon), used to counteract the effects of sedatives or analgesics.

antecubital fossa The depression on the anterior aspect of the elbow.

anthropomorphic Simulating human form.

antibiotic A drug used to treat infections; antimicrobial.

antibodies Blood proteins produced in response to and counteracting a specific antigen.

anticoagulant A drug that prevents the clotting of blood within the vessels.

antidote A drug that treats a toxic effect.

antihistamine A drug used to treat allergic reactions.

antimicrobial A drug used to treat infections; antibiotic.

aorta The largest artery of the body, passing from the heart through the chest and the abdomen.

apex The tip or point of a structure, such as the apex of the heart.

array-beam collimation Dual-energy x-ray absorptiometry system that uses a narrow "slit" x-ray collimator and a multi-element detector. The motion is in one direction only, which greatly reduces scan time and permits supine lateral spine scans. It introduces a slight geometric distortion at the outer edges, which necessitates careful centering of the object of interest.

artifact An erroneous portion of an image or tracing that does not accurately represent the subject of the image or measurement being recorded.

asepsis The process of reducing the probability that infectious organisms will be transmitted to a susceptible individual.

aspiration The process of inhaling a foreign body or substance into the trachea or a bronchus.

assault The threat of touching in an injurious way.

assertive Describes an attitude characterized by the calm, firm expression of feelings or opinions.

asthma A difficulty in breathing caused by constriction of the bronchi.

atelectasis Lung collapse.

atlas The C1 vertebra; a ringlike structure with no vertebral body and a very short spinous process.

atomic number Represents the number of protons in the nucleus of an atom.

atrophy A wasting away; a reduction in size of a tissue, organ, or part.

attenuation Absorption of the x-ray beam in matter, usually the human body.

autoclave An electric steam chamber that achieves high temperatures under pressure for the purpose of sterilization.

automatic exposure control (AEC) An electronic circuit within the x-ray machine that automatically terminates the exposure time when a predetermined quantity of x-rays has been detected.

axilla The armpit.

axis The C2 vertebra; the vertebra on which the atlas rotates so the head can turn from side to side.

bacterium (pl. bacteria) Very small, single-cell microorganism that has a cell wall and an atypical nucleus without a membrane; some are pathogenic.

base number The number that is multiplied times itself to form a mathematical term with an exponent.

battered child syndrome The signs and symptoms characteristic of child abuse.

battery An unlawful touching of a person without consent.

benign Not malignant; not recurrent; favorable for recovery.

benzodiazepine The class of psychoactive drugs known as tranquilizers.

biohazard symbol A warning mark that indicates a substance that may cause harm chemically or biologically.

biohazardous waste Garbage that is a threat to the environment and the organisms within it.

blow-out fracture Traumatic opening between the orbital floor and the maxillary sinus, usually caused by a blow to the eye.

bone densitometry The art and science of measuring the bone mineral content, area, and density of specific anatomic sites or the whole body.

bone mass A general term for the amount of mineral in a bone.

bone mineral content (BMC) A measure of bone mineral in the total area of a region of interest.

bone mineral density (BMD) A measure of bone mineral per unit area of a region of interest.

bone remodeling The process of bone resorption by osteoclasts, followed by bone formation by osteoblasts. The relative rates of resorption and formation determine whether bone mass increases, remains stable, or decreases.

bradypnea Abnormally slow breathing; fewer than 12 breaths per minute.

bremsstrahlung radiation One of two types of x-rays. Bremsstrahlung is created when an electron enters the tungsten anode of the x-ray tube, misses the tungsten electrons, and gets very near the nucleus. The electron suddenly slows down and deviates, and the loss of energy creates an x-ray photon.

brightness The digital term for "density." Describes the overall radiographic image appearance on the display monitor.

bronchus An air passageway that connects the trachea to a lung or portion of a lung.

buccal Inside the cheek; a topical route of drug administration.

Bucky A device that contains a moving grid.

bursitis Inflammation of a bursa.

calcaneus The heel bone.

cannula A tube.

cardiac Pertaining to the heart.

cardiac ischemia Deficiency of blood supply to the heart muscle.

cardiophrenic angles The inferior medial corners of the lungs.

carina A prominent ridge of the lowest tracheal cartilage running anteroposteriorly between the orifices of the two main stem bronchi.

carpal digits The fingers.

carpus, carpal The eight short bones of the wrist; pertaining to these bones.

carrier An individual infected with a pathogenic organism who does not contract the disease but is capable of spreading it to others.

CCMS Abbreviation for "clean-catch midstream specimen"; a method for collecting urine for urinalysis.

CDC Centers for Disease Control and Prevention, a federal agency that monitors and studies the diseases, particularly infectious diseases, that are occurring in the nation; a resource for disease information.

Celsius scale A metric system for measuring temperature.

centigrade scale Old term for the Celsius scale; a metric system for measuring temperature. In this system, water freezes at 0° and boils at 100°.

centrifuge An electric laboratory device that spins test tubes rapidly to separate solids from liquid.

cerebral concussion A blow to the head that causes brief unconsciousness or disorientation.

cerebrovascular accident (CVA) A stroke.

cervical spine The most superior section of the vertebral column; it consists of seven vertebrae with a lordotic curve.

chaperone A female health care worker who is in the same room when a female patient is examined or treated by a male physician or other health care worker, particularly when the examination or treatment involves undraping of the genitals or breasts.

characteristic radiation One of two types of x-ray production. Characteristic radiation is created when an electron enters the tungsten anode of the x-ray tube and knocks out a K-shell electron. This interaction produces an x-ray photon.

chart An extensive compilation of information; the medical record of a patient's care.

charting The process of adding information to a document or medical record.

chronic Persisting over a long period of time.

clavicle The collar bone.

clean-catch midstream specimen A urine specimen obtained in such a way as to prevent bacterial contamination of the specimen.

CNS Central nervous system; the brain and spinal cord.

coccyx The most inferior section of the vertebral column, consisting of three to five vertebral segments; also called the *tailbone*.

code of ethics A document that sets forth professional standards of ethical behavior.

collimation Restricting the size and shape of the radiation beam as it exits the x-ray tube.

colon The large intestine.

common denominator A denominator that is the same for two or more fractions in an expression.

compare feature Software feature of dual-energy x-ray absorptiometry that replicates the size and placement of regions of interest from the reference scan on the follow-up scan.

complementary metal oxide semiconductor (CMOS) A special type of memory chip that uses a small rechargeable or lithium battery to retain information about the computer's hardware while the computer is turned off.

Compton effect One of three interactions of radiation with human body tissues. In this effect, the x-ray photon is scattered from the body rather than going directly through to expose the film. This effect is undesirable in radiographic imaging.

computed radiography (CR) One of the two types of digital imaging systems. CR is *cassette-based* digital imaging because the image of the body part is obtained using storage phosphor plates.

congenital Referring to conditions that are present at birth.

contrast The difference in density between any two adjacent portions of the image.

contrast resolution The ability to distinguish anatomic structures of similar subject contrast such as liver-spleen and gray matter-white matter.

contrecoup injury Brain injury caused by movement of the brain within the cranium that results from a severe blow to the head on the opposite side.

contusion A bruise; an injury of a part without a break in the skin.

cortical bone Dense, compact outer shell of all bones and the shafts of the long bones; it supports weight, resists bending and twisting, and accounts for about 80% of the skeletal mass.

corticosteroid A synthetic hormone drug that acts as an anti-inflammatory agent.

costophrenic angles The inferior lateral corners of the lungs.

CPR Cardiopulmonary resuscitation; basic life support system used to ventilate the lungs and circulate the blood in the event of respiratory or cardiac arrest.

CR reader Unit used in computed radiography to scan and process the latent image. A laser scan is used to release the stored image, which is collected and converted to an electrical signal and is then sent to the computer for viewing.

cranium The eight bones that surround the brain; the brain case.

cubed In mathematics, the description of a number that has been multiplied by itself two times.

cyanotic Having a bluish coloration in the skin that indicates a lack of sufficient oxygen in tissues.

dead pixels Occur when dust, scratches, and interactions between materials result in some defective pixels. As the detector ages, the number of dead pixels increases. Manufacturers make efforts to maintain a standard of less than approximately 0.1% to 0.2%.

decimal A fraction with a denominator of 10, 100, 1000, or any number that consists of a 1 followed by one or more zeros.

decimal point The dot at the left of a decimal fraction.

decubitus ulcer A lesion that develops over bony prominences when pressure is exerted over time.

defamation of character Disclosure of information that reflects negatively on a person's reputation.

defibrillator A device that administers an electric shock to correct a weak and irregular heart rhythm.

degeneration Deterioration or impairment of an organ or body part.

degenerative Tending to cause degeneration; characteristic of degeneration.

dehydration Lack of fluid in the tissues because of insufficient fluid intake.

demineralization Calcium loss in bones that causes them to become more radiolucent.

denominator The lower number of a fraction.

dens A tooth or toothlike structure or process; the odontoid process of the axis.

densitometer A device that measures the optical density on a film.

diabetic coma State of unconsciousness caused by abnormally high blood glucose levels, characterized by a relatively slow onset.

diaphoretic Perspiring.

diaphragm The large sheath of muscle between the chest and the abdomen that expands and contracts with breathing.

diastolic Referring to the point of least pressure in the arterial system.

difference In mathematics, the answer to a subtraction problem.

digital imaging The process of acquiring images of the body using x-rays, displaying them digitally, and viewing and storing them on a computer and in computer files.

Digital Imaging and Communications in Medicine (DICOM) The universally accepted standard for the storage, transmission, and display of medical images.

digital radiography (DR) One of the two types of digital imaging systems. DR is *cassetteless* because these systems do not use a cassette with phosphors. Instead the phosphor is bonded to a flat panel detector built into the x-ray table.

diode An electronic device that permits current to flow in one direction only.

discordance A situation in which a patient has a T-score indicating osteoporosis at one anatomic site but not at another site, or when indicated by one modality but not by another.

disinfection The destruction of pathogens by chemical agents.

diverticula Abnormal small sacs or pouches that form in the walls of the digestive tract, particularly the colon.

diverticulitis Inflammation of colonic diverticula.

dividend In mathematics, the number divided into in a division problem.

divisor In mathematics, the number that is divided into the dividend.

doctrine of the reasonably prudent person The standard that requires a person to perform as any reasonable person would perform under similar circumstances.

droplet contamination Contamination by droplets from an infectious individual's nose or mouth.

dual-energy x-ray absorptiometry (DXA) A bone density measurement technique using an x-ray source separated into two energies. It has good accuracy and precision and can scan essentially any anatomic site, which makes it the most versatile of the bone density techniques.

duodenum The proximal portion of the small intestine.

dynamic range The number of gray shades that an imaging system can reproduce.

dyspnea Difficult breathing.

edema The accumulation of excessive fluid in the subcutaneous tissues.

effective dose (EfD) This value is the limiting system used to calculate the upper limits of occupational exposure permissible.

efficacy Effectiveness.

electrocardiogram (ECG, EKG) The tracing made on paper by an electrocardiograph machine.

electrocardiograph A machine used to assess heart function and diagnose heart disease.

electrocardiograph leads Electrode combinations used to record heart function in electrocardiography. Twelve leads constitute a standard study.

electrode A contact that receives electric signals, such as the contact between the patient and a lead wire of an electrocardiograph.

electromagnetic energy The spectrum of energies that includes radio waves, microwaves, visible light, ultraviolet light, x-rays, gamma rays, and cosmic rays. The energy has both electrical and magnetic properties.

emesis Vomiting.

empathy A sensitivity to the needs of others that allows one to meet those needs constructively.

emphysema A chronic lung condition characterized by obstruction and destruction of the small airways and alveoli of the lungs, which results in the inability to effectively exhale stale air.

endospore A bacterial form that is generated to survive harsh environmental conditions.

enteral Via the digestive tract; refers to method of feeding or medication administration.

epiphysis The growth plate near the end of a long bone; it is active in bone growth in childhood and calcified in adults.

epistaxis Nosebleed.

equation A mathematical declaration that two mathematical statements (groups of numbers, together with their signs or mathematical functions) are equal to each other.

equivalent dose (EqD) The absorbed dose multiplied by a radiation weighting factor. For diagnostic x-rays, the weighting factor is 1; therefore, the absorbed dose and equivalent dose will be the same for diagnostic x-rays.

erythema A reddening of the skin, such as occurs after a large amount of radiation has been received.

esophagus The part of the digestive system that connects the pharynx to the stomach.

ethics Rules that apply values and moral standards to activities within a profession to define professional behavior.

ethnic Relating to races or large groups of people who have the same customs, religion, origin, or nationality.

excretion Elimination from the body, often by way of the urinary tract, but also via the respiratory system, the digestive tract, or as a component of sweat.

exercise tolerance test (stress test) An electrocardiographic test taken during physical activity and used to evaluate cardiac ischemia.

exponent A superscript number that indicates how many times a number is multiplied by itself.

exposure indicator (EI) number A manufacturer-specific number that correlates to the amount of radiation that reaches the digital image receptor.

external auditory (acoustic) meatus (EAM) The opening to the ear canal.

external occipital protuberance (EOP) The palpable bony prominence in the approximate center of the occipital bone.

extravasation Infiltration of a drug into the tissue surrounding an intravenous injection site.

fabella The normal variation of a small sesamoid bone located posterior to the knee.

facet The articular surface of intervertebral joints. Facets are located on each of the four articular processes that extend superiorly and inferiorly from the vertebral arch.

Fahrenheit scale A system for measuring temperature. In this system, water freezes at 32° and boils at 212°.

false imprisonment The unjustifiable detention of a person against his or her will.

fat pad sign Radiographic evidence of displacement of the fat pad in the joint region of the elbow that indicates a fracture involving the elbow joint.

femur The long bone of the thigh.

fibrillation A rapid, weak, and inefficient heartbeat.

fibula The thin, shorter long bone located laterally in the lower leg.

flat-panel detector A detector under the table of a digital radiography table that allows direct conversion of the x-rays to electrical signals, which are then converted to an image.

fluorescence The emission of light from the screen inside the cassette after exposure to x-rays.

fomite An object that has been in contact with pathogenic organisms.

foramen magnum The large round hole in the anterior portion of the occipital bone through which the spinal cord passes.

forced expiration test A common spirometry test used to measure forced expiratory volume and forced vital capacity; a type of pulmonary function test (PFT).

forced expiratory volume (FEV) The quantity of air that can be forcefully exhaled during a specific time period.

forced vital capacity (FVC) The amount of air that can be forced from the lungs following a deep breath.

fraction In mathematics, a number that represents a portion of a whole number.

fragility fracture A nontraumatic fracture resulting from low bone mass, usually at the hip, spinal vertebrae, wrist, proximal humerus, or ribs.

FRAX® A tool developed by World Health Organization to evaluate fracture risk of patients. The FRAX® algorithm gives the 10-year probability of fracture.

fungus (pl. fungi) A yeast or mold; one of a huge class of microorganisms that may be either beneficial or pathogenic.

generic Pertaining to the identifying title of a product that is not a brand or proprietary name.

geriatrics The care of elder adults.

glabella The bony prominence on the frontal bone between the eyebrows.

glans penis The conical tip of the penis.

glenoid process The lateral portion of the scapula that forms the socket of the shoulder joint.

glottic closure Sudden cessation of exhalation caused by closure of the opening to the trachea.

gonion The angle of the mandible.

grand mal seizure Major motor seizure.

Gray (Gy) The SI unit of measure for radiation absorbed dose. It is subdivided into air exposure (Gy_a) and tissue exposure (Gy_t).

HBV Hepatitis B virus.

health care–associated infections (HAI) Infections contracted in the process of receiving health care; nosocomial infections.

Heimlich maneuver Abdominal thrust; a technique for dislodging a foreign object from the throat of a person who is choking.

hematoma An abnormal collection of blood beneath the skin, usually clotted or partially clotted.

hematuria Blood in the urine.

hemolysis The rupture or destruction of red blood cells.

hemoptysis Coughing up of blood.

hemorrhage The continuous abnormal flow of blood.

hepatitis An infectious inflammatory disease of the liver.

hilum A depression or pit at that part of the organ where vessels and nerves enter. The hila of the lungs are located on either side of the carina.

HIV Human immunodeficiency virus, the causative agent of acquired immunodeficiency syndrome (AIDS).

humerus The long bone of the upper arm.

hydration The provision of adequate water to body tissues.

hyperopia Farsightedness.

hyperparathyroidism Disease caused by excessive secretion of parathyroid hormone (PTH) from one or more parathyroid glands resulting in excessive calcium in the blood; it affects cortical bone more than trabecular bone.

hypertension Abnormally high blood pressure.

hyperthermia Fever, pyrexia; abnormally high temperature.

hyperventilation Air hunger with rapid respirations.

hypoglycemia Low blood glucose level.

hypoglycemic agent A drug used to control the level of glucose in the blood.

hypotension Abnormally low blood pressure.

hypothyroidism A condition of abnormally decreased hormone secretion by the thyroid gland, which leads to reduced metabolism and retarded growth in children.

iatrogenic Health care–related, as an infection.

idiosyncratic Unusual or peculiar.

ileum The distal portion of the small intestine that is connected to the large intestine.

ilium The upper portion of the innominate bone.

image receptor (IR) The device that receives the energy of the x-ray beam and forms the image of the body part. The IR may be a screen-film cassette, a computed radiography (CR) imaging plate, or a solid-state digital receptor.

imaging plate A plate with special phosphors used in digital imaging. The plate is housed inside a cassette and stores the x-ray image until it is processed.

immunocompromised patients Patients with weakened immune systems as a result of disease, such as HIV, or treatments, such as radiation therapy or chemotherapy.

improper fraction A fraction with a value greater than 1 in which the numerator is larger than the denominator.

incontinence Loss of bowel or bladder control.

infiltration Condition of intravenous fluid leaking into surrounding tissue.

informed consent The written acceptance of any procedure that is considered experimental or that involves substantial risk.

infusion A method of instilling relatively large quantities of fluids or drugs into the bloodstream intravenously.

innominate bone One of the two composite bones that make up the pelvis.

insulin The hormone that converts blood glucose into usable energy; a drug administered to treat diabetes.

intentional misconduct An action that violates the law or a professional code of ethics and was committed knowingly.

intervertebral disk A pad of fibrocartilage between vertebral bodies that cushions vertebral motion and absorbs shock.

intradermal Referring to shallow injections made between the skin layers.

intramuscular (IM) Referring to injections made directly into muscle tissue.

intravenous (IV) Referring to injections made directly into a vein.

invasion of privacy The failure to maintain confidentiality of information or the improper exposure or touching of the patient's body.

inverse square law A law that states that x-ray intensity is inversely proportional to the square of the distance from the source.

ion A neutral atom that gains or loses an electron.

ionizing radiation Radiation that, when passing through the body tissues, produces positively or negatively charged particles.

ischemia Deficiency of blood in a body part because of functional constriction or actual obstruction of a blood vessel.

ischium The posterior inferior portion of the innominate bone.

Ishihara test A test used to measure color perception.

jejunum The second section of the small intestine.

joint effusion Increased fluid in the joint capsule.

KUB The anteroposterior supine projection of the abdomen. It stands for *k*idneys, *u*reters, and *b*ladder.

kyphotic curve, kyphosis A posterior convex curvature of the spine.

lacrimal bone One of the smallest and most fragile bones of the face, located at the anterior part of the medial wall of the orbit.

lamina Any thin, flat layer of membrane or other bulkier tissue; the right or left posterior portion of the vertebral arch.

larynx Voice box.

latent image The image contained in the film before it is processed.

latitude The term used to describe the range of densities that can be recorded on an x-ray film.

lead (ECG) One of a set of electrodes that produces a specific recording in an electrocardiographic (ECG) study.

lesion A circumscribed area of pathologic tissue; a sore or wound.

libel The malicious spreading of information that results in defamation of character or loss of reputation.

limited operator A general term applied to a person who receives training to perform a limited variety of x-ray examinations. The term *limited x-ray machine operator (LXMO)* is the formal term given to such an individual.

longitudinal quality control Manufacturer-defined procedures performed on a regular basis to ensure that patients are scanned on properly functioning equipment with stable calibration. Scanning must be postponed until identified problems are corrected.

lordotic curve, lordosis An anterior convex curvature of the spine.

lowest terms In mathematics, the form of a fraction in which no number except 1 can be evenly divided into both the numerator and denominator.

lumbar spine The five vertebrae located inferior to the thoracic spine.

lumen The channel within a hollow tubelike structure, such as a catheter or blood vessel.

malignant Tending to become progressively worse and to result in death; said of tumors.

malpractice An act of negligence in the context of the relationship between a professional person and a patient or client.

mandible The lower jaw.

Mantoux test A skin test for tuberculosis; same as the purified protein derivative (PPD) test.

maxilla The upper jaw.

mean A statistic commonly called the *average;* the sum of a set of data values divided by the number of data values.

mediastinum The part of the thoracic cavity that encompasses the space between the lungs.

meniscus The C-shaped cartilage that cushions the articular surface of each femoral condyle.

mental protuberance (point) The prominence in the center of the mandible's lower margin.

metabolism The process by which the body breaks down substances for use and/or elimination.

metacarpal A bone of the hand.

metastasis A growth of pathogenic microorganisms or of abnormal cells distant from the site primarily involved.

metatarsal A bone of the forefoot.

microbe, microorganism A living organism too small to see with the naked human eye.

microbial dilution Reduction of the total number of microorganisms in an area.

mixed number A number consisting of a whole number and a fraction.

moral agent The person responsible for implementing an ethical decision.

morals Beliefs or principles based on familial and societal standards that influence a person's actions.

morphology Shape.

morphometric x-ray absorptiometry (MXA) Lateral scans of the thoracic and lumbar spine using single or dual x-ray absorptiometry to determine vertebral abnormalities or fractures from the shapes of the vertebrae.

multiple myeloma A malignant bone disease that may involve many bones of the body.

myocardium Heart muscle tissue.

myopia Nearsightedness.

nasal conchae Six thin, curved, bony projections that divide the nasal cavities.

nasion The anterior depression in the midline of the skull between the orbits.

nasopharynx The passageway between the nose and the upper throat.

National Osteoporosis Foundation (NOF) The nation's leading voluntary health organization solely dedicated to osteoporosis.

nebulizer A mist applicator for administration of medication by inhalation.

negligence The omission of reasonable care or caution.

NHANES III The third National Health and Nutrition Examination Survey.

nonaccidental trauma (NAT) Another name for battered child syndrome.

normal flora Microorganisms that live on or within the body without causing disease.

nosocomial Pertaining to or originating in a hospital, as in nosocomial disease.

NSAID Nonsteroidal antiinflammatory drug; one of a class of analgesics.

numerator The upper number of a fraction.

obese Accumulation of excess body fat to the extent that health is adversely affected and may lead to reduced life expectancy.

object–image receptor distance (OID) The distance from the patient (object) to the image receptor. Must be kept to a minimum to reduce magnification and increase spatial resolution.

olecranon process A posterior projection at the proximal end of the ulna; the "funny bone" or "crazy bone."

opiate A drug derived from opium.

opioid A drug whose action is similar to that of morphine.

opportunistic infection An infection that occurs when certain microorganisms take advantage of the opportunity to invade in the absence of an immune response.

orbit Eye socket.

organic brain syndrome The term for a large group of disorders associated with brain damage or impaired cerebral function.

orthopnea The inability to breathe while lying down.

orthostatic hypotension A temporary state of low blood pressure that causes patients to feel light-headed or faint when first sitting up.

OSHA Occupational Health and Safety Administration; a federal agency governing safety in the workplace.

osteoarthritis A degenerative joint disease.

osteoblastic Referring to the osteoblasts or a disease that results in increased bone formation.

osteoblasts Bone-building cells that fill the pits left by resorption with new bone.

osteoclasts Bone-destroying cells that break down and remove old bone, leaving pits.

osteolytic Referring to a disease that causes bone destruction.

osteoma A benign bone tumor.

osteomalacia A bone disorder characterized by variable amounts of uncalcified osteoid matrix.

osteomyelitis Inflammation of the bone caused by a pathogenic organism.

osteopenia Calcium loss in bones, causing them to become more radiolucent; demineralization. By World Health Organization criteria, it is a bone mineral density or bone mineral content T-score between −1 and −2.5.

osteophytes Enlarged, deformed portions of the bone, usually caused by arthritis.

osteoporosis Calcium loss in bones, often through aging, that results in bones becoming porous, brittle, and more radiolucent. By World Health Organization criteria, it is a bone mineral density or bone mineral content T-score of less than −2.5.

OTC Over the counter; designation of drugs available without a prescription.

PACS (Picture Archival and Communications System) Systems used in the radiology department to transmit images to remote locations and to store images for long-term use.

Paget disease A disease of the elderly that results in the softening and destruction of the bone, followed by thickening and irregular calcification as the bone is repaired.

palatine bone A part of the roof of the mouth.

parenteral Injected into the body through the skin.

parietal membrane The lining of the body's cavities.

Parkinson disease A degenerative condition of the nervous system that causes tremors.

PASS The acronym for the operating instructions for a fire extinguisher *P*ull the pin. *A*im the nozzle. *S*queeze the handle. *S*weep.

patella The kneecap.

pathogen A microorganism capable of causing disease.

peak bone mass Maximum bone mass, usually achieved between 30 and 35 years of age. Population mean peak bone mass is used as a reference point for the T-score.

pedal digits The toes.

pediatrics The care of children.

pedicle A narrow stalk, stem, or tube of tissue attached to a tumor, skin flap, bone, or organ; the right and left anterior portions of the vertebral arch on either side of the vertebral body.

pencil-beam collimation Dual-energy x-ray absorptiometry system using a circular pinhole x-ray collimator that produces a narrow x-ray stream, which is received by a single detector. It has a serpentine (or raster) motion across or along the length of the body. Modern systems have improved scan time and image quality. Off-centering of the object does not cause geometric distortion.

percent coefficient of variation (%CV) A statistic used to compare standard deviations from different data sets that may have different means; also a measure of precision. It is calculated as the standard deviation divided by the mean, times 100. A smaller %CV indicates better precision.

percentage A form of a fraction with a denominator of 100.

peripheral Situated away from the center or central structure.

peritoneum The double-walled serous membrane sac that contains the abdominal organs.

peritonitis Inflammation of the peritoneum; a life-threatening infection of the peritoneum that can result from rupture of the gastrointestinal tract.

phalanx A long bone of the finger or toe.

pharmacodynamics The effects of drugs on the normal physiologic functions of the body.

pharynx The throat.

photoelectric effect One of three interactions of radiation with human body tissues. In this effect, the x-ray photon is totally absorbed in the body tissues.

photostimulable phosphor (PSP) A phosphor used in computed radiography (CR) plates to absorb the x-ray energy and store it until it is processed by a special unit and laser light.

pledget An alcohol swab or "prep" used to cleanse the skin before injection or venipuncture.

pleura The membrane that covers the lungs and lines the pleural cavities.

pleural effusion An abnormal collection of fluid in the pleural space.

pneumoconiosis A group of chronic occupational lung diseases caused by the inhalation of irritating dust.

pneumonia Inflammatory disease of the lung.

pneumothorax A collection of air or gas in the pleural space associated with lung collapse.

PO Per os; by mouth.

potency Strength.

potential difference The force or strength of the electrons flowing within an electrical circuit. Term is the same as the volt.

power In mathematics, the number of times a number is multiplied by itself, as indicated by the exponent.

PPD test Purified protein derivative test; a skin test for tuberculosis infection.

prehypertension Systolic blood pressure in the range between 120 and 140 mm Hg.

presbyopia Farsightedness that occurs with advancing age.

primary osteoporosis Osteoporosis that is not caused by an underlying disease; classified as type I or type II.

prime factors (of exposure) milliamperage (mA), exposure time (S), kilovoltage (kVp), and source–image receptor distance (SID).

principlism Principle-based ethics, a widely accepted standard for selecting and defending solutions to ethical dilemmas in health care communities.

prions The smallest and least understood of all infectious agents, thought to be infectious proteins.

product In mathematics, the answer to a multiplication problem.

proper fraction A fraction with a value less than 1.

proportion In mathematics, a statement that two ratios are equal to each other.

proprietary name Title of a product that belongs exclusively to the company that produces it.

prosthesis Anatomic replacement.

protozoa Complex, single-cell animals that generally exist as free-living organisms, but some are pathogenic parasites.

pubis The anterior inferior portion of the innominate bone.

pulse The advancing pressure wave in an artery caused by the expulsion of blood when the left ventricle of the heart contracts.

pulse oximeter An electronic device that measures and displays the rate of the pulse and the oxygen saturation of the blood.

pyrexia Fever; hyperthermia; abnormally high temperature.

quantitative ultrasound (QUS) Quantitative measurement of bone properties related to mechanical competence using ultrasound.

quantum mottle A grainy or mottled (spotty) appearance of the image, usually caused by the use of an insufficient radiation exposure for the body part or for the requirements of the image receptor. Quantum mottle is not desirable in creating x-ray images.

quotient In mathematics, the answer to a division problem.

rad A unit measuring the quantity of radiation absorbed in the tissues.

radial deviation Movement of the hand toward the radial side of the wrist.

radiographer A radiologic technologist who has completed and passed the certification examination in radiography given by the American Registry of Radiologic Technologists (ARRT).

radiographic absorptiometry (RA) A technique in which hand x-ray density in an image is visually compared with that of a known standard in the exposure field.

radiologic technologist A general term applied to a person who is certified and qualified to use x-rays, radioactive substances, and radiation therapy to diagnose and treat disease.

radiologist A physician specialist who interprets radiographic images and performs special imaging procedures.

radiolucent Referring to a substance that is easily penetrated by x-rays. The term also refers to an area of the film through which a moderate amount of light from the view box is transmitted.

radius The thick, shorter long bone located laterally in the forearm.

ratio The quotient that results from dividing one number into another.

reagent strip A paper strip containing small pads of absorbent material impregnated with chemical reagents; used for urinalysis and other laboratory evaluations.

reasonably prudent person Legal standard for determining negligence.

recorded detail The sharpness of the structures in the image. The terms detail, sharpness, and resolution are sometimes used to refer to recorded detail. Not used much, being replaced with the term "spatial resolution."

rectification The process of changing alternating current into direct current to produce x-rays.

reference population Large, sex-matched, community-based population used to determine the average bone mineral density and standard deviation at each age.

region of interest (ROI) The defined portion of a bone density scan where the bone mineral density is calculated; it may be placed manually or automatically by computer software.

remainder The number that is left over when one number is divided unequally into another.

remnant radiation The radiation that exits or leaves the patient's body and exposes the film.

respondeat superior The legal doctrine that states that the employer is liable for employees' negligent acts that occur in the course of their work.

roentgen A unit measuring the amount of radiation intensity in the air. It is the amount of radiation measured before it is absorbed in the body.

rule of personal responsibility The rule that states that each individual is liable for his or her own negligent conduct.

sacrum The five vertebral segments inferior to the lumbar vertebrae, which fuse together in adulthood to form a solid bony structure.

scapula The shoulder blade.

scoliosis An abnormal lateral curvature of the spine.

secondary osteoporosis Osteoporosis caused by an underlying disease.

sedative A drug that causes a quieting effect, inducing sleep.

sella turcica The rounded fossa in the center of the anterior superior surface of the sphenoid bone; the location of the pituitary gland.

sensitometer A device that prints a standard gray scale of densities on radiographic film.

serial scans Sequential scans, usually performed 12, 18, or 24 months apart, to measure changes in bone density.

sesamoid bone A small, flat, oval bone within a tendon that is not counted among the bones of the body.

SESIP Sharp with engineered sharps injury protection; Occupational Health and Safety Administration–approved sharp instruments designed to prevent accidental exposure to blood-borne pathogens.

shaken baby syndrome Bleeding within the cranium that can occur when a small child is violently shaken.

sharps Anything that can puncture skin, such as needles, glass tubes, glass slides, or finger lancets.

sharps container A receptacle for needles, syringes, and other contaminated items capable of puncturing the skin.

Shewhart Control Chart rules Classic quality control rules based on comparing a data value to the mean and standard deviation of a set of similar values.

shock A life-threatening condition that occurs when the body does not get enough blood flow.

sievert (Sv) A unit measuring the effective radiation dose to a patient. Bone density doses are measured in microsieverts, where 1 microsievert equals 1 one millionth of 1 sievert.

signal-to-noise ratio (SNR) The ability of the digital system to convert the x-ray input electrical signal into a useful radiographic image.

single-energy x-ray absorptiometry (SXA) A technique for measuring bone density in the peripheral skeleton using a single-energy x-ray source and an external medium.

slander The malicious spreading of information that results in defamation of character or loss of reputation.

smoothing The result of averaging each pixel's frequency with surrounding pixel values to remove high-frequency noise. Also known as *low-pass filtering.*

Snellen alphabet chart A chart for testing distance vision that uses letters of the alphabet.

Snellen E chart A chart for testing distance vision that uses the block letter E in various positions instead of letters of the alphabet.

source–image receptor distance (SID) The distance from the focal spot of the x-ray tube to the image receptor. It should be as long as practical to minimize magnification and maximize spatial resolution.

spatial resolution The ability to distinguish between adjacent structures. Amount of detail or sharpness of an image as seen on the computer monitor.

spectral emission The color of the light emitted by the phosphor of the x-ray screen.

sphincter A round muscle that opens and closes the opening of an organ.

sphygmomanometer A blood pressure cuff and gauge.

spirogram The graph that results from a spirometry test.

spirometer A machine for measuring pulmonary function.

spirometry The measurement of pulmonary function using a spirometer.

spontaneous combustion The occurrence of a chemical reaction in or near a flammable material that causes enough heat to generate a fire.

squared In mathematics, the description of a number that has been multiplied by itself.

square root In mathematics, that portion of a number that, when multiplied by itself, equals the original number.

standard deviation (SD) A measure of the variability of a set of data values about their mean value.

Standard Precautions The use of barriers in anticipation of contact with certain body fluids and extracts. In 1996, the CDC recommended a new system that synthesizes the features of universal precautions (UP) and body substance isolation (BSI). This most recent system is called Standard Precautions.

standardization mark The mark on an electrocardiogram that results from deflection of the stylus by a 1-mV stimulus. The mark is evaluated to ensure that the machine is recording accurately.

standardized BMD (sBMD) The result of converting bone mineral density (BMD) values obtained using equipment from one manufacturer to values that can be compared with those obtained using equipment from other manufacturers by application of mathematic formulas. It is reported in milligrams per centimeter squared (mg/cm^2) to differentiate it from BMD.

standing order Written directions signed by a physician for the use of a specific medication or procedure under certain defined circumstances that may be carried out without further order.

status epilepticus Prolonged or repeated seizures.

stenosis Narrowing of a passageway, such as an intervertebral foramen.

sterilization The destruction of all microorganisms; surgical asepsis.

sternum The breastbone.

stockinette Tubular knitted fabric placed on extremities before the application of a cast.

stridor A harsh, high-pitched sound during respiration caused by obstruction of the bronchi.

stroke Cerebrovascular accident (CVA); a sudden loss of blood supply to a portion of the brain. It may be caused by hemorrhage or blood clot.

stylus The tracing pen on an electrocardiograph machine.

subcutaneous (SC) Referring to injections into the fat layer beneath the skin.

subdural hematoma A collection of blood between the brain and the dura mater membrane, caused by hemorrhage, and producing increased intracranial pressure.

sublingual Under the tongue; a topical route of drug administration.

sum In mathematics, the total or the answer to an addition problem.

supine The position in which a person is lying on the back, face up.

suture A synarthrodial joint that connects the bones of the cranium; a stitch used to close a wound or the material used to close a wound in this way.

syncope Fainting.

synergistic Enhancing the effect of another drug or agent when the two are combined.

syphilis A sexually transmitted disease caused by a spirochete type of bacterium.

systolic Referring to maximum blood pressure, occurring during contraction of the left ventricle.

tachycardia A rapid pulse.

tachypnea Abnormally rapid breathing; more than 20 breaths per minute.

talus The ankle bone.

tarsal bones The five short bones of the midfoot.

TB Tuberculosis.

teamwork Cooperative effort by the members of a group to achieve a common goal.

tendinitis Inflammation of a tendon.

thermionic emission The process by which electrons are "boiled off" from the tungsten filament in the x-ray tube. This occurs when the filament is heated during the x-ray exposure. These electrons are then forced into the anode during the x-ray exposure, creating x-rays.

thoracic spine The dorsal spine, which consists of 12 vertebrae with a kyphotic curve; located inferior to the cervical spine.

thorax The upper portion of the trunk; the chest.

thready pulse A weak and rapid pulse.

tibia The thick, longer long bone located medially in the lower leg.

tonic-clonic seizure Major motor seizure.

topical Referring to medication that is applied to the skin.

tourniquet A rubber strap or tube tied around the arm to facilitate blood collection or access to the vein for injection.

toxic Poisonous.

trabecular bone Delicate, lattice-work structure within bones that adds strength without excessive weight. It supports compressive loading at the spine, hip, and calcaneus and is also found in the ends of long bones such as the distal radius.

trachea The windpipe, which connects the throat to the bronchi.

tranquilizer A drug that reduces anxiety and mental tension.

transient ischemic attack (TIA) An attack with symptoms similar to those of a stroke but of short duration.

tremor Involuntary vibration that may be caused by illness or fear; trembling.

Trendelenburg position The position of the patient in which the head is lowered at least 15 degrees.

T-score The number of standard deviations by which an individual's bone mineral density differs from the average bone mineral density of young, normal, sex-matched individuals with peak bone mass.

tuberculosis A disease of the lungs caused by the acid-fast bacillus *Mycobacterium tuberculosis.*

turbid Describes a liquid that is murky or extremely cloudy.

tympanic Pertaining to the tympanic membrane or eardrum; a route for measuring body temperature by placing a special thermometer in the ear.

type I osteoporosis Primary osteoporosis related to postmenopausal status.

type II osteoporosis Primary osteoporosis related to aging.

ulna The thin, longer long bone located medially in the forearm.

ulnar deviation Movement of the hand toward the ulnar side of the wrist.

urethral meatus The external opening to the urethra; the tube through which urine exits the body.

urinalysis The physical, microscopic, or chemical examination of urine.

urticaria Hives.

valid choices A selection of alternatives, all of which are acceptable.

values The priorities that are placed on the significance of moral concepts.

vector An arthropod in whose body an infectious organism develops or multiplies before becoming infectious to a new host.

vehicle A medium that transports microorganisms.

vena cava The large vein that brings oxygen-depleted blood from the body to the right atrium of the heart.

venipuncture The collection of blood by insertion of a needle into a vein.

vertebra Any one of the 33 bones (26 in the adult) of the spinal column.

vertebral fracture assessment (VFA) Used to denote densitometric spine imaging performed for the purpose of detecting vertebral fractures.

vertigo Dizziness; a condition in which the patient feels as if the room is moving or whirling.

virus Subcellular pathogenic agent. Viruses are responsible for such diseases as influenza, chickenpox, acquired immunodeficiency syndrome, and the common cold.

visceral membrane The covering of the organs.

visible image The image that is displayed on the computer monitor or is seen on radiographic film.

visual acuity Sharpness of perception.

volatile Referring to substances that change readily from a solid or a liquid to a vapor.

vomer The bone that forms the inferior portion of the nasal septum.

wheal A raised area on the skin, similar to an insect bite, that results from an intradermal injection, as in a tuberculin skin test.

WHO World Health Organization.

window level Adjustment of the brightness (or density) of a digital image.

window width Adjustment of the contrast of a digital image.

Z-score The number of standard deviations by which an individual's bone mineral density differs from the average bone mineral density of a sex- and age-matched reference group.

zygoma The cheek bone.

Index

Page numbers followed by *f* indicate figures; *t,* tables; *b,* boxes.